BIOMEDICAL ASPECTS

OF

DRUG TARGETING

BIOMEDICAL ASPECTS

OF

DRUG TARGETING

EDITORS

VLADIMIR MUZYKANTOV, M.D., Ph.D.
University of Pennsylvania
School of Medicine
Philadelphia, PA
USA

VLADIMIR TORCHILIN, Ph.D., D.Sc.
Northeastern University
School of Pharmacy
Boston, MA
USA

KLUWER ACADEMIC PUBLISHERS
Boston/Dordrecht/London

Distributors for North, Central and South America:
Kluwer Academic Publishers
101 Philip Drive
Assinippi Park
Norwell, Massachusetts 02061 USA
Telephone (781) 871-6600
Fax (781) 681-9045
E-Mail: kluwer@wkap.com

Distributors for all other countries:
Kluwer Academic Publishers Group
Post Office Box 322
3300 AH Dordrecht, THE NETHERLANDS
Telephone 31 786 576 000
Fax 31 786 576 474
E-Mail: services@wkap.nl

 Electronic Services < http://www.wkap.nl >

Library of Congress Cataloging-in-Publication Data

A C.I.P. Catalogue record for this book is available
from the Library of Congress.

The Publisher offers discounts on this book for course use and bulk purchases. For further information, send email to mimi.breed@wkap.com.

TABLE OF CONTENTS

SECTION 1: GENERAL PRINCIPLES OF DRUG TARGETING

SECTION 2: CARDIOVASCULAR TARGETING

SECTION 3: TUMOR TARGETING

CONTRIBUTORS

Fariyal Ahmed
Department of Chemical and
Biomolecular Engineering, Departments
of Bioengineering and Mechanical
Engineering and Applied Mechanics,
Institute for Medicine and Engineering,
University of Pennsylvania, Philadelphia,
PA 19104

Michaela Arndt
SAIC Frederick, National Cancer
Institute at Frederick, Frederick, MD
21702

John W. Babich, Ph.D.
Biostream, Inc., Cambridge,
Massachusetts

Frank S. Bates
Department of Chemical Engineering and
Material Science, University of
Minnesota, Minneapolis, MN 55455

Walter A. Blättler
ImmunoGen, Inc., Cambridge, MA
02139

Christoph Bode
Department of Cardiology and
Angiology, University of Freiburg,
Hugstetter Str. 55, 79106 Freiburg,
Germany

Sabine Boeckle
Department of Pharmacy, Chair of
Pharmaceutical Biology – Biotechnology,
Ludwig-Maximilians-Universität
München, Butenandtstraße 5-13,
D-81377 Munich, Germany

Lucy A. Carver
Sidney Kimmel Cancer Center,
San Diego, CA 92121

Ravi V. J. Chari
ImmunoGen, Inc., Cambridge, MA
02139

Gerard D'Souza
Northeastern University, Bouve College of
Health Sciences, School of Pharmacy,
Department of Pharmaceutics, Boston, MA
02115

Sergei M. Danilov
Department of Anesthesiology, University
of Illinois in Chicago, Chicago IL USA

Dennis E. Discher
Department of Chemical and Biomolecular
Engineering, Departments of
Bioengineering and Mechanical
Engienering and Applied Mechanics,
Institute for Medicine and Engineering,
University of Pennsylvania, Philadelphia,
PA 19104

Ruth Duncan
Centre for Polymer Therapeutics, Welsh
School of Pharmacy, Cardiff University,
King Edward VII Avenue, Cardiff
CF10 3XF, UK

Alan L. Epstein
Department of Pathology, Keck School of
Medicine at the University of Southern
California, Los Angeles, CA 90033

Hua Fang
Department of Microbiology, Montana
State University, Bozeman MT 59717

Victor S. Goldmacher,
ImmunoGen, Inc., Cambridge, MA 02139

David S. Halpern
Isotron, Inc. Alpharetta, GA 30022

Ken-ichi Hosoya
Faculty of Pharmaceutical Sciences,
Toyama Medical and Pharmaceutical
University, Sugitani, Toyama, 930-0194,
Japan. CREST of Japan Science and
Technology Corporation (JST)

Peisheng Hu
Department of Pathology, Keck School
of Medicine at the University of Southern
California, Los Angeles, CA 90033

Steven K. Jacobs
New York Medical College, New
Windsor, NY 12553

Ban-An Khaw
Bouve College of Health Sciences,
School of Pharmacy, Department of
Pharmaceutical Sciences, Northeastern
University, Boston, MA 02115

Leslie A. Khawli
Department of Pathology, Keck School
of Medicine at the University of Southern
California, Los Angeles, CA 90033

Alexander L. Klibanov
Cardiovascular Research Center,
Division of Cardiology, University of
Virginia

Juergen Krauss
SAIC Frederick, National Cancer
Institute at Frederick, Frederick, MD
21702

John M. Lambert
ImmunoGen, Inc., Cambridge, MA
02139

Klaus Ley
Cardiovascular Research Center, and
Department of Biomedical Engineering,
University of Virginia

Jonathan R. Lindner
Cardiovascular Research Center,
Division of Cardiology, University of
Virginia

Eng H. Lo
Neuroprotection Research Laboratory,
Dept. of Neurology and Radiology,
Massachusetts General Hospital, and
Program in Neuroscience, Harvard
Medical School

D. Robert Lu
College of Pharmacy, University of
Georgia, Athens, GA 30602

Hiroshi Maeda
Department of Microbiology, Kumamoto
University School of Medicine, Kumamoto
860-0811, Japan

Vladimir R. Muzykantov
Department of Pharmacology, University
of Pennsylvania School of Medicine,
Philadelphia, PA 19104-6068

Dianne L. Newton
SAIC Frederick, National Cancer Institute
at Frederick, Frederick, MD 21702

Manfred Ogris
Department of Pharmacy, Chair of
Pharmaceutical Biology – Biotechnology,
Ludwig-Maximilians-Universität München,
Butenandtstraße 5-13, D-81377 Munich,
Germany

Sumio Ohtsuki
Department of Molecular Biopharmacy and
Genetics, Graduate School of
Pharmaceutical Sciences, and New Industry
Creation Hatchery Center, Tohoku
University, Aoba, Aramaki, Aoba-ku,
Sendai 980-8578, Japan. CREST of Japan
Science and Technology Corporation (JST)

Ranganath Parthasrathy
Department of Chemical and Biomolecular
Engineering, Institute for Medicine and
Engineering, University of Pennsylvania,
Philadelphia, PA 19104

Karlheinz Peter
Department of Cardiology and Angiology,
University of Freiburg, Hugstetter Str. 55,
79106 Freiburg, Germany

Margaret A. Petty
CNS Pharmacology, Aventis
Pharmaceuticals Inc. Route 202-206, P.O.
Box 6800, Bridgewater, New Jersey 08807

Peter Photos
Department of Chemical and Biomolecular Engineering, Institute for Medicine and Engineering, University of Pennsylvania, Philadelphia, PA 19104

Seth H. Pincus
Research Institute for Children, Children's Hospital, LSU Health Sciences Center, New Orleans LA 70118

Laszlo Prokai
Center for Drug Discovery and Department of Pharmaceutics, College of Pharmacy, and the McKnight Brain Institute, University of Florida, Gainesville, FL 32610-0497, USA

Sophia Ran
The University of Texas Southwestern Medical Center at Dallas, 2201 Inwood Road, Dallas, TX 75390-8594

Paul N. Reynolds
Department of Thoracic Medicine, Royal Adelaide Hospital, Adelaide, South Australia 5000

Michael Rosenblum
M.D. Anderson Cancer Center, 1515 Holcombe Boulevard, Box 44, Houston, TX 77030-4009

Susanna M. Rybak
Developmental Therapeutics Program, Division of Cancer Treatment and Diagnosis, National Cancer Institute at Frederick, Frederick, MD 21702

Ranajoy Sarkar
College of Pharmacy, University of Georgia, Athens, GA 30602

Jan E. Schnitzer
Sidney Kimmel Cancer Center, San Diego, CA 92121

Tetsuya Terasaki
Department of Molecular Biopharmacy and Genetics, Graduate School of Pharmaceutical Sciences, and New Industry Creation Hatchery Center, Tohoku University, Aoba, Aramaki, Aoba-ku, Sendai 980-8578, Japan. CREST of Japan Science and Technology Corporation (JST)

Philip E. Thorpe
The University of Texas Southwestern Medical Center at Dallas, 2201 Inwood Road, Dallas, TX 75390-8594

Vladimir P. Torchilin
Department of Pharmaceutical Sciences, Bouve College of Health Sciences, Northeastern University, Boston, MA 02129, USA

Bang K. Vu
SAIC Frederick, National Cancer Institute at Frederick, Frederick, MD 21702

Ernst Wagner
Department of Pharmacy, Chair of Pharmaceutical Biology – Biotechnology, Ludwig-Maximilians-Universität München, Butenandtstraße 5-13, D-81377 Munich, Germany

Volkmar Weissig
Northeastern University, Bouve College of Health Sciences, School of Pharmacy, Department of Pharmaceutics, Boston, MA 02115

Royce Wilkinson
Department of Microbiology, Montana State University, Bozeman MT 59717

John Woodley
Faculté des Sciences Pharmaceutiques, 31500 Toulouse, France

Zhongyu Zhu
SAIC Frederick, National Cancer Institute at Frederick, Frederick, MD 21702

PREFACE

Drugs usually have no natural affinity for the cells, tissues and organs where therapeutic effects are needed, which frequently results in low efficiency and unwanted side effects. This concern is even more profound when using highly potent and cytotoxic anticancer drugs or specific agents, such as enzymes and genetic materials, since their effective and safe action requires precise cellular or even sub-cellular addressing in the target organ. To meet safety, efficiency and specificity requirements, drugs somehow must be targeted to the sites of their expected therapeutic action. The idea of the "magic bullet," or drug targeting, proposed by Erlich a century ago, generates great and continuously growing interest in biomedical, industrial and financial circles.

This book is focused on the strategies designed to target therapeutic or diagnostic agents to the disease sites. In an attempt to include in this volume the set of chapters reflecting both traditional and emerging areas of drug targeting, we have contacted many leading scientists in the field asking for their contributions. Their responses were most favorable and encouraging. As a result, we have succeeded in assembling a series of outstanding contributions reflecting practically all the key areas of drug targeting. The final structure of this book is as follows.

The first section of this book includes two review chapters covering the general means used for and the biological barriers of drug targeting. The second section of this book includes seven chapters addressing the specific area of targeting in the cardiovascular system and discusses such topics as targeting myocardial infarction, thrombi and endothelium. The third section includes six chapters focused on targeting drugs and imaging agents to tumors and discusses such topics as immunotoxins and anti-tumor targeted polymer carriers. This section also discusses the specific features of tumor vasculature permitting the effect of enhanced permeability and retention (EPR) and selective targeting of drugs to tumor endothelium. The fourth section includes four chapters on targeting drugs to brain, with such topics as targeting specific receptors in cerebral blood vessels, brain tumors and stroke. The fifth section provides a diverse collection of seven chapters describing drug delivery to some specific targets, such as infection, HIV-infected cells and gastro-intestinal tract, as well as some new exciting approaches in targeting, such as peptide-mediated transmembrane delivery, polymerosomes and sub-cellular addressing of drugs. In addition to a standard subject index at the end of the book, each chapter has a brief glossary that will help unfamiliar readers to grasp the main terminology.

By the very nature of the research, drug targeting combines knowledge, techniques and ideas from diverse disciplines, including chemistry, pharmacy, pharmacology, vascular biology, cell and molecular biology, immunology, pathology and radiology. Many excellent books and chapters on the subject have been published during the last decade. Some were focused on chemical and pharmaceutical aspects of targeting; some provided protocols and descriptions of specific experimental procedures and results. This level of rigor is necessary to prove the validity of the results and permit their reproduction by peers in laboratories. However, the goal of the present book is to concentrate on biomedical aspects of drug targeting and address the related issues to a wide medical and scientific audience including medical professionals and scientists not working in the field.

Even those directly involved in targeting researches represent quite different professional groups. Many of these researchers have backgrounds in chemistry, bioengineering, pharmaceutical sciences and biotechnology. We appreciate this professional diversity from personal perspectives: by training, one of us is a medical doctor (and teaches in a medical school), while the other is a chemist (and teaches in a school of pharmacy). Not surprisingly, our book does not target a specific scientific audience, but tries to deliver the materials packed in the most digestible form to medical doctors and pharmacists, as well as research scientists, experts in biomedical patents and technology transfer, and managers in academia, research institutions and industry. The book may help these readers to clarify some medical aspects of targeting, such as the anatomy and physiology of important targets and barriers, as well as pathological mechanisms of the diseases. On the other hand, the book presents drug targeting to a wide biomedical community including medical students and faculty. We believe that now is the right time to introduce these concepts to medical professionals (active and in the making) who likely will use them in their future practice.

Some of the strategies outlined in the book are already used in clinical settings, while many strategies are under exploration in laboratories. Almost every year, new, highly promising concepts evolve; yet we realize that, within a few years, some of today's news will look obsolete. Therefore, we did not design the book as a collection of fresh experimental papers, but rather used particular examples (we believe, very exciting ones) to show targeting principles (even at the cost of oversimplifying the details).

Of course, not all related studies, approaches, laboratories and individual researchers are directly presented on the pages of the book. Such incompleteness was inevitable due to restrictions of the book size, inability of some scientists to commit sufficient time in their overloaded schedules and other reasons (objective and subjective, but always important and understandable). In addition, drug targeting is a huge and rapidly progressing area. In one single volume, even with the participation of the leading scientists from the field, one can hardly assemble a set of papers covering all possible aspects of targeted delivery of pharmaceuticals. The editors realize than some potential readers could be disappointed by not finding in this book certain information they might be looking for. However, we had the privilege of gathering a wonderful collective of outstanding researchers who were kind, patient and collaborative during this work. With great pleasure (and the relief of having finished the task) we express our deep gratitude to all contributors.

We strongly believe that everyone working in this exciting field of research, and especially those who just begin their scientific careers, will still be able to use this volume as a helpful source. If this is the case, the contributors for this book are to receive all possible credits, while the editors are ready to take the blame for any omissions and drawbacks. Any comments will be highly appreciated. We hope you will enjoy reading as much as we enjoyed working on this book.

Vladimir Muzykantov, M.D., Ph.D.
University of Pennsylvania
School of Medicine

Vladimir Torchilin, Ph.D., D.Sc.
Northeastern University
School of Pharmacy

ACKNOWLEDGEMENTS

We thank Mimi Thompson Breed and Kluwer Academic Publishing Company for giving us the opportunity to publish this book. We are especially grateful to Mimi for her constant guidance and friendly encouragement during the planning, writing, arrangement and preparation of the book for production. We thank Mrs. Colleen O'Brien (University of Pennsylvania) for her excellent secretarial help. We are indebted to Julie Bookbinder (University of Pennsylvania) for her dedication to this book and her invaluable help and meticulous attention to every detail during technical editing, pagination and formatting the entire book. We thank all our authors who contributed marvelous chapters, as well as publishers who granted us permission to incorporate reproductions of previously published works into the text of our book. Finally, we would like to thank members of our families who tolerated our extra hours of work and encouraged us with love and care.

SECTION 1:

GENERAL PRINCIPLES OF DRUG TARGETING

1

STRATEGIES AND MEANS FOR DRUG TARGETING: AN OVERVIEW

Vladimir P. Torchilin
Department of Pharmaceutical Sciences, Bouve College of Health Sciences, Northeastern University, Boston, MA 02129, USA

INTRODUCTION: THE GENERAL CONCEPT OF DRUG TARGETING

The specificity of pharmaceuticals towards disease sites or individual diseases is usually based on a drug's ability to interfere with local pathological processes or with defective biological pathways, but not on its selective accumulation in the specific intracellular compartment or in the target cell, organ or tissue. Traditional pharmaceutical agents, practically independent of the administration route, distribute evenly (or at least proportionally to a regional blood flow) within the body. In addition, they have to cross many biological barriers to reach the site of disease and can cause undesirable side-effects or be inactivated in organs and tissues not even involved in the pathological process. Consequently, to achieve an effective therapeutic concentration in a desired location, one has to administer the drug in large quantities, which increases the cost of the therapy and the severity of side-effects. Long ago it was hypothesized that the problem may be resolved by achieving so-called targeted drug delivery: the ability of the drug to accumulate in the target organ or tissue selectively and quantitatively, independent of the site and methods of its administration. This type of delivery was expected to increase drug concentration in the target area without any side-effects in normal tissues. For any pharmaceutical, including both therapeutic and diagnostic agents, the following advantages of a targeted delivery drug are evident: (a) simplification of administration protocols; (b) drastic reduction in the cost of therapy and drug quantity required to achieve a therapeutic effect; (c) sharp increase in drug concentration in the required sites without negative effects on non-target areas.

The concept of targeted pharmaceuticals considers a coordinated behavior of several key components: (a) the pharmaceutical agent itself; targeting moiety (immunoglobulins - usually, monoclonal antibodies - primarily of IgG class, are the most promising and widely used targeting moieties); (b) the pharmaceutical carrier used to multiply the number of drug molecules per single targeting moiety (such as soluble polymers, microcapsules, microparticles, cells, cell ghosts, lipoproteins, liposomes, and micelles); (c) a potential target. The recognition of the target can occur on various levels, for example, on the level of a whole organ, on the level of certain cells specific for a given organ, or even on the level of individual components characteristic of these cells, such as cell surface antigens. The recognition on the molecular level is certainly the most universal form of target recognition because each organ or tissue is characterized by a unique set of chemical compounds, among which components (antigens) can be found that are specific to that organ or tissue. With all this in mind, numerous approaches for drug targeting have been developed that are capable of the specific delivery of therapeutic and diagnostic agents to the variety of tissues and organs (refs. 1-3 among others). Some of these approaches do not involve the use of any targeting moieties, but are rather based on certain physical principles and/or some physiological features of the target area. This chapter will briefly consider the main schemes of targeted delivery of pharmaceuticals that are currently in different stages of development.

MAIN APPROACHES TO TARGETED DELIVERY OF PHARMACEUTICALS

Among the principal schemes of targeted delivery of pharmaceuticals, one finds very different approaches, such as: (a) direct application of the drug into the affected zone; (b) "physical" targeting based on abnormal pH and/or temperature in the target zone, such as in a tumor or inflammation (pH- and temperature-sensitive drug carriers), or based on the use of certain external forces, such as magnetic field; (c) passive accumulation of the drug through leaky vasculature (a so-called Enhanced Permeability and Retention - EPR - effect, found to work for tumors, infarcts, and inflammation areas); (d) the use of specific delivery vectors (or certain ligands possessing high specific affinity towards the target areas).

The successful examples of the most straightforward approach – direct drug administration into an affected area - include the intracoronary infusion of thrombolytic enzymes in the therapy of the coronary thrombosis (4), and the intra-articular administration of hormonal drugs for the treatment of arthritis (5). Unfortunately, the applicability of this approach is limited to very few clinical situations.

Certain physical factors are able to mediate targeted delivery of pharmaceuticals. Those factors may be of endogenous and exogenous origin. For example, the targeting may use the known differences in various properties, such as pH and temperature, between pathological areas and normal tissues. Because the areas of inflammation and neoplastic growth usually demonstrate some decrease in the pH value and increase in the temperature, one can load pharmaceutical agents onto stimuli-responsive drug carriers that can disintegrate with the pH decrease or at higher temperature (compared to normal tissues) releasing the pharmaceutical agent. In this case, even though the carrier is evenly distributed within the circulation, it degrades and releases the drug only in the target area (Figure 1).

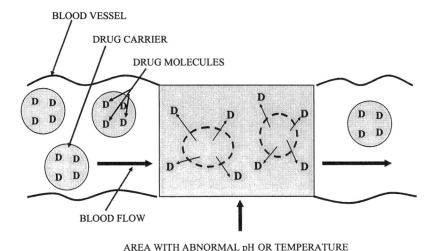

Figure 1. The schematic representation of the physical targeting of drugs/drug carriers. Stimuli-sensitive drug carrier disintegrates in the target zone and releases the drug.

Intravenously administered anti-cancer drug methotrexate accumulated in tumors in mice several times faster when it was incorporated into temperature-sensitive liposomes and the external heat was applied locally onto the tumor area (6). In general, drug-loaded pH-sensitive liposomes are frequently used for experimental delivery of drug and genetic material into a variety of compromised tissues (for review, see ref. 7).

An external physical force such as the magnetic field can also be used for the targeted delivery of pharmaceuticals. If the drug is attached to a drug carrier possessing ferromagnetic properties, one can expect that upon the intravenous administration, the drug-ferromagnetic carrier complex will accumulate within the area to which an external magnetic field is applied. Because of high blood flow velocity (and shear strength) in large blood vessels and high gradient of the magnetic field, the chance of efficient drug accumulation is higher in smaller blood vessels that are located closer to the body surface and have slower blood flow (8). If a strong magnet was positioned externally to the artery, where the thrombus was initiated, the local prevention of thrombosis in arteries of dogs and rabbits was achieved by the intravenous application of the autologous red blood cells loaded with ferromagnetic colloid compound and aspirin (9). If a small permanent magnet was implanted into the tissues next to a vessel in the region of thrombus formation, thrombolytic enzyme streptokinase immobilized on dextran-coated microparticles of iron oxide was successfully used for the targeted thrombus lysis of artificially formed thrombi in carotid arteries of experimental dogs (10). Histological analysis of arterial sections obtained 5 hours after the operation revealed no thrombus formation in the artery with the magnet, while occluding thrombi were formed in control arteries.

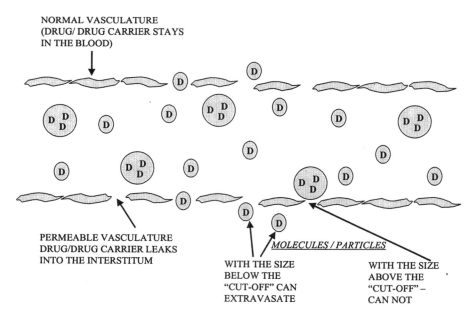

Figure 2. The schematic representation of the "passive" targeting (interstitial accumulation) of drugs and drug carriers through the leaky vasculature and the role of the "cut-off" size.

Under certain circumstances, the blood vessel wall endothelium might become more permeable than in the normal state. For example, the vascular endothelium demonstrates a noticeably increased permeability in many tumors (11) and infarcted areas (12). In such areas, even relatively large particles, such as micelles and liposomes ranging from 10 to 500 nm in size, can extravasate and accumulate inside the interstitial space. If these particles are loaded with a pharmaceutical agent, they can bring this agent into the area with increased vascular permeability where the drug can be eventually released from the carrier. Because the cut-off size of the permeabilized vasculature varies from case to case, the size of a drug carrying particle may be used to control the efficacy of such spontaneous "passive" drug delivery know also as the EPR (13), (see Figure 2 above).

This type of targeted delivery requires the drug carriers used to stay in the blood long enough to provide a sufficient level of target accumulation. The typical way to make drug carriers circulate for a longer time is to graft their surfaces with certain water-soluble polymers that have well-solvated and flexible main chains, such as polyethylene glycol (PEG); some other polymers can also be used (14). These surface-grafted polymers effectively prevent the opsonization of drug carriers and their clearance by the RES. The approach is best developed for liposomes (15), though has a rather broad applicability (16). Anticancer drug doxorubicin incorporated into long-circulating PEG-coated liposomes [PEG is incorporated into the liposomal membrane via PEG-attached phosphatidyl ethanolamine (PE) group], currently used in clinical conditions, demonstrates high efficacy in EPR-based tumor therapy and strongly diminishes side-effects (17) of the therapy with free doxorubicin. Long-circulating polymeric micelles may be used as carriers for drug delivery into tumors with a smaller cut-off size, such as Lewis lung carcinoma (18). Important advantages of prolonged circulation of drugs and drug carriers in the blood flow include: (a) the possibility of maintaining a required concentration of a drug or drug carrier in the blood for a long time after a single administration; (b) the ability to utilize the EPR effect for the accumulation of pharmaceuticals in the areas with leaky vasculature; (c) the possibility of enhancing drug and drug carrier targeting into the areas with limited blood supply and/or low concentration of a target antigen when an extended time is required for a sufficient quantity of a drug to accumulate in the target zone.

TARGETING MOIETIES

Unfortunately, none of the approaches to drug targeting described above can be generally applied. For example, the direct administration of a drug into an affected organ or tissue in a majority of cases is technically quite difficult; on the other hand, many diseases are spread over a variety of cells or tissues. Frequently, a pathological site does not differ much from normal tissues in terms of vascular permeability, temperature or local pH value, which makes the use of pH- or temperature differences-based targeting non-applicable. Magnetic drug delivery also has limitations related to the blood flow rate in the target, and is virtually impossible in large vessels or in "deep" tissues. In many pathological situations, the integrity of vascular endothelium remains non-affected and the EPR opportunity is not available. Eventually, the understanding was developed that the most widely applicable way to target a non-specific drug or drug carrier to a required area is to conjugate this drug with another molecule (usually referred to as a targeting moiety of vector molecule) capable of specific recognition and binding to a target site. The variety of substances that can be used as targeting moieties includes: (a) antibodies and their fragments; (b) lectins; (c) other proteins; (d) lipoproteins; (e) hormones; (f) charged molecules; (g) mono-, oligo- and polysaccharides; (h) some low-molecular-weight ligands, such as folate (1). Still, monoclonal antibodies (and their fragments) against characteristic components of target organs or tissues are the most frequently used vector molecules.

A direct coupling of a given pharmaceutical with a targeting moiety looks like the simplest way to prepare a targeted drug. However, one has to keep in mind that, in this case, each antibody molecule is able to carry just one or, at best, few active drug molecules. This coupling can work only in a limited number of cases, when the drugs used possess a very high specific activity, and only a small number of drug molecules are required in a target area to produce a therapeutic effect. This may be true in case of certain toxins and enzymes. Immunotoxins represent the most vivid examples of this approach (19). An active (toxic) fragment of the molecule can be produced by chemical or enzymatic cleavage from a whole toxin molecule and then conjugated with an appropriate antibody.

As a result, a toxic moiety may be delivered only in those cells that express an appropriate antigen recognized by this antibody (usually, cancer cells are targeted with immunotoxins), while antigen-free cells will not be recognized by the antibody and damaged. Because toxic units of toxins (active part of immunotoxins) are extremely active (a single such moiety can kill a cell by destroying multiple ribosomes), it is still believed that immunotoxins will find a clinical application (Figure 3 below).

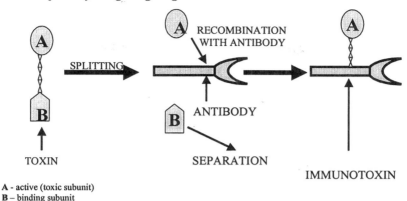

A - active (toxic subunit)
B – binding subunit

Figure 3. The scheme of immunotoxin preparation. A natural toxin is split into active and cell-binding subunits, and the active subunit is recombined with a target-specific monoclonal antibody yielding the immunotoxin.

The attachment of various thrombolytic enzymes to some antibodies specific towards different components of thrombi provides another interesting example of a direct drug-to-vector moiety conjugation. Thrombolytic enzymes by themselves may be inhibited, inactivated or cleared from the blood rather quickly, and their accelerated targeted delivery directly to the thrombosis sites may enhance the outcome of the therapy dramatically. For example, it was clearly demonstrated in hamsters and baboons that the effective thrombolysis may be achieved by using the conjugate between single-chain urokinase-type plasminogen activator and a bispecific monoclonal antibody against this activator and fibrin (20). The data on enzyme-antibody conjugates for thrombolysis as well as on a variety of antibodies used to deliver the thrombolityc therapy directly to the occlusion site are numerous and well reviewed (21). In addition, the special chapter in this book also discusses targeted thrombolytic therapy.

Some interesting attempts have been made to use simple drug-to-antibody conjugates for targeted treatment of malignant lung diseases, such as human small cell lung cancer (SCLC). An antibody against the proliferative compartment of mammalian squamous carcinomas was conjugated with daunomycin and sharply enhanced the potency of the latter in the murine model (22). Murine monoclonal antibody NCC-LU-243 was conjugated with mitomycin C and used for the targeted therapy of nude mice with transplanted antigen-positive cell line of human SCLC (23).

However, in a general case, a single targeting moiety should have a much higher load of a pharmaceutical agent to make the whole approach beneficial and practically applicable.

An alternative approach includes the use of a certain soluble or insoluble carrier, which can be loaded with multiple active moieties and then conjugated additionally with the targeting unit and some other optional groups, according to the principal scheme suggested by Ringsdorf in mid-70s (24), Figure 4.

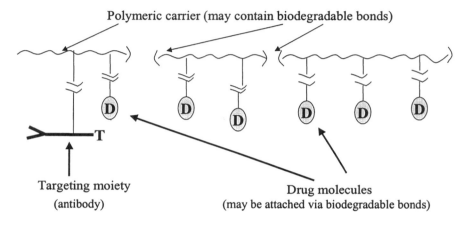

Figure 4. The schematic structure of polymeric drug. According to (24).

Different biocompatible and biodegradable water-soluble polymers containing a sufficient number of reactive groups (to attach drug molecules and targeting moities) can be used as soluble carriers (see the Chapter by Ruth Duncan in this book). The family of insoluble carriers includes microcapsules, nanoparticles, liposomes, micelles and even cell ghosts and whole cells. In general, microreservoir-type systems, such as liposomes or microcapsules, have certain advantages over other delivery systems. The advantages include: (a) a maximum volume at a given surface providing a maximum load of the drug; (b) a small required quantity of a targeting component, because just a few targeting moieties can carry multiple drug moieties loaded into the reservoir; (c) a possibility to easily control composition, size, and even permeability of a microreservoir.

By now, different mechanisms can successfully target various body compartments, such as components of cardiovascular system (blood pool, vascular walls, lungs, heart), reticulo-endothelial system (liver and spleen), lymphatic system (lymph nodes and lymphatic vessels), as well as different individual diseases including tumors, infarcts, inflammations, infections, and areas of transplant rejection. The parameters determining the efficacy of drug targeting include: the size of the target, blood flow through the target, number of binding sites for the targeted drug/drug carrier within the target, number and affinity of targeting moieties on a drug molecule (drug carrier particle), multipoint interaction of a drug/drug carrier with the target, longevity of drug conjugates and drug carriers in the circulation. By varying some of those parameters, one can control physico-chemical and biological properties of targeted drug delivery systems in rather broad limits.

In a single chapter, it is virtually impossible to cover even the most basic aspects of targeted drug delivery. Further, just some important examples of targeted drug carriers and possible fields of their application will be presented. However, one has to clearly understand that the key principles underlying the chosen examples can be applied to all other targeted delivery systems not considered here.

IMMUNOLIPOSOMES AND LONG-CIRCULATING IMMUNOLIPOSOMES

Immunoliposomes

Liposomes, artificial phospholipid vesicles with size varying from 50 to 1000 nm, can be loaded with a variety of water-soluble drugs (which go into their inner aqueous compartments) and water-insoluble drugs (which can be incorporated into the hydrophobic compartment of the phospholipid bilayer) have been considered as promising drug carriers for over two decades (25). However, upon intravenous administration, plain liposomes are very quickly (usually within 15 to 30 min) opsonized and sequestered by cells of the reticuloendothelial system (RES), primarily by the liver (25). From this point of view, the use of targeted liposomes, i.e. liposomes with a specific affinity for the affected organ or tissue, may both increase the efficacy of liposomal drug and decrease the loss of liposomes and their contents in RES.

To obtain targeted liposomes, different methods have been developed to bind corresponding vectors (antibodies) to the liposome surface. These methods are relatively simple and allow the binding of sufficient numbers of antibody molecules to a liposome surface without affecting the liposome integrity and antibody affinity and specificity. At present, 100 or more antibody molecules can be bound to a single 200 nm liposome, allowing for firm multi-point liposome binding with a target. The routine methods for antibody coupling to liposomes include covalent binding to a reactive group on the liposome membrane, and hydrophobic interaction of proteins specifically modified with hydrophobic residues with the membrane (2, 25).

Table 1. The binding of various liposomal preparations with denuded and intact areas of perfused human blood vessels (as a ratio of radiolabeled liposomes accumulated in denuded and intact areas, D/I).

Liposome preparation	D/I ratio
"Plain" liposomes	0.6
Non-specific IgG-liposomes	0.9
Anti-collagen antibody-liposomes	6.1
Fibronectin-liposomes	5.3

Plain liposomes and liposomes bearing non-specific antibodies were used as controls that did not differentiate between normal and denuded areas. Specific liposomes (liposomes bearing anti-collagen antibody or protein fibronectin possessing high affinity towards collagen) clearly demonstrated preferential binding to denuded areas of the vessel wall.

A potentially important problem with liposome (or any other microparticulate drug carrier) targeting is their inability to reach extravascular targets. However, this fact does not affect liposome and immunoliposome abilities to interact with cells and non-cellular components within the circulation system, such as blood components, endothelial cells, subendothelial structures, and ischemic regions of the heart. Several interesting attempts of targeted delivery of immunoliposomes have been performed within the cardiovascular system.

The initial stage of many vessel injuries, including atherosclerosis and thrombosis (coronary ones among them), is a disruption of the vessel wall's endothelial cover integrity, leading to subendothelial denudation, which serves as a strong stimulator of platelet activation and adhesion (26). Naturally, it is tempting to think of early detection of such disruptions of endothelium and direct action at these sites to promote endothelium growth or prevent platelet adhesion onto the exposed collagen. To prove the possibility of using targeted immunoliposomes as specific drug carriers to such areas, conjugates have been obtained between liposomes and antibodies against extracellular matrix antigens - collagen, laminin, fibronectin (27). The data obtained clearly demonstrated that anti-collagen-liposomes and other matrix-specific liposomes could specifically recognize and bind collagen gaps between endothelial cells both in cell cultures and in perfused blood vessels (Table 1 above).

In another set of experiments, liposomes with attached antibody to canine cardiac myosin were used to target the area of myocardial infarction, where intracellular protein myosin becomes exposed to the circulation because of ischemia-provoked cell membrane degradation. This exposure leaves the myosin accessible for the attachment of an antimyosin antibody (28, 29). The *in vivo* studies were performed in dogs with experimental myocardial infarction developed in anesthetized animals by temporary occlusion of the anterior descending coronary artery. After 30 min of reperfusion, antimyosin-liposomes containing inside ^{111}InCl$_3$ were administered intravenously, and infarct imaging was performed on a gamma-camera. Good accumulation of the intraliposomal radioactive marker in the infarct was demonstrated, proving the possibility of immunoliposome targeting into necrotic myocardium for imaging and possible treatment of myocardial infarction.

An interesting example is connected with the targeting of ischemic cells, such as cardiocytes, with cytoskeleton-specific immunoliposomes (see also the chapter by Ban-An Khaw in this book). The approach is based on the known fact that various pathological conditions, including hypoxia and inflammation, induce cell membrane lesions (microscopic holes in the sarcolemma). Certain intracellular proteins of the cytoskeleton (myosin, vimentin) become exposed through these holes to the extracellular milieu. Appropriately radiolabeled antibodies against intracellular cytoskeletal antigens have been described to delineate cell membrane lesions (28).

Hypoxia-provoked membrane disruption cannot be reversed by simple restoration of blood flow to the ischemic zone. It was hypothesized that if the membrane lesions could be sealed to prevent the loss of intracellular molecules, the treated cells should recover and remain viable. With this in mind, the use of antibody-targeted liposomal plugs was proposed (30): a cytoskeletal antigen exposed via a membrane lesion can be used to anchor the immunoliposome directly onto (into) the hole to provide the initial protection (seal) and prevent leakage of the intracellular contents.

The phenomenon of "plug and seal" to prevent the necrotic cell death was demonstrated using myosin as the cytoskeletal target antigen and the corresponding antimyosin antibody as the anchoring device incorporated in the liposomes. It was tested in the model of hypoxic injury of H9C2 rat embryonic cardiocytes (30). The assessment of the viability of the cultured H9C2 cells subjected to the artificial hypoxia was performed after 24 hours of hypoxia by trypan-blue exclusion method or by [^{3}H]-thymidine incorporation. While control preparations provided little to no protection from the hypoxic injury, cytoskeleton-specific immunoliposomes (CSIL) almost completely prevented cell death with cell viability similar to that of normoxic cells (Table 2). CSIL-treated hypoxic cells were growing normally for more than 7 days after the hypoxic event when subsequently cultured under normoxic conditions and were able to replicate normally. Prevention of cell death by the targeted sealing of cell membrane lesions as described could have a significant clinical utility.

Table 2. Assessment of hypoxic cell viability in the presence of different liposomal preparations by Trypan Blue exclusion test (TBET) and by ^{3}H-Thymidin (3HT) uptake

Cells and treatment conditions	Viability by TBET (% of initial cell number)	Viability by 3HT (% of control)
Normoxic cardiocytes (control)	98	100
Hypoxic cardiocytes	13	3
Hypoxic cardiocytes + PL	42	31
Hypoxic cardiocytes + IgL	43	-
Hypoxic cardiocytes + IL	96	89

Viability by TBET was assessed utilizing all cells in each culture flask in triplicates. Viability by 3HT was assessed by incubating myocytes pre-cultured for 24 h under hypoxic or normoxic conditions, for another 24 h under normal conditions with 5µCi of 3HT and with or without liposomes.

The same approach provides an interesting possibility for highly efficient cell transfection and intracellular drug delivery. The fusion of the CSIL with the cell membrane was shown to be an important component of the "plug and seal" effect, which has to be followed by the release of the liposomal contents into the cytoplasm (30). With this in mind, it was suggested that, if the target cells are under artificially imposed hypoxic stress, stress-induced small membrane lesions will allow the attachment of drug- or DNA-loaded CSIL to these lesions with a subsequent fusion and cytoplasmic delivery of CSIL's contents (31).

For *in vitro* targeted gene transfection, transient, reversible hypoxic injury may be induced in the target cells or tissue grafts, and DNA-bearing CSIL could deliver the constructs directly into the cytoplasm with the restoration of the membrane integrity and cell viability. This method was termed as a "CSIL-fection." The very high efficacy of CSIL-fection was demonstrated with H9C2 cardiocytes and CSIL loaded with luciferase pGL2 vector and pSV-β-galactosidase vector (31), Table 3.

Table 3. Expression of luciferase and β-galactosidase in CSIL-fected cardiocytes.

Transfection system	RLUs of luciferase	% of cells expressing β-gal
CSIL – hypoxic cells	72,000	94
CSIL – normoxic cells	3,000	3
Plain liposomes – hypoxic cells	2,000	1
Plain liposomes – normoxic cells	3,000	0
Free DNA – hypoxic cells	3,000	1
Free DNA – normoxic cells	2,000	0

Relative light units (RLUs) produced by firefly luciferase and % of cells expressing β-galactosidase as evidence of the efficiency of transfection by CSILs in normoxic and hypoxic H9C2 cardiocytes. The expression of the transfected genes was also compared to normoxic and hypoxic cells treated with DNA-containing plain liposomes and with naked DNA.

Long-Circulating Immunoliposomes

Despite some promising results with immunoliposomes as pharmaceutical carriers, the whole approach is limited because of the short life-times of liposomes and immunoliposomes in the circulation. The majority of antibody-modified liposomes still end in the liver as a consequence of an insufficient time for the interaction between the target and targeted liposome. This is certainly the case when the target has a diminished blood supply (ischemic or necrotic areas). Even high liposome affinity towards the target could not provide a substantial liposome accumulation because of the small quantity of liposomes passing through the target with the blood. The same lack of targeting can happen if the concentration of the target antigen is very low or if sufficient blood flow (and liposome passage) through the target does not result in good accumulation due to the small number of "productive collisions" between antigens and immunoliposomes. In both cases, better accumulation can be achieved if liposomes can remain in the circulation long enough. This will increase the total quantity of immunoliposomes passing through the target in the first case, and the number of "productive collisions" between immunoliposomes and target antigens in the second. This is why long-circulated (usually, PEGylated) liposomes have attracted so much attention over the last decade (see above).

It was demonstrated (32-34) that unique properties of long-circulating and targeted liposomes can be combined in one preparation. Early experiments (32) have been performed utilizing the direct co-immobilization of an antibody and PEG on the surface of the same liposome. The concern here was that PEG can create steric hindrances to normal antibody-target interaction. However, under certain circumstances, the antibody and PEG (or any other protecting polymer) can act simultaneously. Thus, liposomes were prepared, containing on their surfaces both antimyosin and PEG, therefore possessing both abilities - to recognize and bind the target and to circulate long enough to provide high target accumulation (33). The data on liposome biodistribution and infarct accumulation clearly demonstrate that radiolabeled PEG-coated anti-myosin-liposomes can circulate for a very long time (half-life of PEG-immunoliposomes can reach more than 10 hours compared with 10 min for unmodified liposomes) and effectively accumulate in the infarct zone. Tissue radioactivity for such liposomes (expressed as a % of injected dose per g of tissue) is almost twice as high as for antibody-free PEG-liposomes or PEG-free immunoliposomes and more than ten-fold higher than for plain liposomes. Two different ways have been found for liposome accumulation in the infarcted heart in experimental rabbits - the specific one, which requires the presence of antibodies on the surface of liposomes, and the non-specific one, which proceeds via impaired filtration mechanism in affected tissues and requires many passages of liposomes through the target, i.e. prolonged circulation. The combination of Fab and PEG on the liposome surface gives absolutely maximal radioactivity accumulation in the infarct, because both accumulation mechanisms are working in this particular case, resulting in additive effect (33).

A synergistic effect of PEG and specific antibody on liposomes was also shown by Blume et al. (34), who demonstrated that PEG-coated liposomes with plasminogen coupled to the ends of long PEG chains may both circulate for a sufficiently long time and effectively bind to fibrin, a natural target for plasminogen. A recently described new technique of a single step attachment of specific ligands including monoclonal antibodies to PEGylated liposomes via p-nitrophenylcarbonyl-terminated PEG-PE provides new opportunities for preparing targeted long-circulating liposomes (35).

MICELLES AND IMMUNOMICELLES

Micelles

Micelles [including polymeric micelles (36)] represent so-called colloidal dispersions that belong to a large family of dispersed systems, consisting of particulate matter or dispersed phase distributed within a continuous phase or dispersion medium. In terms of size, colloidal dispersions occupy a position between molecular dispersions with particle size under 1 nm and coarse dispersions with particle size greater than 0.5 µm. More specifically, micelles normally have particle size within 5 to 50-100 nm range. An important property of micelles that has a particular significance in pharmacy is their ability to increase the solubility and bioavailability of sparingly soluble substances. The use of certain special intravenously administered amphiphilic molecules as surfactants can also extend the half-life of micelles in the blood. There are several key micelle properties that are important for the preparation of successful micellar drugs. Those properties include size, CMC, and loading capacity of the hydrophobic core of the micelle. Though some extreme cases are known, the usual size of a pharmaceutical micelle is between 10 and 80 nm, optimal CMC value should be in a low micromolar region, and the loading efficacy towards a hydrophobic drug should be between 5 and 25 % wt.

Three targeting mechanisms can be seen for micelles as for any other pharmaceutical long-circulating drug carrier. The first one is based on micelle spontaneous penetration into the interstitium through the leaky vasculature (EPR effect) and is considered as a "passive targeting" (12, 13, and 17). Thus, it was repeatedly shown that micelle-incorporated anticancer drugs [such as adriamycin, see, for example (37)] accumulate much better in tumors than in non-target tissues (such as the heart muscle), minimizing undesired drug toxicity. In certain cases, it is the small size of micelles which makes them superior compared to other nanoparticulates, including liposomes. The transport efficacy and accumulation of microparticulates, such as liposomes and/or micelles, in the tumor interstitium is to a great extent determined by their ability to penetrate the leaky tumor vascular endothelium (11, 38) (see the schematic representation of this phenomenon on Figure 2). Diffusion and accumulation parameters were recently shown to be strongly dependent on the cutoff size of tumor blood vessel wall, which varies for different tumors. As a result, the use of PEG-PE micelles for the delivery of a model protein drug to a murine solid tumor with a low permeability, Lewis lung carcinoma, provided the best results compared to other particulate carriers (18), (see Table 4).

Table 4. Accumulation of the native protein (soybean tripsin inhibitor, STI) and protein incorporated into liposomes or micelles in Lewis lung carcinoma tumor (LLC) in mice

Preparation	Tumor accumulation (%injected dose/g tumor)
Native STI	0.8
STI in PEG-liposomes	4.1
STI in PEG-PE micelles	7.2

Radiolabeled preparations of STI were injected into the tail vein of experimental mice with subcutanously implanted LLC tumor. Tumor-accumulated radioactivity was estimated one day post-injection.

The second targeting mechanism is based on the fact that many pathological processes in various tissues and organs are accompanied with local temperature increase and/or acidosis (39). Micelles made of thermo- or pH-sensitive components, such as poly(N-isopropylacrylamide) and its co-polymers with poly(D,L-lactide) and other blocks, can disintegrate in such areas releasing the micelle-incorporated drug (40).

Immunomicelles

Specific ligands can be attached to the water-exposed termini of hydrophilic blocks, such as antibodies and/or certain sugar moieties (41, 42). In this case, in order to make micelles targeted without creating any steric hindrances for antibody, the antibody of choice or its fragment can be chemically attached to an activated water-exposed free terminus of a hydrophilic block of micelle-forming polymer. For this purpose, a relatively simple chemistry can be applied, similar to that developed earlier for liposomes (35), and involving the use of amphiphilic PEG-PE with a protein-reactive p-NP group on the distal tip of the hydrophilic PEG block. The optimum protocol for antibody incorporation onto the micelle surface includes a preliminary antibody coupling with a terminus-reactive PEG-lipid conjugate and subsequent mixing of the product obtained with the residual non-activated PEG-lipid. In the case of targeted micelles, a local release of a free drug from micelles in the target organ should lead to the increased efficacy of the drug, while the stability of the micelles en route to the target organ or tissue should contribute drug solubility and toxicity reduction due to fewer interactions with non-target organs.

The approach is at its early stage, however, myosin-specific monoclonal antibody 2G4 and nucleosome-specific monoclonal antibody 2C5 have been coupled to PEG-PE micelles, and the resulting immunomicelles have demonstrated good binding with monolayers of appropriate antigens. Thus, micelles, including polymeric micelles, could be relatively easily made targeted by attachment of antibodies or other specific ligands.

INTRACELLULAR DRUG DELIVERY

With the development of the whole approach, more and more frequently drug and DNA targeting are considered not only on a cellular, but also on a subcellular level. Dr. Weissig's chapter in this book addresses mitochondria-specific targeting. However, mitochondria are just one of intracellular compartments of a special interest for targeted drug delivery technology. For example, a direct delivery of pharmaceuticals into the cell cytoplasm may dramatically enhance the efficacy of anticancer chemotherapy (by bypassing a p-glycoprotein pump involved in the phenomenon of multidrug resistance) or gene therapy (by bypassing the endocytic pathway and preventing lysosomal degradation of a major part of intracellularly delivered DNA).

'Protein transduction' was demonstrated with the trans-activating transcriptional activator (TAT) protein (86-mer polypeptide) from HIV-1 and some other proteins shown to enter a variety of cells when added to the surrounding media (43). Since traversal through cellular membranes represents a major barrier for efficient delivery of macromolecules into cells, the TAT protein may serve to ferry various drugs into mammalian cells *in vitro* and *in vivo*. The authors of a study published in 1999 (44) succeeded in delivering TAT protein-attached β-galactosidase in all tissues in mice, even the brain. Certain small regions of such proteins (10-16-mers) called 'protein transduction domains' (PTDs), and some other natural or synthetic peptides also efficiently traverse biological membranes (see the chapter by Ernst Wagner in this book). This process is receptor-independent and transporter-independent, is not endocytosis-mediated, and may target the lipid layer directly. The use of peptides and protein domains with amphipathic sequences for drug and gene delivery across cellular membranes is getting increasing attention (45). Covalent hitching of proteins, drugs or DNA onto PTDs may circumvent conventional limitations, by allowing transport of these compounds into a wide variety of cells *in vitro* and *in vivo* (46). TAT-peptide chemically attached to various proteins (horseradish peroxidase, β-galactosidase, and some others) was able to deliver these proteins to various cells and even in tissues in mice, resulting in high levels in heart, lung, and spleen (47).

A challenging task is to use PTDs for intracellular delivery of drug carriers, such as micelles, liposomes, and nanoparticles. So far, dextran-coated iron oxide colloidal particles with the size of about 40 nm and containing several attached molecules of TAT-peptide per particle were delivered into lymphocytes much more efficiently than free particles (48). This raises the interesting question of what may be the maximum size of particulate drug carriers that still would be translocated into cells by TAT-peptide if a sufficient number of its molecules are attached to the particle surface.

Recently, we have been able to demonstrate that relatively large 200 nm plain and PEGylated liposomes can be delivered into various cells by multiple TAT-peptide molecules attached to the liposome surface via pNP-PEG-PE (49). This phenomenon was also shown to be energy-independent and did not involve the cell respiratory chain and cytoskeleton. Our further experiments with a set of normal and cancer cells have demonstrated an efficient transfection of these cells with TAT-liposomes complexed with DNA (a plasmide encoding for the Green Fluorescent Protein).

The covalent coupling of TAT-peptides to microparticulate drug carriers may provide an efficient tool for cytosolic delivery of various drugs and drug carriers *in vitro* and *in vivo*.

TARGETED DELIVERY OF IMAGING AGENTS

At least a few words have to be said about the relatively new and highly promising area of targeted pharmaceuticals connected with a target-specific delivery of imaging agents for various imaging modalities (3). The classical example of this approach is the use of monoclonal antibodies for gamma-imaging and magnetic resonance imaging (MRI). A wide range of radioisotopes is now available for labeling antibodies used, first of all, for diagnostic imaging of cancer, myocardial infarction, certain infections, and areas of inflammation (3). 111-Indium and 99m-Technitium are frequently used for gamma-imaging and Gadolinium or Manganese is used for MRI. For rapid and firm attachment of the reporter metal atoms to an antibody molecule, chelating residues are first chemically attached to an antibody. The use of labeled antibodies for targeted *in vivo* imaging should meet several important criteria: (a) the attachment of the chelating moiety as well as metal binding should not affect the affinity and specificity of the antibody; (b) chelating group used should not permit metal detachment (transchelation) or rechelating; (c) high specific radiolabeling should be achievable to provide a good *in vivo* signal; and (d) the removal of non-bound radiolabel should be fast enough to decrease the background signal and thereby provide high target-to-normal ratios.

The optimal results of radiolabeling with metal-chelate complexes can be obtained using an indirect method of antibody modification with chelating groups (50). Synthetic polymers containing numerous chelate residues and a single terminal protein-reactive group have been developed, (see ref. 51 for review). The ability of a polymer to carry a large number of chelating moieties and bind to an antibody via a single point attachment provides a major advancement towards increasing the amount of heavy metal binding sites per antibody molecule. Thus, using chelate-derived polylysines of different molecular weights, several dozens of reporter metal atoms have been bound to a single antibody molecule; the principle of the method is shown in Figure 5. As a result, the amount of radioactive 111-In bound to an antibody Fab fragment via the single-site attached polymeric chelate (DTPA-polylysine) was approximately 15 to 20 times higher than for the same Fab fragment directly modified with a few chelating groups (DTPA).

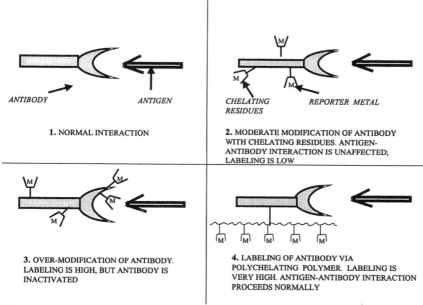

Figure 5. Possible ways to label antibody with a reporter metal via chelating group. Single-point attachment of a polymeric chelate provides the maximum metal load without affecting antibody immunologic properties.

An interesting case of imaging agent targeting is the targeting of the blood pool itself. This case includes diagnostic agents able to stay in the circulation long enough and to provide the information about the status of blood flow in different body compartments. The imaging of the blood pool and determination of functional data of the blood flow are especially important in the diagnosis of cardiovascular and thromboembolic diseases. It may be also useful in the detection of abnormal vascular permeability. Blood pool imaging can be performed in different imaging modalities, such as magnetic resonance imaging, gamma-scintigraphic imaging, and computed tomography (CT). The appropriate imaging agents must circulate for a long enough time in the blood, possess low toxicity and immunogenicity, and exhibit good excretability. Various macromolecular contrast agents have already been suggested for blood pool imaging, such as isotope-labeled polymers, label-loaded liposomes, stabilized magnetite colloids, and iodine-containing nanocrystals. These agents can be used for gamma-, MR, and CT imaging (52).

SHORT CONCLUSION

The author has to repeat again, that in a single chapter is impossible to overview even briefly the huge and continuously growing variety of approaches to targeted delivery of pharmaceutics for both therapeutics and diagnostics. Those approaches differ with respect to targeting methods, types and sites of pathologies targeted, expected outcomes, and "levels" of targeting (organ, cell or intracellular compartment). The goal of this chapter was to provide some general understanding of the field and give several representative examples of current scientific interest.

REFERENCES

1. Gregoriadis, G. (1977) Targeting of Drugs. Nature 165, 407-411.
2. Drug Targeting. Strategies, Principles, and Applications (G.E.Francis and C.Delgado, eds.), Humana Press, Totwa, NJ, 2000.
3. Handbook of Targeted Delivery of Imaging Agents (V.P.Torchilin, ed.), CRC Press, Boca Raton, FL, 1995.
4. Chazov, E.I., Matveeva, L.S., Mazaev, A.V., Sargin, K.E., Sadovskaya, G.V. and Ruda, M.Ya. (1976) Intracoronary administration of fibrinolysin in acute myocardial infarct.
   Ter. Arkh. (Russ.) 48 (4), 8-19.
5. Williams, A.S., Camilleri, J.P., Goodfellow, R.M. and Williams, B.D. (1996) A single intra-articular injection of liposomally conjugated methotrexate suppresses joint inflammation in rat antigen-induced arthritis. Br. J. Rheumatol. 35, 719-24
6. Weinstein, J.N., Magin, R.L., Yatvin, M.B. and Saharko, D. (1979) Liposomes and local hyperthermia: selective delivery of methotrexate to heated tumors. Science 204, 188-191.
7. Torchilin, V.P., Zhou, F. and Huang, L. (1993) pH-Sensitive liposomes. J. Liposome Res. 3, 201-255.
8. Widder, K.J., Marino, P.A., Morris, R.M. and Senyei, A.E. (1983) Targeting antineoplastic agents using magnetic albumin microspheres. In: E. Goldberg (Ed.), Targeted Drugs. John Wiley and Sons, New York, pp. 201-230.
9. Orekhova, N.M., Akchurin, R.S., Belyaev, A.A., Smirnov, M.D., Ragimov, S.E. and Orekhov, A.N. (1990) Local prevention of thrombosis in animal areteries by means of magnetic targeting of aspirin-loaded red cells. Thromb. Res. 57, 611-616.
10. Torchilin, V.P., Papisov, M.I., Orekhova, N.M., Belyaev, A.A., Petrov, A.D. and Ragimov, S.E. (1988) Magnetically driven thrombolytic preparation containing immobilized streptokinase - targeted transport and action. Haemostasis 18, 113-116.
11. Jain, R.K. (1999) Transport of molecules, particles, and cells in solid tumors. Ann. Rev. Biomed. Eng. 1, 241-263.

12. Palmer, T.N., Caride, V.J., Caldecourt, M.A., Twicjler, J. and Abdullah, V. (1984) The mechanism of liposome accumulation in infarction. Biochim. Biophys. Acta 797, 363-368.
13. Maeda, H., Wu, J., Sawa, T., Matsumura, Y. and Hori, K. (2000) Tumor vascular permeability and the EPR effect in macromolecular therapeutics: a review. J. Control. Release 65, 271-284.
14. Torchilin, V.P. and Trubetskoy, V.S. (1995) Which polymers can make nanoparticulate drug carriers long-circulating? Adv. Drug Deliv. Rev. 16, 141-155.
15. Stealth Liposomes (D.D.Lasic and F.Martin, eds.) CRC Press, Boca Raton, FL, 1995.
16. Torchilin, V. P. (1998) Polymer-coated long-circulating microparticulate pharmaceuticals. J. Microencapsul. 15, 1-19.
17. Gabizon, A.A. (1995) Liposome circulation time and tumor targeting: implications for cancer chemotherapy. Adv. Drug Deliv. Rev. 16, 285-294.
18. Weissig, V., Whiteman, K.R. and Torchilin, V.P. (1998) Accumulation of protein-loaded long-circulating micelles and liposomes in subcutaneous Lewis lung carcinoma in mice. Pharm. Res. 15, 1552-1556.
19. Vitetta, E.S., Krolik, K.A., Miyama-Inaba, M., Cushley, W. and Uhr, J.W. (1983) Immunotoxins: a new approach to cancer therapy. Science 219, 644-650.
20. Imura, Y., Stassen, J.M., Kurokawa, T., Iwasa, S., Lijnen, H.R. and Collen, D. (1992) Thrombolytic and pharmacokinetic properties of an immunoconjugate of single-chain urokinase-type plasminogen activator (u-PA) and a bispecific monoclonal antibody against fibrin and against u-PA in baboons. Blood 79, 2322-2329.
21. Haber, E. (1994) Antibody targeting as a strategy in thrombolysis. In: B.A.Khaw, J.Narula and H.W.Strauss (Eds.), Monoclonal Antibodies in Cardiovascular Diseases. Lea and Febiger, Malvern, pp. 187-197.
22. Ding, L., Samuel, J., MacLean, G.D., Noujaim, A.A., Diener, E. and Longenecker, B.M. (1990) Effective drug-antibody targeting using a novel monoclonal antibody against the proliferative compartment of mammalian squamous carcinomas. Cancer Immunol. Immunother. 32, 105-109.
23. Kubota, T., Yamamoto, T., Takahara, T., Furukawa, T., Ishibiki, K., Kitajima, M., Shida, Y. and Nakasubo, H. (1992) Targeting cancer chemotherapy using a monoclonal antibody (NCC-LU-243) conjugated with mitomycin C. J. Surg. Oncol. 51, 75-80.
24. Ringsdorf, H. (1975) Structure and properties of pharmacologically active polymers. J. Polym. Sci. 51, 135-153.
25. Lasic, D.D. Liposomes: from Physics to Applications, Elsevier Science Pulishers, Amsterdam. 1993.
26. Ross, R. (1993) The pathogenesis of atherosclerosis: a perspective for 1990s. Nature, 362, 801-809.
27. Smirnov, V.N., Domogatsky, S.P., Dolgov, V.V., Hvatov, V.B., Klibanov, A.L., Koteliansky, V.E., Muzykantov, V.R., Repin, V.S., Samokhin, G.P., Shekhonin, B.V., Smirnov, M.D., Sviridov, D.D., Torchilin, V.P. and Chazov, E.I. (1986) Carrier-directed targeting of liposomes and erythrocytes to denuded areas of vessel wall. Proc. Natl. Acad. Sci. USA 83, 6603-6607.
28. Khaw, B.A. (1994) Antimyosin antibody for the diagnosis of acute myocardial infarction: experimental validation. In: B.A.Khaw, J.Narula and H.W.Strauss (Eds.), Monoclonal Antibodies in Cardiovascular Diseases. Lea and Febiger, Malvern, pp. 15-29.
29. Torchilin, V.P., Khaw, B.A., Smirnov, V.N. and Haber, E. (1979) Preservation of antimyosin antibody activity after covalent coupling to liposomes, Biochem. Biophys. Res. Commun. 89, 1114-1119.

30. Khaw, B.A., Torchilin, V.P., Vural, I. and Narula, J. (1995) Plug and seal: prevention of hypoxic cardyocyte death by sealing membrane lesions with antimyosin-liposomes, Nature Med. 1, 1195-1198.

31. Khaw, B.A., daSilva, J., Vural, I., Narula, J. and Torchilin, V.P. (2001) Intracytoplasmic gene delivery for in vitro transfection with cytoskeleton-specific immunoliposomes. J. Contr. Release 75, 199-210.

32. Torchilin, V.P., Klibanov, A.L., Huang, L., O'Donnell, S., Nossiff, N.D. and Khaw, B.A. (1992) Targeted accumulation of polyethylene glycol-coated immunoliposomes in infarcted rabbit myocardium. FASEB J. 6, 2716-2719.

33. Torchilin, V.P., Narula, J., Halpern, E. and Khaw, B.A. (1996) Poly(ethylene glycol)-coated anti-cardiac myosin immunoliposomes: factors influencing targeted accumulation in the infarcted myocardium. Biochim. Biophys. Acta 1279, 75-83.

34. Blume, G., Cevc, G., Crommelin, M.D., Bakker-Woudenberg, I.A., Kluft, C. and Storm, G. (1993) Specific targeting with poly(ethylene glycol)-modified liposomes: coupling of homing devices to the ends of the polymeric chains combines effective target binding with long circulation times. Biochim. Biophys. Acta 1149, 180-184.

35. Torchilin, V.P., Levchenko, T.S., Lukyanov, A.N., Khaw, B.A., Klibanov, A.L., Rammohan, R., Samokhin, G.P. and Whiteman, K.R. (2001) p-Nitrophenylcarbonyl-PEG-PE-liposomes: fast and simple attachment of specific ligands, including monoclonal antibodies, to distal ends of PEG chains via p-nitrophenylcarbonyl groups. Biochim. Biophys. Acta 1511, 397-411.

36. Torchilin, V.P. (2001) Structure and design of polymeric surfactant-based drug delivery systems. J. Contr. Release 73, 137-172.

37. Kwon, G.S. and Kataoka, K. (1999) Block copolymer micelles as long-circulating drug vehicles. Adv. Drug Delivery Rev. 16, 295-309.

38. Yuan, F., Dellian, M., Fukumura, M., Leunig, M., Berk, D.A., Torchilin, V.P. and Jain, R.K. (1995) Vascular permeability in a human tumor xenograft: Molecular size dependence and cutoff size. Cancer Res. 55, 3752-3756.

39. Helmlinger, G., Yuan, F., Dellian, M. and Jain, RK. (1997) Interstitial pH and pO2 gradients in solid tumors in vivo: high-resolution measurements reveal a lack of correlation. Nature Med. 3, 177-182.

40. Jones, M.-C. and Leroux, J.-C. (1999) Polymeric micelles – a new generation of colloidal drug carriers. Eur. J. Pharm. Biopharm. 48, 101-111.

41. Cho, C.S., Chang, M.Y., Lee, H.C., Song, S.C., Goto, M. and Akaike, T. (1998) Proc. 25th Intl Symp. Contr. Rel. Bioact. Mater., Contr. Rel. Soc., Inc. 721-722.

42. R.Rammohan, R., T.Levchenko, T., V.Weissig, V., A.Chakilam, A. and V.Torchilin, V. (2001) Proc. 28th Intl Symp. Contr. Rel. Bioact. Mater., Contr. Rel. Soc., Inc. 484-485.

43. Joliot, A., Pernelle, C., Deagostini-Bazin, H. and Prochiantz, A. (1991) Antennapedia homeobox peptide regulates neural morphogenesis. Proc. Natl. Acad. Sci. USA 88, 1864-1868.

44. Schwarze, S.R., Ho, A., Vocero-Akbani, A. and Dowdy, S.F. (1999) In vivo protein transduction: delivery of a biologically active protein into the mouse. Science 285, 1569-1572.

45. Plank, C., Zauner, W. and Wagner, E. (1998) Application of membrane-active peptides for drug and gene delivery across cellular membranes. Adv. Drug Deliv. Rev. 34, 21-35.

46. Gius, D.R., Ezhevsky, S.A., Becker-Hapak, M., Nagahara, H., Wei, M.C. and Dowdy, S.F. (1999) Transduced p16INK4a peptides inhibit hypophosphorylation of the retinoblastoma protein and cell cycle progression prior to activation of Cdk2 complexes in late G1.Cancer Res. 59, 2577-2580.

47. Fawell, S., Seery, J., Daikh, Y., Moore, C., Chen, L.L., Pepinsky, B. and Barsoum, J. (1994) Tat-mediated delivery of heterologous proteins into cells. Proc. Natl. Acad. Sci. USA 91, 664-668.
48. Lewin, M., Carlesso, N., Tung, C.-H., Tang, X.-W., Cory, D., Scadden, D.T. and Weissleder, R. (2000) Tat peptide-derivatized magnetic nanoparticles allow in vivo tracking and recovery of progenitor cells. Nature Biotech. 18, 410-414.
49. Torchilin, V.P., Rammohan, R., Weissig, V. and Levchenko, T.S. (2001) TAT peptide on the surface of liposomes affords their efficient intracellular delivery even at low temperature and in the presence of metabolic inhibitors. Proc. Natl. Acad. Sci. USA, 98, 8786-8791.
50. Torchilin, V.P. and Klibanov, A.L. (1991) The antibody-linked chelating polymers for nuclear therapy and diagnostics. CRC Crit. Rev. Ther. Drug Carriers Syst. 7, 275-308.
51. Torchilin, V.P. (1999) Novel polymers in microparticulate diagnostic agents. CHEMTECH 29, 27-34.
52. Torchilin, V.P., Babich, J. and Weissig, V. (2000) Liposomes and micelles to target the blood pool for imaging purposes. J. Liposome Res., 10, 329-345.

GLOSSARY

Drug targeting: spontaneous (for example, via EPR effect) or targeting moiety-mediated increased accumulation of a drug in the required area of the body compared to other tissues and organs.

EPR effect: increased extravasation and accumulation of macromolecules and microparticulates (including drugs and drug carriers) in certain pathological tissues due to increased permeability of blood vessel walls in these areas.

Imaging agent: imaging or contrast agent represents a certain reporter group capable of increasing the signal from the tissue of interest in various imaging modalities (such as gamma-imaging, magnetic resonance imaging, computed tomography, and sonography).

Immunoliposome: a targeted liposome with a surface-attached specific antibody.

Immunomicelle: a targeted micelle with a corona-attached specific antibody.

Immunotoxin: a therapeutic molecule consisting of a target-specific antibody, which bears a catalytic (toxic) subunit of a natural toxin.

Liposome: a popular drug delivery system that represents an artificial phospholipid vesicle (100 to 1000 nm in size) that can be loaded with various soluble and insoluble drugs (which go into aqueous interior or phospholipid membrane of the liposome, respectively).

Long-circulation drug carrier: drug carriers that are able to stay in the circulation system for hours or even days without being recognized and captured by cells of the reticulo-endothelial system

Micelle: a drug delivery system that represents a microscopic spherical colloidal particle (5 to 50 nm in size) and self-assembles from various amphiphilic molecules. Micelle consists of a hydrophobic core (that solubilizes various water-insoluble drugs) and hydrophilic shell.

PEG: polyethylene glycol, biocompatible and non-toxic polymer that is widely used to extend the circulation time of many drugs and drug carriers and to minimize their side effects.

Polymeric drug: therapeutic structure consisting of multiple drug molecules attached to a biocompatible and biodegradable polymeric carrier, which can additionally bear a targeting moiety.

Targeting moiety: a molecule (usually, antibody) that can specifically recognize and bind certain structures in pathological areas. Being attached to a drug molecule or drug carrier particle, such molecule enhances their accumulation in therapeutic targets.

TAT: or trans-activating transcriptional activator is a 86-mer protein from HIV-1 that is capable of energy- and receptor-independent translocation through biological membranes. TAT and similar proteins as well as certain peptides derived from these proteins can serve as targeting moieties for intracellular drug delivery.

2

BIOLOGICAL BARRIERS FOR DRUG TARGETING

Vladimir R. Muzykantov
Department of Pharmacology, University of Pennsylvania School of Medicine, Philadelphia, PA 19104-6068

INTRODUCTION

Applications of large, complex carriers that deliver powerful, specific and sensitive agents (cytokines, toxins, enzymes and genetic materials) face formidable challenges. Drug targeting strategies have to traverse diverse barriers: biological (e.g., associated with drug delivery, subcellular addressing of a drug, metabolization of carriers, etc), technological (e.g., associated with production, dosing, shelf-life of a drug-carrier complexes) and socio-economical (e.g., price, practical utility and public accessibility of a targeting strategy).

This chapter focuses on the biological barriers associated with drug delivery to a target, including limitations of current administration routes, biocompatibility and bioavailability of drug-carrier complexes, and the side effects and restrictions associated with transport of these complexes through endothelial cells, tissues and target components. Some means proposed to traverse these barriers and, therefore, translate targeting strategies to clinical practice, are briefly reviewed in the chapter.

ADMINISTRATION ROUTES FOR DRUG TARGETING: LIMITATIONS AND OPTIONS

Table 1 (below) briefly outlines major routes useful for drug targeting administration. The oral route of administration is hardly applicable for the drug targeting beyond the gastrointestinal tract, because: i) drug-carrier complexes, especially carrying proteins and DNA, rapidly degrade in the digestive system; and, ii) large size of the complexes (usually in the range of

10-500 nm diameter) precludes their absorption. Theoretically, oral route could be used for systemic drug targeting. For example, M-cells in the Payer's patches absorb and transport large molecules and particles via intestinal walls, for presentation to the immune cells. It is tempting to speculate that this mechanism may be utilized for oral delivery of drug-carrier complexes into the systemic circulation (see Chapter 22).

Intraperitoneal and pleural routes provide formation of local depots releasing drug-carrier complexes that enter blood and/or lymphatic circulation, eventually. Use of slow-release polymers or micro-pumps further prolongs the pharmacokinetics. However, these routes are relatively invasive and prone to infection-associated complications. Only fractions of a drug-carrier complex permeate the pleural and peritoneal barriers and avoid inactivation on route to the circulation.

Table 1. Major routes of administration for drug targeting. See explanations in this and following sections.

Route	Advantages	Limitations
Oral	Well tolerated, easy to dose, low safety concerns	Very low bioavailability due to fast degradation and poor absorption
Peritoneal, Pleural	High access to target cells in the cavities, slower kinetics of drugs in the circulation	Low effectiveness, degradation of drugs on the route to circulation; invasiveness, safety concerns;
Direct, e.g.: Cranial Tumor	High accessibility of target cells and high local drug level in target area	Useful only for targets with known location amenable for challenging surgical access; invasiveness
Vascular Muscular Dermal	Expedited delivery of drugs; good access to diverse targets via circulation	Inactivation of drugs in blood; elimination; RES uptake; systemic side effects
Pulmonary	Targeting to lung cells, non-invasive delivery to blood	Low effectiveness and homogeneity of alveolar delivery, poor absorption

Implantation of a drug-carrier complex in joints, cerebral cavities or in solid tumors provides an invasive route to achieve a high local drug level in certain surgically accessible sites. However, this route cannot be used for drug delivery to disseminated targets and targets with unknown location.

Therefore, intravascular administration is the main route for systemic delivery of drugs to diverse targets with known and unknown location including disseminated cells, tumors, inflammation, brain, thrombi, heart, vascular and immune cells. A necessity for injections and safety concerns represents obvious limitations. Subcutaneous, intra-dermal and intramuscular routes are more tolerable and create short-term depots with a relatively high access to blood or/and lymphatic vasculature. These routes provide less effective delivery, but more prolonged pharmacokinetics than a direct intravascular administration. Micron-scale injection devices that are currently in development promise a more user-friendly, painless use of these routes for either injections or prolonged administrations.

Major efforts have been focused in the last decades on the pulmonary route (e.g., inhalation) that permits relatively effective targeting of drugs and genetic materials to the lung cells and beyond the alveolar barrier, which consists only of thin monolayers of epithelial and endothelial cell separated by the basal membrane (1). Thus, some drugs (e.g., insulin) manage to permeate the barrier and enter blood, although the mechanisms, effectiveness and therapeutic use of this pathway remain to be better characterized. A relatively low effectiveness and high heterogeneity of a drug deposition in the alveoli represent major challenges; the larger the size of a drug-carrier complex, the more difficult it is to achieve high effectiveness and homogeneity. Means to overcome this problem include aerosolization of drugs (including proteins, DNA or liposomes) and use of pulmonary surfactant as an additive to a carrier moiety, in order to provide a more effective mixing with alveolar content and uptake by the alveolocytes.

INACTIVATION AND ELIMINATION OF DRUG-CARRIER COMPLEXES

After entering the bloodstream, even drugs coupled with high affinity carriers require a considerable time in order to accumulate in the target sites. For example, antibodies and their fragments require at least several minutes to accumulate in easily accessible targets, such as blood cells and endothelium. Hours and even days may be needed for them to accumulate in the extravascular sites (e.g., tumors). The larger a drug-carrier complex is, the longer time period required for the targeting.

Therefore, inactivation and elimination, both restricting the half-life of a functionally active drug-carrier complex in circulation, are barriers for targeting. In general, there are two major clearing systems: small (<40 kD) molecules are cleared via renal glomeruli filtration, whereas large molecules and complexes are taken up by reticuloendothelial system (RES) organs, first of all, liver and spleen (2).

Some protein drugs bind to specific receptors that accelerate clearance, especially when a receptor is accessible from blood, such as receptors on blood cells, endothelium, macrophages and renal cells. Thus, certain enzymes and cytokines disappear from the bloodstream within a few minutes due to a receptor-mediated uptake (3). Hepatocytes and macrophages uptake drugs and carriers exposing sugars (e.g., glycoproteins with mannose or galactose terminal groups) via corresponding sugar receptors.

Even prior to elimination, many drugs become impaired, inhibited or completely inactivated in the circulation. Proteases and nucleases in blood and tissues rapidly degrade agents such as proteins and genetic materials (e.g., oligonucleotides and DNA). Liposomes and polymer carriers protect encapsulated cargoes, but affinity moieties and drugs bound to carrier surfaces are exposed to inactivating factors. Liposome-coupled antibodies may bind soluble forms of target antigens or antigen-mimicking molecules. This competitive binding inhibits the targeting. Inhibitors in blood and tissues inactivate therapeutic enzymes, e.g., plasma inhibitors of serine proteases, serpins, impair activity of fibrinolytic enzymes.

Often times, binding of a soluble ligand or an inhibitor accelerates both inactivation and elimination of a drug-carrier complex. Fate of the tissue-type plasminogen activator (tPA, a protease widely used for therapeutic fibrinolysis, see Chapter 5) illustrates the point (4). After intravascular administration, tPA and tPA-containing complexes bind to a specific hepatic receptor that mediates rapid elimination of the drug. In addition, binding of plasminogen activator inhibitor-1 (PAI-1) to tPA or activated urokinase-type plasminogen activator inactivates their fibrinolytic activity and further accelerates hepatic uptake by a receptor that recognizes the tPA/PAI-1 complex via binding of PAI-1.

IMMUNE MECHANISMS OF INACTIVATION AND ELIMINATION

One of the major barriers for drug targeting is associated with immune reactions. For example, natural antibodies against some components of drug-carrier complexes (phospholipids, DNA) exist in the inborn immune repertoire in humans. Antibodies may also be generated in a patient's body as a result of previous administrations of drugs and carriers.

Effects of such antibodies provide yet another example of one of a plethora of scenarios for a combined inactivation and elimination induced by a soluble ligand. Binging of antibodies inactivates drug-carrier complexes (e.g., by steric blocking of therapeutic or affinity moieties), accelerates elimination (via specific mechanisms discussed below) and causes complement activation.

Complement is a cascade of specific plasma proteases and regulating proteins (main components indicated as numbered capital C) that contributes to anti-microbial and anti-tumor host defenses (5). Diverse molecules, particles and surfaces may activate complement via the classical, alternative and lectin-mediated pathways. Deposition of activated complement component C3b on the invaders initiates a series of reactions including lysis by membrane-attacking complex C7-9, phagocytosis and generation of inflammatory peptides C3a and C5a.

The classical pathway is initiated by interaction of C1q component with Fc fragments of antigen-bound antibodies, while sugar-mediated C1q binding to microorganisms and other objects initiates the lectin pathway. Bacteria, lipopolysaccharides, heterologous erythrocytes and DNA initiate the alternative pathway that starts with direct binding of C3b to these objects, which fail to inactivate bound C3b. Normal cells in human body possess specific components in the plasma membrane including decay accelerating factor (DAF) and CD59 that inactivate C3b and C7-9 and prevent self-damaging complement activity (6).

However, unless specific countermeasures are undertaken, certain drugs, carriers and vehicles may activate plasma complement. For example, carrier antibodies may activate complement via classical pathway, since C1q binds to Fc-portion of the antigen-engaged IgG and IgM. Modified red blood cells (that may be used for drug targeting) and certain types of liposomes bind C3b and activate complement (7, 8). Complement activation may lead to destruction of a carrier (hypotonic lysis of liposomes or red blood cells), generation of pro-inflammatory components of activated complement and enhanced uptake by phagocytes. Thus, opsonization, i.e. binding of antibodies or complement to a drug-carrier complex, promotes phagocytosis, accelerates elimination and may cause harmful side effects.

RES macrophages in the liver, spleen and bone marrow have good access to circulation, since the endothelial lining is not continuous in these organs. Thus, even objects with diameter of several microns may contact directly with RES macrophages (e.g., hepatic Kupffer cells) that eliminate drug-carrier complexes. The uptake reduces effectiveness of drug targeting, dictates potentially harmful dose elevations and may cause RES dysfunction (2).

Macrophages possess receptors for Fc-fragment of immunoglobulins and components of complement that serve for docking and endocytosis of foreign objects coated with antibodies or complement components. In addition, engagement of complement receptors (e.g., C3b-receptor) and Fc-receptors activates macrophages and causes release of aggressive proteases and oxidants. Thus, opsonization facilitates both the macropnage uptake and activation.

As noted above, Fc-fragments of antibodies initiate defense reactions including activation of complement and phagocytes. In addition, binding of Fc-fragment to the receptors on lymphocytes and platelets induces acute reactions such as cytotoxicity and thrombosis. Ability to activate Fc-fragment mediated reactions varies for different classes of immunoglobulins: IgM is hyperactive, whereas certain sub-classes of IgG are less potent in terms of Fc-fragment mediated activities.

Free monomeric antibodies do not initiate these reactions. However, interaction with an antigen causes conformational changes in an antibody molecule, permitting Fc-fragment binding to C1q and Fc-receptors. Specific auxiliary molecules (complement components, MHC class molecules, platelet integrin receptors) facilitate cellular responses mediated by Fc-fragment. Multimerization of Fc-fragment, as a result of formation of immune complexes, immunoconjugates, IgG aggregation or coupling to a polymer carrier, also greatly facilitates Fc-fragment mediated reactions.

Therefore, immune defense mechanisms contribute generously to inactivation and elimination of drug-carrier complexes (Figure 1 below). Importantly, they also mediate many side effects of drug targeting and, therefore, are subject of serious safety concerns.

BIOCOMPATIBILITY AND SIDE EFFECTS OF DRUG-CARRIER COMPLEXES

Targeting systems should not cause untoward activation of acute cascades as thrombosis, inflammation, toxicity and immune response. Optimally, they should be biodegradable or cleared by physiological pathways such as pulmonary exhalation, hepatic bile excretion or renal urine filtration (9). Otherwise, a prolonged deposition in tissues may cause necrosis, apoptosis and fibrosis. In addition, overload of RES with poorly degradable carriers may inhibit or kill macrophages and thus compromise the host defense.

Some polymers and drug-carrier complexes (e.g., antibody conjugates, charged liposomes) activate coagulation cascade, platelets and white blood cells. This may cause thrombosis and inflammation, side effects especially dangerous in therapy of the patients predisposed to these pathological conditions.

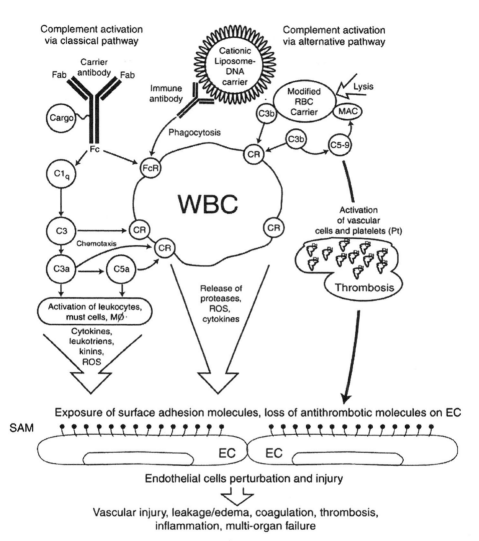

Figure 1. Immune mechanisms of elimination, inactivation and side effects. Carrier antibodies may activate complement via the classical pathway, while liposome and modified red blood cell (RBC) carriers may activate both classical and alternative pathways. Active C3b induces generation of strong pro-inflammatory peptides C3a and C5a, uptake of the complexes by phagocytes (polymorphonuclear neutrophils, PMN, and macrophages) via complement receptors (CR) and lysis of carriers by membrane attacking complex (MAC, C5-9). Phagocytes uptake complexes opsonized by host antibodies, via Fc-receptors (FcR). Engagement of FcR and CR, as well as effect of C3a and C5a, activate phagocytes; hence release of proteases, reactive oxygen species (ROS) and cytokines. C3a and C5a directly activate platelets (Pt) and vascular endothelial cells (EC). Endothelial perturbation, adhesiveness, thrombosis and vascular injury represent possible dangerous outcomes.

The design of athrombogenic biomaterials is critical for successful use of dialysis systems, artificial organs, implantable devices (e.g., stents and vascular prosthesis) and targeting systems (e.g., liposomes). Several means are being developed currently for this purpose, including coating with heparin and other anticoagulants or fibrinolytics (e.g., plasminogen activators).

Activation of complement by drug-carriers complexes may lead to hemolysis of bystander erythrocytes and generation of complement components C3a and C5a, potent mediators of inflammation. These peptides activate white blood cells and tissue macrophages that in turn release cytokines, proteases, toxic peptides and oxidant species. The vicious cycle ensues via production of vasoactive peptides, kinins and chemoattractants that perturb endothelium and further propagate thrombosis, leukocytes adhesion and inflammation. Vascular leakage, tissue injury, systemic cytokine activation and multi-organ failure represent possible and very dangerous outcomes. However, this pro-inflammatory, pro-thrombotic "side effect" of targeting may be useful for anti-tumor therapies (the chapter by Ran and co-authors).

Administration of drug/carrier complexes may elicit immune response and generation of antibodies. This side effect is especially profound in the case of targeting of highly immunogenic drugs, such as proteins and nucleic acids. In addition, carriers can work as an adjuvant, by providing multiple copies of antigenic molecules to antigen presenting cells. Immune response leading to drug inactivation by antibodies and allergic reactions represents one of the major obstacles for multiple administrations of drug-carrier complexes.

MEANS REDUCING INACTIVATION, ELIMINATION, IMMUNE RECOGNITION AND INCREASING THE SAFETY

A powerful means to minimize side effects of antibody-targeted drugs is to use Fab fragments and small hypervariable domains produced by protease cleavage or genetic engineering. This modification eliminates Fc-fragment mediated untoward reactions including activation of complement, immune cells and platelets. On the other hand, this maneuver reduces RES clearance by eliminating Fc-receptor mediated uptake and thus enhances the bioavailability of immunoconjugates.

Singular antigen-binding entities (e.g., monovalent Fab fragments) possess lower affinity to antigens; hence effectiveness of the targeting may be lower than that with whole antibodies. Thus, highly avid mAb must be selected for targeting. On the other hand, relatively small Fab- or sFv-fragment based conjugates may be the subjects of renal clearance. Therefore, blood clearance of such conjugates may be faster than the clearance of conjugates based on intact IgG molecules. Thus, selection of optimal forms of antibody carrier should balance between the safety, affinity, half-life and uptake pathways.

Humanization of murine monoclonal antibodies (insertion of an antigen-binding portion of a murine antibody into human IgG by gene engineering) minimizes inter-species immune reactions. Antibodies' gene engineering permits construction of novel fusion proteins with unique affinity end effector properties (see Chapter 14). However, most targeted drug delivery systems at the present time are designed for a single administration, in order to avoid immune reactions.

Covalent attachment of activated linear polymer, polyethylene glycol (PEG) to proteins, liposomes and polymers forms a "polymer brush" creating a water shell that repels opsonins and phagocytes (10). Thus, PEG-ylation markedly prolongs circulation time of drugs and drug-carrier complexes (Figure 2 below). In some cases, the half-life increases from a few minutes for naïve agents to many hours for PEG-ylated counterparts.

PEG-ylation of antigens masks their immunogenic determinants that otherwise are recognized by immune defenses, thus reducing immune reactions (11). PEG decoration of viruses is currently under exploration, as a means to suppress acute immune reactions to gene therapies. PEG-ylation also enhances ability of liposomes and modified red blood cells to withstand shear stress and thus improves the rheological properties of the carriers (12). Therefore, PEG-ylation represents one of the most powerful and popular approaches to increasing bioavailability and biocompatibility of drug-carrier complexes and reducing harmful side effects associated with immune responses ("stealth targeting"). Feasibility, safety and applicability of diverse regimens of PEG-ylated stealth liposomes, including their repetitive administration, are the subjects of current pre-clinical animal studies (13).

Studies of PEG-ylated immunoliposomes revealed critical importance of an order in which a carrier antibody and PEG polymer are coupled to liposomes. PEG-ylation of antibody-carrying liposomes yields very stable, long-circulating and safe "stealth" liposomes, but markedly reduces the affinity to targets. The latter unfavorable effect is due to masking of antibodies by PEG moieties. However, conjugation of antibodies to liposome-coupled PEG molecules yields high-affinity stealth immunoliposomes.

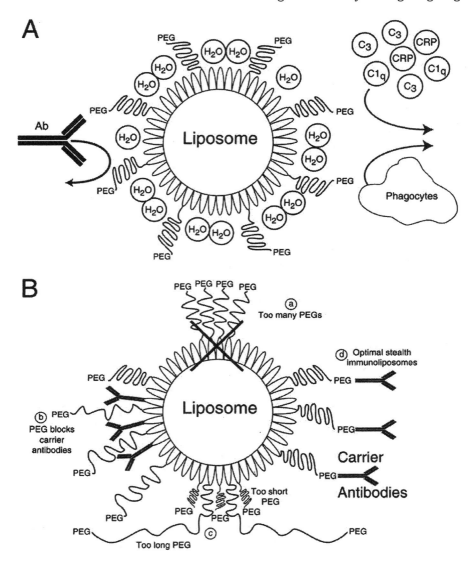

Figure 2. Stealth approach with PEG-modification (see explanation in the text). Panel A: Covalent attachment of PEG forms a water shell around carriers and drugs that repels opsonins and masks the complexes from immune recognition. Panel B: Technical aspects of PEG stealth technology. a, attachment of too many PEG molecules per liposome destabilizes lipid membrane; b, coupling of PEG after carrier antibodies diminishes their accessibility to targets; c, coupling of too long PEG polymers compromises biodegradation, whereas too short polymers fail to protect liposomes; d, stealth immunoliposomes possessing carrier antibodies coupled to the end groups of PEG molecules of optimal length.

Moreover, antibodies attached to extended and flexible PEG polymers enjoy practically unlimited steric freedom that facilitates interaction with insoluble antigens. Thus a resulting effective affinity to the targets increases (14).

Protecting effects of PEG-ylation increase with both the polymer length and number of PEG molecules attached. PEG-5000 is one of the most popular PEG derivatives for stealth targeting. Theoretically, the denser the PEG-brush is, the more profound the protective effect. However, an excessive decoration with PEG leads to inactivation of proteins, while incorporation of large number of PEG molecules in liposomes destabilizes lipid bilayer. Synthesis of long PEG-lipid derivatives and design of synthetic totally PEG-coated vesicles ("polymerosomes") represents an interesting novel technology to produce inert, long-circulating vehicles for drug targeting (see Chapter 24).

Genetic and chemical modifications of drugs, especially therapeutic proteins used for the targeting, represent powerful tools to minimize inactivation and elimination. For example, chimeric recombinant tPA mutants lacking domains recognized by tPA receptor and PAI-1 circulate in the bloodstream for a prolonged circulation in active form. Accordingly, PAI-1-resistant derivatives of plasminogen activators represent preferential agents for thrombi targeting (see Chapter 5).

Decoration of drugs or drug vehicles and carriers with biological "repellents" that elude the host defense is also an attractive avenue for improving biocompatibility of drug targeting systems. For example, coupling or incorporation of complement inhibitors, DAF and CD59, represents an interesting specific approach to reduce the lysis and, to some extent, formation of C3a and C5a peptides (6). Coupling or incorporation of negatively charged glycosides or syalic acid residues masks the complexes from recognition by immune mechanisms and markedly prolongs their bioavailability, in part due to suppression of the binding to negatively charged cell surfaces, including luminal surface of the vascular endothelium.

ENDOTHELIAL BARRIER FOR THE EXTRAVASCULAR TARGETING

A monolayer formed by endothelial cells lining the luminal surface of the blood vessels separates compounds circulating in the blood from the extravascular tissues, including such important targets as tumors. Rates of extravasation of molecules and particles vary in different tissues. For example, endothelium in RES (e.g., in spleen and liver) is fenestrated, i.e. has micron-size openings, which permit a relatively free passage of large objects to the tissues (2). In contrast, endothelial cells in the brain form an extremely tight monolayer with specific features preventing drugs entry into the brain (blood-brain barrier, BBB: see in details in the Chapters 16-19).

However, in most organs (e.g., heart, and lung) only small molecules easily traverse continuous endothelium, while transendothelial passage of large molecules is restricted and occurs normally at slow rates. In order to overcome this barrier and to accelerate accumulation of drugs or imaging agents in the extravascular targets, pre-targeting strategies utilizing sequential injection of small ligands following injection of modified affinity antibodies are being explored (15).

However, the endothelial barrier is not completely impermeable for large molecules and microparticles. Thus, even sub-micron lipoprotein particles reach smooth muscle cells, fibroblasts and macrophages localized in the subendothelial layers. There is a constant passage of plasma proteins, including relatively large ones (e.g., 800 kD IgM) into the extravascular compartments such as tissues, peritoneum and alveoli.

There has been a decade-long discussion about whether intercellular or transcellular pathway provides the main physiological passage of large molecules across the endothelial barrier. The jury is still out; it seems be fair to say that both mechanisms likely operate in the vasculature, but their contributions varies in different organs and at different conditions. For example, diverse pathological conditions facilitate extravasation, mainly by the opening of inter-endothelial junctions and elevation of pericellular transport. The intimate molecular mechanisms of this process that mediates tissue edema involve complex signaling and reorganization of cytoskeleton and cell junction components, as well as proteolytic modification of the elements of endothelial extracellular matrix. However, inflammation, angiogenesis and tumor growth are associated with increased extravascular filtration that in many cases is initiated by binding of the vasoactive agents histamine, substance P, VEGF and other growth factors to specific receptors on endothelial cells.

Targeting tumors and inflammation takes advantage of this natural pathological mechanism (see Chapters 10-13). On the other hand, specific interventions, including local hyperthermia, application of ultrasound and substances increasing vascular permeability (e.g., bradykinin, VEGF), are explored as means to facilitate extravascular targeting (16). However, the mechanisms, therapeutic applicability and safety of these interventions remain to be better characterized.

Transcellular transport via endothelium also represents an important pathway for the drug targeting (Figure 3). Endothelial cells have well-developed machinery for endocytosis (clathrin-coated pits) and transcytosis (caveoli). Caveoli represent structurally and functionally distinct invaginations in cholesterol-enriched domains of endothelial plasma membrane that serve as mechano-sensing, signaling and transport compartment of endothelial cells. Very importantly, certain surface determinants are concentrated in the caveoli and their ligands seem to traverse endothelial cells very effectively. Therefore, targeting caveoli promises a novel modality for permeation of the endothelial barrier.

This newly discovered paradigm is of great importance for the drug targeting strategies. For example, gp-60 (albumin-binding protein 60 kD, or albondin) seems to be a good determinant for transendothelial targeting. Antibodies directed against gp-60 bind to the endothelial cells, stimulate transcytosis via caveoli and appear on the basolateral surface of endothelium (17). Alternatively, a newly described monoclonal antibody directed against a non-identified caveoli-associated antigen, gp 90, permits an extremely effective accumulation of conjugated tracer compounds in subendothelial compartment in the pulmonary vasculature after intravenous injection in intact rats (18) (see Chapter 6).

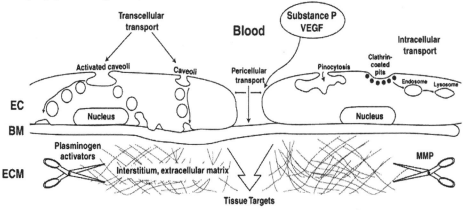

Figure 3. Permeation of the endothelial barrier (see explanations in the text). VEGF – vascular endothelial growth factor; EC – endothelial cells, scissors: MMP (matrix metalloproteinases) and plasminogen activators degrade extracellular matrix.

TRANSPORT IN THE TISSUES AND PENETRATION OF THE TARGETS

Even after extravasation, transport of drugs in the tissues and within certain targets is subject to additional limitations. Under normal circumstances, diffusion in the interstitial compartment is slow. Rate of tissue filtration and diffusion is reversibly proportional to size of a drug-carrier complex. In addition, transport of charged compounds (e.g., DNA and DNA polyplexes) is further impeded by binding to proteoglycans and other charged components of extracellular matrix.

Some pathological processes accelerate transport in the extravascular compartment. Hemorrhages, blood leakage from the vessels, represent a "semi-specific" pathological mechanism for transport of drugs (e.g., stimulants of normal reparation) into the affected organ. Inflammation activates tissue metalloproteinases that disorganize dense structure of extracellular matrix, whereas tissue edema facilitates solute diffusion. However, certain areas of pathological foci remain poorly accessible to the targeting. For example, diffusion of drugs to the core of solid tumors represents a well-recognized problem (19).

High affinity carriers provide the specificity of targeting, but affinity carrier-driven drugs poorly penetrate even relatively small (hundreds of micron to a fraction of centimeter) targets. Such carriers bind to antigens on the surface and superficial layers of targets and, therefore, their diffusion is slower than that of non-targeted counterparts. Targeting of blood clots illustrates the paradoxical problem of "affinity retention and depletion": the higher affinity of a fibrinolytic to specific clot antigens (fibrin or activated platelets), the slower delivery of drugs into the deep layers of clots and less effective resulting lysis (20).

SIDE EFFECTS ASSOCIATED WITH DRUG-CARRIERS INTERACTION WITH TARGETS

In addition to side effects induced by non-intended interactions with reactive systems on the route to the target discussed above, specific interactions with targets may cause potentially harmful effects. For example, local activation of complement, phagocytes and lymphocytes by the target-bound antibodies via Fc-fragment mediated mechanisms may cause immune damage to the target cells. Elimination of Fc-fragment helps to prevent this untoward effect. However, in the case of anti-tumor therapies, this effect represents an important benefit.

Even in the absence of Fc-fragment mediated activities, binding of drug-carrier complexes to some determinants may cause specific side effects due to their conformational alterations, function inhibition or activation, masking and enhanced shedding or internalization (21). Importantly, effects of carriers (e.g., monoclonal antibodies or monovalent Fab-fragments) may differ from those of multivalent, large, complex carrier-drug compounds. Engagement or cross-linking of surface determinants may cause redistribution of the plasma membrane domains, activate endocytosis and ignite signal transduction pathways leading to either cell activation or apoptosis.

The functional consequences of binding many affinity carriers to their targets are understood relatively poorly. In the case of anti-tumor targeting, such "secondary" effects may be beneficial (blocking and/or inactivation of the receptors for angiogenic and growth factors) (see Chapter 12). In other cases, blocking of a target determinant may cause harmful side effects. Targeting to thrombomodulin, which may inhibit the anti-thrombotic activity of this endothelial glycoprotein and thus provoke vascular thrombosis, illustrates the point (Chapter 7). Depending on the pathological context, therapeutic goals and individual reactions of patients, intervention in functions of the same target determinant may cause either beneficial or harmful effects. Therefore, effects induced, mediated or modulated by interactions with target determinants represent potential barriers that must be rigorously studied and accounted for in every application of the targeting.

CONCLUSIONS AND PERSPECTIVES

The problems of biological barriers are not new for the targeted drug delivery strategies. In fact, many of the barriers described in this chapter impede pharmacotherapy with regular drugs. However, the size, complexity, immunogenicity and powerful side effects of the targeted drug-carrier compounds magnify the problems that require adequate solutions in order to translate promising laboratory studies into clinically applicable treatments.

Bioengineering and biotechnology means are utilized very actively to overcome the biological barriers. Certain carriers themselves help to overcome biological barriers for drug targeting. Thus, encapsulation protects against inactivation, whereas high-affinity carriers reduce time required for the targeting and thus alleviate the problem of elimination. Novel means for immune masking and improved delivery via vascular and other routes are being explored. Gene engineering of antibodies and production of small affinity carriers including peptides fused directly to effector moieties promises even better control over delivery features and potential side effects of targeting systems.

Progress of drug targeting is inseparable from that of other fields of biomedicine. Better understanding of the mechanisms of immune recognition and reactions, endothelial transport and functional consequences of engaging of the target determinant greatly support our efforts to achieve safe, effective, specific and powerful treatments utilizing drug targeting.

ACKNOWLEDGEMNTS

This work was supported by NIH SCOR in Acute Lung Injury (NHLBI HL 60290, Project 4), NHLBI RO1 (HL/GM 71175-01) and American Heart Association Bugher-Stroke Award and the Department of Defense Grant (PR 012262).

REFERENCES

1. D.Edwards, A.Ben-Jebria and R.Langer (1998) Recent advances in pulmonary drug delivery using large, porous inhaled particles. *J.Appl.Physiol.*, 84:379-385
2. M.Poznansky and R.Juliano (1984) Biological approaches to the controlled delivery of drugs: A critical review. *Pharmacol. Reviews*, 36(4):277-336
3. Y.Yabe, M.Nishikawa, A.Tamada, Y.Yakakura and M.Hashida (1999) Targeted delivery and improved therapeutic potential of catalase by chemical modification: combination with superoxide dismutase. *J.Pharm.Exp.Ther.*, 289:176-184
4. M.Narita, G.Bu, J.Herz and A.Schwartz (1995) Two receptor systems are involved in the plasma clearance of tissue-type plasminogen activator (t-PA) in vivo. *J. Clin. Invest.*, 96:1164-1168
5. M.Walport (2001) Complement. *New Engl.J.Med.*, 344:1058-1066
6. M.Medof, T.Kinoshita and V.Nussenzweig (1984) Inhibition of complement activation on the surface of cells after incorporation of decay-accelerating factor (DAF) into their membranes *J. Exp. Med.*, 160:1558-1578
7. J.Szebeni (1998) The interaction of liposomes with the complement system. *Crit. Rev.Ther.Drug Carrier Systems*, 15:57-88
8. V.Muzykantov and J.C.Murciano (2002) Streptavidin-mediated coupling of therapeutic proteins to carrier erythrocytes. In: Erythrocyte engineering for drug delivery and targeting (M.Maniani, Ed.), Landes Bioscience-Eurekah, TX, 37-67
9. B.Jeong, Y.Bae, D.Lee and S.Kim (1997) Biodegradable block copolymers as injectable drug-delivery systems. *Nature*, 388:860-862
10. A.Abuchowski, J.R.McCoy, N.C.Palczuk, T.van Es and F.F.Davis (1977) Effect of covalent attachment of polyethylene glycol on immunogenecity and circulating life of bovine liver catalase. *J. Biol. Chem.*, 252(11):3852-3586
11. M.Scott, K.Murad, F.Koumpouras, M.Talbot and J.Eaton (1997) Chemical camouflage of antigenic determinants: Stealth erythrocytes. *Proc. Natl. Acad. Sci. USA*, 94:7566-7571
12. J.Armstrong, H.Meiselman and T.Fisher (1997) Covalent binding of poly(ethylene glycol) (PEG) to the surface of red blood cells inhibits aggregation and reduces low shear blood viscosity. *Am. J. Hematol.*, 56:26-28
13. P.Laverman, M.Carstens, O.Boerman, E.Dams, W.Oyen, N.Rooijen, F.Corstens and G.Storm (2001) Factors affecting the accelerated blood clearance of PEG-liposomes upon repeated injections. *J.Pharm.Exp.Ther.*, 298:607-612
14. CB Hansen, GY Kao, EH Moase, S Zalipsky and TM Allen (1995) Attachment of antibodies to sterically stabilized liposomes: evaluation, comparison and optimization of coupling procedures. *Biochim.Biophys.Acta.* 1239:133-44
15. D.Goodwin, C.Meares and M.Osen (1998) Biological properties of biotin-chelate conjugates for pretargeted diagnosis and therapy with the avidin/biotin system. *J. Nucl. Med.*, 39:1813-1818

16. J.Rosenecker, W.Zhang, K.Hong, J.Lausier, P.Geppetti, S.Yoshihara, D.Papahadjopoulos and J.Nadel (1996) Increased liposome extravasation in selected tissues: effect of substance P. *Proc.Nath.Acad.Sci.USA*, 93:7236-41

17. S.Vogel, R.Minshall, M.Pilipovic, C.Tiruppathi and A.Malik. Albumin uptake and transcytosis in endothelial cells in vivo induced by albumin-binding protein. *Am J Physiol Lung Cell Mol Physiol.*, 2001; 281(6):L1512-22

18. McIntosh, D.P., X.Y.Tan, P.Oh and J.E.Schnitzer (2002) Targeting endothelium and its dynamic caveoli for tissue-specific transcytosis in vivo: a pathway to overcome cell barriers to drug and gene delivery. *Proc.Natl.Acad.Sci.USA*, 99:1996-2001

19. R.Jain. Transport of molecules, particles, and cells in solid tumors (1999) *Annu.Rev. Biomed.Eng.* 1:241-263

20. D.Sakharov and D.Rijken (1995) Superficial accumulation of plasminogen during plasma clot lysis. *Circulation*, 92:1883-1890

21. V.Muzykantov (1998) Immunotargeting of drugs to the pulmonary endothelium as a therapeutic strategy. *Pathophysiology*, 5:15-33

GLOSSARY

Alternative pathway of complement: mechanism of complement activation initiated by binding of C3 component directly to an invader's surface and forming an active C3b component.

Caveoli: highly specialized endothelial organelles that are localized on the luminal surface and control signaling, internalization and transcellular transport.

Classical pathway of complement: mechanism of complement activation initiated by binding of the first component, C1q, to Fc-fragment of immunoglobulins.

Complement: a cascade of plasma proteases and regulating proteins that destroys invading cells by making hydrophilic pores in their membranes (hypotonic lysis), as well as attracting and activating leukocytes.

Decay Accelerating Factor (DAF): a surface glycoprotein expressed in most human cells that binds and inactivates activated C3b component of complement and thus protects against self-inflicted injury of the host cells.

Endothelium: a monolayer lining inner surface (lumen) of the blood vessels formed by the highly specialized endothelial cells that control vascular permeability, anti-thrombotic activities and many other functions of cardiovascular system. In many organs, endothelium prevents effective passage of macromolecules, liposomes and cells to the tissues.

Fc-fragment: a constant part of immunoglobulins that, upon interaction with an antigen or IgG multimerization, becomes accessible for binding/activation of the complement and Fc-receptors.

Fc-receptors: a family of glycoproteins expressed in all immune cells (macrophages, lymphocytes, leukocytes) and some other cell types (e.g., platelets) that bind immunoglobulins via their Fc-fragment. In most cases this causes activation of Fc-receptor bearing cells.

Hepatic uptake: binding and internalization (and, in most cases, eventually degradation) of molecules, complexes, liposomes, aggregates and cells by hepatic macrophages (Kupffer cells) and hepatocytes.

Opsonization: deposition of activated components of complement, antibodies and other plasma components on the surface of invading cells, microorganisms and artificial objects (e.g., liposomes) that facilitates binding to and phagocytosis by white blood cells and macrophages.

Polyethylene glycol (PEG): a linear organic polymer. PEG conjugation to proteins, liposomes and cells forms a hydrophilic shell around these objects that repels opsonins and defense cells. PEG-ylation reduces immune reactions and elimination of the injected materials ("stealth technology").

Renal clearance: a size-dependent elimination of molecules (usually smaller than 50 kDa) from the bloodstream via glomerular filtration in the kidneys.

Reticulo-endothelial system, RES: macrophages and other cells involved in active phagocytosis and immune signaling (lymphocytes, endothelial cells) in liver, spleen, bone marrow and lymphoid tissues. RES cells have good access to blood and play a key role in elimination of foreign cells and other objects. These cells also activate systemic defense reactions by production of cytokines.

Vascular Endothelial Growth Factor (VEGF): a multifunctional protein that facilitates vascular permeability and stimulates vascular proliferation and angiogenesis.

SECTION 2:

CARDIOVASCULAR TARGETING

3

TARGETING THE PATHOLOGICAL MYOCARDIUM

Ban-An Khaw, PhD.
Bouve College of Health Sciences, School of Pharmacy, Department of Pharmaceutical Sciences, Northeastern University, Boston, MA 02115

INTRODUCTION

The rationale for targeting the pathological myocardium is to enable development of better diagnostic modalities or to enhance therapeutic interventions. Since the heart is an end-differentiated organ that has no substantial regenerative properties, any injury to the heart could potentially lead to high morbidity and mortality. The causes of myocardial injury are varied. Acute myocardial infarction results in oncotic myocardial cell death, whereas cardiomyopathies are now believed to be associated primarily with apoptotic myocardial cell death. If these myocardial disorders can be targeted specifically for early diagnosis, then morbidity and mortality may be reduced and novel therapeutic interventions may result in decreasing the injury to the heart. This chapter will focus primarily on targeting the oncotic myocardium. Targeting the apoptotic myocardium will not be considered in detail, but an introduction to the latest advances will be provided.

TARGETING THE ONCOTIC MYOCARDIUM

Acute myocardial infarction is a coronary artery disease that results in myocardial oncosis within a few hours from the onset of chest pain. Although 17 million people in the US have coronary heart disease, and 8 million patients visit the emergency departments throughout the country annually for chest pain of various etiology, only 1.5 million of them would suffer acute myocardial infarction (1). Yet $1/3^{rd}$ to $1/4^{th}$ of the patients with acute myocardial infarction will be misdiagnosed by the traditional diagnostic methods (2). Therefore, there is a need for target specific diagnosis of acute myocardial infarction.

Monoclonal antimyosin antibodies

Radiolabeled antimyosin antibody was initially developed as a target specific non-invasive imaging agent for detection of acute myocardial infarction (3). The rational for the specific targeting is as follows: normal myocardial cells with intact cell membrane will prevent extracellular macromolecules from entering the cell (Figure 1). Necrotic myocardial cells with cell membrane disruption can no longer prevent the influx of

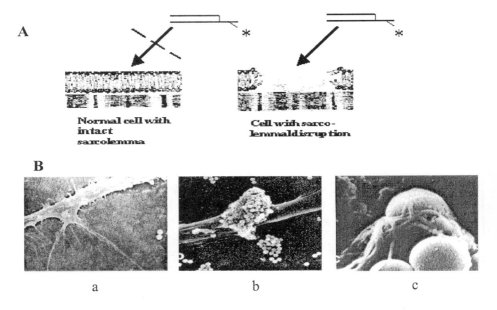

Figure 1. (A) Diagrammatic representation of the mechanism of antimyosin localization in the oncotic myocardium. * represents appropriate signal ligand. Arrow denotes the direction of the antibody Fab to bind to the intracellular myosin (right). The arrow with the dashed line through it denotes the inability of the antibody to bind to the intracellular myosin.
(B) Scanning electronmicrographs of (a) normal neonatal myocyte with antimyosin beads away from the cell, (b) oncotic neonatal myocyte with antimyosin beads attached through the membrane lesions and (c) 100,000 x magnification of the antimyosin beads interacting with the myofilaments.

extracellular macromolecules, or egress of intracellular components. Therefore, an antibody specific for an intracellular cardiac protein that is insoluble in the physiological fluid should be able to enter the cardiac cells with cell membrane disruption, and bind to the homologous antigen. Since myosin is an insoluble component of the contractile myofibrils, it will not be washed out of the necrotic cell (3). If a specific antibody such as antimyosin antibody were introduced into the extracellular milieu, the antibody should be able to bind with the now exposed cardiac myosin. If the antimyosin an insoluble component of the contractile myofibrils, it will not be washed out of the necrotic cells (3). If a specific antibody such as antimyosin antibody were introduced into the extracellular milieu, the antibody should be able to bind with the now exposed cardiac myosin. If the antimyosin antibody were appropriately radiolabeled, then one should be able to target the regions of cell membrane disruption by external gamma camera imaging (Figure 1 A).

The earliest demonstration of the specificity of radiolabeled antimyosin antibody for targeting the oncotic myocardium in experimental acute myocardial infarction was performed with I-125 and I-131 labeled antimyosin $F(ab')_2$ and non-specific IgG $F(ab')_2$ (4). Later, imaging studies were employed to show that the oncotic myocardium can be visualized only with radiolabeled monoclonal antimyosin Fab but not with radiolabeled non-specific monoclonal antibody Fab (Figure 2, A) (5).

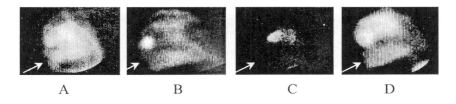

A   B   C   D

Figure 2. Left lateral gamma images of dogs with acute experimental myocardial infarction imaged with In-111 labeled control Fab (A), In-111 labeled R11D10 (B), I-123 labeled 2G42D7(C) and In-111 labeled 3H3 (D). Arrows denote the areas of experimental myocardial infarction with no infarct localization in A and D, but showed myocardial infarct activity in B and C.

Furthermore, when radiolabeled specific antimyosin Fab was injected into sham operated non- infarcted dogs, myocardial targeting of the radioactivity was not observed. Not only is targeting the oncotic myocardium dependent on the specificity of the antibody, we demonstrated that it is also dependent on its affinity. By using Fab fragments of three monoclonal antimyosin antibodies with different apparent affinities; R11D10 (B) (Ka = 1.5-2.5 x 10^9 liters/mole), 2G42D5 (C) (Ka = 3 x 10^9 liters/mole) and 3H31E6 (D) (Ka = 3-6 x 10^5 liters/mole) (5), the role of affinity in *in vivo* targeting was demonstrated. Figure 2B and C show left lateral gamma images of two dogs injected with the high affinity antimyosin Fab (R11D10 and 2G42D7). In these two images, the infarcted myocardium can be visualized unequivocally. However, when the low affinity antimyosin 3H3 Fab was used in the imaging studies, no infarct could be visualized (Fig 2D). Infarct (I) to blood (B) activity ratios from computer planimetry of the gamma images of dogs with acute myocardial infarction injected with high or low affinity antimyosin Fabs showed that both high affinity antimyosin antibodies had similar mean I/B ratios (1.501 $\pm$ 0.267, and 1.701$\pm$0.376, p =NS). These mean I/B ratios were significantly higher than the mean I/B ratio of the low affinity antimyosin Fab (0.85 ± 0.115, $p<0.0001$), which was similar to that of non-specific control Fab (0.7605 ± 0.0148) (5). Therefore, specificity of antimyosin antibodies alone is not a sufficient condition for successful *in vivo* gamma imaging of acute myocardial infarction. High enough affinity is a necessary condition. Due to the roles of specificity and high enough affinity of antimyosin antibody for targeting the oncotic myocardium, antimyosin imaging of acute myocardial infarction is rendered doubly specific.

Necessity of cell membrane lesion development for targeting with antimyosin

Specificity and sufficiently high affinity of antimyosin antibodies have been established as necessary and sufficient conditions for targeting acute myocardial infarction. Yet another condition that remains to be verified is the necessity of the dissolution of cell membrane integrity to enable antimyosin antibody to target the infarcted myocardium. Hypoxic neonatal murine myocytes in primary cultures treated with antimyosin antibody attached covalently to 1 micron diameter polystyrene beads were used to show that these beads attached only to myofilaments through the lesions in the cell membrane (Figure 1B, b)(6). Normal myocytes with intact sarcolemma prevented accumulation of these antimyosin beads (Figure 1B, a). Higher magnification of the necrotic cells at 100,000x enabled visualization of the binding of the antimyosin beads to the myofilaments containing cardiac myosin (Figure 1B, c) (6). Therefore, both *in vivo* and *in vitro* data confirmed the specificity of antimyosin antibody for targeted delineation of myocardial cells with cell membrane disruption associated with myocardial oncosis.

Relationship between antimyosin localization and other markers of myocardial injury

Radiolabeled antimyosin Fab is a highly specific delineator of the oncotic myocardium. Therefore, there should be some correlation to other radiopharmaceuticals used for diagnosis of myocardial injury. Tl-201 is an analogue of potassium and therefore is sequestered by the myocardium with normal blood flow. However, antimyosin is an infarct avid agent and localizes in most severely injured myocardium where blood flow is insufficient to maintain myocardial viability. Therefore, there should be an inverse correlation between these two radiopharmaceuticals. An inverse relation between antimyosin uptake and Tl-201 distribution was observed (7). Radiolabeled Sestamibi, another myocardial perfusion agent, also demonstrated an inverse relationship to radiolabeled antimyosin localization (8). Thus it appears that when there is normal blood flow in the myocardium, there is no antimyosin uptake whereas when perfusion drops significantly to result in myocardial oncosis, antimyosin uptake occurs.

Clinical studies

Based on the hypothesis that localization of radiolabeled monoclonal antimyosin Fab in the region of the myocardium is due to the presence of myocardial oncosis, studies have been undertaken in acute myocardial infarct patients with and without thrombolytic therapy. In the run of the mill acute myocardial infarction, interpretation of the gamma images obtained with In-111 antimyosin Fab is relatively straightforward (9). The radioactivity is localized to the discrete regions corresponding to the territories of the culprit coronary vessels (Figure 3). Localization of the infarcts appears to be independent of thrombolytic therapy since both successfully reperfused and non-reperfused myocardial infarcts were delineated by antimyosin immunoscintigraphy (9). However, reduced tracer uptake has been observed by Johnson et al in myocardial infarct patients having no collateral circulation (10). Another problematic area is in the interpretation of antimyosin images of patients with minimal myocardial injury. The presence of residual blood

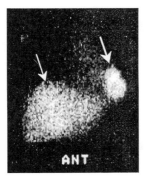 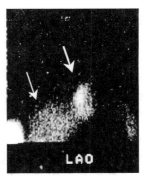

Figure 3. Anterior (left) and left anterior oblique 45° (right) gamma images of a patient with anterior acute myocardial infarction. The images were obtained approximately 24 h after In-111 antimyosin Fab administration. Thick arrows point to the infarct activity and the thin arrows point to the liver activity.

pool activity even at 24 h may be interpreted as originating from the myocardium. Re-imaging at 48 h in such a situation would normally resolve the dilemma (9).

The sensitivity of radiolabeled antimyosin Fab for diagnosis of Q-wave acute myocardial infarction has been reported to be between 87 and

98%. In a multicenter trial of 50 patients, Johnson et al (11) reported positive antimyosin delineation of the infarcts in 46 patients (sensitivity 92%). In a larger phase III trial of 492 patients, undertaken at 26 centers (12), 190 out of 202 patients with Q-wave MI were positive by antimyosin imaging (94% sensitivity) and 48 of 57 patients (84% sensitivity) with non-Q-wave MI. A specificity of 93% was reported in patients with chest pain but no clinical evidence of infarction. Specificity of In-111 antimyosin antibody imaging for detection of acute myocardial infarction was further demonstrated by Jain et al (13) and Hendel et al (14) in case reports of antemortem confirmation of antimyosin infarct delineation to the postmortem histochemically and histologically demarcated infarction.

Although antimyosin imaging of acute myocardial infarction is highly specific and sensitive, a major draw back exists in its application for diagnosis of myocardial infarction acutely. Since antibodies are proteins, the clearance from the blood is rather slow with a mean $T_{1/2}$ of about 4 h for Fab (9). In-111 labeled Fab has a biexponential clearance with the $T_{1/2}$ α of 0.8 h and $T_{1/2}$ β of 12 h thereby leaving substantial myocardial blood pool activity for greater than 6 h. This prolonged half-life of the antimyosin Fab makes it sub-optimal for acute diagnosis of myocardial infarction, yet it is highly useful for definitive diagnosis of equivocal MI. Jain et al (15) studied 75 patients with suspected acute MI with antimyosin imaging. Seven of 75 had no ECG changes diagnostic of acute MI. However all 7 were positive for the presence of myocardial necrosis by antimyosin imaging criteria. Figure 4 shows one such example from our study (9) where the diagnosis was equivocal by ECG and serum enzyme methods but the patient was diagnosed to have had a posterior MI only after antimyosin imaging.

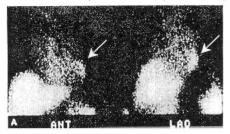 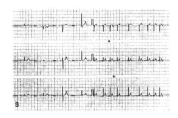

Figure 4. Anterior (ANT) and left anterior oblique (LAO) In-111 antimyosin Fab gamma images of a patient with equivocal acute myocardial infarction. The ECG was non-diagnostic for myocardial infarction (right panel), but the gamma images showed posterior MI particularly in the LAO view (arrow). In the anterior view, the arrow points to the infarct activity.

Due to the specificity and sensitivity of antimyosin immunoscintigraphy for detection of acute myocardial oncosis, antimyosin has also been used for the detection of right ventricular (RV) infarction. Right ventricular infarction is reported to occur in up to 50% of patients dying of inferior MI. Since diagnosis of right ventricular infarction is difficult unless right ventricular dysfunction occurs from extensive RV MI, or ST-segment elevation occurs in right ventricular precordial leads, use of Tc-99m labeled pyrophosphate scintigraphy has been recommended. Tc-99m pyrophosphate imaging may confirm presence of right ventricular infarction but a negative pyrophosphate scan does not necessarily exclude diagnosis of RV MI. Johnson et al (16) studied 34 patients with posteroinferior MI with In-111 antimyosin and Tl-201 simultaneous imaging by Single Photon Emission Tomography (SPECT). RV MI was detected in 12 patients; only 3 had ECG evidence of right ventricular MI. In one patient, diagnosis of RV MI was made solely on the basis of the antimyosin scans. This patient was misdiagnosed as an anterior wall ischemia due to ST-segment elevation in leads V1-3.

Despite the high sensitivity and specificity of antimyosin imaging for acute myocardial infarction, the delay of 12-24 h between radiotracer administration and unequivocal diagnostic image acquisition poses the most serious obstacle for routine use of antimyosin. This delay places the diagnostic time outside the window for maximal patient benefit from thrombolytic therapy. On the other hand, if a qualitative diagnostic end-point is the desired result, infarcts may be detected earlier than 18 to 24 h. Infarcts can be visualized over and above the blood pool activity anywhere from 6 to 14 hours after IV administration of antimyosin.

Antimyosin imaging for post-operative MI

Another potential application of antimyosin imaging is in the diagnosis of postoperative myocardial infarcts (MI) (17). Five percent of patients undergoing coronary by-pass surgery develop postoperative MI based on the appearance of new Q-waves and in 40% on ST-T change (18). Bulkley and Hutchins (19) observed that of the 58 patients who died within 30 days after coronary bypass surgery, 48 had evidence of sub-endocardial contraction band necrosis in the areas of the patent bypass grafts. Therefore, antimyosin may provide a diagnostic means early after the surgery when serum enzymes and ECG are not functional. Antimyosin scintigraphy was performed by van Vlies and co-workers on 23 stable angina patients who underwent coronary bypass surgery and who had no history of MI. Antimyosin uptake was observed in 19 patients, diffuse uptake in 7 and localized uptake in 12. Although 14 of the 19 patients had ST segment changes, no postoperative pathologic Q waves were observed (17).

Thus, it appears that antimyosin is highly specific for delineation of irreversibly injured myocardium with sensitivity averaging in the 95%. However, as an agent for early diagnosis of acute myocardial infarction for directing thrombolytic therapy, it does not appear to be adequate. Since thrombolytic therapy is most effective if initiated during the first 6 h of chest pain, a delay of 6-7 h to obtain a rule-in diagnosis may not be appropriate especially in light of the reports that if thrombolysis were initiated within 2 h, left ventricular function can be preserved and mortality reduced by 50% (20, 21). Therefore, an agent that can delineate the infarcted myocardium within a few hours after intravenous administration, whose diagnostic images can be used to direct thrombolytic therapy and post thrombolytic care, would be highly desirable.

Tc-99m Glucaric acid

Glucaric acid is a natural six-carbon dicarboxylic acid sugar that is found in high concentrations in certain green vegetables and can be labeled with Tc-99m (22). It was developed by Pak and co-workers as a transchelator for radiolabeling Fab' fragments of antibodies with Tc-99m (22). Serendipitously, it was observed that Tc-99m labeled glucaric acid localized in reperfused canine experimental myocardial infarcts within minutes after intravenous administration (23). Glucaric acid, being a small molecule with a molecular weight of 210 daltons, clears from the blood with a very short $T_{1/2}$. This may permit development of a target to background ratio that enables early visualization. The preliminary results of Fornet et al. suggested that Tc-99m glucaric acid might identify both zones of reversible and irreversible myocardial injury (24). However, subsequent study by Orlandi and co workers (25), as well as by us (26), established unequivocally that Tc-99m glucarate is not sequestered by the ischemic myocardium. Orlandi et al. reported that 20 minutes of ischemia (no histochemical triphenyl tetrazolium chloride stained infarction) in dogs did not cause Tc-99m glucaric acid localization (25). This was confirmed by Narula et al. using 5 and 15 min of ischemia induced by occlusion of the left descending coronary artery in a rabbit model (26).

In the canine reperfused myocardial infarct model reported by Orlandi et al, Tc-99m glucaric acid uptake was positive as early as 3 hours of reperfusion, was significantly higher at 48 hours but no uptake was seen at 10 days (25). We, however, were able to visualize canine reperfused acute myocardial infarction within 4 – 10 min after intravenous administration of Tc-99m glucarate (23). Visualization of non-reperfused rabbit infarcts required about 1-hour delay, whereas reperfused rabbit infarcts were visualized within 30 minutes. In non-reperfused acute MI in rats, optimal uptake occurred acutely at 4 hours of persistent coronary artery occlusion with diminishing localization after 24 hours and no localization of Tc-99m glucarate at 75 hours and 7 days (27). These studies all indicate that glucaric acid may be useful as a hyper acute diagnostic reagent in reperfused as well as non-reperfused acute myocardial infarction.

Narula et al. reported that Tc-99m glucaric acid can be used for hyperacute localization and visualization of experimental myocardial infarcts in reperfused and non-reperfused rabbit infarct models (26). When uptake of Tc-99m glucarate and In-111 antimyosin Fab, which were administered simultaneously into rabbits with acute MI, were compared, a direct correlation was obtained in either non-reperfused or reperfused infarcts. Target to non-target ratios of Tc-99m glucaric acid were substantially higher than the corresponding In-111 AM-Fab uptake ratios in the same tissue samples (26). When uptake ratios of Tc-99m glucaric acid were compared to In-111 AM-Fab uptake ratios in the canine reperfused myocardial infarct model, a direct correlation was also obtained (r^2 = 0.98) (23). Since antimyosin is highly specific for delineation of myocardial oncosis, and a direct correlation was obtained between Tc-99m glucarate and In-111 antimyosin Fab, the former must also be delineating acute myocardial oncosis. Since the correlation coefficient is almost 1 (0.98), the two infarct-avid agents must be delineating the same infarcted tissues. However, Tc-99m glucaric acid generated higher target to non-target ratios than In-111 antimyosin Fab within the same time period, in the same tissue samples.

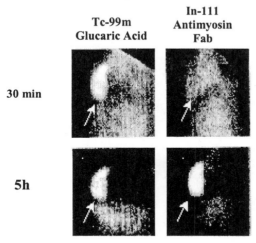

Figure 5. Left lateral gamma images obtained at 30 min (top panels) and 5 h (bottom panels) after intravenous administration of a mixture of In-111 antimyosin Fab (right panels) and Tc-99m glucaric acid (left panels). Top left panel shows the delineation of the infarct very clearly (arrow) at 30 min after intravenous administration of Tc-99m glucaric acid. With In-111 antimyosin Fab, only blood pool was seen at the same time (top right panel, arrow). However, by 5 h, both reagents were just as effective in the delineation of the infarcts respectively (bottom left and right panels).

Therefore, it stands to reason that visualization of the infarct should occur faster with Tc-99m glucaric acid than with In-111 AM-Fab. Figure 5 shows that Tc-99m glucaric acid already delineated the infarct as early as 30 minutes post radiotracer administration (left top panel), whereas the simultaneously administered In-111 AM-Fab showed only blood pool activity at that time (right top panel). By 5 hours both radiotracer showed unequivocal infarct delineation in canine reperfused myocardial infarcts (23).

The mechanism by which Tc-99m glucaric acid localizes in the oncotic myocardium is believed to be due to its affinity for the histones of the oncotic myocytes (26, 28). When the radioactivity from the infarcted tissues at 1 and 3 h after iv administration of Tc-99m glucaric acid were fractionated into nuclear, mitochondrial and cytosolic fractions, >75% of the infarct radioactivity was associated with the nuclear fraction. Further fractionation of the nuclear activity into nucleoproteins and DNA demonstrated that the predominant radioactivity was associated with the nucleoproteins that consisted primarily of histones (28). Therefore, it appears that when acute myocardial oncosis occurs, the nucleohistones become accessible to Tc-99m glucaric acid. The initial entry of Tc-99m glucaric acid into the infarct zone appears to be via collateral circulation and or diffusion. However, the highly basic nucleohistones may act as a sink for concentrating the acidic glucaric acid once the integrity of the sarcolemma has been lost. The high avidity of Tc-99m glucaric acid for the nucleohistones together with the fast blood clearance should allow development of target to background ratios that permit early visualization of the infarcted myocardium. This very acute localization capability of Tc-99m glucaric acid has also been seen in patients.

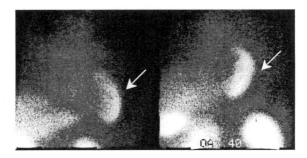

Figure 6. Anterior (left panel) and LAO 40° (right panel) images of a patient with acute myocardial infarction imaged at about 4 h after Tc-99m glucaric acid administration. The arrows point to the infarct delineated by Tc-99m glucaric acid.

Figure 6 shows the anterior and left anterior oblique images of a patient who underwent successful thrombolysis within 3.5 hours of chest pain. Tc-99m glucaric acid was administered at 4.5 hours of chest pain (29). To date studies from Europe have demonstrated that hyperacute visualization of acute MI is feasible with Tc-99m glucaric acid. Large MIs can be visualized earlier than small MIs. Nevertheless, Mariani and co-workers observed that diagnostic results of small non-reperfused MIs are visualized within 3 hours of intravenous administration of this reagent (29). Furthermore, it appears that Tc-99m glucaric acid is highly specific for acute MI but not for MI older than 2-3 days. This observation is consistent with the avidity of Tc-99m glucarate for the nucleoproteins since it appears that at 2 to 3 days, the targets of Tc-99m glucaric acid may no longer be present due to autolysis in the infarct. However, the exact duration for Tc-99m glucarate positivity in patients with acute MI is not known. Mariani et al observed that in reperfused MIs positivity wanes after peak serum Creatine Kinase levels have been reached (29). Whether the same time will hold for non-reperfused MI must await additional studies.

Therefore, it appears that, Tc-99m glucaric acid may provide a very acute myocardial infarct imaging modality. Large MIs should be visualizable by gamma imaging within an hour after intravenous administration and small MI should be detectable by 3 h. This diagnostic time frame may be compatible for directing thrombolytic therapy in the emergency department.

Targeting the apoptotic myocardium

Cardiomyopathies are currently believed to be due to apoptotic myocardial cell death. Although the process of apoptosis is believed to be very fast, reaching completion within hours, there appears to be sufficient number of cell deaths in myocarditis, dilated cardiomyopathy, heart transplant rejection and other cardiomyopathies to enable antimyosin imaging to target the cardiomyopathic hearts.

To date there are two radiopharmaceuticals that can be used to target apoptotic myocardial cell death. In-111 labeled antimyosin has been proven to be effective in the non-invasive diagnosis of myocardial cell deaths. Tc-99m labeled Annexin V has been demonstrated to be able to target the clinical heart transplant rejection (30).

Irrespective of the targeting reagents used, it appears that both antimyosin and Annexin V can target both apoptotic and oncotic myocardial cell deaths. If the pathophyosiology of the disorder were suspected, then use of either reagent would permit diagnosis of the disorder. However, to date, one would be hard-pressed to find a targeting agent that can definitively define apoptotic form oncotic myocardial cell deaths.

TARGETED THERAPY

Targeting the necrotic myocardium with immunoliposomes and long circulating immunoliposomes

Due the ability of specific targeting of the necrotic myocardium with radiolabeled antimyosin antibody, we proposed that liposomes could also be made myocardial target specific if monoclonal antimyosin antibody were to be incorporated into the liposomes. These immunoliposomes might then serve as targeted therapeutic drug delivery vehicles. To demonstrate that *in vivo* targeting of the necrotic myocardium is possible with immunoliposomes, we developed antimyosin immunoliposomes by covalent attachment of antimyosin Fab to liposomes containing phosphotidylethanolamine as a target for antibody attachment (31). The antibody was attached to the amine of the phosphotidylethanolamine by carbodiimide activation. In-111 labeled bovine serum albumin (BSA) was used as the signaling agent that was entrapped in the intraliposomal space. Although the infarct was targeted and visualized by gamma imaging, the myocardial activity was not optimal. The liver activity was greater than that of the target activity. Therefore, to ensure greater target activity, we also developed long circulating antimyosin immunoliposomes containing polyethyleneglycol as a component of the liposomal surface moiety.

Furthermore, In-111 was labeled to DTPA-phosphiotidylethanolamine that was incorporated into the liposomal bilayer. Thus the In-111 labeled long circulating liposomes were prepared and dogs with reperfused acute myocardial infarction were injected with this preparation. Localization of the In-111 labeled long circulating immunoliposomes in acute canine experimental infarction was feasible in about 8 hours. Since the PEG-modified liposomes are long circulating liposomes, the development of target to background ratios consistent with gamma scintigraphic visualization was delayed. However, it concomitantly enabled greater delivery of the immunoliposome into the infarcted myocardium. Injection of the long circulating immunoliposomes into sham operated dogs showed no radiotracer accumulation in the region of the heart. Since there was no region of myocardial infarction, as expected, there was no radiotracer accumulation in the myocardial region.

Another factor that affected the *in vivo* distribution and targeting of these long circulating immunoliposomes is the concentration of polyethylene glycol. Utilizing a rabbit model of acute myocardial infarction, we demonstrated that when 10% mole PEG was incorporated into antimyosin immunoliposomes, its blood clearance was the slowest with a $T_{1/2}$ of 1000 minutes. Whereas, $T_{1/2}$ of standard immunoliposomes was 40 minutes, that of 4% mole PEG liposomes was 300 minutes, and 4% mole PEG antimyosin immunoliposomes was 200 minutes. The immunoliposome preparation with the greatest half life provided the highest absolute target activity, however, the target to non-target ratios were greater with 4% mole PEG immunoliposomes than with 10% mole PEG immunoliposomes. This is most probably due to faster blood clearance of the 4% mole PEG immunoliposomes than the 10% mole PEG immunoliposomes (32).

Such a targeted delivery system could be envisioned for delivery and establishment of a depot of therapeutic drugs at the sites of tissue injury after the acute injury event. As the process of scar tissue formation and fibroblast infiltration proceeds, the slow release of transfection vectors containing myogenic genes, such as myogenin or myoD genes, could transfect the fibroblasts and transform them into cardiocytes, if such a depot of these vectors were established in the region of myocardial oncosis. Although experimentally, transformation of fibroblasts into myocytes has been achieved *in vitro*, transformation into skeletal myoblasts has been the only successful achievement. Nevertheless, advancements in molecular genetics and molecular engineering may render such applications feasible.

Preserving the myocardial viability with immunoliposomes

Another application of antimyosin immunoliposomes that we have envisioned is in preserving the myocardial viability in the therapy of acute myocardial infarction (33). Imaging studies with radiolabeled antimyosin Fab have established that the hallmark of myocardial cell death is the development of sarcolemmal lesions. We have also demonstrated that antimyosin immunoliposomes could be generated and that these immunoliposomes could target sites of sarcolemmal lesions in acute myocardial infarction (31). It has been established that due to the similarity in the lipid bilayer composition of liposomal membrane and cell membrane, fusion of liposomes with cells occurs (34). Therefore, we proposed that using antimyosin immunoliposomes, one could target the myocardial membrane lesions induced by ischemia, physical or chemical injuries. The liposomal antimyosin antibody would interact with the cytoskeletal myofilaments containing myosin through cell membrane lesions. If the targeting of the lesions occurs before the diameter of the lesions becomes larger than the diameter of the immunoliposomes, the immunoliposomes should be able to plug the lesions and prevent additional loss of intracellular macromolecules. This should provide the initial step in the intervention. As more antimyosin antibodies on the immunoliposome bind to the myosin molecules in the cytoskeletal myofilaments (Figure 7A), the immunoliposome should be wedged tighter into the lesion. This should ultimately cause fusion of the liposomal membrane with the cell membrane resulting in the sealing of the cell membrane lesion. We propose that such a mechanism of cell membrane lesion sealing would provide a novel therapeutic intervention for preservation of myocardial viability. Due to the mechanism of cell lesion sealing, one should also be able to deliver drugs of choice such as therapeutic genes, directly into the cytoplasm of the compromised cardiocytes and thereby achieve more efficient transfection relative to other non-viral methods.

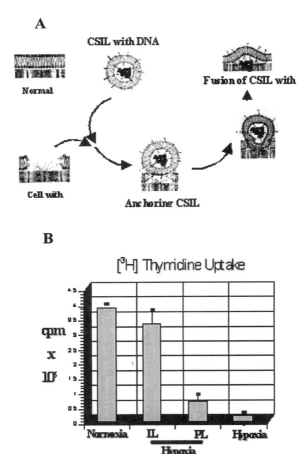

Figure 7. (A) Diagrammatic representation of the proposed mechanism of intracellular gene delivery using cytoskeleton-specific immunoliposomes (CSIL). The hypothetical drug is represented by the intraliposomal structure. It could be pharmaceuticals or gene constructs for intracytoplasmic delivery. (B) Myocyte viability determined by ³H-thymidine uptake. IL= cytoskeletal antigen specific immunoliposomes, PL= plain liposomes.

To demonstrate the utility of antimyosin immunoliposomes for preservation of myocardial cell viability, rat embryonic cardiocytes H9C2 cells in culture were made severely hypoxic in an atmosphere of N_2 for 24 h. Hypoxic cardiocytes treated with antimyosin immunoliposomes had viability similar to that of normoxic controls determined by trypan blue exclusion test. Cardiocytes treated with plain liposomes or non-specific IgG-liposomes had significantly less viable cells. Untreated control hypoxic cells were almost all non-viable. ^{3}H-thymidine uptake studies confirmed that severely hypoxic cardiocytes treated with antimyosin immunoliposomes had ^{3}H-thymidine uptake similar to that of normoxic cardiocytes (Figure 7B), whereas, hypoxic cardiocytes treated with plain liposomes or not treated at all were observed to contain significantly less viable cells. Since, ^{3}H-thymidine uptake in cells represent DNA replication, it provided a more stringent evidence of cell viability than that by trypan blue exclusion criteria.

To further determine the mechanism of cell membrane lesions sealing, rhodamine labeled lipids were included in the preparation of the liposomes. Hypoxic cardiocytes treated with antimyosin immunoliposomes were observed by epifluorescent microscopy to have fluorescent confluent cells whereas plain liposome treated hypoxic cells had only scattered minimally fluorescent cells debris. When these cells were examined by confocal microscopy, antimyosin immunoliposome treated hypoxic cells retained normal cell morphology and fluorescent liposome incorporation

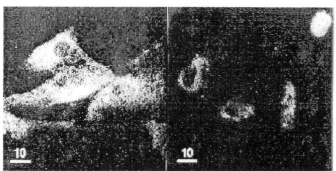

Figure 8.   Confocal micrographs showing hypoxic cardiocytes treated with rhodamine antimyosin immunoliposomes (left) and those treated with rhodamine plain liposomes. The micrographs were in color but have been made into black and white display. The liposomes appear as white regions.

into the cell membranes could be visualized (Figure 8). Again, cells treated with plain liposomes without the normal cell morphology (right panel) were rounded and only scattered non-specific adsorption of fluorescent plain liposomes on very few nonviable cells were observed.

To determine whether there is actual fusion of the antimyosin immunoliposomes with the hypoxic cardiocytes, antimyosin liposomes and plain liposomes were also prepared so that silver grains are entrapped in the intraliposomal space.   When hypoxic cells treated with silver grains impregnated antimyosin immunoliposome or plain liposomes were examined by transmission electron microscopy, silver grains were observed intracellularly in cells treated with antimyosin immunoliposomes.   Cells treated with plain liposomes were mostly nonviable, but few viable cells were detected and they showed no inclusion of silver grains in the cytosol.   The silver grains were observed in the extracellular space with cellular debris.

These studies supported the hypothesis that cytoskeleton specific immunoliposomes can be used to preserve myocardial viability. Preservation of cell viability is due to cell membrane lesion sealing with antimyosin immunoliposomes and that the immunoliposomes fuse with cell membrane thereby delivering the intraliposomal contents directly into the cytosol.

Targeting the myocardium with immunoliposomes for targeted gene delivery

Due to the mode of cell membrane lesion sealing with antimyosin immunoliposomes and the demonstration that silver grains entrapped in the immunoliposomes can be delivered directly into the cytoplasm, we also proposed that genetic constructs should also be amenable to intracellular delivery by the same method (34).   To achieve this, we used pSV-beta-galactosidase vector from Promega. When the hypoxic H9C2 cardiocytes were treated with immunoliposomes prepared with 50 µg /ml vectors, almost all cells were transfected with the vector as evidenced by presence of blue chromogens in almost every cell in the field of view (Figure 9, left). Normoxic cells treated with the same immunoliposome vectors showed no transfections.   Similarly, no transfection was observed with IgG liposomes. However, cationic liposomes showed some transfected cells (Figure 9 right).

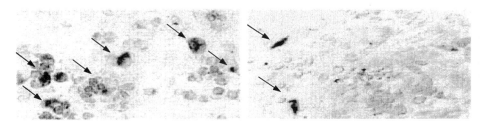

Figure 9. X-gal stained micrographs of hypoxic cardiocytes treated with CSIL (antimyosin immunoliposomes) containing pSV-beta-galactosidase vectors (left) and cardiocytes treated with cationic liposomes containing pSV-beta-galactosidase vectors.   Beta-galactosidase expression is seen in CSIL transfected cells as dark stained regions (arrows denote only some regions of most intense gene expression) (left panel) In the cationic liposome transfected cardiocytes (right panel), only two cells show gene expression (arrows).

When the vector concentration was increased by 3 folds to 150 microgram per ml of the immunoliposomes, more intense rate of transfection with beta-galactosidase vectors was obtained. Thus not only can antimyosin immunoliposomes serve to preserve myocardial viability in acute myocardial infarction, it may also be used for gene therapy with very high efficiency.

SUMMARY

The pathological myocardium can be targeted with antibodies to intracellular antigen that is exposed only during oncotic and apoptotic myocardial cell deaths. Antimyosin antibody is the first of its kind used targeting the oncotic as well as the apoptotic myocardium. Although there are other radiopharmaceuticals that are used to target the oncotic myocardium, only antimyosin appears to be highly specific. Subsequently, radiolabeled glucaric acid was observed to be able to target the oncotic myocardium. Its advantage is the short time it takes to obtain a diagnostic image.

Subsequent to targeting the oncotic myocardium, targeting of the apoptotic myocardium was envisioned. Initial studies showed that antimyosin was avid for targeting the apoptotic myocardium associated with various cardiomyopathies. Subsequently, Annexin V has been promoted as the next radiopharmaceutical for imaging apoptotic tissues.

Having the capability to detect oncotic myocardium has lead to the development of novel cell membrane lesion sealing technology. Due to its mechanism of cell membrane lesion sealing, it was also observed that drugs and gene constructs might be delivered directly into the cytoplasm of cardiocytes that have been treated with cytoskeleton-specific immunoliposomes. Whether this novel approach to cell viability preservation and gene transfer will become a general method for therapy must await additional investigation and acceptance by the scientific community.

REFERENCES

1   Pasternak RC, Braunwald E. Acute myocardial infarction. In Harrison's Principles of Internal Medicine. Eds. Isselbacher KJ, Braunwald E, Wilson JD, Martin JB, Fauci AS, Kasper DL. McGraw-Hill Inc. New York. 13th edition. 1994:1066.
2   McCaarthy BD, Beshansky JR, D'Agostino RB, Selker HP. Missed diagnosis of acute myocardial infarction in the emergency department: Results from a multicenter study. Ann Emerg Med. 1993;22:579- .
3   Khaw BA, Beller GA, Haber E, Smith TW. Localization of cardiac myosin-specific antibody in myocardial infarction. J Clin Invest. 1976; 58:439-446.

4   Khaw BA, Gold HK, Leinbach RC, Fallon JT, Strauss HW, Pohost GM, Haber E.
         Early imaging of experimental myocardial infarction by intracoronary administration
         of ^{131}I-labeled anticardiac myosin (Fab')$_2$ fragments. Circulation. 1978; 58:1137-
         1142.

5   Khaw BA, Petrov A, Narula J. Complementary roles of antibody affinity and
         specificity in *in vivo* diagnostic cardiovascular Targeting: How specific is
         antimyosin for irreversible myocardial damage? J Nucl Cardiol 1999;6:316-23.

6   Khaw BA, Scott J, Fallon JT, Haber E, Homcy C. Myocardial injury: Quantitation
         by cell sorting initiated with anti-myosin fluorescent spheres.   Science. 1982;
         217:1050-1053.

7   Khaw BA, Strauss HW, Pohost GM, Fallon JT, Katus HA Haber E. The relationship
         of immediate and delayed thallium-201 distribution to localization of I-125-
         antimyosin antibody in acute experimental myocardial infarction.   Am J Cardiol.
         1983; 51:1428-1432.

8   Khaw BA, Mousa S.   Comparative Assessment of Experimental Myocardial
         Infarction with Tc-99m Hexakis-t-Butyl-Isonitrile (Sestamibi), In-111 antimyosin
         and Tl-201. Nuclear Medicine Communications. 1991;12:853-863..

9   Khaw BA, Yasuda T, Gold HK, Leinbach RC, Johns JA, Kanke M, Barlai-Kovach
         M, Strauss HW, Haber E.   Acute myocardial infarct imaging with Indium-111-
         labeled monoclonal antimyosin Fab. J Nucl Med. 1987; 28:1671-1678.

10   Johnson LL, Seldin DW, Becker LC, LaFrance ND, Liberman HA, James C, Mattis
         JA, Dean RT, Brown J, Reiter A, Arneson V, Cannon PJ, Berger HJ. Antimyosin
         imaging in acute transmural myocardial infarction: results of a multicenter clinical
         trial. J Am Coll Cardiol 1989;13:27.

11   Johnson LL, Seldin DW, Becker LC, LaFrance ND, Liberman HA, James C, Mattis
         JA, Dean RT, Brown J, Reiter A, Arneson V, Cannon PJ, Berger HJ. Antimyosin
         imaging in acute transmural myocardial infraction: results of a multicenter clinical
         trial. J Am Coll Cardiol 1989;13:27-35.

12   Berger H, Lahiri A, Leppo J, Makler T, Maddahi J, Mintz G, Strauss HW.
         Antimyosin imaging in patients with ischemic chest pain: initial results of phase III
         multicenter trial. J Nucl Med 1988; 28: 805 (Abstract).

13   Jain D, Lahiri A, Crawley JCw, Raftery EB. Indium-111 antimyosin imaging in a
         patient with acute myocardial infarction: postmortem correlation between
         histopathologic and autoradiographic extent of myocardial necrosis.   Am J Card
         Imaging. 1988; 2:158-161.

14   Hendel RC, McSherry BA, Leppo JA. Myocardial uptake of indium-111 =-labeled
         antimyosin in acute subendocardial infarction: clinical, histochemicaland
         autoradiographic correlation of myocardial necrosis. J Nucl med. 1990; 31:1851-
         1853.

15   Jain D, Lahiri A, Raftery E. Immunoscintigraphy for detecting acute myocardial
         infarction without electrocardiographic changes. Br Med J. 1990;300:151-153.

16   Johnson LL, Seldin DW, Tresgallo ME, et al. Right ventricular infarction and
         function from dual isotope indium-111 antimyosin/thallium-201 SPECT and gated
         blood pool scintigraphy [abst]. J Nucl Med. 1991; 32:1018.

17   van Vlies B, van Royen ED, Visser CA, et al. Frequency of myocardial indium-111
         antimyosin uptake after uncomplicated coronary bypass surgery.   AM J Cardiol
         1990;66:1191-1195.

18   Hultgren HN, Shettigar UR, Pfeifer JF, Angell WW. Acute myocardial infarction
         ischemic injury during surgery for cornary artery disease. Am Heart J. 1977;94:146-
         153.

19   Bulkley BH, Hutchins GM. Myocardial consequences of coronary artery bypass
         graft surgery: the paradox of necrosis in areas of revascularization. Circ. 1977;
         56:906-913.

20   Califf RM, Topol EJ, George BS, et at. One-year outcome after therapy with tissue plasminogen activator-, Report from the Thrombolysis and Angioplasty in Myocardial Infarction trial. *Am Heart J* 119;1990;777.

21   The TIMI Study Group. Comparison of invasive and conservative strategies after treatment with intravenous tissue plasminogen activator in acute myocardial infarction: Results of the Thrombolysis in Myocardial Infarction (TIMI) Phase 11 trial. *N Engi J Med* 320;1989,618.).

22   Pak KY, Nedelman MA, Kanke M, Khaw BA, Mattis JA, Strauss HW, Dean RT, Berger HJ. An Instant Method for Labeling Antimyosin Fab' with Technetium-99m: Evaluation in an Experimental Myocardial Infarct Model. J Nucl Med. 1992; 33(1): 144-149.

23   Khaw BA, Nakazawa A, O'Donnell, Pak KY, Narula J. Avidity of ^{99m}Tc-glucarate for the necrotic myocardium: *In vivo* and *in vitro* assessment. J Nucl Cardiol 1997;4:283-290.

24   Fornet b, Yasuda T, Wilkinson R, Ahmed M, Moore R, Khaw BA, Fischman AJ, Strauss HW. Detection of acute cardiac injury with technetium-99m glucaric acid. J nucl Med. 1989;30:1743.

25   Orlandi C, Crane PD, Edwards DS, Platts SH, Bernard L, Lazewatsky J, Thoolen MJ. Early scintigraphic detection of experimental myocardial infarction in dogs with technetium-99m-glucaric acid. J Nucl Med. 1991; 32:263-268.

26   Narula J, Petrov A, Pak KY, Lister BC, Khaw BA. Very early noninvasive detection of acute experimental non-reperfused myocardial infarction with technetium-99m-labeled glucarate. Circ 1997; 95:1577-1584.

27   Ohtani H, Callahan RJ, Khaw BA, Fischman AJ, Wilkinson RA, Strauss HW. Comparison of technetium-99m-glucarate and thallium-201 for the identification of acute myocardial infarction in rats. J Nucl Med. 1992; 33:1988-1993.

28   Khaw BA. daSilva J, Petrov A, Hartner W. In-111 antimyosin and Tc-99m glucaric acid for non-invasive identification of oncotic and apoptotic myocardial necrosis. J Nucl Cardiol. (Submitted).

29   Mariani G, Villa G, Rossettin PF, Spallarossa P, Bezante GP, Brunelli C, Pak KY, Khaw BA, Strauss HW. Detection of acute myocardial infarction with 99mTc-labeled D-glucaric acid: imaging in patients presenting with acute chest pain. J Nucl Med. 1999;40:1832-1839.

30   Narula J, Acio ER, Narula N, Samuels LE, Fyfe B, Wood D, Fitzpatrick JM, Raghunath PN, Tomaszewski JE, Kelly C, Steinmetz N, Green A, Tait JF, Leppo J, Blankenberg FG, Jain D, Strauss HW. Annexin-V imaging for noninvasive detection of cardiac allograft rejection. Nat Med 2001 Dec;7(12):1347-52

31   Torchilin VP, Khaw BA, Smirnov VN, Haber E. Preservation of antimyosin antibody activity after covalent coupling to liposomes. Biochem Biophys Res Comm. 1979; 89:1114-1119.

32   Torchilin VP, Klibanov AL, Huang L, O'Donnell S, Nossiff ND, Khaw BA. Targeted accumulation of PEG-coated immunoliposomes in infarcted myocardium in rabbits. FASEB J. 1992; 6: 2716-2719.

33   Khaw BA, Torchilin VP, Vural I, Narula J. Plug and Seal: Prevention of Hypoxic Cardiocyte Death by Sealing Membrane Lesions with Antimyosin-Liposomes. Nature Medicine 1995; 1(11):1195-1198.

34   Khaw BA, daSliva J, Vural I, Narula J, Torchilin VP. Intracytoplasmic gene delivery for *in vitro* transfection with cytoskeleton-specific immunoliposomes. J Cont. Release, 2001;75:199-210.

GLOSSARY

2G42D7: Monoclonal antimyosin antibody, IgG1 subclass, Ka $\simeq$ $3x10^9$ Liters/mole.

3H3: Monoclonal antimyosin antibody, IgG1 subclass, Ka $\simeq$ $5x10^5$ Liters/mole.

AMI: Acute Myocardial Infarction, or (in common terms), a heart attack.

Anterior view: The gamma camera is placed anterior to the patient or subject to collect the counts of the radioisotope.

Apoptosis: Suicide mode of cell death that is initiated from the nucleus outward with the cell membrane remaining intact until very late stages of cell death. This mode of cell death is involved in the embryonic differentiation and homeostasis.

Fab: Papain digested fragment of intact antibody with a molecular weight approximately 50,000 daltons.

Glucaric acid: 6 carbon dicarboxylic acid also known as saccharic acid.

I/B ratios: Infarct activity to blood activity ratios.

I-125, I-131 and I-123: Radioisotopes of iodine. I-125 has a half life of 60 days; I-131 has T1/2 of 8days and I-123 T1/2 of 13 hours.

Left anterior oblique (LAO): The camera is placed to the left at various degrees form the anterior position.

Left lateral: Image obtained by positioning the gamma camera to view from the left side.

Necrotic: Originally referred to cell death now designated oncotic. The present designation of necrosis encompasses both oncotic and apoptotic cell deaths.

Oncosis: Method of cell death due to external stimuli homologous to homicide mode of death where cell membrane disruption is a necessary condition.

R11D10: Monoclonal antimyosin antibody, IgG2b subclass, Ka$\simeq$$2x10^9$ Liters/mole.

Radiolabeled: Attachment of radioisotope to a compound such as proteins, carbohydrates, etc.

RV: Right ventricular.

SPECT: Single photon emission computed tomography.

4

TARGETING ATHEROSCLEROTIC PLAQUES

Ban-An Khaw, PhD.
Bouve College of Health Sciences, School of Pharmacy, Department of Pharmaceutical Sciences, Northeastern University, Boston, MA 02115

INTRODUCTION

Clinical imaging of atherosclerotic plaques is based on anatomical demonstration of the narrowing of the involved artery (1). Angioscopy (2) and intravascular ultrasound (3) can demonstrate the precise location of the lesions, the extent of luminal narrowing and plaque thickening. However, both methods are invasive and cannot provide the composition or the metabolic status of the atherosclerotic lesion (4). Plaques rich in macrophages and foam cells may denote high risk of plaque rapture (5) whereas fibrous plaques may denote slowly emergent lesions. Lesions rich in actively proliferating smooth muscle cells may be an indication of accelerated luminal diameter reduction (6). Other targets that might have potential applications may be associated with neoantigens that are expressed due to microvascular injury inherent in atherogenesis. Therefore, targeting macrophage, foam cell hyper-accumulation or hyperactivity intravascularly, neoexpression or hyperexpression of various vascular adhesion molecules, or the metabolites that may be incorporated into the cellular components of the atherosclerotic lesions may provide novel and specific diagnostic and therapeutic applications.

Atherogenesis involves interaction between components of the blood vessel walls and blood (7). It is usually initiated by endothelial injury. The initiation of this injury is multifactorial. Some risk factors are hypertension, hyperlipidemia, cigarette smoking and genetic predisposition. Irrespective of the initial cause of the endothelial injury, it leads monocyte adhesion probably due to enhanced expression of adhesion molecules (8) and the secretion of chemokines (7). Exposure of the thrombogenic subendothelium also leads to platelet aggregation. Monocytes and low-density lipoproteins (LDL) from the blood can then permeate into the region of the injured vessel. Monocytes then ingest the LDL that have been oxidized by the endothelial cells (9). The oxidized LDL with high avidity for a receptor on endothelial cells and macrophages (10) is toxic to proliferating cells. These processes lead to a continuation and a vicious cycle of cell injury, macrophage accumulation and oxidized LDL accumulation.

Growth factors derived from platelets, as well as from the macrophages cause differentiation of the contractile smooth muscle cells of the media into the synthetic phenotype. These synthetic phenotypic smooth muscle cells migrate to the intima and proliferate in the subendothelial region. Loss of growth inhibitors such as prostacyclin and heparin-like molecules locally may also promote the neointimal proliferation.

Due to the mechanisms involved in atherogenesis, many potential targets may be envisioned. Investigators have targeted the accumulation of oxidized LDL (11), platelet aggregation (12), macrophages and foam cells as well as smooth muscle cell proliferation (13) and the neoexpression of receptors on differentiated smooth muscle cells (14).

TARGETING OF THE ATHEROSCLEROTIC LESIONS

Targeting LDL accumulation

The regenerating injured endothelium is more permeable than uninjured normal endothelium leading to subintimal accumulation of lipoproteins. Roberts et al. used radiolabeled low density lipoproteins (LDL) to demonstrate LDL accumulation in deendothelialized rabbit descending aorta (11). It was proposed that the use of radiolabeled LDL accumulation in the endothelium could permit evaluation of lipoprotein metabolism associated with atherosclerotic lesion (15). Subsequently, studies in three patients with I-125 labeled LDL were performed. At thirty-six hours after radiotracer injection, the carotid lesions were detected by gamma imaging (16). However, the target to background ratios ranged from 1.5 to 3 times resulting in very poor quality spatial resolution images. Subsequent studies with Tc-99m labeled LDL were somewhat better for detection of carotid, iliac and femoral vessel lesion (17). Nevertheless, coronary lesions were not unequivocally visualized. These studies with radiolabeled LDL suggest that such an approach for imaging atherosclerotic lesions has potential.

Monocytes/macrophages in atherosclerotic lesions

Targeting with autologous monocytes

Vascular inflammation, with or without denudation of the endothelial lining, leads to accumulation of circulating monocytes. These monocytes migrate into the vascular subendothelial space where the following ingestion of the oxidized LDL leads to the formation of foam cells. Virgolinin et al. labeled autologous monocytes with In-111 oxine and attempted to image carotid and femoral lesions. In 5 of 13 symptomatic patients such lesions were visualized within 1 to 4 h of radiolabeled autologous monocyte injections. However, the primary site of indium-111 monocyte accumulation was the spleen, with transient lung accumulation initially (18).

Targeting Fc receptors on monocytes

Targeting the Fc receptors that are ubiquitous on monocytes can also localize monocytes that accumulate in the vascular lesions. Fishman et al. demonstrated that radiolabeled polyclonal IgG localized in experimental atherosclerotic lesions in rabbits (19). Subsequently Fc fragments of polyclonal IgG were also demonstrated to be able to localize atherosclerotic lesions whereas similarly radiolabeled Fab of polyclonal IgG showed only minimal targeting in the same experimental model. Clinical study in 4 patients with 12 angiographically confirmed atherosclerotic lesions with In-111 labeled polyclonal human IgG enabled visualization of the lesion at 9 sites (20). Earlier detection was better than re-imaging at 24 h after radiotracer administration. Only 7 of the initial 9 targets were still positive at 24 H.

Targeting monocytes with specific antibodies

Accumulation of macrophages is well documented in experimental (21) and clinical lesions (22). Gown et al. observed that fibro-fatty lesions consisted almost exclusively of macrophages and lymphocytes, whereas fibrous plaques consisted predominantly of smooth muscle cells and advanced plaques consisted of a varying admixture of macrophages and smooth muscle cells (23). Therefore, it stands to reason that targeting macrophage accumulation in atherosclerotic lesions should provide diagnostic information on the type of lesions that are existent *in vivo*. Yet, to date no study has supported the contention that anti-macrophage antibodies can be used to image macrophage rich fibro-fatty lesions. This may be due to the ubiquitous presence of macrophages *in vivo* and the unavailability of foam cell specific monoclonal antibodies. Yet it is hoped that such an approach to targeting may permit differentiation of the different forms of atherosclerotic lesions.

Platelet aggregation or clots

Since atherogenesis involved vascular endothelial injury, platelet aggregation and fibrin deposition must necessarily follow. Therefore, targeting atherosclerotic lesions with radiolabeled autologous platelets (12), antiplatelet antibody (24) or radiolabeled fibrinogen (25) may be envisioned.

Targeting platelet aggregation

Davis et al. studied 34 patients with cerebrovascular disease with In-111 labeled autologous platelets. In 16 patients, 33 angiographically confirmed lesions were compared to In-111 labeled platelet imaging results (12). Only 20 lesions were detected by In-111-platelet imaging. However, 3 other sites were observed without angiographic abnormality. In another study, involving 60 patients with transient ischemic carotid artery disease, the study was repeated in 36 patients 3 to 4 days after carotid endarterectomy (26). No correlation was observed between the scintigraphic imaging results and symptomatic status of the patients, the interval between ischemic attacks and severity of stenosis, or plaque morphology and antiplatelet therapy. Due to this lack of correlation, as well as the necessity to manipulate blood products for radiolabeling, the utility of radiolabeled autologous platelet imaging is not very attractive.

Targeting with antiplatelet antibody

The rationale for using antibodies to activated platelets for imaging atherosclerotic lesions stems from the observation that there is platelet aggregation at atherosclerotic lesions. Miller et al used Tc-99m labeled monoclonal antibody S12 specific for activated platelets to demonstrate aortic lesions at sites of percutaneous transluminal aortic angioplasty (24). S12 is specific for the α-granule membrane protein P-selectin (GMP-140) that redistributes to the platelet surface during activation. *In vivo* anterior gamma images and ex vivo images of the descending aorta containing the regions of the lesions corresponded to the angiographically defined regions of the stent placement and the gross specimen showing thrombi accumulation in the region. Due to non-target organ activities, the lesions could not be visualized *in vivo*. However, in the ex vivo image of the descending aorta, radiotracer accumulation could be discerned quite clearly. Imaging of the aortic lesion one week after angioplasty showed decreased radiotracer accumulation indicating that imaging with radiolabeled antiplatelet antibody might be best performed during the acute phase of vascular injury.

Targeting clots

Fibrin deposition usually follows initial platelet aggregation. Therefore, use of radiolabeled fibrinogen to target sites of platelet aggregation at the atherosclerotic lesions is a rational outcome. Mettinger et al used I-123 labeled fibrinogen to target atherosclerotic plaques in patients with carotid lesions (25). Increased radiotracer uptake was observed in the carotid arteries with lesions but not at the non-diseased arteries. However, radiotracer accumulation was only transient with no localization detected by 20 h post injection.

Although the potential for targeting endothelial injury associated with atherogenesis via platelet and/or blood clot accumulation has been investigated, no viable clinical diagnostic approach has emerged.

Targeting proliferating smooth muscle cells of atherosclerotic lesions

Monoclonal antibody Z2D3

Since two out of three kinds of atherosclerotic plaques, the fibrous and the advanced plaques, contain smooth muscle cells that are actively proliferating, and even the fibro-fatty lesions are never totally devoid of smooth muscle cells (23), scientists of Scotgen (Menlo Park, CA) reasoned that antibodies to proliferating smooth muscle cells may provide a specific technique for imaging atherosclerotic lesions. Thus a monoclonal antibody designated Z2D3 was developed using human atherosclerotic lesion homogenate as immunogen. This murine IgM monoclonal antibody was specific for a complex lipid antigen associated with the proliferating smooth muscle cells (27). Figure 1 shows the immunoperoxidase stained frozen sections of human and rabbit atheroscloretic lesions (4, 13). Serial sections of human atheroma stained with Z2D3 antibody (b) and anti-macrophage antibody (c) showed that Z2D3 stained regions corresponded to the unstained regions with anti-macrophage antibody (c). These micrographs indicated that the regions stained with Z2D3 were different from the regions of macrophage/foam cell accumulation. Z2D3 was also observed to cross-react with rabbit atherosclerotic lesion (d). The region of Z2D3 positivity in experimental atherosclerotic lesions was observed to correspond to the region of cellular proliferation as demonstrated by staining with anti-proliferating cell nuclear antigen (PCNA) (e). Furthermore, it was observed that Z2D3 did not stain the smooth muscle cells in the tunica media that were of the contractile phenotype. These immunohistochemical-staining studies indicated that Z2D3 is specific for smooth muscle cells that are actively proliferating and therefore are of the synthetic phenotype. To enable better *in vivo* targeting potential, the murine IgM Z2D3 was subsequently class switched and genetically engineered to produce a murine-human chimeric Z2D3 of the IgG1 subclass (13). This chimeric Z2D3 also stained the rabbit atheroma similar to the parent IgM antibody (f).

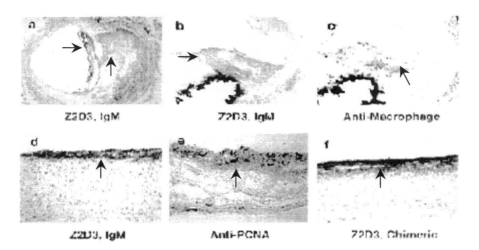

Figure 1. Immunohistochemical staining of (a and b) human atheroma with Z2D3 IgM, (c) serial section to b stained with anti-macrophage antibody, (d) experimental rabbit atheroma stained with Z2D3 IgM, (e) experimental rabbit atheroma stained with anti-PCNA antibody and (f) rabbit experimental atheroma stained with chimeric ZeD3. Arrows denote immunoperoxidased stained regions of atherosclerotic lesions.

In vivo imaging with murine Z2D3 antibody

Initial feasibility studies were performed with murine IgM Z2D3 labeled with In-111 in rabbits with deendothelialized descending aorta (28). Atherosclerotic lesions were detected by *in vivo* gamma imaging in most of the rabbits (7). Control In-111 labeled IgM did not show localization in the lesions. Localization of the radiolabeled Z2D3 was observed to be in the healing edges of the lesions that simulated human atheroma where proliferating smooth muscle cells predominated. Evans Blue stain demarcated the denuded from the regenerating endothelium. The healing endothelium showed no staining. Control non-specific IgM also labeled with In-111 did not show uptake in rabbits with similar experimental atherosclerotic lesions. Use of IgM Z2D3 rendered high bone, liver, kidney and other non-target organ activities, resulting in high background and non-target organ activities. Therefore, subsequent studies switched to the use of $F(ab)_2$ fragments of murine-human chimeric genetically engineered Z2D3.

Imaging with chimeric Z2D3

To simulate human atherosclerotic lesions more accurately, we then switched to the use of modified rabbit model of hyperlipidemic diet and endothelial denudation (13). The rabbits were put on 6% peanut oil and 2% cholesterol diet for 12 weeks. One week after the initiation of this diet, the descending aorta from below the diaphragm to the bifurcation of the femoral arteries was denuded of the endothelium with a balloon catheter. After 10 to 12 weeks of hyperlipidemic diet and endothelial denudation, the descending aorta was observed to have extensive atherosclerotic lesions in the region of the endothelial denudation as well as spontaneous lesions in the aortic arch. Such lesions simulated human lesions more accurately with more proliferating smooth muscle cells (SMCs) albeit with less fatty streaks. Although the area of the experimental lesion was extensive, the intima involved was only a few cell layers thick resulting in a model of atherosclerosis that was less severe than that encountered in a clinical situation. Nevertheless, this model enabled *in vivo* visualization of the experimental atherosclerotic lesions with In-111 labeled chimeric Z2D3 $F(ab')_2$. Chimerization of the parental IgM to murine-human Z2D3 (cZ2D3) was achieved by ligation of the constant region genes of human IgG1 to the murine variable heavy chain gene of the parental murine IgM Z2D3 (13). The intact cZ2D3 antibody was digested with pepsin to produce $F(ab')_2$. This cZ2D3 $F(ab')_2$ labeled with In-111 was used to image experimental atherosclerotic lesions produced by endothelial denudation and hyperlipidemic diet in New Zealand White rabbits. However, lesions were observed only after 48 h of blood pool activity clearance (Figure 2, second panel from left). In the earlier images, the lesion activity could not be differentiated from the aortic blood pool activity (left-most panel). Localization of In-111 labeled cZ2D3 F(ab')$_2$ in the gamma image of the excised aorta (middle image) was observed to correspond to the region of the lesions in the necropsy specimen (Figure 2). cZ2D3 F(ab')$_2$ uptake was 6 times greater than that in the adjacent normal aorta of the same animal. No uptake was observed with In-111 cZ2D3 F(ab')$_2$ in normal aorta of control normal rabbits, nor were there any radiotracer uptake in rabbits with experimental atherosclerotic lesion injected with In-111 labeled non-specific human IgG1 F(ab')$_2$.

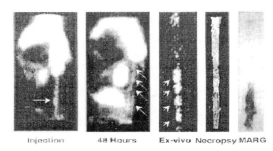

Injection   48 Hours   Ex-vivo Necropsy MARG

Figure 2. Left lateral gamma images of a rabbit with atherosclerotic lesions induced by endothelial denudation and hyperlipidemic diet obtained at the time of injection (Left most panel, arrow indicates the blood pool activity in the descending aorta, the sites of endothelial denudation) and 48 h after injection (next panel to the right, the arrows indicate the regions of atherosclerotic lesion showing radiotracer accumulation). The ex vivo gamma image is shown in the center panel. The arrows correspond to the regions demarcated by the arrows in the *in vivo* 48 h image. The gross pathological specimen is shown in the next panel to the right. The right end panel shows the macroautoradiograph (MARG) of the descending aorta.

Image enhancement with negative charge modified cZ2D3 F(ab')$_2$

We have previously demonstrated that non-specific background activity of antibodies may be decreased *in vivo* by negative charge modification of the antibody (28). Subsequently, others have also observed that decreasing the isoelectric points of the antibody molecules resulted in decreased background activity and increased target to background ratios (29-31). Therefore, we modified cZ2D3 F(ab')$_2$ with highly negatively charged chelating polymers (13). This modification rendered the antibody with low isoelectric point of about 4-5 and the capability to chelate a large number of In-111 per antibody molecule. The polymer is modified with a large number of chelate molecules (diethylene triamine pentaacetic acid, DTPA), providing high chelating potential as well as imparting approximately 4 carboxylic groups per DTPA attached to the polymer. The efficacy of this negative charge modification to reduce non-target organ and background activity was based on the hypothesis that antibodies are basic molecules and the cell surfaces and ground substances that constitute the extracellular matrix, are rich in acidic residues that could lead to non-specific ionic interaction. However if the charge of the antibodies were modified to be negative, then there should be repulsion due to like negative charges between the modified antibody and the cell surfaces or the ground substances (32). The presence of chelating polymer on the antibody also allowed chelation of In-111 to the modified antibody with high specific radioactivity. The standard DTPA-F(ab')$_2$ has a specific radioactivity of about 10 mCi / mg . The negative charged-polymer modified F(ab')2 had specific radioactivity of 50-100 mCi/mg. A 25 µg aliquot (~650 µCi) of charge-modified Z2D3 F(ab')$_2$ in rabbits with experimental atherosclerotic lesions enabled visualization of the lesion by 24 h (33). No lesions were visualized with negative charge modified non-specific IgG F(ab')$_2$. We also investigated whether higher dose of radioactivity would allow earlier visualization of the lesions by injecting rabbits with atherosclerotic lesions with 125 µg negatively charge modified Z2D3 F(ab')$_2$ (~3mCi). With the high dose of radioactivity, lesions were visualized by 3 h after intravenous administration of the negatively charge modified Z2D3 (33). The lesions visualized in the *in vivo* images were confirmed by the ex vivo images of the excised aorta.

Similarly, Johnson et al used the negatively charge modified Z2D3 F(ab')$_2$ to visualize lesions in a swine model of atherosclerotic lesions induced by stent placement in the coronary arteries (34).

Clinical application of charge-modified Z2D3 F(ab')$_2$

Following the preclinical studies that showed the safety and feasibility of imaging atherosclerotic lesions, Phase I studies were undertaken at two European Centers at Sant Pau Hospital, Barcelona, Spain and Bufalini Hospital, Cesena, Italy. Sterile and apyrogenic kits containing negative charge-modified Z2D3 F(ab')$_2$ (250 µg) were labeled with In-111 and 5 mCi aliquots were administered into 9 patients with angiographically confirmed carotid atherosclerosis (35). Planar and single photon emission computed tomographic (SPECT) images were obtained at 4, 24, 28 and 72h. The contralateral carotid arteries without the lesions constituted internal controls. All lesions in nine patients were detected either by planar or SPECT at 4 h after radiotracer administration. No adverse effects were observed after In-111 negative charge-modified Z2D3 F(ab')$_2$ administration. Figure 3 shows a pair of anterior planar images of a patient before and after endarterectomy. In panel A, a diffused region of radiolabeled antibody activity can be seen in the region of the left carotid (arrow). The image of a normal patient (panel B) showed no radiotracer accumulation. The coronal SPECT image of another patient with a right carotid artery lesion is shown in Figure 4. The corresponding arteriogram on the left shows the lesion that was visualized in the SPECT image (right). Carrio et al. reported that antibody Z2D3 specific for an antigen produced by the proliferating smooth muscle cells could be used to image atherosclerotic lesions by gamma immunoscintigraphy (35).

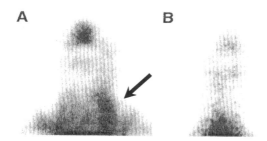

Figure 3.   Anterior gamma images of In-111 labeled negative-charged modified Z2D3 F(ab')$_2$ in a patient with left carotid lesion (arrow) (A) and a patient with no carotid lesion (B) (Carrio et al. J Nucl Cardiol. 1998;5:551-557 with permission).

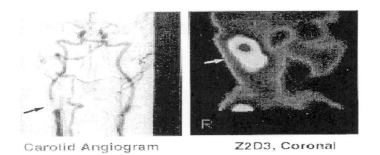

Figure 4.   Carotid angiogram of a patient with right carotid lesion (arrow) (left panel) and the corresponding coronal SPECT image showing In-111 labeled negative charge-modified Z2D3 F(ab')$_2$ localization (right panel, arrow) (Carrio et al. J Nucl Cardiol. 1998; 5:551-557 with permission).

Targeting the upregulated purine receptors on proliferating smooth muscle cells in atherosclerotic lesions

Smooth muscle cell proliferation is an integral component of atherosclerotic lesions. Although they are present in minor concentrations in fibro-fatty lesions, smooth muscle cells constitute the predominant type in fibrous and advanced plaque (14). Furthermore, the phenotype of intimal smooth muscles cells is of the synthetic form. The cells have dedifferentiated from the contractile to the synthetic form. It has been observed in cultured smooth muscle cells that such dedifferentiated cells also acquire different adenosine receptor phenotypes. There appears to be upregulation of the expression of P2U and P2D purine receptors on the synthetic phenotypic smooth muscle cells (36). Diadenosine polyphosphates have higher avidity for P2U and P2D purine receptors. Therefore, use of radiolabeled diadenosine polyphosphate may enable targeting and visualization of the proliferating smooth muscle cell component of the atherosclerotic lesions. Elmaleh et al labeled diadenosine tetraphosphate (AP4A) with Tc-99m and imaged rabbit atherosclerotic lesions induced by descending aorta endothelial denudation and hyperlipidemic diet as previous described (13). In 6 atherosclerotic rabbits, Tc-99m labeled AP4A enabled visualization of the lesions as early as 30 minutes after intravenous administration of the radiotracer (Figure 5).

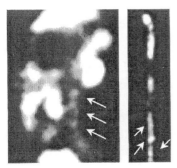 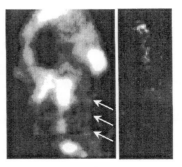

Figure 5. Left lateral gamma image of an atherosclerotic rabbit injected with Tc-99m labeled AP4A (left panel, left image, arrows indiate atherosclerotic lesions) and the image of the excised atherosclerotic aorta (left panel right image). Left lateral gamma image of a normal rabbit (right panel, left image) injected with Tc-99m labeled AP4A (arrows indicate region of the descending aorta) and the image of the excised aorta (right panel, right image)(Elmaleh et al. Proc Nat Acad Sci. USA. 1998; 95:691-695, with permission).

No localization was seen in the 3 normal control rabbits also injected with the same radiotracer. Ex vivo radiotracer accumulation in the lesions was approximately 7.5 times greater than the activity seen in normal aorta. The radiotracer distribution also corresponded to the regions of histological lesions. This study demonstrated that upregulated purinoceptors in proliferating smooth muscle cells might allow development of very early targeting of atherosclerotic lesions by non-invasive gamma imaging.

CONCLUSIONS

Atherosclerotic lesions can be imaged with radiolabeled autologous blood cells and or blood components. However, due to the nonspecificity of the localization of these reagents, imaging of atherosclerotic lesions is only marginally successful. Monoclonal or chimeric antibody to an antigen specific for the proliferating smooth muscle cells appears to be more avid for targeting atherosclerotic lesions. More specific *in vivo* localization is achieved with negative charge-modified Z2D3 antibody, enabling gamma imaging at 24 h after intravenous administration of the radiotracer. Even earlier imaging was achieved with high dose, high specific radioactivity preparations of negative charge-modified Z2D3. Faster targeting and visualization of experimental atherosclerotic lesions is achieved with radiolabeled diadenosine tetraphosphate that localizes in the upregulated purine receptors (P2U and P2D) of the proliferating smooth muscle cells in experimental atherosclerotic lesions.

Of the above-mentioned methods, autologous blood cells and components have been tested in clinical trials. Z2D3 has also reached Phase I clinical trials. However, to date there is no one leading candidate that can claim supremacy for imaging the metabolic status of the atherosclerotic lesions. Future imaging targets may involve foam cells, apoptotic cells of the atherosclerotic lesions, upregulated adhesion molecules or other neoantigens that are as yet untested. It would be important to elucidate and assess the metabolic status of the lesions as indicators of success or failure of therapeutic interventions. Even though the current approaches to targeting atherosclerotic lesions have been encouraging, newer, faster and more specific methods for diagnosis would be highly desirable.

REFERENCES

1. Sones FM, Shirley EK. Cine coronary arteriography. Mod Concepts Cardiovascl Dis 1962; 31:735-751.
2. Sherman CT, Litvack F, Grundfest W, et al. Coronary angioscopy in patients with unstable angina pectoris. N Engl J Med. 1986; 315:913-919.
3. Tardif JC, Pandian NG. Intravascular ultrasound imaging in peripheral arterial and coronary artery disease. Curr Opin Cardiol. 1994;9:627-633.
4. Khaw BA, Carrio I, Pieri PL, Narula J. Radionuclide imaging of the synthetic smooth muscle cell phenotype in experimental atherosclerotic lesions. Trends in Cardiovascular Med. 1996; 7:226-232.
5. Falk, E, Shah P, Fuster V. Coronary plaque disruption. Circulation 1995; 92:657-671.

6. Holmes DR Jr, Vliestra RE, Smith HC, et al. Restenosis after percutaneous transluminal coronary angioplasty (PTCA): a report from PTCA registry of the HHLBI. Am J Cardiol. 1984; 53:77C-81C.

7. Narula, J, Ditlaow C, Chen F, Khaw BA. "Monoclonal antibodies for the detection of atherosclerotic lesions." In: *Monoclonal antibodies in cardiovascular diseases.* Khaw BA, Narula J, Strauss HW, ed. Lea and Febiger, Philadelphia. 1994; pp 206-215.

8. DiCorleto PE, Chisolm GM. Participation of the endothelium in the development of the atherosclerotic plaque. Prog Lipid Res 1986;25:365-374.

9. Parthasarthy S, Steinbrecher UP, Barnett J, Witztum JL, Steinberg D. Essential role of phospholipase A2 activity in endothelial cell-induced modification of low density lipoprotein. Proc Natl Acad Sci USA 1985; 82: 3000-3004.

10. Goldstein JL, Ho YK, Basu SK, Brown MS,. Binding site on macrophages that mediates uptake and degredation oof acetylated low density lipoprotein, producing massive choletsterol deposition. Proc Natl Acad Sci UAS 1979;76:333-337.

11. Roberts AB, Lee AM, Lees RS, Strauss HW, Fallon JT, Taveras J, Kopiwoda S. Selective accumulation of low dsensity lipoproteins in damaged arterial wall. J Lipid Res. 1983;24:1160-1167.

12. Davis HH, Siegel BA, Joist JH, Heaton WA, Mathias CJ, Sherman LA, Welch MJ. Scintigraphic detection of atherosclerotic lesions and venous thrombi in man by In-111 labeled autologous platelets. Lancet 1978;1:1185-1187.

13. Narula J, Petrov A, Bianchi C, Ditlow CC, Dilley J, Pieslak I, Chen FW, Torchilin VP, Khaw BA. Noninvasive localization of experimental atherosclerotic lesions with mouse/human chimeric Z2D3 antibody specific for the proliferating smooth muscle cells of human atheroma: Imaging with conventional antibody and image enhancement with negative charge-modified antibody. Circulation 1995; 92:474-484.

14. Elmaleh DR, Narula J, Babich JW, Petrov A, Fischman AJ, Khaw BA, Rapaport E, Zamecnik PC. Rapid noninvasive detection of expertimental atherosclerotic lesions with novel ^{99m}Tc-labeled diadenosine tetraphosphates. Proc Nat Acad Sci. USA. 1998;95:691-695.

15. Moerlein SM, Daugherty A, Sobel BE, Welch MJ. Metabolic imaging with ^{68}Ga and ^{111}In-labeled LDL. J Nucl Med 1991;32:300-307.

16. Lees RS, Lees AM, Strauss HW. External imaging of human atherosclerosis. J Nucl Med 1983;24:154-156.

17. Lees AM, Lees RS, Schoen FJ, Issachsohn JL, Fischman AJ, McKusick KA, Strauss HW. Imaging human atherosclerosis with Tc-99m-labeled LDL. Atherosclerosis 1988;8:461-470.

18. Virgolino I, Muller F, Fitscha P, Chiba P, Sinzinger H. Radiolabeling autologous monocytes with ^{111}In oxine for reinjection in patients with atherosclerosis. Prog Clin Biol Res 1989;355:271-280.

19. Fischman AJ, Rubin RH, Khaw BA, Kramer PB, Wilkinson R, Ahmad M, Needelman M, Locke E, Nossiff ND, Strauss HW. Radionuclide imaging of experimental atherosclerosis with non-specific polyclonal immunoglobulin G. J Nucl Med. 1989; 29:1095-1100.

20. Fischman AJ, Rubin RH, Delvecchio A, Ahmed M, Khaw BA, Callahan RJ, LaMuraglia GM, Strauss HW. Imaging of atheromatous lesions in the iliac and femoral vessels: preliminary experience with indium-111-IgG in human subjects. J Nucl Med. 1989; 30(5):817.

21. Watanabe T, Hirata M, Yoshikawa Y, Nagafuchi Y, Toyoshima H, Watanabe T. Role of macrophages in atherosclerosis. Sequential observations of cholesterl-induced rabbit aortic lesion by the immunoperoxidasse technique using monoclonal antimacrophage antibody. Lab Invest 1985; 53(1):80-90

22. Aqel NM, Ball RY, Waldmann H, Mitchinson MJ. Identification of macrophages and smooth muscle cells in human atherosclerosis using monoclonal antibodies. J Pathol 1985; 146:197-204.

23. Gown AM, Tsukada T, Ross R. Human atherosclerosis. II. Immunocytochemical analysis of the cellular composition of human atherosclerotic lesions. Am L Pathol 1986;125:1910297.

24. Miller DD, Boulet AJ, Tio PO, Garcia OJ, Guy DM, McEver RP, Palmer JC, Pak KY, Neblock DS, Berger HJ. *In vivo* ^{99m}Tc S12 antibody imaging of platelet alpha granules in rabbit endothelial neointimal proliferation after angioplasty. Circulation 1991;83:224-236.

25. Mettinger KL, Ericson K, Larson S, Casseborn S. Detection of atherosclerotic plaques in carotid arteries by the use of ^{123}I fibrinogen. Lancet 1978;1:242-244.

26. Minar E, Ehringer H, Dudczak R, Schofl R, Jung M, Koppensteiner R, Ahmadi R, Kreschmer G. ^{111}In-labeled platelet scintigraphy in carotid atherosclerosis. Stroke 1989;20:27-33.

27. Harrison DC, Calenoff E, Chen F, Parmley W, Khaw BA, Ross R. Plaque-Associated Immune Reactivity as a Tool for the Diagnosis and Treatment of Atherosclerosis. Proceedings of the American Clinical and Climabiological Association. Trans Am Clin Climatol Assoc. 1992; 103:210-217.

28. Khaw BA, Calenoff E, Chen F, O'Donnell SM, Nossiff ND, Strauss HW. Localization of Experimental Atherosclerotic Lesion with Monoclonal Antibody Z2D3. J Nucl Med. 1991; 32(5):1005.

29. Sharifi J, Khawli LA, Hornick JL, Epstein AL. Improving monoclonal antibody pharmacokinetics via chemical modification. Q J Nucl Med 1998 Dec;42(4):242-9

30. Colcher D, Pavlinkova G, Beresford G, Booth BJ, Choudhury A, Batra SK. Pharmacokinetics and biodistribution of genetically-engineered antibodies. Q J Nucl Med 1998 Dec;42(4):225-41

31. Khawli LA, Glasky MS, Alauddin MM, Epstein AL. Improved tumor localization and radioimaging with chemically modified monoclonal antibodies. Cancer Biother Radiopharm 1996;11:203-15.

32. Khaw BA, Klibanov A, O'Donnell SM, Siato T, Nossiff N, Slinkin MA, Newell JB, Strauss HW, Torchilin VP. Gamma imaging with negatively charge-modified monoclonal antibody; Modification with synthetic polymers. J Nucl Med. 1991; 32:1742-1751.

33. Narula J, Petrov A, Ditlow C, Pak KY, Chen FW, Khaw BA. Maximizing radiotracer delivery for scintigraphic localization of experimental atherosclerotic lesions with high-dose negative-charge-modified Z2D3 antibody. J Nucl Cardiol; 1997; 4:226-233.

34. Johnson LL, Schofield LM, Verdesca SA, Sharaf BL, Jones RM, Virmani R, Khaw BA. In-vivo uptake of radiolabeled antibody to proliferating smooth muscle cells in a swine model of coronary stent restenosis. J Nucl Med.2000; 41:1535-1540.

35. Carrió I, Pieri PL, Narula J, Prat L, Riva P, Pedrini L, Pretolani E, Caruso G, Sarti G, Estorch M, Berná L, Riambau V, Matías-Guiu X, Pak C, Ditlow C, Chen F, Khaw BA. Noninvasive localization of human atherosclerotic lesions with In-111-labeled monoclonal Z2D3 antibody specific for proliferating smooth muscle cells. J Nucl Cardiol 1998; 5: 551-557.

36. Pintor J, Miras-Portugal MT. Diadenosine polyphosphates (ApxA) as new neurotransmitters. Drug Dev Res 1993;28:259-262.

GLOSSARY

AP4A: Diadenine tetraphosphate.

F(ab')$_2$: Divalent pepsin digest fragment of intact antibody, molecular weight approximately 100,000 daltons.

LDL: Low density lipoprotein.

MARG: Macroautoradiograph.

P2D and P2U: Purine receptors that are expressed on smooth muscle cells after they have undergone dedifferentiation form the contractile to the synthetic phenotypes.

S12: Monoclonal antibody specific for P-selectin.

SMC: Smooth muscle cells.

SPECT: Single photon emission computed tomography.

Z2D3: Murine monoclonal IgM antibody to a complex lipid antigen produced by proliferating smooth muscle cells in atherosclerotic lesions. Subsequently, it was class switched to IgG1 and then chimerized with human IgG1 constant region.

5

THROMBUS TARGETING OF PLASMINOGEN ACTIVATORS AND ANTICOAGULANTS

Karlheinz Peter, Christoph Bode
Department of Cardiology and Angiology, University of Freiburg, Hugstetter Str. 55, 79106 Freiburg, Germany

INTRODUCTION

Large-scale studies with mortality endpoints comparing fibrinolytic therapy with placebo in patients with acute myocardial infarction (AMI) have documented the benefit of timely dissolution of coronary arterial thrombi by intravenous infusion of plasminogen activators (Fig. 1). (1)

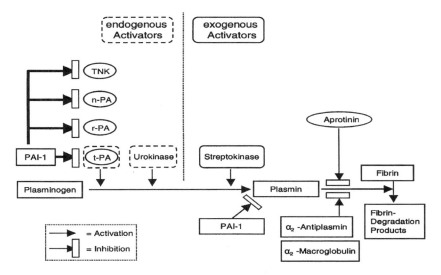

Figure 1. Fibrinolysis: Activators and Inhibitors. Plasminogen is cleaved and thereby activated to plasmin by the endogenous activators urokinase and tissue-plasminogen activators and its mutants (r-PA: reteplase, n-PA: lanoteplase, TNK: tenecteplase) and the exogenous activators streptokinase. Plasmin lyses clots by cleaving fibrin-to-fibrin degradation products. Plasmin is inhibited by aprotinin, α_2-Antiplasmin, and α_2-Makroglobulin.

The GUSTO-1 trial (2), comparing four thrombolytic strategies, showed a small but noteworthy improvement (1.0%) in survival among patients treated with recombinant tissue-type plasminogen activator (t-PA) compared with streptokinase (SK). Equally important with this incremental improvement in survival was the finding that there is a direct correlation between early and complete reperfusion and survival. (2) These data are consistent with the hypothesis that fibrin-specific thrombolytic agents (such as t-PA) achieve lower mortality by lysing coronary thrombi more rapidly and more completely. The results of the GUSTO trial thus appear to give reasonable direction to researchers involved in the design of plasminogen activators for the improvement of potency and specificity by clot targeting of fibrinolytic agents.

Significant limitations, even of the most advanced thrombolytic regimens, at present fail to achieve some reperfusion in 15% - 20% and complete reperfusion in 35% - 45% of patients within 90 min after start of therapy. (2, 3) The failure rate at earlier time points is even higher. In addition, an early re-occlusion rate of 5%—15% limits the benefits of therapy in initially successfully treated patients. Furthermore, 3% - 10% of patients experience bleeding episodes that necessitate transfusions. In 0.3% - 0.7% of patients, intracerebral hemorrhage occurs. It has to be emphasized, that the above data refers to patients who have been carefully selected for thrombolytic therapy and who constitute only a "low risk" fraction of all patients with AMI.

New fibrinolytic agents, mainly deletion and point mutants of t-PA, have been developed (Fig. 2 below). Nevertheless, in comparison to t-PA, mortality in patients with acute myocardial infarction was not significantly improved by these new agents. (4) Very recently the combination of fibrinolysis and GP IIb/IIIa blockade, which has demonstrated increased and earlier patencies, has been tested in large clinical trials. (5) However, mortality in patients with the combination of fibrinolysis and GP IIb/IIIa blockade was not improved compared to fibrinolysis alone. Furthermore, the rate of bleeding complications significantly increased with the combinational therapy.

Overall, there is a need to enhance the efficacy, speed, and freedom from side effects of thrombolytic therapy. This chapter describes novel approaches for the development of agents that either dissolve clots or prevent clot formation that are based on the strategy to target fibrinolytics or anticoagulants to the thrombus.

THE PRINCIPLE OF ANTIBODY TARGETING

Antibody targeting for the treatment or prevention of thrombosis entails the engineering of a bifunctional molecule that contains both a highly specific antigen-binding site, that concentrates the molecule at the desired target, and an effector site that either initiates thrombolysis or prevents additional thrombus formation.

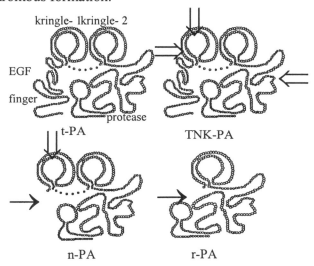

Figure 2. Fibrinolytic Agents: t-PA and its Mutant/Deletion Variants. Schematic drawing of the molecular structure of t-PA (alteplase), TNK-PA (tenecteplase), n-PA (lanoteplase), and r-PA (reteplase) with the main determinants (finger domain, EGF-like domain, kringle-1 and kringle-2 domain and protease (plasminogen) domain). Variants are created by deletions (→) and point mutations (⇒). The variants differ mainly in fibrin specificity and plasma clearance.

The repertoire of potential antibody specificities allows for the selection of monoclonal antibodies that can differentiate among very similar antigens. Thus, it is possible to target to fibrin but not fibrinogen or to recognize the activated form of the platelet integrin receptor glycoprotein (GP) IIb/IIIa, but not its inactive conformation. Obviously, the effectiveness of a clot-specific antibody is dependent on a lack of cross-reactivity between the desired epitope and all non-thrombus epitopes on endothelial or other vascular cells.

Anti-Fibrin Antibodies

Our most extensive experience has been gained with fibrin-specific antibody 59D8. The antibody was raised by immunizing Balb/C mice with a synthetic peptide containing the sequence of the thrombin-generated amino terminus of the fibrin β-chain, coupled to a carrier protein. (6) Monoclonal antibody 59D8 binds to fibrin with high affinity (0.77 nmol/l) but does not bind to fibrinogen. In contrast, the binding constant of t-PA for fibrin is 0.16 µmol/l. Other groups have used different antibodies specific for fibrin.

Anti-Platelet Antibodies

Platelets undergo structural changes as they aggregate and are incorporated into a thrombus. The integrin GP IIb/IIIa ($\forall_{IIb}\exists_3$) on the platelet membrane functions as a receptor for fibrinogen. As such the complex has a role in crosslinking platelets not only to one another, but also to fibrin, thereby stabilizing the thrombus. The humanized antibody fragment c7E3 (abciximab) binds to and inhibits GP IIb/IIIa, thus inhibiting platelet aggregation. The antibody has been shown to be a useful adjunct to thrombolysis, PTCA, and stenting. (7, 8) For our purposes, c7E3 provides a model vehicle for targeting plasminogen activators or anti-thrombin agents to an epitope expressed on platelet-rich, arterial thrombi. The disadvantage of 7E3 as a targeting antibody is that it interacts with GP IIb/IIIa on both activated and resting platelets; thus targeting the thrombus only with relative selectivity. Others have used the monoclonal antibody Fab-9 directed against GP IIb/IIIa that was subsequently optimized by mutagenesis and affinity maturation, using phage display techniques. (9)

Chemical Conjugates or Recombinant Fusion Proteins

Chemical conjugation between antibody and effector molecule is the fastest and easiest method to create a model bifunctional molecule. Recombinant fusion proteins have the advantage of a uniform and large-scale preparation of protein material and they avoid the low-yield of chemical cross-linking. Also, recombinant fusion molecules are not limited like chemical conjugates to recombination of whole proteins or domains that can be generated by enzymatic digestion. Rather, the needed regions of proteins can be fused and, if necessary, cleavage sites for different enzymes can be introduced (see below) to endow the molecules with additional specificity. Thus, while chemical conjugates are suitable to explore the general concept, only recombinant fusion molecules can be tailored with suitable sophistication in order to endow them as powerful new therapeutic agents.

Synthesis, Purification, and Characterization of Chemical Antibody-Plasminogen Activator Conjugates

Synthesis

The method for chemically cross-linking plasminogen activators to antibodies has initially been established in our laboratories. (10) The general approach is to generate stable disulfide or thio-ester bonds between the two proteins of interest. One of the most useful strategies is to link two proteins using the cross-linking reagent, N-succinimidy 3-(2-pyridyldithio)propionate (SPDP). This is a heterobifunctional reagent: the attachment and cross-linking steps of the reaction are separate and it is possible to use either the same or different functional groups on each protein. In order to prevent the formation of aggregates and to increase the yield of the 1:1 conjugate it is essential to establish conditions that allow modification of a single amino group on each protein. Alternatively, free sulfhydryl groups can be generated on one of the proteins under reducing conditions. This approach has been very effectively used in coupling Fab'-fragments of the targeting antibody using the reduced inter-heavy chain disulfide bonds of the hinge-region as reactive sulfhydryl groups and reacting these with SPDP-modified plasminogen activator. A third commonly used approach is to modify the proteins to be coupled with two different cross-linking reagents. It is thus possible to control conditions in a way that the favored reaction is between the two desired species.

Purification

Although the methodology described in this section was first developed for purification of chemically coupled conjugates, similar methods are used for purification of recombinant hybrid molecules. In principle, purification strategies are employed, that select for size (a 1:1 molar ratio of the antibody and plasminogen activator is the desired product) and also for biological activity of both the antibody and the enzyme. Thus, gel filtration is usually implemented to separate the desired 1:1 conjugate from uncoupled reactants as well as higher molecular weight polymers. Even a very pure peak that contains a 1:1 molar ratio of antibody and plasminogen activator, as assessed by SDS-polyacrylamide gel electrophoresis, does not guarantee that all conjugates contain biological activity for both the antibody and plasminogen activator. Sequential affinity chromatography with appropriate immobilized ligands can be used to select for biologically active conjugates or fusion proteins. The first affinity step selecting for active urokinase (UK) or tissue plasminogen activator (t-PA) involves benzamidine immobilized on Sepharose that specifically binds to (and inhibits) the intact active center of serine proteases. The benzamidine-Sepharose column does not retain uncoupled antibody or Fab'-fragment or inactivated enzyme that is washed out. Elution by pH-change yields both conjugated material with an active plasminogen activator domain and free plasminogen activator that was not coupled initially.

The second affinity step selects for molecules with an intact antibody portion. For example, anti-fibrin antibody 59D8 can be bound to a Sepharose matrix to which the peptide is coupled against which the antibody was initially raised (β-peptide). When the eluate from the benzamidine-Sepharose column purification step is further purified on a β-peptide-column, any conjugates with antibody unable to bind to its antigen will not bind to the column. Also, uncoupled plasminogen activator will not bind to the β-peptide-Sepharose column. The eluted final product from this column will thus be a 1:1 conjugate containing biologically active plasminogen activator and antibody domains. For antibodies or plasminogen activators [e. g., single-chain urinary-type plasminogen activator (scuPA)] for which suitable ligand-Sepharose columns are not available, immunoaffinity chromatography, using antibody-Sepharose columns, have been used successfully. Ideally, the immobilized antibody only recognizes and binds to the active form of plasminogen activator or antibody in the conjugate or fusion protein. If such an antibody is unavailable, less efficient alternatives include the use of immobilized antibodies which cannot distinguish active from inactive antibody or plasminogen activator or the use of immobilized protein A or G.

Characterization

Characterization of chemical conjugates as well as of recombinant fusion proteins includes assessment of molecular size by SDS gel electrophoresis under reducing and non-reducing conditions, antigenicity studies by Western-blot and analysis of the functional status of the antibody combining site (compared to native antibody) and of the plasminogen activator enzymatic properties (compared to native plasminogen activator). The focus of this review will be on functional characterization in terms of enhancement of fibrinolytic and thrombolytic potency of conjugate versus native plasminogen activator *in vitro* and *in vivo*.

Further insight can be gained by comparing fully functional conjugates to conjugates in which one partner is inactive. Control conjugates with plasminogen activator (e.g., urokinase) coupled to irrelevant antibodies (e.g., specific for digoxin) have been used to discriminate between enhancement of activity due to increase in molecular weight (and reduced clearance of conjugate versus native plasminogen activator) and enhancement due to targeting of the enzyme by the specific antibody combining site.

Anti-Fibrin-UK Conjugates

Chemical conjugates between anti-fibrin antibody 59D8 and urokinase (UK) were 100 - 250 times as potent as uncoupled UK and 10 times as potent as t-PA in an *in vitro* fibrinolytic screening assay with purified components (fibrin-Sepharose assay). (10) In an assay that monitored the lysis of fresh human thrombus in a human plasma bath, the UK-anti-fibrin conjugate proved to be 2.2 - 4.4 times as efficient as urokinase alone. In both assays, conjugates of whole (bivalent) anti-fibrin IgG and those of (monovalent) anti-fibrin Fab fragments performed equally well. Based on the promising results with chemical anti-fibrin-UK conjugates a recombinant approach with an anti-fibrin single chain antibody was chosen.

Anti-Fibrin-t-PA Conjugates

Tissue-type plasminogen activator is more difficult to handle than urokinase in conjugation experiments because it is less soluble at higher concentrations. The t-PA-anti-fibrin conjugate was 10 times as efficient as uncoupled t-PA in the *in vitro* screening assay with purified components (fibrin-Sepharose assay) and it was 3.2 times more potent than t-PA in the human plasma clot assay. (11) *In vivo*, in a rabbit jugular vein model of thrombolysis, the conjugate proved to be 3.0-9.6 times as potent as t-PA alone. (12) Both, *in vitro* and *in vivo*, the t-PA anti-fibrin conjugate increased fibrinolytic potency without sacrificing specificity: fibrinogen, plasminogen and α_2-anti-plasmin consumption were lower relative to that obtained with t-PA alone, indicating that the increase in potency was the result of an increase in selectivity.

Anti-Fibrin-scuPA Conjugates

Although scuPA has no affinity for fibrin it is a relatively fibrin selective agent through other mechanisms. The prospect of being able to improve the plasminogen activating properties of scuPA by adding fibrin affinity, i.e., through a second mechanism of fibrin selectivity, appeared particularly interesting. In an assay with purified components the fibrinolytic potency of the conjugate proved to be 230 times greater than that of scuPA, 420 times greater than that of urokinase, and 33 times greater than that of t-PA. (13) Subsequent studies *in vitro* in human plasma showed enhanced lysis in terms of speed completeness and specificity *In vivo* in the rabbit jugular vein model, anti-fibrin-scuPA was 29 times more efficacious than its natural counterpart.

Anti-Platelet-Urokinase Conjugates

Arterial thrombi contain a high concentration of activated platelets. As such, platelet-rich thrombi appear to be particularly resistant to thrombolysis. Thus, massive platelet participation in thombogenesis may be a major reason for the limited success rate of thrombolytic therapy in patients with AMI and they also appear to play a major role in early re-occlusion after initially successful thrombolysis. Antibody 7E3, which binds specifically to the platelet GP IIb/IIIa receptor which mediates platelet aggregation, has been shown to be a useful adjunct to thrombolysis, PTCA, and stenting. It was of particular interest to determine whether the targeting of a plasminogen activator to the GP IIb/IIIa receptor through 7E3 would enhance the antibody's ability to block platelet aggregation. In addition to blocking access of the GP IIb/IIIa receptor to fibrinogen by virtue of 7E3's binding to the receptor, the high local concentration of plasmin achieved through targeting the plasminogen activator to platelets was thought to lyse fibrin and (locally) fibrinogen responsible for aggregating the platelets. A urokinase-7E3-Fab'-conjugate bound to purified GP IIb/IIIa and intact activated platelets and also exhibited plasminogen activator activity. At the concentrations tested, urokinase showed very little activity against the clots, whereas the conjugate was 970 times more active. An equimolar mixture of urokinase and 7E3 was no more effective than urokinase alone. (14) The rate of lysis was dependent upon the concentration of platelets in the clot and no enhancement in lysis by the conjugate over urokinase was apparent in platelet-free clots. On the other hand, the conjugate was substantially more potent in inhibiting platelet aggregation when compared to antibody 7E3 alone. Thus, urokinase targeted to GP IIb/IIIa by conjugation to antibody 7E3 accounted for enhanced lysis and improved inhibition of platelet aggregation when compared to the parent molecules alone.

Anti-Platelet-scuPA Conjugates

Similar results were obtained for a conjugate between 7E3 and scuPA. No advantage in using scuPA over urokinase was observed. (14) Using different antibodies, Dewerchin et al. (15) confirmed and extended our observations by showing that an anti-platelet-scuPA conjugate was more effective than scuPA in lysing platelet-rich thrombi *in vivo* in a hamster model of pulmonary embolism.

Targeting with Bifunctional Antibodies

Principal Considerations

In naturally occurring bivalent IgG antibodies, both antigen combining sites are identical in structure and specificity. An alternative to a chemical conjugate or a fusion protein that contains segments of two proteins of different function is a bifunctional antibody that is able to bind both thrombus (e.g., fibrin) and an effector protein (e.g., a plasminogen activator) without diminishing its physiologic function (e.g.. enzyme activity). Such a bifunctional antibody would serve as an "adapter molecule" bringing the plasminogen activator into close proximity with fibrin, without the need to manipulate the enzyme chemically. Also, a bispecific antibody can be used by itself to enhance the potency of endogenous enzymes (e.g., t-PA). By using chemical methods it is possible either to cross-link intact antibodies of different specificities or to produce bispecific (Fab')2 molecules. A better method for producing bispecific antibodies on a larger scale is the hybrid-hybridoma approach, specifically somatic cell fusion of two monoclonal antibody-producing hybridoma cell lines.

Bispecific IgG (Intact Antibodies)

It was anticipated that an antibody specific for both fibrin and t-PA would bind to the fibrin matrix of thrombi and also to circulating t-PA, thereby increasing the concentration of t-PA at the surface of thrombi. The feasibility of this approach was first tested by chemically cross-linking SPDP-modified anti-fibrin antibody 59D8 with an iminothiolane-modified antibody specific for t-PA. In an *in vitro* quantitative fibrinolysis assay, the relative fibrinolytic potency of t-PA bound to the bispecific antibody was 13 times greater than that of t-PA and 200 times greater than that of urokinase. When fibrin was treated with bispecific antibodies before being mixed (loaded) with t-PA, the relative fibrinolytic potency of t-PA was enhanced 14-fold. (16) This capture of t-PA also occurred when the concentration of t-PA present in the assay was less than the concentration of t-PA present in normal human plasma. In human plasma clot assays, samples containing both the bispecific antibody and t-PA exhibited significantly more lysis than did samples containing t-PA alone. Despite of the increased clot lysis effected by the bispecific antibody, there was no significant increase in fibrinogen or α_2-anti-plasmin consumption at equal t-PA concentrations. The ability of the bispecific antibody to concentrate exogenous t-PA *in vivo* was examined in the rabbit jugular vein model. Systemic infusion of a small amount of t-PA produced no significant increment in thrombolysis over the level of spontaneous lysis (14%). However, simultaneous infusion of t-PA and bispecific antibody resulted in 42% lysis. These results suggest that bispecific antibodies can enhance thrombolysis by capturing endogenous or exogenous t-PA. Other examples of the same approach include the synthesis of anti-platelet-anti-t-PA bispecific antibodies and of anti-fibrin-anti-UK bispecific anti-bodies. (17, 18)

Bispecific (Fab')2

As a potential pharmacologic agent, a bispecific (Fab')2 has several advantages over a bispecific IgG: (1) The (Fab')2 lacks the Fc region of the IgG, which is responsible for nonspecific effector functions such as complement activation; (2) The molecular weight of the (Fab')2 is just 100 kD as opposed to 300 kD for IgG; (3) The (Fab')2 complex does not contain cross-linking residues; (4) The final product is uniform because the constituent Fab' molecules have only one alternative to form (Fab')2.

A bispecific (Fab')2 molecule was constructed by linking the monovalent Fab' from monoclonal anti-fibrin antibody 59D8 to the Fab' from monoclonal anti-t-PA antibody TCL8 by means of inter-heavy-chain disulfide bonds. An immunochemical complex composed of the bispecific (Fab')2 molecule bound to t-PA was then generated and purified. Its molecular weight was 170 kD, corresponding to the sum of (Fab')2 and t-PA. The t-PA-bispecific (Fab')2 complex was 8.6 times more efficient in fibrinolysis than t-PA alone and 94times more potent than urokinase. (19) This enhancement in the fibrinolytic potency suggests that this (compared to bispecific IgG) pharmacologically preferable molecule is capable of binding both fibrin and t-PA with similarly high affinity as bispecific IgG.

Bispecific Antibodies by Hybrid-Hybridoma Technique

An alternative method that yields larger quantities of uniform and stable bi-specific antibody is the hybrid-hybridoma technique. A thymidine kinase-deficient clone from the hybridoma producing the anti-fibrin antibody was subjected to somatic cell fusion with a hypoxanthine guanine phosphonbosyl transferase-deficient clone of the hybridoma producing the anti-t-PA antibody. Surviving clones were selected in hypoxanthine aminopterm thymidine medium. The resulting bispecific antibodies were as effective as their chemically synthesized counterparts in concentrating t-PA to fibrin. (20)

Double Targeting

In an effort to increase further the potency of plasminogen activators, urokinase was chemically linked to a bispecific antibody or bispecific (Fab')2 with specificity for fibrin (by means of a Fab'-fragment from antibody 59D8) and platelets (by means of a Fab'-fragment from antibody 7E3). (17) These ternary complexes were tested in several assays that revealed an increase of fibrinolytic potency of double-targeted urokinase over single antibody-UK conjugates, but only if the epitope targeted by the UK-conjugate was present in the clot. *In vitro* clot lysis of platelet-rich and fibrin-rich plasma clots demonstrated an up to 5-fold higher potency of the conjugate compared to the parent molecule. *In vitro* platelet aggregation was effectively inhibited by the hybrid molecule, whereas urokinase had no effect. Thus, the bispecific anti-fibrin-anti-platelet urokinase conjugate has the ability to lyse both fibrin-rich and platelet-rich thrombi with high efficacy and also inhibits platelet aggregation that occurs regularly on the surface of a fresh thrombus.

Expression and Characterization of Recombinant Anti-Fibrin-Plasminogen Activator Fusion Proteins

Anti-Fibrin-SK Constructs

In order to add fibrin selectivity to SK, Goldstein et al. (21) have constructed a chimeric SK molecule that consists of the Fab'-fragment of the anti-fibrin antibody 59D8 and a full length SK sequence 1 - 414. An expression plasmid containing the cDNA encoding the heavy-chain variable region from 59D8 and the coding region of a genomic clone of SK was electroporated into a 59D8 light-chain producing hybridoma cell line. The chimeric SK was purified by affinity chromatography over the immobilized octapeptide ligand for 59D8. The 59D8-SK fusion protein increased clot lysis only twofold compared to SK but exhibited changed activator properties. It was relatively inactive in human plasma but lysed clots slowly and completely, whereas SK lysed clots rapidly but incompletely. (21)

Anti-Fibrin-t-PA Constructs

Following successful construction of chemically conjugated antibody-plasminogen activator hybrids, recombinant DNA methodology was used to produce similar recombinant hybrid molecules. In theory, producing antibody-plasminogen activator hybrids by recombinant methods should allow much more flexibility in the design of hybrid molecules, as well as improve purity and yield. A number of different recombinant antibody-plasminogen activator hybrid molecules have been constructed. The first such molecule was an anti-fibrin (59D8) t-PA fusion protein. (22) It was found not to be an ideal construct, because the activity of t-PA depends largely on fibrin-stimulation and this mechanism is impaired by the presence of an antibody at the N-terminus. (23)

Smith and collaborators (9) used a different approach. They replaced amino acid sequence 63—71 in the epidermal growth factor (EGF) region of human t-PA with a peptide containing the CDR3 region of the heavy chain of Fab-9, an antibody with nanomolar affinity for β_3-integrins. The modified activator, LG-t-PA, had full enzymatic activity and the presence of fibrin enhanced plasminogen activation by the modified t-PA to the same degree as wild-type t-PA. LG-t-PA bound in a specific and saturable fashion to GP IIb/IIIa exhibited a K_D of approximately 0.9 nmol/l. Unfortunately the construct also bound to integrin $\alpha_V\beta_3$ receptor on endothelial cells, thereby loosing clot selectivity.

Anti-fibrin-scuPA Constructs

Pro-UK (scuPA) was found more suitable for integration into fusion proteins for the following reasons: first, scuPA does not require fibrin binding for activation, second, scuPA is a relatively fibrin-specific plasminogen activator even though it does not bind to fibrin (so we could anticipate enhanced specificity after endowing the molecule with high fibrin affinity through the antibody), and third, scuPA is resistant to inactivation by plasminogen activator inhibitor-1 (PAI-1). An expression plasmid containing DNA coding for the antibody 59D8 heavy chain variable, first constant domains, and the catalytic domain of scuPA was transfected into a "heavy chain loss variant" of the hybridoma cell originally secreting antibody 59D8. The light chain of antibody 59D8, which was still produced in the variant hybridoma cell line, assembled with the chimeric molecule (heavy chain and plasminogen activator) within the variant hybridoma cells. A molecule was secreted that contained both an antigen binding site of predefined specificity (from antibody 59D8) and a catalytic site capable of cleaving plasminogen (from scuPA). In the original construct only the Fab part of the antibody had been included in the molecule in an effort to limit the mass of the chimera to its essential components. In a similar vein, the kringle and growth factor domains of scuPA were omitted and only the sequence corresponding to low molecular weight (LMW); 32kD scuPA was used. The recombinant 59D8-scuPA fusion molecule that was used in the assays and experiments described below contained the heavy chain from residues 1-351 and a native light chain of antibody 59D8 and, in contiguous peptide sequence on the heavy chain, residues 144-411 of scuPA. (24)

r-scuPA-59D8 was characterized in functional assays comparing it to the two parent molecules. The scuPA part did not differ from native scuPA in terms of the conversion of plasminogen to plasmin and the fibrin binding ability did not differ between the parent antibody molecule 59D8 and r-scuPA-59D8. In human plasma, clot lysis assays r-scuPA-59D8 was six times more potent than scuPA. *In vivo*, in a rabbit jugular vein model, the r-scuPA-59D8 fusion molecule compared with native scuPA showed a 20-fold increase in potency. In a thrombolysis model in which thrombi are preformed *in vivo* in juvenile baboons, r-scuPA-59D8 lysed thrombi six times more rapidly than scuPA and t-PA and reduced the rate of new thrombus formation far more than comparable doses of the other activators. At equivalent thrombolytic doses rscuPA-59D8 produced fewer anti-hemostatic effects than either t-PA or scuPA. Overall, r-scuPA-59D8 may not only be more potent than other plasminogen activators but has the potential for greater safety as well. (25)

In continuation of the work above, we designed a recombinant plasminogen activator consisting of a single-chain antibody specific for fibrin and a low-molecular-weight form (residues leu144–leu411) of single-chain urokinase-type plasminogen activator (scuPA, Fig. 3) (26).

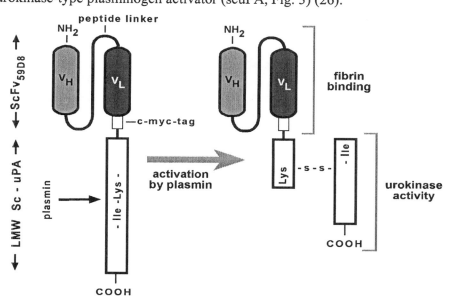

Figure 3. A design of a thrombus-targeted fibrinolytic consisting of an anti-fibrin single chain antibody and the low molecular weight form of single chain urokinase. Proteolysis of the single chain form to the two-chain form of urokinase by plasmin increases plasminogen activating activity. In addition to the antibody targeting, this activation by plasmin transfers relative thrombus specificity to this new fibrinolytic agent.

The variable regions of the heavy and light chains of a fibrin-specific antibody were amplified by polymerase chain reaction (PCR) using hybridoma 59D8 cDNA as template. The cDNA of scuPA was produced by reverse transcription of endothelial (ECV) cell mRNA, amplified by PCR and genetically fused to the C-terminus of the variable region of the light chain (Fig. 3).

The fusion protein was produced in E. coli, purified by affinity chromatography, and characterized by its size on SDS-Page (56 kDa) by western blotting and by its binding to the fibrin specific epitope B∃15-22. Both, fibrin targeting and plasminogen activation, could be demonstrated. In direct comparison to equimolar amounts of native urokinase a 6-8 fold higher efficiency in the lysis of ^{125}I-labeled fibrin clots in human plasma could be demonstrated. (26) Thus, the newly designed fusion protein demonstrated a fibrin targeted plasminogen activation and was highly efficient in clot lysis. Therefore, an efficient clot lysis with a low risk of bleeding complications may be achieved. The efficient and fast production at low cost in bacteria should facilitate the further evaluation and potential clinical use of this new fibrinolytic agent.

Collen and co-workers (27, 28) have pursued similar studies with a different fibrin-specific antibody and reached similar conclusions.

Yang et al. (29) have modified the scuPA catalytic domain of the rscuPA-59D8 molecule described above. ScuPA has many cleavage sites. Among the various sites, there is a thrombin sensitive site between Arg[156] and Phe[157] that results in an inactivated molecule upon cleavage. Between Lys[158] and Ile[159] is the plasmin-sensitive site that results, after cleavage, in the enzymatically active two-chain UK. The deletion of Phe[157] and Lys[158] creates a thrombin-sensitive cleavage site that results, after cleavage, in an active two-chain plasminogen activator. Thus, upon activation by thrombin, this molecule converts plasminogen to plasmin and effects efficient clot lysis. Activation of the molecule can be inhibited by hirudin and the heparin/anti-thrombin complex, both thrombin inhibitors. These observations suggest that the thrombin-activatable form of r-scuPA-59D8 has the potential to lyse selectively fresh clots (which are thrombin rich) more effectively than older clots (which are poorer in thrombin). In a clinical situation like AMI a fresh coronary thrombus is most likely the causative agent that needs to by lysed whereas older thrombi that function as hemostatic plugs are best left intact in order to prevent hemorrhage. Thus, this variant of r-scuPA-59D8 may add extra safety features to the concept of antibody targeting in a clinical setting.

Alternative Approaches of Targeting Plasminogen Activators to Thrombi

Several approaches have been used to target plasminogen, t-PA, scuPA, or staphylokinase to fibrin, platelets, P-selectin, or annexin V without the use of antibodies or Fab fragments. Yamada et al. (30) have substituted the amino sequence 148—151 of a loop in kringle 1 of the human t-PA with the integrin-specific sequence Arg-Gly-Asp (RGD). The mutant t-PA maintained full enzymatic activity compared to wild-type t-PA and bound in a specific and saturable fashion to GP IIb/IIIa.

Dawson et al. (31) have altered the plasminogen cleavage site Arg[561] - Val[562] by substituting the P_3, P_2, and P_1 residues with sequences from thrombin cleavable proteins in an attempt to target the plasminogen to clot bound thrombin. Rapid and efficient lysis of *in vitro* clots could be achieved by these constructs.

Wan and collaborators (32) have engineered a recombinant chimeric urokinase construct that consists of a humanized monoclonal antibody (SZ-5lHu) directed against P-selectin (highly expressed on the surface of activated platelets) and the UK sequence 1-411. With *in vitro* human plasma/platelet clots and in a hamster pulmonary embolism model, lysis was 4 to 8 times enhanced by the conjugate compared to the parent urokinase. Fibrinogen breakdown using the construct was minimal.

The peptide Gly-Pro-Arg (GPR) that corresponds to the amino-terminal portion of the fibrin α-chain after release of the fibrinopeptide A prevents the polymerisation of fibrin monomers. This peptide also binds to fibrinogen and to fibrin fragment D. Addition of proline to the tripeptide significantly increases binding and the inhibitory activity. Hua et al. (33) have examined whether a construct of Gly-Pro-Arg-Pro fused to LMW-UK (Leu[144] - Leu[411]) improved its efficacy as a thrombolytic agent. The construct exhibited a six-fold greater affinity for fibrin and had a two- to three-fold greater fibrinolytic potency in *in vitro* clot lysis assays. Fibrinogen degradation was much lower during clot lysis compared to that produced by wild-type LMW-UK.

Annexin V is a human protein that binds with high affinity to the abundant phosphatidyl serine molecules exposed on activated platelets. Binding to quiescent platelets *in vitro* is minimal. Maximally stimulated platelets contain approximately 200 000 annexin V binding sites, substantially exceeding the number of approximately 70 000 GP IIb/IIIa receptors. Tait et al. (34) have fused full-length scuPA (amino acids 1-411) or LMW-scuPA (amino acids 144-411) to full length annexin V. Both constructs, after activation by plasmin, had similar amidolytic activities and activated plasminogen marginally better than wild-type scuPA. *In vitro* both constructs lysed platelet-rich clots as well but not better than LMW-scuPA. No *in vivo* experiments have been published so far.

Van Zyl and collaborators (35) produced a multivalent staphylokinase construct. Staphylokinase, a highly fibrin specific thrombolytic agent was fused via a factor Xa cleavable linker to the cDNA of an anti-thrombotic peptide of 29 amino acids comprising: (1) an Arg-Gly-Asp (RGD) sequence to prevent binding of fibrinogen to platelets, (2) a portion of fibrinopeptide A, an inhibitor of thrombin, and (3) the tail of hirudin, a potent direct thrombin inhibitor. The fibrinolytic potential of PLATSAK (Platelet-Anti-Thrombin-Staphylokinase) was slightly lower than that of the parent molecule. PLATSAK markedly lengthened the thrombin time and the aPTT, thereby indicating inhibition of thrombin activity. It had a negligible effect on platelet aggregation, possibly due to inaccessibility of the RGD peptide in the tertiary structure of PLATSAK.

Targeting the Thrombin Inhibitor Hirudin to Fibrin

General Considerations

The intent of this design is the inhibition of further fibrin deposition at the site of thrombosis while avoiding systemic anticoagulation. Antibody 59D8 is a particularly attractive targeting agent for a thrombin inhibitor because the epitope on fibrin (that the antibody binds to) becomes exposed after thrombin has cleaved fibrinopeptide B off the fibrinogen β-chain. Thus, the inhibitor is concentrated at the very site of thrombin action.

Chemical Conjugates

Chemical conjugates of the antibody fragment 59D8-Fab' or of intact 59D8 and hirudin were constructed, purified, and tested in an *in vitro* assay measuring the deposition of fibrin on the surface of a standard clot. The 59D8 Fab'-hirudin conjugate was 10 times more potent than hirudin alone or a mixture of hirudin and 59D8-Fab' in inhibiting fibrin deposition, presumably because of anti-thrombin concentration on the surface of the clot. (36) The potency of fibrin-targeted hirudin was also compared *in vivo* with that of uncoupled recombinant hirudin in a baboon model of thrombus formation. Fibrin-targeted hirudin was 10 times more potent than hirudin in inhibiting platelet deposition and thrombus formation. (37) These data indicate that targeting a thrombin inhibitor and presumably also other anticoagulants to an epitope present in thrombi such as fibrin or the platelet IIb/IIIa receptor results in significantly increased anti-thrombotic potency.

Recombinant Fusion Protein

Since the production of recombinant antibodies in hybridoma cells is expensive and is often hampered by low yields we chose to produce a single chain antibody for fibrin targeting. Single chain antibodies are produced in bacteria and are accessible for mutagenesis and coupling with effector molecules using well established molecular biology techniques. Furthermore, production of single chain antibodies is inexpensive and can be performed on a large-scale basis. Overall, the single chain antibody technology provides several features that are advantageous for industrialized production of pharmaceutical agents.

To obtain a recombinant anti-fibrin single chain antibody, mRNA was prepared from the hybridoma cell line secreting the IgG antibody 59D8. (6) The variable regions of the heavy and light chain of the 59D8 antibody were amplified by PCR using cDNA prepared by reverse transcription of 59D8 mRNA. To obtain a functional single chain antibody (scFv), a linker region consisting of $(Gly_4Ser)_3$ was introduced by overlap PCR (Fig. 4 below).

After ligating the scFv clones with DNA encoding, the pIII protein of the M13 phage high affinity clones were selected by 10 rounds of panning on the fibrin-specific peptide B∃15-22 (∃-peptide). Hirudin was genetically fused to the C-terminus of the variable region of the light chain. To release the functionally essential N-terminus of hirudin at the site of a blood clot a factor Xa recognition site was introduced between $scFv_{59D8}$ and hirudin (Fig. 4 below). The fusion protein was characterized by its size on SDS-PAGE (36 kDa), Western blotting, by its cleavage into a 29 kDa (single chain alone) and 7 kDa (hirudin) fragment, by its binding ∃-peptide and by thrombin inhibition after Xa cleavage. Finally, the fusion protein inhibited appositional growth of whole blood clots *in vitro* more efficiently than native hirudin. (38)\

The constructed fusion protein anti-fibrin single chain antibody, factor Xa cleavage site, hirudin promises to be only active at the site where its effects are needed (Fig. 4). Since hirudin needs a free N- as well as a free C-terminus to be fully active, an intact fusion protein would be inactive. Factor Xa cleaves the C-terminus of the recognition sequence and liberates active hirudin. Because factor Xa is a constituent of thrombi, this approach also adds specificity in limiting the action of hirudin to the surface of a thrombus and hopefully will decrease the risk of bleeding complications.

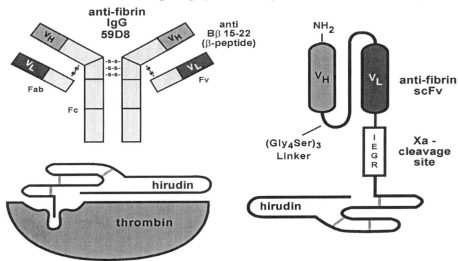

Figure 4. Design of a thrombus-targeted anticoagulant consisting of an anti-fibrin single chain antibody and the direct thrombin inhibitor hirudin. Hirudin in its fused form is an inactive molecule, since it needs a free N-terminal end for effective thrombin inhibition. The inclusion of a factor Xa cleavage site in the fusion protein allows liberation of active hirudin. Because factor Xa is a constituent of thrombi, this approach also adds specificity in limiting the action of hirudin to the surface of a thrombus and together with the thrombus targeting by the anti-fibrin antibody will hopefully decrease the risk of bleeding complications.

Table 1. Targets and Properties of Fusion Proteins (chemical/recombinant coupling)

Target	Property
Fibrin	
anti-fibrin antibody	urokinase activity (10)
	t-PA activity (11,12,22,23)
	scuPA activity (13,24,25-28)
	streptokinase activity (21)
	hirudin (36-38)
bifunctional antibodies	capture of t-PA (16,20)
	anti-t-PA antibody
	capture of urokinase (17,18)
	anti-urokinase antibody
fibrin-binding peptide (GPR)	urokinase (33)
Platelet	
anti-GP IIb/IIIa antibodies urokinase (14,15)	
	scuPA (14,15)
inclusion of CDR3 of an anti-GP IIb/IIIa antibody	t-PA (9)
inclusion of RGD anti-GP IIb/IIIa	t-PA (30)
anti-P-selectin	scuPA (31)
annexin V	scuPA (34)

Table 1 (above) shows examples of conjugation of anti-thrombotic agents with affinity carriers, i.e., antibodies directed against fibrin and platelets. Plasminogen activators (tPA and urokinase) conjugates are used for fibrinolysis (therapy), whereas hirudin conjugates are used to prevent thrombosis (thromboprophylaxis).

CONCLUSION

Antibody targeting is an attractive approach to enhance the potency and specificity of effector molecules. The approach has been used in cancer research and was first applied to the field of thrombolysis in the 1980s. Since then, chemical conjugates have been substituted by recombinant fusion proteins and the tools of molecular biology have allowed to minimize the size of the fusion partners as well as to overcome largely the antigenicity of the antibody fragments by "humanization," a problem avoidable in the future by screening human antibody libraries. Promising results have been obtained *in vitro* and were substantiated by *in vivo* experiments in rabbits and non-human primates. Great efforts are currently being undertaken to simplify the expression of fusion proteins by developing single-chain antibodies, both specific for fibrin, platelets, or to the pulmonary vasculature (39) and in the development of other means (such as the incorporation of small peptide into a protein loop) for targeting plasminogen activators to fibrin (33) or platelet constituents (30) in a thrombus. The impressive results of antibody application in the treatment of acute coronary syndromes and adjunctive therapy to intracoronary interventions with the GP IIb/IIIa inhibitor c7E3 show the promise of antibody treatment alone which may well be enhanced by using this antibody (as described above) or a single-chain Fv-fragment of an even more specific anti-platelet-antibody. Similar applications with different antibodies such as against P-selectin may also prove useful. Only the surface of the potential of the general concept has been scratched at present. Confirmation of the concept of antibody targeting in cardiovascular disease now awaits clinical trials.

REFERENCES

1. Armstrong PW, Collen D (2001) Fibrinolysis for acute myocardial infarction: Current status and new horizons for pharmacological reperfusion, Circulation 103:2862-66
2. The GUSTO Angiographic Investigators (1993) The effects of tissue plasminogen activator, streptokinase, or both on coronary-artery patency, ventricular function, and survival after acute myocardial infarction. N Engl J Med 329:1615— 1622
3. Bode C, Smalling RW. Berg O, Burnett C, Lorch O, Kalbfleisch JM, Chernoff R, Christie LG, Feldman RL, Seals AA. Weaver WD. for the RAPID II Investigators (1996) Randomized comparison of coronary thrombolysis achieved with double-bolus reteplase (recombinant plasminogen activator) and front-loaded, accelerated alteplase

(recombinant tissue plasminogen activator) in patients with acute myocardial infarction. Circulation 94:891—898

4. Assessment of the Safety and Efficacy of a New Thrombolytic Investigators (1999) Single-bolus tenecteplase compared with front-loaded alteplase in acute myocardial infarction: the ASSENT-2 double-blind randomized trial. Lancet 354:716-22

5. The GUSTO V Investigators (2001) Reperfusion therapy for acute myocardial infarction with fibrinolytic therapy or combination reduced fibrinolytic therapy and platelet glycoprotein IIb/IIIa inhibition: the GUSTO V randomized trial. Lancet 357: 1905-1914

6. Hui KY, Haber E, Matsueda GR (1983) Monoclonal antibodies to a synthetic fibrin-like peptide bind to human fibrin but not fibrinogen. Science 222:1129— 113211.

7. Califf RM (2000) Combination therapy for acute myocardial infarction: fibrinolytic therapy and glycoprotein IIb/IIIa inhibition. Am Heart J 139 Suppl:S33—S37

8. Topol EJ, Byzova TV, Plow EF (1999) Platelet GPIIb-IIIa blockers. Lancet 353: 227-31

9. Smith JW, Tachias K, Madison EL (1995) Protein loop grafting to construct a variant of tissue-type plasminogen activator that binds platelet integrin aIIbß3. J Biol Chem 270:30486—30490

10. Bode C, Matsueda GR, Hui KY, Haber E (1985) Antibody-directed urokinase: a specific fibrinolytic agent. Science 229:765—767

11. Runge MS, Bode C, Matsueda GR, Haber E (1988) Conjugation to an antifibrin monoclonal antibody enhances the fibrinolytic potency of tissue plasminogen activator *in vitro*. Biochemistry 27:1153—1157

12. Runge MS, Bode C, Matsueda GR, Haber E (1987) Antibody-enhanced thrombolysis: Targeting of tissue plasminogen activator *in vivo*. Proc Natl Acad Sci USA 84:7659-7662

13. Bode C, Runge MS. Schönermark S, Eberle T, Newell JB. Kübler W. Haber E (1990) Conjugation to antifibrin Fab' enhances fibrinolytic potency of single-chain urokinase plasminogen activator. Circulation 81:1974—1980

14. Bode C, Meinhardt G, Runge MS, Freitag M, Nordt T. Arens M. Newell JB, Kübler W. Haber E (1991) Platelet-targeted fibrinolysis enhances clot lysis and inhibits platelet aggregation. Circulation 84:805—813

15. Dewerchin M, Lijnen HR. Stassen JM. De Cock F, Quertermous T, Ginsberg MH, Piow EF, Collen D (1991) Effect of chemical conjugation of recombinant single-chain urokinase-type plasminogen activator with monoclonal antiplatelet antibodies on platelet aggregation and on plasma clot lysis *in vitro* and *in vivo*. Blood 78:1005—1018

16. Bode C, Runge MS. Branscomb EE, Newell JB. Matsueda GR. Haber E (1989) Antibody-directed fibrinolysis. An antibody specific for both fibrin and tissue plasminogen activator. J Biol Chem 264:944—948

17. Ruef J, Nordt TK, Peter K, Runge MS, Kübler W, Bode C (1999) A bispecific antifibrin-antiplatelet urokinase conjugate (BAAUC) induces enhanced clot lysis and inhibits platelet aggregation. Thromb Haemost 82:109-114

18. Charpie JR, Runge MS, Matsueda GR, Haber E (1990) A bispecific antibody enhances the fibrinolytic potency of single-chain urokinase. Biochemistry 29:6374—6378

19. Runge MS, Bode C, Savard CE. Matsueda GR, Haber E (1990) Antibody-directed fibrinolysis: a bispecific (Fab')2 that binds to fibrin and tissue plasminogen activator. Bioconjug Chem 1:274—277

20. Branscomb EE, Runge MS, Savard CE. Adams KM, Matsueda GR. Haber E (1990) Bispecific monoclonal antibodies produced by somatic cell fusion increase the potency of tissue plasminogen activator. Thromb Haemost 64:260—266

21. Goldstein J, Matsueda GR, Shaw S-Y (1996) A chimenic streptokinase with unexpected fibrinolytic selectivity. Thromb Haemost 76:429—438

22.   Schnee JM, Runge MS. Matsueda GR, Hudson NW, Seidman JG, Haber E, Quertermous T (1987) Construction and expression of a recombinant antibody-targeted plasminogen activator. Proc Natl Acad Sci USA 84:6904—6908

23.   Love TW, Quertermous T, Runge MS, Michelson KD, Matsueda GR, Haber E (1994) Attachment of an antifibrin antibody to the amino terminus of tissue-type plasminogen activator impairs stimulation by fibrin. Fibrinolysis 8:326—332

24.   Runge MS, Quertermous T, Zavodny PJ, Love TW, Bode C. Freitag M, Shaw S-Y, Huang PL. Chou C-C, Mullins D, Schnee JM, Savard CE, Rothenberg ME, Newell JB, Matsueda GR. Haber E (1991) A recombinant chimeric plasminogen activator with high affinity for fibrin has increased thrombolytic potency *in vitro* and *in vivo*. Proc Nat Acad Sci USA 88:10337—10341

25.   Runge MS, Harker LA, Bode C, Ruef J, Kelly AB. Marzec UM; Allen E. Caban R, Shaw S-Y, Haber E. Hanson SR (1996) Enhanced thrombolytic and antithrombotic potency of a fibrin-targeted plasminogen activator in baboons. Circulation 94:1412—1422

26.   Peter K , Tovic I, Graeber J, Weirich U, Bauer S, Ruef J, Nordt T, Bode C (2001) Construction and functional evaluation of a new fibrin-targeted fibrinolytic: a recombinant fusion protein with an anti-fibrin single-chain antibody and a low molecular weight form single-chain urokinase. Circulation 104:SII-96

27.   Dewerchin M, Vandamme AM. Holvoet P, De Cock F, Lemmens G. Lijnen HR. Stassen JM. Gollen D (1992) Thrombolytic and pharmacokinetic properties of a recombinant chimeric plasminogen activator consisting of a fibrin fragment D-dimer specific humanized monoclonal antibody and a truncated single-chain urokinase. Thromb Haemost 68:170—179

28.   Holvoet P, Laroche Y, Stassen JM, Lijnen HR, Van Hoef B, De Cock F, Van Houtven A, Gansemans Y, Matthyssens G, Collen D (1993) Pharmacokinetic and thrombolytic properties of chimeric plasminogen activators consisting of a single-chain Fv fragment of a fibrin-specific antibody fused to single-chain urokinase. Blood 81:696—703

29.   Yang W-P. Goldstein J, Procyk R, Matsueda GR. Shaw S-Y (1994) Design and evaluation of a thrombin-activable plasminogen activator. Biochemistry 33:2306—2312

30.   Yamada T, Shimada Y. Kikuchi M (1996) Integrin-specific tissue-type plasminogen activator engineered by introduction of the Arg-Gly-Asp sequence. Biochem Biophys Res Commun 228:306—311

31.   Dawson KM, Cook A, Devine JM. Edwards RM, Hunter MG. Raper RH. Roberts G (1994) Plasminogen mutants activated by thrombin. Potential thrombus-selective thrombolytic agents. J Biol Chem 269:15989—15992

32.   Wan H, Liu Z. Xia X, Gu J, Wang B. Liu X. Zhu M. Li P, Ruan C (2000) A recombinant antibody-targeted plasminogen activator with high affinity for activated platelets increases thrombolytic potency *in vitro* and *in vivo*. Thromb Res 97:133—141

33.   Hua Z-C, Chen X-C, Dong C, Zhu D-X (1996) Characterization of a recombinant chimeric plasminogen activator composed of Gly-Pro-Arg-Pro tetrapeptide and truncated urokinase-type plasminogen activator expressed in Escherichia coli. Biochem Biophys Res Commun 222:576—583

34.   Tait JF, Engelhardt S, Smith C, Fujikawa K (1995) Prourokinase-annexin V chimeras. Construction, expression, and characterization of recombinant proteins. J Biol Chem 270:21594-21599

35.   van Zvl WB. Pretorius GHJ. Hartmann M. Kotze HF (1997) Production of a recombinant antithrombotic and fibrinolytic protein, PLATSAK, in Escherichia coli. Thromb Res88:419—426

36.   Bode C, Hudelmayer M, Mehwald P, Bauer S, Freitag M, von Hodenberg E. Newell JB, Kübler W, Haber E, Runge MS (1994) Fibrin-targeted recombinant hirudin inhibits fibrin deposition on experimental clots more efficiently than recombinant hirudin. Circulation 90:1956—1963

37.   Bode C, Hanson SR, Schmedtje JF Jr. Haber E, Mehwald P, Kelly AB. Harker LA, Runge MS (1997) Antithrombotic potency of hirudin is increased in nonhuman primates by fibrin targeting. Circulation 95:800-804

38.   Peter K, Graeber J, Kipriyanov S, Zewe-Welschof M, Runge MS, Kübler W, Little M, Bode C (2000) Construction and functional evaluation of a single-chain antibody fusion protein with fibrin targeting and thrombin inhibition after activation by factor Xa. Circulation 101:1158-1164

39.   Muzykantov VR, Barnathan ES, Atochina EN, Kuo A, Danilov SM, Fisher AB (1996) Targeting of antibody-conjugated plasminogen activators to the pulmonary vasculature. J Pharmacol Exp Ther 279:1026—1034

GLOSSARY

59D8: A fibrin-specific IgG mouse antibody that was raised by immunizing mice with a synthetic peptide containing the sequence of the thrombin generated amino terminus of the fibrin β-chain

Abciximab: A chimeric human/mouse antibody fragment (c7E3) specific for platelet integrin GP IIb/IIIa

Bispecific antibodies: Antibodies that possess two binding sites of two different antibodies

Fibrinolysis: Proteolytic degradation of fibrin by plasmin resulting in destabilization of the fibrin meshwork and dissolution of the thrombus

GP IIb/IIIa: Platelet integrin receptor $\forall_{IIb}\exists_3$ (CD41/CD61) mediating fibrinogen binding and therefore platelet aggregation

Hirudin: A direct thrombin inhibitor isolated from the salivary gland of the European leech, Hirudo medicinalis

Plasminogen activators: Natural (urokinase, streptokinase, tPA) or recombinant proteases (tenecteplase, reteplase) that cleave plasminogen to plasmin, which then cleaves fibrin

Single chain antibody: A single chain fusion protein consisting of the variable regions of the heavy and light chain fused via a linker region

Thrombus targeting: Enrichment of effector molecules at the thrombus (e.g., by antibodies)

6

TISSUE-SPECIFIC PHARMACODELIVERY AND OVERCOMING KEY CELL BARRIERS IN VIVO: VASCULAR TARGETING OF CAVEOLAE

Lucy A. Carver and Jan E. Schnitzer
Sidney Kimmel Cancer Center, San Diego, CA 92121

INTRODUCTION

Molecular medicine has discovered many new therapeutic modalities using state-of-the art techniques in molecular biology. High through-put, in vitro assays that screen for pharmacological actions on the cell type of interest are frequently used in the design of new drugs. Although the potential for such agents is great and certainly justified by their success in vitro, they frequently perform much less effectively in vivo where the agent must reach its target cells in a tissue in sufficient quantities to be potent, while sparing bystander organs. Depending on the route of administration, the endothelium and/or epithelium form significant barriers that greatly limit the in vivo accessibility of many drugs, antibodies, and gene vectors to their intended target sites of pharmacological action, namely specific cells inside the tissue (1, 2). For example, poor tissue penetration has hindered the ability of many monoclonal antibodies to reach their cell-specific antigens and thus to achieve effective tissue- or cell-directed pharmaco-delivery in vivo (1-3). Understanding general and selective transport across key cell barriers to pharmaco-delivery in vivo is fundamental to achieving effective directed therapy. Moving the target from the tissue cell surface to the surface of the cell barrier, such as the vascular endothelium, has many theoretical advantages in tissue-specific delivery (4-7). The newly discovered molecular heterogeneity of endothelia among different tissues invites a new strategy of vascular targeting. Yet, this vascular targeting strategy still requires both validation in vivo and, to be useful for many therapies, a means by which to cross the vascular wall for access to underlying tissue cells (4). This chapter will not focus on all the elements and requirements for the "ideal" drug delivery system (for review, see (1)) but will be limited to an essential and critical component of access and getting intravenously injected agents specifically to a single tissue as well as inside the tissue across the endothelial cell border to the intended target cells.

RATIONALE FOR SITE-SPECIFIC DELIVERY

The design of traditional therapeutic agents has focused primarily on the immediate interaction between a drug and its intended pharmacological site of action. Because the "bull's eye" is usually a specific cell type inside a tissue, the target cell must first be accessible in vivo to the drug, which, for instance, when administered intravenously, must overcome the endothelial cell barrier either by percolating directly through the plasma membrane, by moving through intercellular junctions between the cells, or by special vesicular transport into and across the cell (5). For many small molecules, accessibility normally does not pose a problem because the drug readily moves across the endothelial cell barrier primarily via paracellular transport from the blood stream across intercellular junctions to gain access to underlying tissue cells. For epithelial cell barriers and select endothelial cell barriers (i.e. in brain and testes), the intercellular junctions can be very tight and thereby restrict the passage of very small molecules. For example, glucose requires a specific glucose transport protein to cross the brain microvascular endothelium. The ability of drugs to diffuse throughout many tissues of the body can be quite disadvantageous because accessing to many tissues increases the effective volume of distribution within the body, which can dilute drug potency and contribute significantly to unwanted pharmacological side effects. On the other hand, large molecules, such as proteins, antibodies, or gene vectors, lack access in many organs because they are unable to readily cross the blood vessel endothelium to reach its target receptor. For large and small molecules, selective delivery to the desired tissue of pharmacological action is expected to improve pharmaco-efficacy at lower dosages and to limit systemic side effects caused by drug uptake by healthy cells.

The idea of site-specific drug delivery has developed largely as an attempt to circumvent the unacceptable toxic effects on non-target cells. It has been defined as "achieving the maximal potential intrinsic activity of drugs by optimizing their exclusive availability to their pharmacological receptor(s) in a manner that affords protection both to the drug and to the body alike" (1). That is, with exclusive and rapid delivery to the specific intended target compartment, most frequently a specific tissue, ingress is better achieved to previously inaccessible sites at a lower effective dose which inherently provides better protection of the drug and body from unwanted nonspecific deposition leading to possible deleterious side effects. One of the areas in which site-directed delivery has garnered the most attention is in cancer research where much effort has been expended in finding specific targets on tumor cells that can be used in the development of tumor cell-targeted drug therapies usually in the form of antibodies linked to toxins. Localizing toxins by selectively targeting tumor cells would not only increase drug efficacy in vivo but also reduce drug toxicity in normal tissues. In addition, tumor cell targets could potentially be useful in detecting primary and metastatic disease as well as for staging and prognostic purposes.

VASCULAR TARGETING

The concept of site-specific drug delivery has evolved considerably since it was first proposed at the turn of the century. In the last ten years, the development of monoclonal antibody technology provided a means of achieving some form of target recognition. Currently, talk of "magic bullets" abounds but in many cases the "bull's eye" has been missed, largely because delivery considerations in vivo have been ignored. For example, when injected into the blood stream, although antibody-drug conjugates demonstrate increased immunospecificity and improved site-directed delivery compared to non-targeted drug delivery, they frequently do not perform as well as suggested by the successful preclinical drug discovery experiments performed on populations of cells grown in culture. Usually, the accumulation of antibodies targeting cells in solid tissues is less than 1% of the injected intravenous (IV) dose, even after 24 hrs (1, 3). The reason for this unfortunate "reality" in vivo is that pharmaco-accessibility is not adequately attained in the body. For instance, in many tissues, there is a lack of appropriate extravasation from the vascular compartment to the underlying tissue cells (3). The endothelium can be a key physical barrier to drug and gene delivery to intended target cells in vivo (1, 3). Therefore, in order to achieve effective site-directed delivery, we need to better understand what some of the normal barriers in the body are that hinder directed drug distribution in vivo and how they may be overcome to provide the access necessary for proper effectiveness.

In recent years, the focus of targeted therapy research has altered to include the development of strategies for targeting the accessible luminal endothelial cell surface of blood vessels that feed tissue cells rather than the tumor- or tissue-cells themselves (Fig. 1). Moving the target from inside the tissue on the other side of the vascular wall to the blood vessel surface in contact with the circulating blood can theoretically achieve inherent accessibility to allow much improved tissue-directed targeting in vivo.

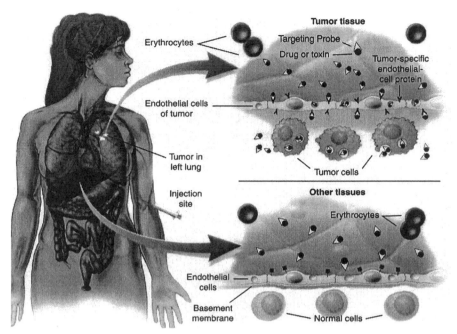

Figure. 1. Tumor vascular targeting strategy. The heterogeneity of the endothelial cell surface may allow specific binding of injectable anti-cancer drugs. Monoclonal antibodies specifically targeting tumor-induced endothelial cell surface markers may be useful for tumor-specific drug delivery for solid tumor ablation. By specifically targeting the endothelial cell surface, the systemic side effects of cancer drugs may be avoided. By targeting caveolae, drugs may also be transcytosed across the endothelial cell barrier to the underlying tumor cells.

Reproduced with permission from Schnitzer, J. E. Vascular targeting as a strategy for cancer therapy. N Engl J Med 1998; 339: 472-4. Copyright ©1998 Massachusetts Medical Society. All rights reserved.

    Such tissue-specific vascular targeting may be useful in the treatment of many diseases, including solid tumors (4, 8). This "vascular targeting" strategy is quite distinct from current anti-angiogenesis therapies for solid tumor therapy because the goal of vascular targeting is not stasis by preventing tumor blood vessel growth but rather infarction of the tumor by rapid and selective destruction of the vasculature supplying the tumor. A new addition to the vascular targeting strategy is the potential utility of a vesicular transport pathway, specifically non-coated plasmalemmal vesicles called caveolae that are abundant in certain endothelium, for selectively overcoming this key cell barrier to facilitate directed delivery of therapeutic agents to underlying tumor- or tissue cells (9).

CELLULAR TRANSPORT PATHWAYS

A critical interface in all systems is the immediate barrier that is in contact with the drug after it enters the body. For drugs injected intravenously, the critical barrier preventing access to the tissue is the luminal endothelial cells lining the blood vessels, whereas for drugs applied topically or as an inhaled aerosol, the interfaces are the dermal and alveolar epithelial cells, respectively. Thus, in order for a drug molecule to reach its target receptor, it must cross a cellular barrier, usually a cell monolayer, whose function is to keep it out.

Different tissue types have evolved various pathways to overcome their natural barriers to allow for the exchange of solutes necessary to maintain the tissue. Paracellular pathways can range in permeability from very leaky, such as those found in the discontinuous or sinusoidal endothelia, to highly restrictive, such as the tight junctions found between continuous microvascular endothelial cells of the brain or testes. The paracellular pathways can be either unregulated (comprised of obvious cellular discontinuities) or highly regulated. In addition, specialized vesicular pathways function to carry proteins into and across cells. Epithelial and endothelial cells in many ways have the same vesicular transport mechanisms for transporting molecules into and across the cells. The clathrin-coated pit pathway is the most well-known and is comprised of plasmalemmal vesicles marked by a fuzzy electron dense coat of clathrin polymers. These structures play an important role in direct and indirect transcellular transport. They are abundant in many cell types, including many epithelial cells, hepatocytes, and the reticular-endothelial system (i.e. liver and spleen). Another pathway that is receiving increasing attention is the caveolar transport pathway. Caveolae are small, omega-shaped, smooth plasmalemmal vesicles abundant in continuous endothelia lining the vasculature of many organs, such as lung and heart but not in liver, brain or testes. Endothelial cells harbor both clathrin-coated vesicles and caveolae in varied proportions, e.g. lung endothelium has abundant caveolae but few clathrin-coated vesicles whereas liver endothelium has virtually no caveolae yet many clathrin-coated vesicles. Although the accessibility issues discussed in this chapter are applicable to both endothelial- and epithelial cells, our focus and experience is primarily with endothelial cells and will be discussed here as such.

THE ENDOTHELIAL CELL BARRIER AND ITS TRANSPORT PATHWAYS

The most efficient route of drug entry into the body is via intravenous injection. The attenuated layer of endothelial cells lining the blood vessels forms a critical barrier controlling the exchange of molecules from the blood to the interstitial fluid. The selectivity of the endothelial barrier varies in different vascular beds and is strongly dependent on the structure and type of endothelium lining the microvasculature (10). As with any cellular barrier, the lipid cell surface membrane tends to restrict transmembrane transport of both small and large circulating molecules including water, ions, and proteins because of electrostatic, steric, and/or hydrophobic exclusion forces. As depicted in Fig. 2, several pathways exist for the transport of blood molecules across continuous endothelium: (a) intercellular junctions are highly regulated structures that form the paracellular pathway for the pressure-driven filtration of water and small solutes; (b) caveolae transcytose plasma macromolecules adsorbed from blood apparently by shuttling their contents from the luminal to antiluminal aspect of the endothelium (5); and (c) transendothelial channels may form transiently in very attenuated regions of the cell by the fusion of two or more caveolae each located on apposing plasma membranes to provide a direct conduit for the exchange of both small and large plasma

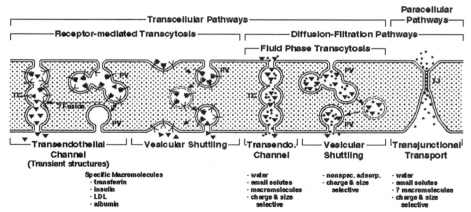

Figure 2. Summary of potential transport pathways across continuous endothelium.
PV, plasmalemmal vesicles; TC, transendothelial channels; TJ, transjunctional

molecules. The transcellular pathway may include both fluid-phase and receptor-mediated transcytosis. Although there has been much research over the last half century on how molecules cross the endothelial cell barrier, there has been little general agreement on the pathways and mechanisms of transendothelial transport of macromolecules (10, 11). Biophysical transport studies indicated that macromolecules cross the endothelium through a hydraulically conductive pathway, modeled simply as pores or filtration slits usually assumed to be located at intercellular junctions. Ultrastructural studies using electron microscopy to take snap shots of molecular transport implicate the abundant population of caveolae in the transendothelial transport of macromolecules. The bias of particular groups of scientists with regards to transcellular vs. paracellular transport reflects in most cases not only the limitations of the techniques used to examine transport (ultrastructural studies vs. permeability measurements) but also a lack of means to examine or to prevent transport selectively.

ROLE OF CAVEOLAE IN ENDOTHELIAL TRANSPORT

Vesicular transport plays a fundamental role in cellular function. The transport of proteins by specific vesicular carriers is well documented in a variety of cells for intracellular trafficking, exocytosis, synaptic neurotransmission, receptor-mediated endocytosis, and transcytosis. Caveolae may deliver ligands, such as cholera toxin, tetanus toxin and albumin-gold complexes, to specific destinations within the cell, such as endosomes and lysosomes (5, 12-15). In addition, caveolae may mediate not only fluid-phase, adsoptive, and receptor-mediated endocytosis but also equivalent transcytosis, at least in vascular endothelium (15). Specific receptors on the surface of various endothelia play a significant role in the transendothelial exchange of a variety of plasma molecules, including insulin, transferrin, ceruloplasmin, albumin (5, 13), orosomucoid, and low density lipoproteins (LDL). When perfused through the microcirculation, probes such as albumin, ferritin and even gold-tagged blood proteins can enter luminal endothelial caveolae and, with time, are found in abluminal caveolae and the interstitium. In all of these cases, the labeling within caveolae, especially those apparently free in the cell, has been interpreted as indicative of transport by caveolae. Thus, it appears that for certain endothelia, specific receptor-mediated processes are necessary for transvascular molecular transport, apparently via caveolae.

Other morphological studies have challenged the data supporting receptor-mediated transendothelial transport by caveolae. Because of the racemose structure of caveolae, wherein many vesicles link to each other in a chain to form a grape-like branching "cave" penetrating deep into the cell, conventional sections for electron microscopy can show about 50% of the caveolae apparently free in the cytoplasm. However, serial ultrathin sectioning reveals that ≤1% exist as discrete structures unattached to other membranes (16). Based on these data, some investigators have logically concluded that: (a) caveolae are not dynamic but rather static elements and (b) the observed transport to the interstitium is primarily mediated by the paracellular pathway with the probe accumulating in the interstitium for entry into the abluminal aspect of a static, branched caveolar system (the "back-filling" model) (16). These past ultrastructural studies with limited probes unfortunately cannot prove definitively that caveolae function in transport nor can they ascertain whether caveolae do or do not form discrete carrier vesicles capable of delivery. To definitively determine whether and how caveolae function in cell transport, high affinity probes targeting caveolae exclusively will be required along with appropriate control probes that do not target but yet are otherwise physically identical.

Molecular mechanism of caveolae budding, docking and fusion

To address the function of caveolae in transport in endothelium, new strategies have been developed (reviewed in (17)). A key advance has been the development of new subfractionation procedures that allow isolation of caveolae from luminal endothelial cell plasma membranes to a high degree of purity (discussed in detail below). Moreover, new assays have been developed for measuring endothelial transport, including intact and permeabilized cultured cell assays (transcytosis/endocytosis), transfected cell systems, in situ assays (involving tissue perfusion), and reconstituted cell free systems. Pharmacological agents have been identified, such as filipin and N-ethylmaleimide (NEM), which inhibit the endocytosis and transcytosis of select ligands that preferentially bind within caveolae and provide new evidence in favor of caveolae functioning as carrier vesicles. In addition, specific molecular machinery have been defined that mediate the budding, docking, and fusion of caveolae as transport vesicles (17). Several key proteins are concentrated in caveolae, including SNAP (soluble NSF attachment protein), VAMP (vesicle-associated membrane protein), small and large GTP binding proteins; the calcium-dependent, lipid binding proteins annexin II and VI; and NSF (NEM-sensitive factor), which form a complex that may mediate docking and fusion. Caveolae require intact VAMP-2 for efficient targeted transport of cholera toxin B subunit to intracellular organelles such as endosomes. Thus, caveolae appear to have the molecular machinery necessary to function as endocytic, and possibly transcytotic, vesicles.

A cell-free assay for reconstituting the budding of caveolae directly from plasma membranes under physiological conditions shows that caveolae can be dynamic vesicles capable of budding from the cell surface (15). The budding process specifically requires cytosol and GTP hydrolysis and the budded vesicles are easily isolated by centrifugation as low density, caveolin-rich vesicles. These budded, free caveolar vesicles are rich in VAMP, albondin and G_{M1} but lack glycosylphosphatidyl inositol (GPI)-anchored proteins and cytoskeletal proteins, such as β-actin (15, 18).

Dynamin has been found to be the GTPase mediating the fission of caveolae (19). Dynamin concentrates in caveolae at the cell surface both in vivo and in cultured cells and appears to be both necessary and sufficient to drive caveolar budding at a step probably at or very near the final budding to release the vesicle from the plasma membrane (19). Immunogold electron microscopy on ultra-thin frozen sections of rat lung tissue confirmed the presence of dynamin in caveolae and revealed that dynamin localizes to the neck of endothelial caveolae, in contrast to clathrin-coated vesicles where it resides in the clathrin-coated bulb region (19). Expression of dynamin in cytosol as well as purified recombinant dynamin alone supports GTP-induced caveolar fission in the cell-free budding assay, whereas its removal from the cytosol or the presence of antibodies to dynamin inhibits caveolar fission (19). Overexpression of a dominant negative mutant form of dynamin, which does not hydrolyze GTP normally, inhibits GTP-induced budding of caveolae and prevents caveolae-mediated internalization of caveolae-targeted agents in intact and permeabilized endothelial cells (19, 20). Thus, dynamin apparently oligomerizes to form a structural collar around the neck of caveolae, where, upon activation, it hydrolyzes GTP to drive neck extension resulting in the fission of caveolae to form free transport vesicles in vascular endothelium in vivo.

Rapid endocytosis of caveolae-targeting antibodies

Even with the new molecular data, it still could not be established definitively that caveolae mediates the transcytosis of macromolecules in vivo because of a lack of proper probes with a high enough specificity, affinity, and level of exclusivity to target caveolae selectively to assess possible caveolar transport in vivo. Recently, two new monoclonal antibody probes, TX1.228 and TX3.406, were generated which are highly specific for caveolar proteins (X-Y. Tan, P. Oh, and J. Schnitzer, unpublished). We used these probes as caveolar-targeting probes in "warm up" internalization assays to examine the possible role of caveolae in endocytosis using endothelial cells (T. Horner, P. Oh, and J. Schnitzer, unpublished). Intact rat lung microvascular endothelial cells incubated with TX1.228 or TX3.406 for 60 min at 4°C were warmed to 37°C for various times, fixed and permeabilized, and labeled with fluorescence-conjugated reporter antibodies. Analysis by fluorescence confocal microscopy revealed that at 4°C, both antibodies exhibit a fine punctate staining pattern distributed evenly over the cell surface. After 10 min at 37°C, much of the antibody appears internalized with staining redistributed to large intracellular clusters primarily at the cell periphery. By 30 min, TX1.228 and TX3.406 appear completely internalized and concentrate in large vesicular structures in the perinuclear region of the cell. Control cells kept at 4°C for the additional 10 to 30 minutes maintain their punctate cell surface caveolar staining with no apparent internalization. Moreover, control antibodies targeting non-caveolar proteins located in lipid rafts exhibit a very slow turnover at the cell surface. Even after 2 hours, a weak, generalized staining of intracellular membranes was seen that remained even after 5 hours. Thus, antibodies targeting caveolae directly are transported rapidly into the cell, consistent with caveolae internalizing their targeted molecular cargo from the cell surface.

Transcytosis of caveolae-targeting antibodies

To test the hypothesis that caveolae can function as carrier vesicles in transcytosis across the endothelial cell barrier, we used a newly generated monoclonal antibody, TX3.833, that is both tissue- and caveolae-specific as detailed by immunogold electron microscopy and subcellular fractionation (9). TX3.833 specifically recognizes a 90 kDa protein specifically in the lung and no other tested organs. Lung tissue subfractionation shows that this protein is enriched greatly in isolated luminal endothelial cell plasma membranes relative to whole tissue homogenate and is primarily concentrated in caveolae (>225-fold over lung homogenate).

We tracked caveolar targeting as well as possible transcytosis of TX3.833 in lung tissue via electron microscopy after intravascular administration of TX3.833 conjugated to gold particles (9) (Fig. 3). TX3.833 specifically targets the lung endothelial caveolae with uptake within 2-3 min (top panel) followed by transport across the endothelium for release by caveolae now on the abluminal surface in just 5-10 min (middle panel). Once transcytosed, the probe accumulates in the interstitium where it can percolate through the basement membrane and then be internalized by the caveolae of the underlying tissue cells, namely lung alveolar epithelium. After 15 min, the antibody is found in the alveolar space as well as inside endosomes. Control antibodies do not similarly enter nor traverse the endothelium so that almost no gold is detected in the interstitium even after 15 min. Thus, two important cell barriers in vivo, the endothelium and epithelium, can be overcome sequentially in a tissue-specific manner with an antibody specifically targeting the caveolar trafficking pathway.

Interestingly, our data showed that the movement of TX3.833-Au across the endothelial cell barrier primarily occurs in a quantal fashion. Fig. 3 shows high magnification views of entry caveolae loaded with ~ 6-7 TX3.833-Au and similar quanta of gold particles exiting emptying caveolae on the other side of the endothelial cell. These findings are not readily predicted by transcellular channels where a continuous stream of molecules is driven by fluid flow and concentration gradients through a pore formed by a chain of caveolae. Occasional transient transendothelial channels probably do co-exist and may contribute to nonspecific and some targeted transendothelial transport. Yet, these channels cannot account for the observed quantal unloading of probe from emptying abluminal caveolae. It seems unlikely,

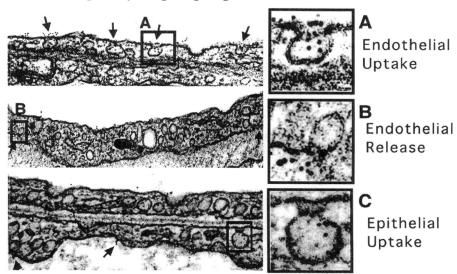

Figure. 3. Electron microscopy of TX3.833-Au binding and transcytosis from the circulating blood to the underlying normal lung tissue. Gold particles conjugated to TX3.833 target and enter the alveolar caveolae of the microvascular endothelium within 2-3 min (**A**) where they cross the endothelium by transcytosis for release to the subendothelial space in 5-10 min (**B**). The transported gold particles also cross the basement membrane (**C**) and in 15 min enter caveolae of alveolar epithelium for transport into and across this cell barrier.

therefore, that continuous transendothelial channels are the primary pathway for targeted transport through the endothelium. Thus, transcytosis of select molecular cargo in the caveolae probably occurs primarily as discrete packages.

TX3.833 targets, and is carried by, dynamic caveolae capable of budding from the endothelial cell surface to form free transport vesicles. We have perfused biotinylated TX3.833 through the rat lung and, after 10 min, isolated luminal endothelial cell plasma membranes in order to perform a reconstituted caveolae budding assay (15). In the presence of GTP, the fission of caveolae from isolated luminal endothelial cell plasma membranes occurs to form free, floating vesicles that were collected as low density caveolar vesicles. These budded caveolae contain the injected TX3.833 as well as caveolin and TX3.833 antigen but not actin nor the lipid raft marker, 5'nucleotidase (9). In the absence of GTP, no caveolae budding is detected and these proteins remain at the plasma membrane. This fission of dynamic caveolae occurs in the presence of cytosol containing normal but not mutant K44A dynamin (19). Thus, TX3.833 can indeed bind its antigen located in dynamic caveolae that require GTP hydrolysis by dynamin for their fission from the plasma membrane to form free transport vesicles carrying the targeted cargo, TX3.833. These data, as well as the quantal transendothelial transport of TX3.833-Au observed by electron microscopy, support a transcytosis model where caveolae function as discrete vesicular carriers capable of budding, docking, and fusion to move molecular cargo into and across the cell.

MAPPING THE MOLECULAR HETEROGENEITY OF THE VASCULAR ENDOTHELIA

The vascular system is lined with a greatly attenuated monolayer of highly differentiated endothelial cells that are strategically located to form the critical barrier in many organs regulating the exchange of water, solutes, macromolecules, cells and even drugs from the circulating blood to the underlying tissue cells. Endothelial cells are quite responsive to the local tissue environment and may modulate their barrier function in accordance with the needs of the underlying tissue cells. There is considerable heterogeneity among the endothelia lining the microvascular beds of different organs. Some differences are even quite apparent by electron microscopy of tissue specimens and can be grouped readily into three distinct morphological types: continuous (found in tissues such as heart, lung, brain and skeletal muscle), fenestrated (kidney glomerulus, intestinal mucosa and endocrine glands) and discontinuous or sinusoidal (liver, spleen and bone marrow).

The extensive phenotypic differentiation of endothelia between organs reflects the influence of the local tissue environment and provides for considerable differences in endothelial cell barrier functions. If one transplants blood vessels from one tissue to another, the endothelia adopt the morphological phenotype of the local tissue (21). The fenestrated phenotype can be modulated by the extracellular matrix and by specific growth factors, such as vascular endothelial growth factor (VEGF), which are expressed by tissue cells. Endothelia of the continuous type vary considerably in their barrier function depending on which organ they reside. Most of them have an abundance of caveolae that function as vesicular carriers for blood proteins into and across the cell. These characteristic vesicles can constitute 50-70% of the cell surface plasma membrane and occupy 10-15% of the total cell volume (about 500-600 vesicles/μm^3). Other continuous endothelia located at the blood brain barrier form a very restrictive barrier by having few, if any, caveolae and elaborating epithelial-like, tight junctions that prevent small solute transport. Brain endothelia must express specific transport proteins to meet the metabolic demands of the brain tissue cells even for small molecules as glucose and amino acids.

In order to fulfill the theoretical promise of the vascular targeting strategy, it is necessary to identify useful targets on the endothelial cell surface of the blood vessels that are specific for the vascular bed of the desired tissue or tumor. The most direct way to accomplish this is to generate a molecular map of the vascular endothelium of the blood vessels supplying various organs and tumor tissue. One reason for the paucity of molecular information about the endothelium in tumors as well as normal organs and the lack of known vascular targets may be related to methodological inadequacies in examining endothelium in vivo not only for identifying endothelial surface proteins but also for purifying them for sequencing and probe production. Even in highly vascularized tissue, the endothelium represents only a very small percentage of the cells constituting the tissue and its membrane proteins exposed directly to circulating the blood are only a small fraction of the total proteins of the tissue. Thus, classic techniques for isolating plasma membranes from tissues will yield endothelial cell membranes, but only as a small percentage of the total membrane isolated. This makes detection, identification, and purification of endothelial- and caveolae-specific proteins very difficult and would make comparisons between normal and neoplastic tissues nearly impossible.

It is not surprising that many researchers have opted for in vitro models using isolated endothelial cells grown in culture. Membranes isolated from cultured cells have been used for molecular mapping studies using genomic analysis (such as DNA microarray technology) as well as creating antibody libraries of endothelial cell proteins. Unfortunately, it is clear that endothelial cells are very sensitive to microenvironmental factors in tissue and therefore change considerably when moved from their native environment in tissue for isolation and growth in culture (8). They lose many of their distinctive characteristics found in vivo including expression of tissue-specific proteins as well as the usual abundance of caveolae, which decreases 30-100-fold in cultured endothelial cells (8). Thus, for the purposes of defining useful vascular target sites, cultured endothelial cells offer limited utility.

A second approach to mapping the vascular endothelium has been to use peptide phage display to identify accessible targets on the luminal endothelial cell surface in vivo. Peptide probes, owing to their size and relatively low complexity, can be synthesized directly and conjugated to many kinds of reagents using a large variety of coupling reagents, and are easily integrated with other recombinant proteins. In vivo screening of highly complex peptide phage libraries has allowed the detection of a number of peptides with improved targeting to a variety of tissues as well as to specific tumor vasculature (22, 23). Unfortunately, the vascular targets recognizing these peptides remain elusive, probably because such small peptides lack the specificity and affinity necessary for purifying a single target molecule (4). Moreover, because of their low specificity and binding affinity, the level of tissue- and tumor-specific targeting and accumulation of the peptides in vivo is rather modest (4). In reported experiments (22, 23), only 0.2% or less of the injected dose of organ- and tumor-specific peptides was found in the target tissue and the desired tissue accumulation was only 2-7-fold more than in the control brain tissue whose highly restrictive endothelium should greatly minimize any nonspecific uptake.

Another interesting methodology has been developed that perfuses rat lungs with low-strength formaldehyde solution to create outside-out membrane vesicles that can be collected from the tissue and used to create antibodies (24). In this manner, multiple monoclonal antibodies were created that inhibit adhesion of lung-metastatic cancer cells to the vesicles and recognize endothelia from lung capillaries, splenic venules and renal medullary vasa recta (24). In fact, the most compelling evidence for the existence of organ-specific markers on the accessible surface of the endothelium comes from the observations of preferential homing of metastatic tumor cells and leukocytes to specific organs in vivo (25-27). In some cases, inducible adhesion molecules appear to mediate this effect (27).

Because the endothelial cell surface is inherently in contact with all elements of the circulating blood, it appears logical to learn more about this surface as it exists in vivo. One may get useful information by combining subfractionation of tissue to isolate the luminal endothelial cell plasma membranes and attached caveolae with highly sensitive proteomic approaches to identifying cell surface proteins. We have developed a method for purifying luminal endothelial cell membranes and caveolae directly from normal organs and solid tumors. In this technique, the tissue microvasculature is perfused in situ with a positively charged colloidal silica solution to coat the luminal endothelial cell membrane normally exposed to the circulating blood,

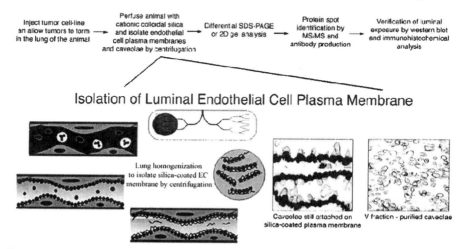

Figure. 4. Tumor model system and subcellular fractionation scheme. Tumors are created by IV injection of tumor cells into rats, which seed and grow in the lung. The luminal endothelial plasma membrane and caveolae are isolated from normal and tumor-bearing tissues for proteomic analysis to identify tumor-induced proteins.

thereby creating a stable adherent silica pellicle marking this specific membrane of interest (8, 18). This coating increases the density of the plasma membrane and is so strongly attached that even after tissue homogenization, large sheets of silica-coated endothelial cell plasma membrane with their attached caveolae are readily isolated from other cellular membranes and debris by centrifugation through a high density medium (Fig. 4, above). The isolated luminal endothelial cell plasma membranes display ample enrichment for endothelial cell surface markers such as caveolin and angiotensin converting enzyme (ACE) (>30-fold), whereas proteins of intracellular components (cytochrome oxidase and ribophorin) and even the plasma membrane of other tissue cells (i.e. fibroblast surface protein) are markedly depleted (>15-fold) (18). Thus, this technique provides a high yield (80%) of luminal endothelial cell plasma membranes with little contamination (8, 18).

This laboratory has been successful in subfractionating isolated luminal endothelial cell plasma membranes to isolate caveolae separately from other plasmalemmal microdomains, including those rich in GPI-anchored proteins or cytoskeletal elements (18). In our characterization of isolated luminal endothelial cell plasma membranes, we observed by electron microscopy that many caveolae were still attached to the membrane on the side opposite to the silica coating. The silica coating appears to stabilize the noncaveolar flat aspects of the plasma membrane so that when subjected to shearing, only the caveolae are physically detached. The detached caveolae are purified by flotation away from any other membranes during centrifugation to yield a homogeneous population of morphologically distinct small caveolin-coated plasmalemmal vesicles with diameters of <90nm, typical for caveolae in vivo (18). Biochemical analysis shows that the isolated caveolae represent specific microdomains of the cell surface with their own unique molecular topography (18, 28). The caveolae are enriched in seven known caveolar markers localized to the endothelial caveolae in vivo by electron microscopy: caveolin, Ca^{++}-ATPase, GM_1, dynamin, VAMP, endothelial nitric oxide synthase (eNOS), and inositol 1,4,5-trisphosphate receptor. Other cell surface markers, including 5'nucleotidase, ACE, Band 4.1, and β-actin, were markedly depleted to absent from the isolated caveolae in spite of being amply present in the silica-coated membranes. Both electron microscopy and biochemical analysis reveal that the caveolae have been removed from the silica-coated membranes yielding a highly purified fraction of caveolae. Without the silica-coating, contamination from other microdomains with similar physical characteristics can occur.

Using these isolated membranes as starting materials, proteomic techniques can be applied to create a reasonably complete molecular map of the endothelium of any perfusable organ or tumor-bearing tissue (Fig. 4). We have compared the proteins in isolated luminal endothelial cell plasma membranes and caveolae isolated from normal tissues and various tumors from humans, rats, mice, rabbits, and rhesus monkeys by 2-D gel analysis.

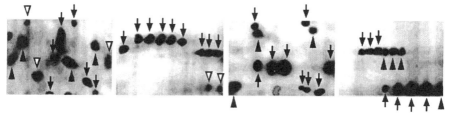

Figure. 5: Tumor Induced Vascular Endothelial Cell Surface Proteins Identified by 2-D gel analysis. We used spot analytical software to identify potential vascular targets in 2-D gels of endothelial cell plasma membranes isolated from lung tumors. In the above four areas, a matching region of silver-stained gels of normal and tumor P proteins have been super-imposed. Arrowheads, more in tumor; empty arrowhead, less in tumor; arrow, only in tumor.

Notably, when 2-D gels maps from many independent animals are compared, we find that they are quite consistent and reproducible. Multiple proteins are detected in isolated luminal endothelial cell plasma membranes from a tumor with little, if any, expression in normal luminal endothelial cell plasma membranes (Fig. 5 above). These apparently tumor-induced endothelial cell surface proteins are not readily detected in the tumor homogenate. Even prominent spots easily detected in isolated luminal endothelial cell plasma membranes by 2-D analysis are not detected in the homogenate. Numerous differences are also detected between tumor and normal endothelial caveolae. Interestingly, many of the proteins that appear to be tumor-induced exist primarily in caveolae. This is also true for other tissue-specific proteins. It appears that the vast majority of the proteins in the tissue and tumor homogenates are neither endothelial nor caveolae in origin so that subfractionation is required to unmask these proteins, including many tissue-specific and tumor-induced proteins. Thus, these isolated membranes are good starting materials for comparative proteomic analysis.

2-D gel electrophoresis followed by analysis by mass spectrometry (MS) and database searching is a widely used method for protein identification. By resolving proteins in two dimensions, hundreds of proteins in luminal endothelial cell plasma membranes and caveolae can be rapidly compared in order to reveal those well-separated protein spots highly enriched in a subset of organs or in tumors vs. normal tissues for MS analysis. One caveat to this method is that some protein groups are under-represented in 2D gels, so that proteins of interest may be missed. These include proteins that do not efficiently pick up the silver or other protein stains and proteins that do not enter the gel in the first dimension (isoelectric focusing), as is well known for integral membrane proteins. Low-abundance proteins and proteins with extremes in molecular weight (<10 kDa or >100 kDa) or pI (isoelectric points >10) are poorly detected. These problems can be partially resolved by solubilizing the proteins in the presence of chaotropes, such as thiourea, which theoretically opens hydrophobic proteins to facilitate their analysis by

2D gel electrophoresis. Alternatively, these limitations can be overcome by replacing the 2D gels with 1-D SDS-PAGE gels where all proteins are essentially solubilized; however, resolving power is reduced, thereby making it more difficult to detect differences between samples. Finally, analyzing differences between 2-D gels requires the isolation and analysis of each protein spot individually and thus can be rather laborious and time-consuming.

A second approach to proteomic analysis that has been recently developed is MS analysis of whole membrane preparations using **Multi-dimentional Protein Identification Technology (MudPIT) (29)**. In this approach, the proteins in the various membrane fractions from tissues are solubilized and this complex peptide mixture is subjected to MS analysis followed by automated analysis of peptide product spectra against spectra obtained with known proteins in available databases. This strategy provides a high throughput, fully automated system that readily identifies membrane proteins and proteins of low abundance that may not be detected in 2-D gels. Because protein separation by cation exchange- and reversed phase chromatography is rather straightforward, all groups of proteins are equally represented (29). Unfortunately, when analyzing a very complex mixture of proteins such as isolated membranes, the higher the abundance of the protein in the mixture, the more peptides may be detected from that protein, thereby possibly obscuring proteins of lower abundance. Even so, by not depending on gel electrophoresis, this method promises to be a valuable complement to the other two techniques described above to identify additional proteins not detected by them.

A proteomics-based analysis offers important advantages over DNA microarray or other genome technology because it allows preferential identification of targets specifically expressed on the luminal cell surface of the tumor endothelium. Even when coupled with more specific approaches such as laser capture microdissection, genomic techniques examine cellular mRNA expression that does not necessarily correlate with protein expression and clearly provides little detail regarding subcellular localization. Because genome-based technology does not distinguish between intracellular and accessible plasma membrane localization, it contributes much less toward solving target accessibility problems. A proteomic strategy coupled with appropriate subfractionation to isolate the desired endothelial cell membranes directly from the tissue greatly narrows our target discovery to a subset of proteins that are actually expressed and directly exposed to the blood circulation. Tissue subfractionation to isolate the membranes containing accessible targets promotes the unmasking, from the thousands of proteins in the tissue, the subset of proteins (hundreds or less) that can be targeted by IV injection in vivo. Such analysis goes beyond the gene and even the product of the gene, the protein, to the actual site where the target protein resides and functions.

TISSUE-SPECIFIC VASCULAR TARGETING WITH AN ORGAN- & CAVEOLAE-SPECIFIC ANTIBODY

New data shows that targeting of endothelium, especially its caveolae, can achieve delivery to a single tissue in vivo (9). We have injected radio-iodinated TX3.833 as well as isotype-matched control IgG into rat tail veins (all IgG$_1$) and find that TX3.833 does indeed provide site-directed delivery *in vivo* with lung accumulation reaching as high as 89% in just 30 min (mean 75%) (9). The control IgG remains primarily in the blood with low uptake in all tissues. The lung tropism of TX3.833 is specific because unlabeled TX3.833, but not control IgG, inhibits lung accumulation by 89% and increases blood levels by >15-fold. Even 24 hours after injection, 46% of the injected dose of TX3.833 still remains in the lung tissue. In experiments where TX3.833 has been conjugated to potential drugs or toxins, their delivery and even bioefficacy can become quite selective for the lung with tissue-specific targeting at levels up to 170-fold greater than controls (9). Thus, TX3.833 appears to have the tissue- and cell-specificity to validate, for the first time, the vascular targeting strategy by achieving high levels of tissue targeting and bioefficacy in vivo that clearly approach theoretical expectations.

Past reports describe various targeting monoclonal antibodies requiring up to 1 week to achieve a maximal tissue uptake of 0.2-4% of the injected dose (1). A lung-targeting monoclonal antibody has been reported (30) but the antigen was subsequently found to be thrombomodulin, which is expressed by many different cell types including the endothelial cell surface of several organs. Improved delivery has been obtained using biotinylated antibodies to ACE complexed to streptavidin (31). These probes conjugated to superoxide dismutase (SOD) and catalase (Cat) via a streptavidin bridge are able to deliver 4-5% of the injected dose (12-20-fold over control IgG) to the lung within one hour. Unfortunately, these probes significantly accumulate in the kidney (7% of the injected dose for SOD conjugate) and spleen (5% of the injected dose for Cat conjugate) as well (31). Similar results have been observed using the pan-endothelial marker, PECAM. Antibodies to PECAM show improved delivery to the lung from the usual <1% to nearly 4% of the injected IV dose (2-4-fold over liver delivery) but only when the antibody is biotinylated and complexed with streptavidin (32). Efforts to target and overcome the blood brain barrier have likewise achieved limited success. Targeting the transferrin receptor provides modest brain accumulation and transcytosis at levels of 0.3-3% injected dose/gram tissue (33, 34).

Unfortunately, transferrin receptors are expressed in other tissues, e.g. hepatocytes in the liver. Tissue-homing peptides have also moderately increased tissue targeting to < 1% of the injected dose in the target tissue with relative targeting indices of 6-20-fold more local delivery than to the brain (22, 23). Using these same criteria, TX3.833 targeting index is >1000-fold (lung/brain).

The work (described above and in (9)) demonstrating specific tissue accumulation and caveolae-mediated transcytosis (Fig. 3) of TX3.833 shows that proteins expressed in caveolae can indeed be accessible by IV injection not only for tissue-specific delivery in vivo but also, perhaps more importantly, for transcytosis occurring within the endothelial cell barrier with delivery to underlying tissue cells. Likewise caveolae also provide a trafficking pathway across epithelial cell barriers. These studies appear promising and consistent with the hypothesis that caveolae function in transendothelial and transepithelial cell transport and that targeting caveolae may be useful for drug and gene delivery in vivo.

CONCLUSION

It is clear that the endothelium, far from being a passive, cellophane-like barrier, is a highly dynamic structure that exhibits many tissue-specific qualities, including protein expression. From a practical standpoint, it has been shown that tissue-specific endothelial cell surface proteins can be used as vascular targets to achieve the theoretical expectation of tissue-specific delivery of antibody-drug conjugates reaching high levels in a single tissue within 60 minutes. Importantly, proteins expressed in endothelial cell plasma membrane subdomains called caveolae can provide useful accessible tissue-specific vascular targets as well as a pathway and mechanism to overcome the endothelial barrier for delivery to underlying tissue cells. The data so far appears encouraging and should motivate the completion of the mapping of the vascular endothelium under native conditions in tissues, in essence, to define the accessible vascular proteome in vivo. With this molecular data, it is now clear that we will be able to define quite concretely the extent to which the vascular targeting strategy will work for drug, and possibly gene, delivery in vivo. Although much work remains to be done, vascular targeting promises to become a very powerful strategy for realizing the goal of site-directed pharmacodelivery.

REFERENCES

1. Tomlinson, E. Theory and practice of site-specific drug delivery. Advanced Drug Delivery Reviews 1987; 1: 87-198.

2.   Jain, R. K. The next frontier of molecular medicine: delivery of therapeutics. Nat Med 1998; 4: 655-7.

3.   Dvorak, H. F., Nagy, J. A. and Dvorak, A. M. Structure of solid tumors and their vasculature: implications for therapy with monoclonal antibodies. Cancer Cells 1991; 3: 77-85.

4.   Schnitzer, J. E. Vascular targeting as a strategy for cancer therapy. N Engl J Med 1998; 339: 472-4.

5.   Schnitzer, J. E. Update on the cellular and molecular basis of capillary permeability. Trends in Cardiovasc. Med. 1993; 3: 124-30.

6.   Denekamp, J. Vasculature as a target for tumour therapy. Progr. Appli. Microcirc. 1984; 4: 28-38.

7.   Burrows, F. J. and Thorpe, P. E. Vascular targeting--a new approach to the therapy of solid tumors. Pharmacol Ther 1994; 64: 155-74.

8.   Schnitzer, J. E. *"The endothelial cell surface and caveolae in health and disease."* in *Vascular Endothelium: Physiology, Pathology and Therapeutic Opportunities,* G.V.R. Born and C.J. Schwartz, ed. Stuttgart, Schattauer, 1997.

9.   McIntosh, D. P., Tan, X.-Y., Oh, P. and Schnitzer, J. E. Targeting endothelium and its dynamic caveolae for tissue-specific transcytosis in vivo: A pathway to overcome cell barriers to drug and gene delivery. Proc Natl Acad Sci U S A 2002; 99: 1996-2001.

10.   Renkin, E. M. Capillary transport of macromolecules: pores and other pathways. J. Appl. Physiol. 1985; 134: 375-82.

11.   Schnitzer, J. E. *"Transport functions of the glycocalyx, specific proteins and caveolae in endothelium."* in *Capillary Permeation, Cellular Transport and Reaction Kinetics,* J.B. Bassingthwaighte, C.A. Goresky and J.H. Lineham, ed. London, Oxford Press, 1997.

12.   Montesano, R., Roth, J., Robert, A. and Orci, L. Non-coated membrane invaginations are involved in binding and internalization of cholera and tetanus toxins. Nature 1982; 296: 651-53.

13.   Schnitzer, J. E., Oh, P., Pinney, E. and Allard, J. Filipin-sensitive caveolae-mediated transport in endothelium: reduced transcytosis, scavenger endocytosis, and capillary permeability of select macromolecules. J. Cell. Biol. 1994; 127: 1217-32.

14.   Schnitzer, J. E., Oh, P., Pinney, E. and Allard, J. NEM inhibits transcytosis, endocytosis and capillary permeability: implication of caveolae fusion in endothelia. Am. J. Physiol. 1995; 37: H48-55.

15.   Schnitzer, J. E., Oh, P. and McIntosh, D. P. Role of GTP hydrolysis in fission of caveolae directly from plasma membrane [publisher's erratum appears in Science 1996 Nov 15;274(5290):1069]. Science 1996; 274: 239-42.

16.   Bundgaard, M. Vesicular transport in capillary endothelium: does it occur? Federation Proc. 1983; 42: 2425-30.

17.   Schnitzer, J. E. Caveolae: from basic trafficking mechanisms to targeting transcytosis for tissue-specific drug and gene delivery in vivo. Adv Drug Deliv Rev 2001; 49: 265-80.

18.   Schnitzer, J. E., McIntosh, D. P., Dvorak, A. M., Liu, J. and Oh, P. Separation of caveolae from associated microdomains of GPI-anchored proteins. Science 1995; 269: 1435-39.

19.   Oh, P., McIntosh, D. P. and Schnitzer, J. E. Dynamin at the neck of caveolae mediates their budding to form transport vesicles by GTP-driven fission from the plasma membrane of endothelium. J Cell Biol 1998; 141: 101-14.

20.   Oh, P. and Schnitzer, J. E. Dynamin-mediated fission of caveolae from plasma membranes. Mol. Biol. Cell 1996; 7: 83a.

21.   Stewart, P. A. and Wiley, M. J. Developing nervous tissue induces formation of blood-brain barrier characteristics in invading endothelial cells: a study using quail-chick transplantation chimeras. Develop Biol 1981; 84: 183-92.

22.   Pasqualini, R. and Ruoslahti, E. Organ targeting *in vivo* using phage display peptide libraries. Nature 1996; 380: 364-66.

23.   Arap, W., Pasqualini, R. and Ruoslahti, E. Cancer treatment by targeted drug delivery to tumor vasculature in a mouse model. Science 1998; 279: 377-80.

24.   Johnson, R. C., Zhu, D., Augustin-Voss, H. G. and Pauli, B. U. Lung endothelial dipeptidyl peptidase IV is an adhesion molecule for lung-metastatic rat breast and prostate carcinoma cells. J Cell Biology 1993; 121: 1423-32.

25.   Auerbach, R., Lu, W. C., Pardon, E., Gumkowski, F., Kaminska, G. and Kaminski, M. Specificity of adhesion between murine tumor cells and capillary endothelium: an *in vitro* correlate of preferential metastasis *in vivo*. Cancer Res 1987; 47: 1492-96.

26.   Nicolson, G. L. Cancer metastasis: tumor cell and host organ properties important in metastasis to specific secondary sites. Biochim Biophys Acta 1988; 948: 175-224.

27.   Springer, T. A. Traffic signals for lymphocyte recirculation and leukocyte emigration: the multistep program. Cell 1994; 76: 301-14.

28.   Schnitzer, J. E., Liu, J. and Oh, P. Endothelial caveolae have the molecular transport machinery for vesicle budding, docking and fusion including VAMP, NSF, SNAP, annexins and GTPases. J. Biol. Chem. 1995; 270: 14399-404.

29.   Washburn, M. P., Wolters, D. and Yates, J. R., 3rd Large-scale analysis of the yeast proteome by multidimensional protein identification technology. Nature Biotechnology 2001; 19: 242-47.

30.   Hughes, B. J., Kennel, S. K., Lee, R. and Huang, L. Monoclonal antibody targeting of liposomes to mouse lung *in vivo*. Cancer Res 1989; 49: 6214-20.

31.   Muzykantov, V. R., Atochina, E. N., Ischiropoulos, H., Danilov, S. M. and Fisher, A. B. Immunotargeting of antioxidant enzyme to the pulmonary endothelium. Proc Natl Acad Sci U S A 1996; 93: 5213-8.

32.   Scherpereel, A., Wiewrodt, R., Christofidou-Solomidou, M., Gervais, R., Murciano, J. C., Albelda, S. M. and Muzykantov, V. R. Cell-selective intracellular delivery of a foreign enzyme to endothelium in vivo using vascular immunotargeting. Faseb J 2001; 15: 416-26.

33.   Shin, S. U., Friden, P., Moran, M., Olson, T., Kang, Y. S., Pardridge, W. M. and Morrison, S. L. Transferrin-antibody fusion proteins are effective in brain targeting. Proc Natl Acad Sci U S A 1995; 92: 2820-4.

34.   Lee, H. J., Engelhardt, B., Lesley, J., Bickel, U. and Pardridge, W. M. Targeting rat anti-mouse transferrin receptor monoclonal antibodies through blood-brain barrier in mouse. J Pharmacol Exp Ther 2000; 292: 1048-52.

GLOSSARY

Caveolae: Small, flask-shaped smooth plasmalemmal vesicles abundant in continuous endothelia lining the vasculature of many organs that play an important role in endocytosis and transcellular transport. By targeting caveolae, drugs or genes may be transported across the endothelial cell barrier to the underlying tissue cells.

Continuous endothelia: A type of capillary endothelium comprised of endothelial cells that lack fenestrations, have uniform intercellular spacing, a continuous basement membrane, and tight junctions between cells to form an unbroken barrier between the blood and the underlying tissue.

Endothelial heterogeneity: The molecular and morphological differences between endothelial cells derived from different organ vascular beds. These differences are influenced by the local tissue environment reflecting, and changing, according to the need of the underlying tissue and result in significant differences in endothelial cell barrier functions between various organs.

Endothelium: An attenuated layer of endothelial cells lining the blood vessels that forms a critical barrier whose function is to control the exchange of molecules from the blood to the underlying tissue.

MudPIT Multidimensional Protein Identification Technology: A relatively unbiased method for rapid and large- scale proteome analysis of whole cell lysates or membrane preparations via multidimensional liquid chromatography, tandem mass spectrometry, and database searching.

Proteomic analysis: the study of all proteins expressed in a cell type, organism, or specific subcellular location within a specified time frame, including the study of protein-protein interactions occurring in vivo.

Site-specific drug delivery: Exclusive and rapid delivery of drugs (or genes) to a particular intended target compartment, usually a specific tissue.

Tandem mass spectrometry (MS/MS): A technique for identifying proteins whereby individual tryptic peptides are fragmented and analyzed to gain amino acid sequence information that can be used to search a database of known protein sequences. Mass spectrometry combined with protein database searching is the major technology used for protein identification in proteomic analyses.

Transcytosis: The transport of molecules from the blood across continuous endothelium to the underlying tissue via vesicular transport mechanisms, transcellular channels or intercellular junctions.

Vascular targeting: A strategy for site-directed drug delivery that targets the accessible luminal endothelial cell surface of blood vessels that feed tissue cells rather than the tissue-cells themselves. This approach for targeting the vascular wall to the blood vessel surface in contact with the circulating blood can theoretically achieve much improved tissue-directed targeting in vivo.

Vesicular transport: The shuttling of molecules into and across the cell as packets of material enclosed within a small, membranous sac.

7

TARGETING PULMONARY ENDOTHELIUM

Vladimir R. Muzykantov
Department of Pharmacology, University of Pennsylvania School of Medicine, Philadelphia, PA 19104-6068

INTRODUCTION

The pulmonary endothelium maintains vital functions including control of thrombosis, inflammation, vascular permeability and blood pressure. Endothelial cells in the lung blood vessels are vulnerable to oxidative, thrombotic and inflammatory insults and represent an important target for therapies. However, despite the huge surface and high accessibility of this target to blood, only a minor fraction of circulating therapeutics is adequately delivered to the pulmonary endothelium. Effective, safe and specific delivery of drugs, enzymes and genetic materials to this target may help to improve current modalities in therapies and prophylaxis of pulmonary hypertension, oxidative stress, embolism, edema, acute lung injury, and other disease conditions.

Affinity carriers, such as monoclonal antibodies and endothelial surface determinants, may permit targeting and proper sub-cellular addressing of drugs in the pulmonary vasculature. Vascular immunotargeting may also provide secondary therapeutic benefits due to blocking of the target antigens, such as surface adhesion molecules involved in inflammation or angiotensin-converting enzyme involved in hypertension. This chapter describes features of the pulmonary endothelium as a therapeutic target, outlines principles, methodologies, the current status of vascular immunotargeting to the pulmonary endothelium, and gives specific examples of delivery systems that show promising results in pre-clinical animal studies.

Pulmonary Endothelium as a Therapeutic Target

Pulmonary endothelial cells, as well as the endothelium in other organs, form a cellular monolayer on the luminal surface of blood vessels and control vascular permeability, blood-tissue exchanges, blood pressure and fluidity, interactions between blood cells and tissues, as well as other important normal and pathological functions of the vascular system.

The endothelium produces and controls synthesis of agents that cause either vasorelaxation (e.g., nitric oxide, NO, and prostacyclin) or vasoconstriction (peptides, endothelin, angiotensin II, Ang II). Peptidases and proteases exposed on the surface of endothelial cells activate vasoactive pro-peptides. For example, angiotensin-converting enzyme, ACE, converts Ang I into Ang II and inactivates bradykinin and substance P (Erdos et al., 1990). Thus, blood perfusion through the lungs serves both gas exchange purposes and enables the conversion of numerous peptides that regulate blood pressure and vascular permeability.

The endothelium helps to prevent thrombosis. In concert with plasma protein C, endothelial transmembrane glycoprotein thrombomodulin converts thrombin into an anti-coagulant enzyme (Esmon, 1989). Among other anti-thrombotic factors, endothelium secretes NO that suppresses platelet aggregation as well as urokinase and tissue type plasminogen activators that dissolve blood clots via generation of a fibrin-degrading protease plasmin.

The endothelium controls inflammation, a process that is often intertwined with thrombosis. Under normal circumstances, endothelial cells provide very limited, if any, support for activities of pro-inflammatory cells (e.g., white blood cells). However, pathological mediators, including cytokines, reactive oxygen species, growth factors and abnormal shear stress, induce endothelial secretion of chemoattractants and exposure of adhesion molecules leading to leukocyte attraction, adhesion and transmigration (see schema of vascular inflammation in Chapter 2).

Endothelial cells play an important role in normal and pathological vascular redox mechanisms. They produce reactive oxygen species (ROS) including superoxide anion (O_2^-) and H_2O_2 via enzymatic pathways that can be further activated by pathological mediators. ROS apparently play an important role in cellular signaling. However, their overproduction leads to vascular oxidative stress, inactivation of NO by O_2^-, lipid peroxidation and tissue injury (Freeman and Crapo, 1987).

In the lungs, most of endothelial cells belong to the alveolar capillaries that are constitutively exposed to relatively high oxygen levels and vulnerable to pro-inflammatory and damaging effects of alveolar macrophages activated by inhaled agents (e.g., dust and pathogens). Pulmonary vasculature is a target of pathological remodeling and fibrosis associated with many forms of heart diseases, drug toxicity, radiation injury and primary pulmonary hypertension. Alveolar capillaries represent a filter, collecting activated leukocytes, metastasizing tumor cells and clots from the venous blood.

The pulmonary endothelium is affected by hyperoxia, hypertension, smoke, dust inhalation, pneumonia, cardiac failure, sepsis, thrombosis, diabetes, cancer and many other pulmonary and systemic disease conditions. Endothelial injury leading to a vicious cycle of pulmonary thrombosis, inflammation and edema underlies the pathogenesis of some forms of Acute Lung Injury (ALI) or Adult Respiratory Distress Syndrome (ARDS), a life-threatening condition associated with trauma, sepsis and hemorrhage that cause a high mortality.

Theoretically, adequate (i.e., effective, specific, safe and directed to a proper sub-cellular compartment) delivery of therapeutics (e.g., drugs, proteins or genes encoding these proteins) could improve treatment of these disease conditions. For example, targeting of NO-donors, NO-synthase or gene encoding NOS could be useful for treatment of pulmonary hypertension. In addition, targeting of anti-oxidant and anti-inflammatory agents might help to manage pulmonary oxidative stress and inflammation, whereas targeting of anti-thrombotic agents might prevent thrombosis or facilitate dissolution of thrombi.

Immunotargeting to the Pulmonary Endothelium: An Overview

The pulmonary vasculature is the first major capillary network encountered by drugs after intravenous injection. It contains roughly one third of endothelial cells in the body, filters the whole cardiac output of venous blood, and represents a privileged target for vascular drug delivery (Danilov et al., 2001). Thus, cationic liposomes and many viruses accumulate in the lungs due to blood filtration. It should be noted, however, that the specificity and safety of this strategy remain to be more rigorously characterized.

Unless drugs are coupled to high-affinity carriers, even after local infusion via vascular catheters, the perfusion removes drugs and their derivatives rapidly. Devices allowing a transient cessation of blood flow in the site of catheter placement have been designed in order to attain a high local concentration and a more effective prolonged interaction of the infused material with endothelium. However, blood flow interruption may lead to ischemia and vascular injury. The lack of a viable means for the effective, rapid, and safe targeting of therapeutic molecules to the endothelium represents an important biomedical problem.

Vascular immunotargeting, a strategy utilizing coupling of drugs to antibodies or antibody fragments to endothelial determinants, promises such a means of delivery of drugs and genetic materials to the pulmonary endothelium (Muzykantov, 1998). The requirements that should be met in order to achieve immunotargeting to pulmonary endothelium include the following:

- Target antigens should be abundant on the endothelium to permit robust targeting. When a transiently expressed antigen is used as a target, the identified time window should be adequate for drug delivery.

- Target antigens should not be present in blood or in non-endothelial cells that are accessible to blood. For example, endothelial cells have transferin receptors; however, they are also abundantly expressed in hepatic and other cells accessible to blood. Therefore, transferin-targeted drugs accumulate mostly in the liver (and, to some extent, in the brain, since cerebral endothelium is enriched in transferin receptors), with a relatively modest uptake in lungs. Plasma or blood cells' antigens' drug delivery detracts from delivery to the endothelium.

- The level of antigen expression by endothelial cells should not be suppressed upon conditions at which targeting is desirable.

- Depending on the therapeutic goal, an antibody-drug complex should be either retained on the cell surface or undergo trafficking to a proper sub-cellular compartment.

- The binding of antibody-drug complexes to an antigen should not cause harmful or uncontrolled side effects.

- Ideally, binding of an antibody-drug complex to a target antigen should cause therapeutically beneficial side effects.

- Theoretically, recognition of specific types of endothelial cells and even certain parts of an endothelial cell body is possible.

The results accumulated within the last decade indicate that monoclonal antibodies to angiotensin-converting enzyme, surface adhesion molecules, and caveoli-associated antigens represent potentially useful carriers for immunotargeting pulmonary endothelium. In the following sections, we briefly discuss methodology of the studies and several selected examples of the immunotargeting.

Methodological aspects of the vascular immunotargeting

Several experimental models are used to study targeting of the pulmonary endothelium. Endothelial cell cultures provide a useful model to determine the affinity of binding, mechanisms of intracellular uptake, and targeting effects under defined conditions with practically unlimited variables and number of measurements. Tracings of radiolabeled compounds, as well as fluorescent and electron-microscopy imaging, provide abundant and easily interpretable data (Figure 1, below). However, the identity of the cultivated cells to their counterparts *in vivo* is questionable (especially at high culture passages) and cells in culture lack adequate environmental factors such as extracellular matrix, physical stress, as well as neuronal and hormonal regulation.

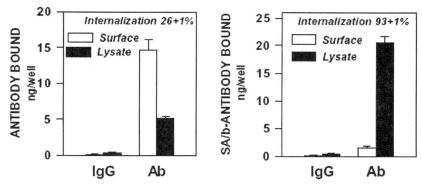

Figure 1. Binding and internalization of radiolabeled PECAM-1 monoclonal antibodies (left panel) and anti-PECAM streptavidin conjugates (SA/b-antibody, right panel) in human umbilical vein endothelial cell cultures (HUVEC). Analysis of the surface-associated and internalized radioactivity was performed using acidic glycin elution. Anti-PECAM and anti-PECAM/SA (both indicated as Ab), but not IgG counterparts specifically bind to the endothelial cells, which constitutively express PECAM. Anti-PECAM remains mostly associated with the cell surface whereas SA/b-anti-PECAM conjugate is internalized at 37°C (Adapted from Muzykantov et al, PNAS USA 1999, with permission, see comments in the section describing PECAM targeting).

Perfusion of isolated lungs represents a unique model that eliminates many artifacts of cell cultures and permits the use of diverse perfusion and ventilation conditions (variable flow rate, temperature, gases, and blood components) to study interactions of circulating agents with pulmonary endothelium in the absence of confusing systemic effects. This model allows confirmation of the specificity and kinetic parameters of the targeting, as well as identification of subcellular addressing of cargoes and effects of the targeting (Muzykantov et al., 1999; Danilov et al., 2001; see also Chapter 6 by Carver and Schnitzer).

Animal studies ultimately evaluate targeting under normal or pathological states. Injections of a mixture of immune and non-immune conjugates labeled with different isotopes (e.g., [125]Iodine and [131]Iodine) permit the most accurate measurement of several parameters of targeting (Figure 2). Percent of injected dose uptake in an organ (%ID) shows biodistribution in the body and robustness of delivery to a target organ. Secondly, %ID normalized per gram of tissue (%ID/g) permits comparison of uptake in different organs and tissue selectivity of the uptake. This parameter also permits comparison of the data obtained in different animal species. Ratio between %ID/g in an organ and in blood gives the Localization Ratio, LR. This parameter compensates for a difference in blood level of circulating radiolabeled antibody (e.g., due to different rate of uptake by clearing or target organs). The Immunospecificity Index (ISI) ratio of the pulmonary uptake of immune and non-immune counterparts provides the most objective measure of targeting specificity.

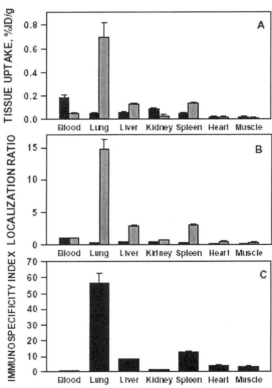

Figure 2. Distribution of ^{131}I-IgG (closed bars) and anti-PECAM/^{125}I-streptavidin (hatched bars) in the organs 1 hr post-systemic intravenous injection in pigs. A. Absolute values of the isotopes uptake normalized per weight. B. Ratio of radioactivity per gram of tissue to that in blood (Localization Ratio). C. Immunospecificity Index of anti-PECAM uptake in the organs calculated as ratio of LR for [125]Iodine and [131]Iodine. Note that the anti-PECAM conjugate, but not the non-immune control counterpart, preferentially accumulates in the lungs (Adapted from Scherpereel et al., JPET 2002, with permission).

SELECTED EXAMPLES OF PULMONARY TARGETING

No universal or ideal carrier that suits all therapeutic needs exists. Specific therapeutic goals require different secondary effects mediated by binding to the target, drug targeting to different populations of endothelial cells (e.g., resting *vs.* inflammation-engaged), and diverse cellular compartments. Table 1 shows endothelial determinants useful for experimental and, perhaps, therapeutic targeting pulmonary endothelium.

Table 1. Endothelial determinants: candidate targets. EC – endothelial cells, ACE – angiotensin-converting enzyme, TM - thrombomodulin, PECAM - platelet-endothelial adhesion molecule, ICAM - intercellular adhesion molecule; gp - glycoproteins.

Target	Function and Localization	Targeting Advantages	Potential Problems
ACE	Peptidase, converts Ang I into Ang II and cleaves bradykinin. ACE enriched in the lung capillaries.	Selective targeting to lung EC. Intracellular delivery. Vasodilating and anti-inflammatory effects of ACE inhibition.	Inflammation suppresses targeting. ACE inhibition may be dangerous.
TM	Binds thrombin and converts it into anti-coagulant enzyme. Enriched in the lungs.	Intracellular delivery to EC useful for modeling of lung injury in animals.	Inflammation suppresses targeting. Thrombosis due to TM inhibition.
PECAM	Facilitates transmigration of leukocytes. Stably expressed in EC borders.	Intracellular delivery of anti-PECAM conjugate may also suppress inflammation	PECAM-signaling and side effects are not understood
ICAM	Mediates leukocyte adhesion to EC. Stably expressed by EC, and up-regulated by pathological agents.	Similar to PECAM, but inflammation enhances targeting.	Similar to PECAM
E-selectin	Supports leukocytes adhesion. Expressed only on altered EC.	Intracellular targeting to EC in inflammation	Targeting is not robust. Transient expression.
P-selectin	Similar to E-selectin	Similar to E-selectin	Similar to above. Targeting platelets
gp90	Function unknown. Localized in EC cavoli.	Transendothelial targeting.	Human analogue and side effects are not known.
gp95	Function unknown. EC avesicular zone in alveolar capillaries.	Targeting to the EC surface	Similar to above
gp60	EC caveoli	Untested	Unknown

Angiotensin-converting enzyme (ACE)

Angiotensin-converting enzyme, a transmembrane glycoprotein expressed on the luminal surface of endothelial cells, is one of the key components of the renin-angiotensin system. Importantly, pulmonary vasculature is markedly enriched in ACE; nearly 100% endothelial cells in the alveolar capillaries are strongly positive for ACE, whereas only 10-15% of endothelial cells in the extra-pulmonary capillaries are ACE-positive (Danilov et al., 2001). In late eighties, Sergei Danilov and co-authors proposed utilizing anti-ACE as an affinity carrier for drug targeting to the endothelium and showed that radiolabeled anti-ACE accumulates selectively in the pulmonary vasculature after intravascular and intraperitoneal injections in rats, hamsters, cats and primates (Danilov et al., 1991; Muzykantov and Danilov, 1995). The following studies showed that endothelial cells internalize anti-ACE that may be used for intracellular drug delivery (Muzykantov et al., 1996a). Diverse reporter compounds and drugs (e.g., antioxidant enzyme catalase) conjugated with anti-ACE accumulate selectively in the lungs after intravenous injection in rats (Muzykantov and Danilov, 1995; Muzykantov et al., 1996b).

ACE converts Ang I into Ang II (Erdos, 1990), a potent vasoconstricting peptide that also has pro-oxidant and pro-inflammatory activities. On the other hand, ACE inactivates bradykinin, a peptide stimulating endothelial production of NO (see Figure 3 below), an important vascular mediator that causes relaxation of vascular smooth muscle cells and suppression of platelet aggregation. Superoxide anion produced by endothelial cells in response to pro-inflammatory agents (including Ang II), inactivates NO and generates peroxinitrite, a potent oxidant. Therefore, inhibition of ACE by anti-ACE causes vasorelaxation and attenuates inflammation and oxidative stress. This effect represents a potential secondary benefit of ACE immunotargeting in certain pathological settings. In patients with acute hemorrhaging and hypotension, this effect may be rather dangerous due to a high probability of causing vascular collapse.

Some ACE antibodies are inhibitory due to the blocking of the active site; yet even non-inhibitory antibodies may suppress ACE activity in the endothelium due to facilitation of its shedding from the plasma membrane. The latter effect is epitope-specific and varies for different monoclonal antibodies (Danilov, 1994; Balyasnikova et al., 2001). Theoretically, ACE antibodies against diverse epitopes may be used for either ACE-inhibiting or non-inhibiting immunotargeting of drugs, thus providing an additional flexibility to the strategy and further advancing its therapeutic applicability.

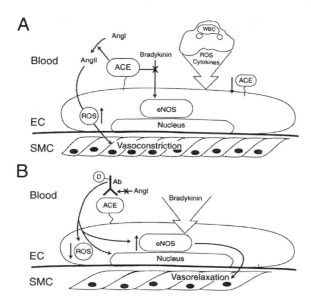

Figure 3. Immunotargeting to ACE (see explanations in the text). EC – endothelial cells, SMC – smooth muscle cells, eNOS – endothelial NO synthase, WBC – white blood cells; ROS – reactive oxygen species, Ab – monoclonal antibody (anti-ACE) conjugated with drugs (D). Panel A: ACE is normally expressed on the endothelial surface (left part), but inflammatory factors (e.g., ROS and cytokines released from activated leukocytes) down-regulate ACE surface density on endothelium (right part). Panel B: Anti-ACE delivers drugs to endothelium and undergoes internalization. This paradigm can be utilized for delivery of antioxidant enzymes (to intercept intracellular ROS) or genetic materials. In addition, anti-ACE inhibits ACE. This attenuates Ang I conversion, protects bradykinin (both of these effects lead to vasorelaxation), and suppresses pro-oxidative effects of Ang II.

Potential therapeutic applications of ACE targeting include intracellular delivery of active enzymes and genetic materials. For example, anti-ACE-conjugated catalase, an antioxidant enzyme that degrades H_2O_2, has been shown to accumulate in the perfused rat lungs and protect the pulmonary endothelium against oxidative stress (Atochina et al., 1998). Recently, ACE immunotargeting has been used for re-targeting of viruses to the pulmonary endothelium (see Chapter 9 by Reynolds and Danilov).

ACE immunotargeting is highly tolerable; anti-ACE does not induce acute harmful reactions in laboratory animals and human volunteers (Muzykantov and Danilov, 1995). One potential problem associated with targeting ACE is that endothelial expression of ACE is suppressed upon many pathological states, including hyperoxia, inflammation, oxidative stress and sepsis (likely due to effects of the cytokines, ROS and other pro-inflammatory factors) (Muzykantov and Danilov, 1995). This effect may compromise the robustness of therapeutic targeting to ACE. However, ACE is one of the premier candidate targets for drug delivery to the pulmonary endothelium, for example, for a prophylactic use.

Platelet-Endothelial Cell Adhesion Molecule (PECAM-1)

PECAM is a pan-endothelial, immunoglobulin superfamily transmembrane glycoprotein, which is predominantly localized in the sites of cellular contacts in the endothelial monolayer. Platelets and white blood cells also express PECAM, but in lesser quantities. The larger portion of the PECAM molecule (extracellular domain) in endothelial cells is exposed to the lumen and serves as a counterpart for leukocytes, thus supporting their transendothelial migration in the sites of inflammation (Newman, 1997). In addition to this function, as documented in many experimental models (Vaporcyian et al, 1993), PECAM apparently may be involved in endothelial signaling and activation, but this aspect of its function remains to be better understood (Newman, 1997).

PECAM is abundant in endothelial cells that express millions of binding sites for anti-PECAM (Muzykantov et al., 1999). In addition, PECAM is a stable endothelial antigen; cytokines and ROS do not down-regulate its expression and surface density on the endothelial cells. These features suggest that PECAM-targeted drug delivery will be robust and can be used for either prophylaxis or therapies, i.e., drug delivery to either normal or pathologically altered vasculature (see Figure 4 below).

Initial studies revealed that although endothelial cells in culture avidly bind anti-PECAM, the antibodies poorly accumulate in the animal lungs after intravenous administration. In addition, endothelial cells did not internalize anti-PECAM. However, anti-PECAM conjugation (e.g., by streptavidin cross-linker) provides multimeric anti-PECAM complexes that are readily internalized by endothelial cells (see Figure 1) and accumulate in the animal lungs after vascular administration (see Figure 2) (Muzykantov et al., 1999). Size of the anti-PECAM conjugates controls their intracellular uptake: neither monomolecular anti-PECAM, nor large (>500 nm diameter) conjugates undergo internalization. Conjugates within 100-300 nm size range are readily internalized by endothelium (Wiewrodt et al., 2002).

This paradigm, facilitation of the internalization and pulmonary targeting by forming 100-300 nm anti-PECAM conjugates, has been employed to achieve an effective, intracellular targeting of diverse cargoes to endothelial cells in cell cultures, perfused rat lungs and in intact animals. For example, an active reporter enzyme, beta-galactosidase conjugated to anti-PECAM, has been shown to accumulate intracellularly in the pulmonary endothelium as soon as 10 min after intravenous injection in mice and pigs (Scherpereel et al, 2002). Anti-PECAM/DNA conjugates provide specific transfection of endothelial cells in culture (Wiewrodt et al., 2002) and in animals (Li et al., 2000).

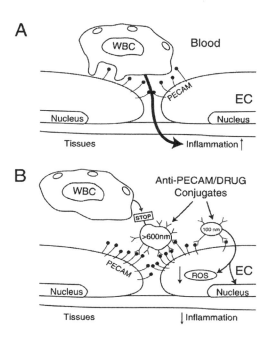

Figure 4. Immunotargeting to PECAM-1 (see explanations in the text). WBC – white blood cells, EC – endothelial cells; ROS – reactive oxygen species. Panel A. PECAM-1 constitutively expressed by endothelium, predominantly in the intercellular contacts, supports WBC transmigration and facilitates inflammation in the tissues. Panel B: Large (>600 nm diameter) anti-PECAM conjugates poorly internalize in the endothelial cells, whereas smaller counterparts (100-300 nm diameter) enter the cells and can be used for intracellular delivery of genetic materials and anti-oxidant enzymes to detoxify ROS. In addition, anti-PECAM conjugates may suppress inflammation via blocking WNC transmigration.

Glucose oxidase (GOX, an enzyme generating H_2O_2 from glucose) has been conjugated to anti-PECAM and tested in cell cultures and mice. In both models, the conjugate demonstrated highly effective and specific binding to the endothelium, internalization, generation of H_2O_2 inside the cell, and acute oxidative stress that lead to a severe edematous lung injury in mice (Christofidou et al, 2002). This result, targeting of active ROS-generating enzymes *in vivo*, confirms that vascular immunotargeting to constitutive endothelial antigens provides biologically significant effects. In addition, anti-PECAM/GOX can be used to model oxidative stress and vascular pulmonary injury in laboratory animals (Christofidou et al., 2002). Theoretically, targeting of GOX or other ROS-generating enzymes to the antigens presented on tumor cells or in the tumor vasculature promises a complementary approach for tumor eradication.

Potential therapeutic applications of anti-PECAM targeting are similar to that of ACE: intracellular delivery of enzymes and genetic materials. For example, anti-PECAM-conjugated catalase binds to endothelial cells, enters the cells, protects them against oxidative stress and accumulates in animal lungs after intravenous injection (Muzykantov et al., 1999). The pilot studies showed that anti-PECAM/catalase affords significant protective effects in animal models of oxidative stress including acute lung transplantation injury, likely due to attenuation of the ischemia/reperfusion syndrome. However, pending applications anti-PECAM and anti-ACE strategies are not identical: the former can be used for both prophylaxis and therapy (including pathological conditions that suppress ACE targeting). In addition, blocking of PECAM-mediated leukocyte extravasation may suppress inflammation, thus providing an important secondary therapeutic benefit in certain groups of patients.

Inter-Cellular Adhesion Molecule, ICAM-1

ICAM-1 (CD54) is an Ig superfamily surface glycoprotein with a short cytoplasmic domain, a transmembrane domain, and a large extracellular domain (Diamond et al., 1990). It is constitutively expressed by the endothelium at a relatively high surface density ($2x10^4$-$2x10^5$ copies per cell). Other cell types also express ICAM (e.g., alveolar epithelial cells, macrophages); however, the major fraction of ICAM accessible to the bloodstream is exposed by the luminal surface of endothelium. Pathological stimuli, such as ROS, cytokines, abnormal shear stress, and hypoxia, stimulate expression of ICAM by the endothelium and thus elevate the ICAM surface density in pulmonary vasculature.

As a counter-receptor for integrins, ICAM supports leukocytes' firm adhesion to the endothelium and facilitates inflammation. In addition, ICAM serves as a natural ligand for certain viruses and serves as a signaling molecule; yet the exact mechanisms, specificity, and significance of this signaling in different cell types remains to be more fully understood. Antibodies (including humanized murine mAbs) directed against ICAM-1 (anti-ICAM) suppress leukocyte adhesion, thus producing anti-inflammatory effects in animal models and clinical pathological settings associated with vascular injury, such as acute inflammation, ischemia/reperfusion, and oxidative stress (DeMeester et al., 1996).

Accumulating data indicate that: (a) ^{125}I-anti-ICAM binds to endothelium *in vivo*; (b) accumulates in highly vascularized organs (first of all, lungs); and (c) inflammation facilitates both processes (Panes et al., 1995; Villanueva et al., 1998). Therefore, ICAM-1 is a good candidate determinant for drug targeting to normal and inflammation-engaged endothelia, especially in the lungs. The published data on *in vivo* effects of anti-ICAM conjugates are rather limited. However, in the model of isolated perfused rat lung, catalase conjugated with anti-ICAM provides a protective effect similar to that of catalase conjugate with anti-ACE (Atochina et al., 1998).

The data on anti-ICAM internalization is fragmentary and controversial. Several laboratories reported that the epithelium and leukocytes internalize ICAM ligands, while data from other groups implies that other cell types internalize anti-ICAM rather poorly (Almenar-Queralt et al., 1995; Mastrobatista et al., 1999). Our preliminary data indicate that the endothelium poorly internalizes monomeric anti-ICAM, as well as large (>500 nm diameter) anti-ICAM conjugates, while 100-300 nm conjugates are internalized via a mechanism that resembles anti-PECAM conjugates uptake. The pilot results show that large anti-ICAM/tissue-type plasminogen activator conjugates accumulate in the lungs, are retained on the endothelial surface, and facilitate fibrinolysis in the pulmonary vasculature.

Collectively, the available data reveal important unique features of ICAM as a target and suggest that anti-ICAM can be used for targeted delivery of diverse drugs to the endothelium:

i)   ICAM-1 is presented on the endothelial surface at high density and easily accessible to drugs circulating in the bloodstream, while its level in blood (i.e., plasma ICAM) is low, thus permitting a robust and specific binding of anti-ICAM conjugates to endothelium in the vasculature.

ii)   Endothelial ICAM-1 is stably expressed and, in contrast with other constitutive endothelial surface antigens, its surface density is increased in pathological conditions. Thus, one could anticipate an effective or even facilitated targeting to pathologically altered endothelium.

iii)   Inhibition of ICAM-1 function by targeting (blockage of leukocyte adhesion to endothelium) may suppress inflammation, a benefit for treatment of vascular oxidative and thrombotic stress. The anti-inflammatory effect of anti-ICAM conjugates may be even more potent.

iv)   Depending on the size of anti-ICAM conjugates, they may target
        active cargoes either to the endothelial surface (e.g., plasminogen
        activators) or to the intracellular compartment (e.g., catalase).

Anti-ICAM is reported to deliver liposomes and other cargoes to the
vascular endothelium (Atochina et al., 1998; Bloeman et al., 1998; Villanueva
et al., 1998). The preliminary data from our laboratory strongly suggest that
anti-ICAM can deliver fibrinolytics to the surface of the pulmonary
endothelium for facilitation of anti-thrombotic potential of the pulmonary
vasculature in cases of high risk of thromboembolism.

Endothelial selectins

Two types of selectin molecules are found in the endothelium: E- and
P-selectins. Both types serve as counterparts for specific sugars on the white
blood cells and support the first phase of their adhesion ("rolling") to the
endothelial cells in the sites of inflammation. Selectin molecules are not
normally expressed on the luminal surface in the vasculature. Resting
endothelial cells store P-selectin in the intracellular vesicles (i.e., Weibel-
Palade bodies) and do not synthesize E-selectin. However, pathological
mediators stimulate rapid mobilization of P-selectin to the endothelial surface,
as well as synthesis and surface expression of E-selectin.

These determinants theoretically may provide a good means for
specific targeting of drugs to the inflammation-engaged endothelium.
Radiolabeled E-selectin antibodies accumulate in the sites of vascular
inflammation (Keelan et al., 1994). Most likely, the targeting might produce a
secondary anti-inflammatory effect due to blocking of leukocyte rolling, yet
this hypothesis has yet to be proven in animal models. Importantly, E-selectin
is an internalizable molecule (Kujpers et al., 1994) that permits intracellular
uptake of the targeted conjugates liposomes and viruses (Spragg et al., 1997;
Harrari et al., 1999). A relatively low surface density of selectins on the
surface of activated endothelial cells, the transient nature of their expression,
and presence of P-selectin on platelets has generated concerns about the
robustness, applicability, and specificity of the targeting. However, targeting
selectins represents an exciting and promising area that is discussed in some
detail in Chapters 8 and 20.

Thrombomodulin, caveoli-associated antigens and other determinants

Thrombomodulin (TM) is a transmembrane endothelial glycoprotein
that binds thrombin, and, in concert with protein C, changes thrombin

substrate specificity and thus converts it from a pro-coagulant enzyme into an anticoagulant one that inactivates coagulation factors (Esmon, 1989). Endothelial cells in the pulmonary capillaries are rich in thrombomodulin, which apparently plays an important role in anti-thrombotic protection of the lung vasculature that collects blood clots from the venous circulation. Steve Kennel and co-authors explored monoclonal antibodies against thrombomodulin as an affinity carrier for targeting the pulmonary endothelium and reported that anti-TM diverse cargoes, including radiolabels and liposomes, accumulated in the murine lungs (Maruyama et al., 1990). However, targeting compromises thrombomodulin function and might predispose or even provoke thrombosis (Christofidou et al., 2002). Therefore, clinical application of anti-TM is questionable due to obvious safety concerns related to the pulmonary thrombosis, yet this delivery system has an important application as an animal model.

Caveoli represent a specialized domain in the endothelial plasma membrane involved in intracellular and trans-cellular trafficking, cellular signaling, and sensing of flow. The pulmonary endothelium is rich in caveoli; several caveoli-associated antigens are being explored as potential determinants for the targeting and intracellular delivery of therapeutic cargoes. One such determinant is gp60, or endothelial albumin-binding protein. Malik and co-workers found that binding of ligands to this protein induces internalization and may permit intracellular delivery (Tirrupati et al., 1997). Schnitzer and co-workers have produced a monoclonal antibody against another caveoli-associated antigen, gp90, (McIntosh et al., 2002) that binds to endothelial cells in the rat pulmonary vasculature, enters the cells, and provide intracellular and trans-cellular targeting of radiolabels and tracer cargoes (see Chapter 6 by Carver and Schnitzer). Theoretically, targeting caveoli represents an exciting avenue that may extend targeting towards sub-endothelial layers, pending identification of functions and human counterparts of these proteins, as well as validation of the targeting and effects of therapeutic agents in animal models.

Recently, a novel endothelial surface determinant, a transmembrane glycoprotein gp85, has been found in a unique area of pulmonary capillary endothelium, namely, the avesicular zone – a thin part of an endothelial cell that lacks major organelles and, together with the thin Type I alveolar epithelium and the basal membrane, separates alveolar and vascular compartments (Ghitescu et al., 1999). Interestingly, a monoclonal antibody against this determinant displays very selective and robust accumulation in the pulmonary vasculature in rats without significant internalization (Murciano et al., 2001). Therefore, this determinant might be considered as a target for the pulmonary delivery of anti-thrombotic agents. However, the function, human counterpart, therapeutic and side effects of targeting gp85 remain to be characterized in order to evaluate its applicability for the targeting pulmonary endothelium.

There are several other endothelial surface determinants identified in the pulmonary vasculature, including Thy-1.1 antigen (Danilov et al., 2001). However, their functions and the effects of targeting remain to be addressed in order to evaluate whether they can be used for targeting.

CONCLUSIONS AND PERSPECTIVES

The pulmonary endothelium represents an important therapeutic target. Many endothelial determinants that are potentially useful for drug delivery have been identified recently using diverse methodologies, including administration of radiolabeled monoclonal antibodies and phage display library *in vivo* (Danilov et al., 1991; Muzykantov et al., 1996; Rayotte et al., 1997; Muzykantov, 1998; Danilov et al., 2001; McIntosh et al., 2002). Some determinants, such as ACE, ICAM and PECAM, can be used for targeting either normal (i.e., prophylaxis) or pathologically altered (i.e., therapy) endothelium, whereas selectins permit specific recognition of pathological endothelium. Targeting caveoli provides an exciting avenue for intracellular and transcellular targeting in the pulmonary vasculature, whereas modulation of the antibody-drug conjugate size provides a novel paradigm for control of intracellular uptake and trafficking of the cargoes. Targeting of active reporter and therapeutic cargoes, including enzymes, genes and viruses, has been recently achieved in intact animals, thus providing a good basis for pre-clinical evaluation of the strategy. Many targeting systems promise unique advantages for delivery of specific therapeutic agents in diverse clinical settings and, therefore, must be carefully tested in terms of the robustness, effectiveness, specificity and effects of the targeting (including the effects mediated by intervention in the functions of target determinants). Based on the current progress rate in the field, it would be not too unrealistic to expect that immunotargeting to the pulmonary endothelium will be in the clinical studies during this decade.

ACKNOWLEDGEMENTS

This work was supported by NIH SCOR in Acute Lung Injury (NHLBI HL 60290, Project 4), NHLBI RO1 (HL/GM 71175-01) and the Department of Defense Grant (PR 012262).

REFERENCES

1. Almenar-Queralt A, Duperray A, Miles LA, Felez J, Altieri DC. Apical topography and modulation of ICAM-1 expression on activated endothelium. *Am.J.Pathol.* 1995;147:1278-88.
2. Atochina EN, Balyasnikova IV, Danilov SM, Granger DN, Fisher AB, Muzykantov VR. Immunotargeting of catalase to ACE or ICAM-1 protects perfused rat lungs against oxidative stress. *Am. J. Physiol.* 1998;275:L806-L817.
3. Balyasnikova IV, Karran EH, Albrecht RF II, and Danilov SM (2002) Epitope-specific antibody-induced cleavage of angiotensin-converting enzyme from the cell surface. *Biochem. J.* 362:585-595
4. Bloemen PG, Henricks PA, van Bloois L, van den Tweel MC, Bloem AC, Nijkamp FP, Crommelin DJ, Storm G. Adhesion molecules: a new target for immunoliposome-mediated drug delivery. *FEBS Lett.* 1995;357:140-4.
5. Christofidou-Solomidou M, Kennel S, Scherpereel A, Wiewrodt R, Solomides CC, Pietra GG, Murciano JC, Shah SA, Ischiropoulos H, Albelda SM, Muzykantov VR. Vascular immunotargeting of glucose oxidase to the endothelial antigens induces distinct forms of oxidant acute lung injury: targeting to thrombomodulin, but not to PECAM-1, causes pulmonary thrombosis and neutrophil transmigration. *Am J Pathol.* 2002;160:1155-69.
6. Danilov SM, Muzykantov VR, Martynov AV, Atochina EN, Sakharov I, Trakht IN, Smirnov VN. Lung is the target organ for a monoclonal antibody to angiotensin-converting enzyme. *Lab Invest.* 1991;64:118-24.
7. Danilov, S., E.Atochina, H.Hiemish, T.Churakova, A.Moldobayeva, I.Sakharov, G.Deichman, U.Ryan, and V.R.Muzykantov. 1994. Interaction of monoclonal antibody to angiotensin-converting enzyme (ACE) with antigen *in vitro* and *in vitro* and *in vivo:* antibody targeting to the lung induces ACE antigenic modulation. *Intern. Immunol.*, 6:1153-1160
8. Danilov SM, Gavrilyuk VD, Franke FE, Pauls K, Harshaw DW, McDonald TD, Miletich DJ, Muzykantov VR. Lung uptake of antibodies to endothelial antigens: key determinants of vascular immunotargeting. *Am J Physiol Lung Cell Mol Physiol.* 2001;280:L1335-47.
9. Diamond MS, Staunton DE, de Fougerolles AR, Stacker SA, Garcia-Aguilar J, Hibbs ML, Springer TA. ICAM-1 (CD54): a counter-receptor for Mac-1 (CD11b/CD18). *J Cell Biol.* 1990;111:3129-39.
10. DeMeester SR, Molinari MA, Shiraishi T, Okabayashi K, Manchester JK, Wick MR, Cooper JD, Patterson GA. Attenuation of rat lung isograft reperfusion injury with a combination of anti-ICAM-1 and anti-beta2 integrin monoclonal antibodies. *Transplantation.* 1996;62:1477-85.
11. Erdos E. (1990) Angiotensin-converting enzyme and the changes of our concept through the years. *Hypertension*, 16:363-370
12. Esmon C. (1989) The role of protein C and thrombomodulin in the regulation of blood coagulation. *J.Biol.Chem.*, 264:4743-4746
13. Everts M., R.J.Kok, S.A.Asgierdottir, B.N.Melgert, T.J.M.Moolenaar, G.A.Konig, M.A.Van Luyn, D.K.F.Meijer, G.Molema (2002) Selective intracellular delivery of dexamethasone into activated endothelial cells using an E-selectin-directed immunotargeting. *J.Immunol.*, 168:883-889
14. Ghitescu, L., B.Jacobson and P.Crine. 1999. A novel, 85-kDa endothelial antigen differentiates plasma membrane macrodomain in lung alveolar capillaries. *Endothelium*, 6:241-250
15. Freeman B and Crapo JD (1987) Free radicals and tissue injury. *Lab Invest* 47:412-426

16. Harari OA, Wickham TJ, Stocker CJ, Kovesdi I, Segal DM, Huehns TY, Sarraf C, Haskard DO. Targeting an adenoviral gene vector to cytokine-activated vascular endothelium via E-selectin. *Gene Ther.* 1999;6:801-7.

17. Keelan ET, Harrison AA, Chapman PT, Binns RM, Peters AM, Haskard DO. Imaging vascular endothelial activation: an approach using radiolabeled monoclonal antibodies against the endothelial cell adhesion molecule E- selectin. *J Nucl Med.* 1994;35:276-81.

18. Kuijpers TW, Raleigh M, Kavanagh T, Janssen H, Calafat J, Roos D, Harlan JM. Cytokine-activated endothelial cells internalize E-selectin into a lysosomal compartment of vesiculotubular shape. A tubulin-driven process. *J Immunol.* 1994;152:5060-9.

19. Li S, Tan YD, Viroonchatapan E, Pitt BP and Huang L (2000) Targeted gene delivery to pulmonary endothelium by anti-PECAM antibody. *Am J Physiol Lung Cell Mol Physiol* **278**:L504-L511

20. Maruyama K., Kennel S, and Huang L. (1990) Lipid composition is important for highly efficient target binding and retention of immunoliposomes. *Proc.Natl.Acad.Sci.USA*, 87:5744-5748

21. Mastrobattista E, Storm G, van Bloois L, Reszka R, Bloemen PG, Crommelin DJ, Henricks PA. Cellular uptake of liposomes targeted to intercellular adhesion molecule-1 (ICAM-1) on bronchial epithelial cells. *Biochim Biophys Acta.* 1999;1419:353-63.

22. McIntosh DP, Tan XY, Oh P, Schnitzer JE. Targeting endothelium and its dynamic caveolae for tissue-specific transcytosis *in vivo*: a pathway to overcome cell barriers to drug and gene delivery. *Proc Natl Acad Sci U S A.* 2002;99:1996-2001.

23. Murciano JC, Harshaw DW, Ghitescu L, Danilov SM, Muzykantov VR. Vascular immunotargeting to endothelial surface in a specific macrodomain in alveolar capillaries. *Am J Respir Crit Care Med.* 2001;164:1295-302.

24. V.Muzykantov and S.Danilov (1995) Targeting of radiolabeled monoclonal antibody against ACE to the pulmonary endothelium. *Targeted delivery of imaging agents* (V.Torchilin, Ed.) CRC Press, Boca Raton, Fl., 465-485

25. Muzykantov VR, Atochina E, Kuo A, Barnathan E, Notarfrancesco K, Shuman H, Dodia C and Fisher AB (1996a) Endothelial cells internalize monoclonal antibody to angiotensin-converting enzyme. *Am J Physiol (Lung Cell Mol Physiol 14)* 270:L704-L713

26. Muzykantov VR, Atochina E, Ischiropoulos H, Danilov S and Fisher AB (1996b) Immunotargeting of antioxidant enzymes to the pulmonary endothelium. *Proc Natl Acad Sci USA* 93:5213-5218

27. Muzykantov VR (1998) Immunotargeting of drugs to the pulmonary vascular endothelium as a therapeutic strategy. *Pathophysiology* 5:15-33

28. Muzykantov VR, Christofidou-Solomidou M, Balyasnikova I, Harshaw DW, Schultz L, Fisher AB, Albelda SM. Streptavidin facilitates internalization and pulmonary targeting of an anti-endothelial cell antibody (platelet-endothelial cell adhesion molecule 1): a strategy for vascular immunotargeting of drugs. *Proc Natl Acad Sci USA.* 1999; 96:2379-84.

29. Newman, P.J. 1997. The Biology of PECAM-1. *J.Clin.Invest.*, 99(1):3-7

30. Panes J, Perry MA, Anderson DC, Manning A, Leone B, Cepinskas G, Rosenbloom CL, Miyasaka M, Kvietys PR, Granger DN. Regional differences in constitutive and induced ICAM-1 expression *in vivo. Am J Physiol.* 1995;269:H1955-64.

31. Rajotte, D., W.Arap, M.Hagedorn, E.Koivinen, R.Pasqualini and E.Ruoslahti. 1998. Molecular heterogeneity of the vascular endothelium revealed by *in vivo* phage display. *J.Clin.Invest.*, 102:430-437

32. Scherpereel A, Rome JJ, Wiewrodt R, Watkins SC, Harshaw DW, Alder S, Christofidou-Solomidou M, Haut E, Murciano JC, Nakada M, Albelda SM,

Muzykantov VR. Platelet-endothelial cell adhesion molecule-1-directed immunotargeting to cardiopulmonary vasculature. *J Pharmacol Exp Ther.* 2002;300:777-86.

33. Spragg DD, Alford DR, Greferath R, Larsen CE, Lee KD, Gurtner GC, Cybulsky MI, Tosi PF, Nicolau C, Gimbrone MA, Jr. Immunotargeting of liposomes to activated vascular endothelial cells: a strategy for site-selective delivery in the cardiovascular system. *Proc Natl Acad Sci U S A.* 1997;94:8795-800.
34. Tiruppathi, C., W.Song, M.Bergenfeldt, P.Sass and A.B.Malik. 1997. gp60 activation mediates albumin transcytosis in endothelial cells by tyrosine kinase-dependent pathway. *J.Biol.Chem.*, 272:25968-25975
35. Vaporician, A.A., DeLisser, H.M., Yan, H.C., Mendiguren, I., Thom, S.R., Jones, M.L., Ward, P.A., Albelda, S.M. 1993. Platelet-endothelial cell adhesion molecule-1 (PECAM-1) is involved in neutrophil recruitment *in vivo. Science,* 262:1580-1582
36. Villanueva FS, Jankowski RJ, Klibanov S, Pina ML, Alber SM, Watkins SC, Brandenburger GH, Wagner WR. Microbubbles targeted to ICAM-1 bind to activated coronary artery endothelial cells. *Circulation.* 1998;98:1-5.
37. Wiewrodt R, Thomas AP, Cipelletti L, Christofidou-Solomidou M, Weitz DA, Feinstein SI, Schaffer D, Albelda SM, Koval M, Muzykantov VR. Size-dependent intracellular immunotargeting of therapeutic cargoes into endothelial cells. *Blood.* 2002; 99:912-22.

GLOSSARY

Alveolar capillaries: Small (5-25 micron diameter) blood vessels surrounding pulmonary alveoli that are involved in gas exchange and metabolization of vasoactive peptides. The alveolar endothelium is a privileged vascular target that represents roughly 30% of total endothelial surface in the human body.

Angiotensin-converting enzyme (ACE): A transmembrane endothelial glycoprotein, an ectopeptidase that controls activity of vasoactive peptides angiotensin and bradykinin. ACE is a candidate determinant for targeting pulmonary endothelium.

Angiotensin I and II: An octapeptide Ang II, produced by ACE from a decapeptide Ang I, induces vasoconstriction and exerts pro-oxidant activity.

Bradykinin: A vasoactive peptide that elevates endothelial permeability and stimulates endothelial production of NO.

Catalase: An enzyme that detoxifies H_2O_2 and could be used as a drug. One of the candidate therapeutic cargoes for vascular immunotargeting to protect the endothelium and treat an acute pulmonary oxidative stress.

Caveoli: A specialized cholesterol-rich domain in the endothelial plasma membrane that forms characteristic flask-shape invaginations and serves as sensing, signaling and endocytotic compartments. Caveoli represent a unique and highly promising target for endothelial drug delivery.

Intercellular adhesion molecule-1 (ICAM-1): A transmembrane endothelial glycoprotein that facilitates leukocytes' adhesion. ICAM-1 is a candidate determinant for targeting pulmonary and systemic endothelium

Localization Ratio: The ratio between the uptake of a drug or a reporter molecule in an organ of interest and its blood level. Comparison of this parameter in different organs and tissues helps to characterize tissue selectivity of the targeting.

Nitric Oxide, NO: A small gaseous molecule produced by endothelial cells that diffuses in blood and vascular tissues and exerts strong vasorelaxing and anti-thrombotic properties.

Platelet-Endothelial Adhesion Molecule-1 (PECAM-1): A transmembrane endothelial glycoprotein that facilitates leukocytes' transmigration from blood to tissues. PECAM-1 is a candidate determinant for targeting pulmonary and systemic endothelium.

Reactive oxygen species (ROS): Pro-oxidant molecules such as superoxide anion and H_2O_2 that are produced in the vasculature normally at low levels. Massive overproduction of ROS under pathological conditions causes oxidative stress and tissue injury.

Selectins: Selectins P and E are surface adhesion molecules involved in leukocyte adhesion to the endothelium, transiently expressed on the surface of pathologically altered endothelial cells, for example, in inflammation foci. The selectins represent candidate determinants for selective targeting pathological endothelium.

Thrombomodulin (TM): A transmembrane endothelial glycoprotein that indirectly suppresses coagulation and thus helps to prevent intravascular thrombosis. The pulmonary endothelium is enriched in TM that can be useful for experimental targeting; yet clinical applications of TM antibodies are questionable due to potential thrombosis.

Vascular immunotargeting: A strategy for delivery of therapeutics to vascular cells (e.g., endothelium) using antibodies or their fragments as affinity carriers.

8

TARGETING INFLAMMATION

Jonathan R. Lindner [1,2] Alexander L. Klibanov[1,2] and Klaus Ley[1,3]
[1]*Cardiovascular Research Center,* [2]*Division of Cardiology, and* [3]*Department of Biomedical Engineering, University of Virginia*

INTRODUCTION

To target sites of inflammation for diagnostic or therapeutic purposes, suitable molecular targets, target-binding molecules, coupling mechanisms and vehicles must be considered. The current technology for detecting sites of inflammation uses isolated, radiolabeled neutrophils and gamma imaging (1). This method is cumbersome because it requires obtaining blood from the patient to isolate and short-term culture neutrophil, radiolabeling (usually with [99m]Technetium) and intravenous injection of the radiolabeled cells in order to detect their accumulation in the inflamed tissue by gamma camera imaging. There is potential for inadvertently introducing infectious agents, and the use of radioactivity is undesirable for certain groups of patients. Hence, radiolabeled neutrophils are rarely used as a primary diagnostic tool and are reserved as a method for cases in which the inflammatory focus cannot be found by other means. Consequently, inflammatory sites are not routinely imaged or treated with targeted agents.

The need for targeting sites of inflammation is based on both diagnostic and therapeutic considerations. In recent years, many cardiovascular diseases including atherosclerosis, myocardial infarction and stroke have been identified as essentially inflammatory in nature, secondary to the influx of oxidized lipids in the case of atherosclerosis and to the ischemic insult in the cases of myocardial infarction, and stroke. Although the inflammatory response after ischemia is the beginning of the healing process, unchecked influx of inflammatory cells can cause as much or more damage than the original insult. Diagnostically, it would be desirable to image the extent and size of an infarct or stroke. Some therapeutic interventions for post-ischemic inflammation are available and experimental treatments are under investigation. Some therapeutic agents would benefit from being applied in a targeted fashion because they have undesired systemic side effects including immunosuppression, or because they are expensive to produce. Many recent clinical trials of anti-adhesion molecule therapies have been disappointing, possibly because of the lack of targeted delivery. It would also be of interest to detect atherosclerotic plaque, potentially distinguishing between stable and vulnerable plaque. If a vulnerable plaque is detected, it could be treated by percutaneous coronary intervention or aggressive treatment of risk factors before it ruptures.

Targeting inflammation is also useful for inflammation outside cardiovascular indications. For example, in rheumatoid and other forms of arthritis it is often difficult to objectively assess the effect of therapeutic interventions until much later, when bone and cartilage manifestations are evident by X-ray. Contrast agents targeted to sites of inflammation could provide a significant diagnostic tool and could also improve the power of clinical trials of new therapeutic interventions. Crohn's disease is a chronic relapsing disease that causes immense suffering in approximately 1 million patients, most of them young or middle-aged. A contrast agent targeting the inflamed wall of the small intestine could provide a diagnostic tool far more powerful and less invasive than the currently used barium enemas or colonoscopy. The indication for surgical intervention could be determined before the patient presents with complications, or surgery may be prevented entirely by just-in-time treatment with steroids, antibiotics, or antibodies to tumor necrosis factor-α (TNF-α).

From these examples, it is clear that targeting inflammation is desirable for both diagnostic and therapeutic reasons. The remainder of this chapter will focus on the principles and the specifics of such targeting. Beginning with the identification of suitable molecular targets, we will discuss the specific example of ultrasound contrast agents, successful targeting strategies, coupling chemistry, and prospects for drug and gene delivery for therapeutic purposes.

ENDOTHELIAL ADHESION MOLECULES

Suitable targets for imaging or treating inflammation must be accessible from the vascular system. This includes inducible endothelial adhesion molecules. Some of these molecules are selectively expressed in certain inflammatory sites, and others are generally expressed at most or all sites of inflammation. Both classes can be used for targeting, depending on the intended area of delineation or treatment. Inducible endothelial adhesion molecules are particularly suitable because many of them are expressed at very low levels on resting endothelium, providing excellent specificity and selectivity (for example, E-selectin), and many are expressed at robust levels of hundreds of thousands of copies per endothelial cell (for example, intercellular adhesion molecule-1, ICAM-1). Other surface molecules may also be considered as targets, like secreted and surface-bound chemokines or G-protein coupled receptors. Surface-bound chemokines may not be anchored firmly enough in the endothelial glycocalyx to support adhesion of diagnostic or therapeutic particles under flow, although this has not been tested systematically. G-protein coupled receptors are usually expressed at low copy numbers and present little sequence on the outside of the cell. No successful targeting to such agents has been reported, and hence these molecules will not be considered here. However, it is possible that future advances of targeting technology may make such molecules practical targets.

During inflammation, a wide variety of cell-cell interactions are important, including leukocyte-leukocyte, leukocyte-endothelium, leukocyte-platelet, leukocyte-vascular smooth muscle cell, leukocyte-extracellular matrix, and leukocyte-interstitial cell interactions. The proteins mediating these interactions, adhesion molecules, belong to four major families: (i) selectins; (ii) selectin ligands; (iii) integrins; and (iv) members of the immunoglobulin family (2). The function of these adhesion molecules is to promote and regulate leukocyte recruitment from the vasculature into tissue through a series of events, including leukocyte rolling along the endothelial cell surface, firm adhesion and activation, and extravasation into the tissue. The expression of the adhesion molecules relevant to inflammatory cell recruitment is regulated at several levels including transcription, translation, surface expression, proteolytic modification, glycosylation, sulfation, and conformational changes. Most known endothelial leukocyte adhesion molecules are preferentially or exclusively expressed on the venular endothelium (3, 4). This means that targeting to endothelial adhesion molecules will usually result in accumulation of the targeted carriers in postcapillary venules, but not in capillaries or arterioles. In addition, the expression of endothelial adhesion molecules varies among organs, possibly allowing targeting to organ-specific inflammatory processes.

Selectins

Activated endothelial cells express P-selectin and E-selectin. Selectins have in fact been proposed for targeting liposomes to sites of inflammation (5), although binding was only tested in vitro and no animal or patient data are available. In vivo, mild surgical trauma is sufficient to cause mast cell degranulation leading to increased expression of P-selectin on the endothelial surface (3). The inflammatory reaction in response to tissue trauma is reduced with time, but does not disappear completely. This inflammatory response is mild, leading to a transient increase in the number of intravascular leukocytes due to rolling and (some) firm adhesion. In some tissues like the skin, P-selectin is constitutively expressed on the surface of venules (6) even without tissue trauma. In atherosclerotic vessels (7), P-selectin is expressed near the shoulder region of the lesions and appears to be involved in monocyte recruitment into the vessel wall. Injection of radiolabeled antibodies showed a six-fold up regulation of P-selectin in the lung, nine-fold in pancreas, and six- to 12-fold in the mesenteric microcirculation in response to systemic injection of TNF-α in mice. This method reports the sum total of P-selectin expressed on the endothelial surface and activated platelets. P-selectin was also found upregulated by bacterial lipopolysaccharide (LPS) in the mesentery, small intestine, caecum, and colon and by allergic inflammation in striated muscle, but not in skin microcirculation (8). Recently, P-selectin was successfully used as a targeting molecule, directing ultrasound contrast microbubbles to inflamed kidney following ischemia and reperfusion (9).

E-selectin is expressed on inflamed endothelial cells in response to treatment with inflammatory cytokines (10). In mice, E-selectin expression is often, but not always associated with P-selectin expression (8). E-selectin is constitutively expressed in skin microvessels (11), which could potentially interfere with targeted delivery via E-selectin. Liposomes coated with sialyl Lewis^x, a tetrasaccharide that binds to E-selectin, were used to target liposomes to cultured endothelial cells and deliver antisense oligonucleotides (12). A study using radiolabeled antibodies to E-selectin found eight-fold upregulation in the lung, six-fold in the heart, and 10- to 20-fold in the mesenteric circulation after injection of TNF-α in mice. Upregulation of E-selectin was also found in response to LPS, ischemia-reperfusion injury, and an ovalbumin-induced model of allergic inflammation (8). In the latter model, E-selectin upregulation was seen in microvessels in the skin, but not in striated muscle (8). These examples may serve to emphasize that precise knowledge of the induced expression of adhesion molecules at the intended site and under the inflammatory conditions to be probed is necessary to optimize targeted delivery to sites of inflammation.

Inflamed endothelial cells also express ligand function for L-selectin expressed on most leukocytes. However, the identity of this molecule has remained elusive and is not suitable for targeting at this time. None of the L-selectin ligands found in high endothelial venules of peripheral lymph nodes are expressed in inflamed venules.

Immunoglobulin-like adhesion molecules

Leukocyte adhesion and transmigration are mediated by integrins and members of the immunoglobulin superfamily (2). Inflamed endothelial cells express several members of the immunoglobulin superfamily of type I transmembrane proteins, which have a series of repeating extracellular IgG-like domains, a transmembrane region, and a short cytoplasmic tail. Endothelial adhesion molecules in this family include intercellular adhesion molecules-1 and -2 (ICAM-1, -2), platelet endothelial cell adhesion molecule-1 (PECAM-1), and vascular cell adhesion molecule-1 (VCAM-1). The expression of VCAM-1 and ICAM-1 increases after stimulation of endothelium by inflammatory cytokines (13); PECAM-1 and ICAM-2 are constitutively expressed on resting endothelial cells.

ICAM-1 (CD54) is expressed on endothelial cells even under baseline conditions, both in vitro and in vivo. Expression is upregulated by interleukin-1 (IL-1), TNF-α or LPS, and the expression increase is further enhanced by interferon-gamma (IFN-γ) (2). This pattern would suggest that ICAM-1 expression is highest during inflammation regulated by T-helper-1 (Th1) lymphocytes, because IFN-γ is a Th1 cytokine. ICAM-1 has been used as an experimental target for imaging agents, both in magnetic resonance imaging (MRI) (14) and ultrasound (15) applications.

VCAM-1 (CD106) shows little or no expression on endothelial cells outside the bone marrow under baseline conditions. Endothelial expression of VCAM-1 is highly upregulated in many inflammatory diseases including arthritis, ileitis, colitis, psoriasis, diabetes, and hypercholesterolemia. VCAM-1 is a very attractive molecule for targeted delivery because it shows a high dynamic range and a high level of expression. However, targeting of contrast agents or drug delivery vehicles to VCAM-1 has not been reported so far.

MAdCAM-1 is a transmembrane protein and constitutively expressed in the intestine, colon, Peyer's patch, and mesenteric lymph nodes. In addition, MAdCAM-1 expression can be significantly enhanced by administration of inflammatory cytokines like IL-1 or TNF-α. MAdCAM-1 is the main ligand for $\alpha_4\beta_7$ integrin and may also bind L-selectin. MAdCAM-1 expression on peripheral lymph node HEV is lost in late fetal to early neonatal life, but is maintained in Peyer's patch HEV, mesenteric lymph nodes and on endothelial cells of lamina propria venules. MAdCAM-1 is also expressed in chronically inflamed venules of the choroid plexus and the pancreatic endothelium, which suggests possible targeting to inflamed brain stem and inflamed pancreas.

$\alpha_v\beta_3$ integrin

The integrin $\alpha_v\beta_3$ was initially identified as a receptor for vitronectin and is widely distributed in vascular tissues. $\alpha_v\beta_3$ is expressed on endothelial cells, especially during active angiogenesis, and smooth muscle cells, on T-cells, neutrophils, and on monocyte-derived macrophages. $\alpha_v\beta_3$ is a very promiscuous integrin with a rather relaxed binding specificity. Ligands include vitronectin, fibrinogen, fibronectin, thrombospondin, osteopontin, von Willebrand factor, and several collagens. Characteristically, all these ligands carry the RGD tripeptide sequence, which is recognized by $\alpha_v\beta_3$. $\alpha_v\beta_3$ is involved in a variety of functions within the vasculature including cell adhesion, proliferation, and migration.

ATHEROSCLEROTIC LESIONS

Atherosclerotic lesions are attractive targets for imaging agents or therapeutic interventions, with particular interest in targeting vulnerable plaque to prevent a heart attack or stroke. In human atherosclerotic lesions, strong expression of P-selectin was detected on the endothelium overlying active atherosclerotic plaques but not on normal arterial endothelium or on endothelium overlying inactive fibrous plaques (7). Expression of ICAM-1 was detected on endothelial cells, macrophages, and smooth muscle cells of plaques with an increase after vascular injury. Normal arterial endothelial cells and intimal smooth muscle cells outside plaques gave weaker or negative reactions. Unlike E-selectin and ICAM-1, VCAM-1 staining of surface endothelium only occurred in fibrous and lipid-containing plaques.

Expression of adhesion molecules was also detected on established lesions in animal models of atherosclerosis. Hypercholesterolemia induced atherosclerotic lesion formation in rabbits, as well as LDL-receptor-deficient (LDLR-/-) and apolipoprotein E-deficient (apoE-/-) mice. Immunohistochemical staining revealed that VCAM-1 and ICAM-1 were expressed in endothelial cells at and adjacent to lesion borders (44). In aortas of normal chow-fed wild-type mice and rabbits, VCAM-1 and ICAM-1, but not E-selectin, were expressed by endothelial cells in regions predisposed to atherosclerotic lesion formation. En face confocal microscopy of the mouse ascending aorta and proximal arch demonstrated that VCAM-1 expression was increased on the endothelial cell surface in lesion-prone areas. By contrast, ICAM-1 expression extended into areas protected from lesion formation. When mice were fed a western diet to cause hypercholesterolemia, VCAM-1 was expressed in groups of endothelial cells in lesion-prone sites in apoE-/- mice, but not control mice.

Taken together, these findings suggest that VCAM-1 and P-selectin have potential as targets for directed delivery of contrast agents and therapeutic agents to atherosclerotic lesions. The knowledge of quantitative adhesion molecule expression is insufficient at this time to predict whether and how vulnerable plaque could be targeted successfully.

ADHERENT LEUKOCYTES

Inflammation is characterized by the accumulation of white blood cells in postcapillary venules and in the inflamed tissue. Although the latter are not readily accessible to targeted contrast agents, the former present adhesion molecules to the blood compartment that can be used for targeted delivery. In acute inflammation, most adherent leukocytes are neutrophils. Although they express hundreds of surface markers, adhesion molecules and a few other highly expressed molecules are the most attractive targets, because they exist in sufficient copy numbers and present a sufficiently large extracellular protein domain to be useful for docking. Importantly, the issue of regulated expression is not of key importance here, because the presentation is regulated at the level of leukocyte-endothelial interactions. Therefore, even constitutively expressed leukocyte antigens are potentially good targets to specifically delineate inflamed areas.

Leukocyte integrins

The β_2 class of integrins is specifically expressed on leukocytes and leukocyte-derived microglia cells. The four known β_2 integrins share a common β_2-chain (CD18) and four different α-chains termed α_L (CD11a), α_M (CD11b), α_x (CD11c), and α_D (CD11d). This results in the formation of four different heterodimers: LFA-1 ($\alpha_L\beta_2$), Mac-1 or CR3 ($\alpha_M\beta_2$), p150.95 ($\alpha_x\beta_2$) and $\alpha_D\beta_2$.

LFA-1 or lymphocyte function-associated antigen ($\alpha_L\beta_2$ integrin) is expressed on virtually all mature leukocytes. LFA-1 binds ICAM-1, -2 and -3, which belong to the immunoglobulin superfamily of adhesion molecules. Binding of LFA-1 to its various ligands is dependent on its activation state. In non-activated leukocytes, LFA-1 is in a resting, non-adhesive state. Activation of leukocytes by agonists that bind to diverse receptor classes can increase the adhesiveness of LFA-1 and other β_2 integrins.

Mac-1 or complement receptor 3 (CR3) is expressed on mature neutrophils, monocytes, macrophages, NK cells and certain subsets of T- and B-lymphocytes. Mac-1 is stored in secretory granules and transported to the cell surface upon activation with a variety of stimuli. Mac-1 is the most promiscuous of the integrins and can bind a large number of different ligands including complement C3bi. C3bi binding leads to complement-triggered phagocytosis of the cell by neutrophils or macrophages. Mac-1 also interacts with elements of the coagulation system such as coagulation factor Xa and fibrinogen. p150.95 ($\alpha_x\beta_2$) is minimally expressed on neutrophils and $\alpha_D\beta_2$ is not expressed.

Both LFA-1 and Mac-1 are expressed at high copy numbers approaching or exceeding 50,000 per activated neutrophil. The broad ligand specificity of Mac-1 includes denatured proteins, specifically denatured albumin. Therefore, albumin-shelled microbubbles bind to adherent leukocytes via Mac-1 (18). This is desirable for targeting sites of inflammation, but also creates increased background when other disease processes are targeted.

Neutrophils also express several complement receptors. Phospholipid-shelled ultrasound contrast agents bind to adherent neutrophils through a complement-dependent mechanism that requires C3 (18). The precise nature of the neutrophil complement receptor involved was not identified. Other possible targeting molecules expressed on leukocytes include Fc receptors, P-selectin glycoprotein ligand-1 (PSGL-1), and L-selectin. Since most L-selectin is lost by proteolytic shedding upon leukocyte activation and adhesion, this molecule may not be a suitable target for imaging or therapeutic agents.

The $\alpha_4\beta_1$ integrin (VLA-4) is highly expressed on T-lymphoblastoid cell lines. α_4 also associates with β_7 subunits to form $\alpha_4\beta_7$ integrin. $\alpha_4\beta_1$ integrin (VLA-4) is expressed on hematopoietic stem cells, monocytes, eosinophils, NK cells, lymphocytes, and (at low levels) on neutrophils. VLA-4 is the major monocyte adhesion molecule responsible for their accumulation at atherosclerosis-prone sites. The expression pattern of α_4 integrins suggest that they could be potential targets for imaging certain forms of inflammation including conditions involving eosinophil or monocyte accumulation, but no therapeutic or diagnostic targeting to α_4 has been reported so far.

PLATELETS

At sites of inflammation, activated platelets can accumulate, predominantly through platelet P-selectin binding to leukocyte PSGL-1. Platelets are not specific markers of inflammation, because thrombi also contain activated platelets that present P-selectin to the blood compartment. Platelets express the integrin $\alpha_{IIb}\beta_3$. Integrin $\alpha_{IIb}\beta_3$ is expressed at high levels and could be a target for delivery to sites of thrombus formation and inflammation.

IMAGING INFLAMMATION WITH CONTRAST ULTRASOUND

There has been substantial progress in the development of methods for non-invasively imaging adhesion molecule expression and leukocyte recruitment using contrast-enhanced ultrasound. Ultrasound imaging relies on the transmission and reception of acoustic energy. Sound can be defined as a wave or a series of cyclic pressure changes that result in compression and rarefaction of the medium insonified. Sound waves may be characterized in terms of the amplitude of the pressure fluctuations, the wavelength of each cycle, and the cycle frequency. The product of the latter two factors describes the sound wave velocity through tissue or a medium. Ultrasound is sound at a frequency of >20,000 cycles per second (20 kHz), just above the audible range for humans. For diagnostic applications, ultrasound is usually generated at frequencies of 1-12 MHz as continuous or pulsed waves by a beam-forming piezoelectric transducer. Returning signals received by the same transducer are digitally processed and displayed according spatial orientation, amplitude, and frequency information. Ultrasound has been applied in the clinical setting for over 3 decades for the real-time assessment of anatomy, function of certain organs (such as the contractile function of the heart), and blood flow within large vessels or the cardiac chambers.

Contrast-enhanced ultrasound relies on the detection of microbubble contrast agents for the enhancement of the blood pool and for the assessment of microvascular perfusion in organs amenable to ultrasound imaging.

Microbubbles generally have a mean diameter of 2-4 μm, which allows them to transit the microcirculation unimpeded. Most agents in clinical use possess an outer shell composed of lipids, denatured albumin, monosaccharides, or polymers (such as polylactides or cyanoacrylate). Encapsulation improves the intravascular stability of microbubbles. Many of the agents contain gases such as perfluorocarbons and sulfur hexafluoride, which imparts further stability by their low diffusion and solubility constants.

Most microbubbles are compressible by acoustic pressure waves and possess a diameter smaller than the wavelength of ultrasound. Because of these characteristics, microbubbles oscillate within the ultrasound field by alternate compression and expansion during pressure peaks and nadirs, respectively. Microbubble resonance results in the emission rather than just reflection of acoustic energy. When acoustic power is high, microbubble oscillation becomes non-linear, meaning that the microbubble size is non-linearly related to the pressure. Non-linear responses produce harmonic frequencies, which are multiples of the transmitted frequency. Since non-linear responses from tissue are minimal, filtering all received signals except those that at a harmonic frequency have been shown to markedly enhance the signal-to-noise ratio for microbubble contrast agents. At very high acoustic powers, exaggerated microbubble oscillations result in not only strong harmonic signals but also in microbubble destruction.

Microbubbles have been considered ideal contrast agents for the assessment of perfusion since they are pure intravascular tracers and their rheology in the microcirculation is very similar to that of red blood cells. In tissue that is injured or inflamed, certain albumin and lipid-shelled microbubbles may not behave like red cells and may instead be retained within the microcirculation. This behavior was first noted by persistent myocardial contrast effect during imaging of myocardium injured either by ischemia and reperfusion, or by hyperkalemic crystalloid cardioplegic solutions (19). Although in vitro flow studies with cultured endothelial cells have demonstrated that albumin microbubbles can attach to the extracellular matrix of activated endothelial cells, direct in vivo observations of the microcirculation with intravital microscopy indicate that microbubble persistence in injured tissue is due primarily to their attachment to activated leukocytes adherent to the venular endothelium (Figure 1) (18). Both albumin and lipid microbubbles bind to leukocytes in skeletal muscle following ischemia-reperfusion injury or exposure to pro-inflammatory cytokines such as TNF-α (18). The number of albumin or lipid microbubbles retained correlates with the extent of inflammation determined by the number of adherent leukocytes, indicating that quantitative assessment of inflammation may be possible by the intensity of the acoustic signal.

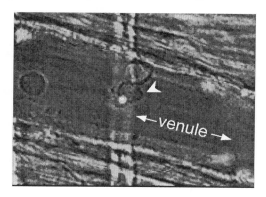

Figure 1. Intravital microscopy images of a venule from the cremaster muscle of a mouse treated with TNF-α demonstrating a fluorescein-labeled albumin microbubble (white) attaching to one of several activated leukocytes adherent to the venular endothelium (arrowhead). From (18) with permission.

Flow cytometry of suspensions of microbubbles mixed with leukocytes have been used to determine the mechanisms responsible for their interactions. The leukocyte β_2-integrin Mac-1 (CD11b/CD18) that binds to immunoglobulin receptors on the endothelium and is known to bind denatured albumin, is primarily responsible for attachment of microbubbles with shells composed of albumin to neutrophils and monocytes (18). In genetically engineered mice deficient for Mac-1 (CD-18 knockout mice), in vivo retention of albumin microbubbles is almost entirely inhibited. For lipid microbubbles, circulating complement proteins become activated and deposited on the shell surface (opsonization), and are then recognized by complement receptors primarily on the surface of neutrophils and monocytes (18). While the mechanisms of attachment for albumin and lipid microbubbles may differ, they both require cell surface expression of specific receptors that occurs upon leukocyte adhesion in the microvessels of regions of inflammation.

Enhancement of microbubble retention in inflamed tissue has been achieved by altering the lipid shell constituents in order to increase the avidity of microbubbles for activated leukocytes. This has been accomplished by the addition of a small amount of phosphatidylserine (PS) to the lipid shell. This strategy was inspired by PS-mediated macrophage recognition and reticuloendothelial clearance of apoptic or senescent cells. Anionic phospholipids such as PS are actively sequestered to the inner leaflet of the cell membrane of viable eukaryotic cells. Translocation of PS to the outer leaflet of the membrane is one of the first manifestations of apoptosis. Recognition of the presence of PS on the cell surface triggers attachment and subsequent phagocytosis by macrophages or, for blood cells, clearance from the circulating blood pool by the reticuloendothelial system. There are a variety of mechanisms by which the presence of PS can potentially trigger macrophage recognition including amplification of classical pathway opsonization, direct interactions with scavenger receptors, thrombospondin-mediated binding of α_v-integrins, or interactions with non-complement serum proteins such as β_2-glycoprotein I. The presence of PS in the membranes of lipid microbubbles has similarly been shown to enhance their retention within inflamed tissue due to increased avidity for activated leukocytes (20). The strong ultrasound signal enhancement that results from retention of PS-containing microbubbles has been used to assess post-ischemic inflammatory responses in the kidney and in the myocardium.

Similar to apoptotic cells, microbubbles that attach to leukocytes in regions of inflammation are phagocytosed within minutes (21), (Figure 2). These microbubbles remain intact for >20 minutes. Since the generation of an ultrasound contrast signal relies on microbubble oscillation, the degree of damping from the surrounding cellular milieu becomes an important issue for the detection of phagocytosed microbubbles. Optical observations of microbubble responses to ultrasound have demonstrated that despite their phagocytosis, microbubbles may still oscillate and be destroyed with high acoustic power ultrasound, although at a rate slower than that of free microbubbles (21). Destruction implies oscillation and, hence, generation of an acoustic signal from these microbubbles.

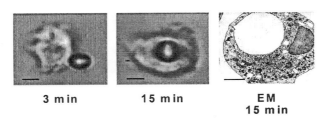

3 min   **15 min**   **EM**
                                    15 min

Figure 2. Light microscopy and electron microscopy (EM) images demonstrating attachment (3 min) and phagocytosis (15 min) of intact lipid microbubbles by activated neutrophils. Scale bars = 2.5 μm. From (18) with permission.

Ultrasound contrast agents can also be retained in inflamed tissue by targeted them to activated endothelial cells. Targeting in this fashion has been achieved by conjugating ligands for endothelial cell adhesion molecules to the surface of microbubbles or other acoustically active microparticles. This strategy is particularly attractive since endothelial cell adhesion molecules are expressed in relatively high concentrations within the vessel lumen during inflammation, and are either not expressed or are expressed at very low levels under normal conditions. Moreover, microbubbles should not be phagoyctosed, which may result in a stronger ultrasound signal than leukocyte-targeted agents.

Ultrasound contrast agents have been targeted to inflammation by covalent conjugation of monoclonal antibodies against ICAM-1 to the shell of perfluorocarbon gas-filled lipid microbubbles (22). In a perfusion chamber, these microbubbles have been shown to bind to activated cultured endothelial cells with minimal attachment to non-activated cells. A similar strategy has been investigated using acoustically-active liposomes composed of small non-gaseous multilamellar lipid vesicles. Monoclonal antibodies against ICAM-1 have been conjugated to the surface of these liposomes and the in vivo binding capacity and resulting acoustic signal for this agent have been evaluated in an inflammatory carotid atherosclerotic model in pigs (15). After their direct intra-arterial injection, anti-ICAM-1 liposomes attach to the endothelium overlying atherosclerotic plaques. Since the inflammatory phenotype of endothelium at sites of atherosclerosis may be valuable for predicting vulnerability of plaque rupture, these findings may be important for the development of a method to assess prognosis based on vessel phenotype.

The ability to detect early inflammatory responses in vivo with intravenous injection of microbubbles has been demonstrated with an agent targeted to endothelial P-selectin (9). For this purpose, antibodies against P-selectin were conjugated to lipid microbubbles using a polyethyleneglycol (PEG) molecular spacer, which improves binding affinity. Each 2-4 µm microbubble contains over 30,000 antibody molecules conjugated to the shell surface. Intravital microscopy has revealed abundant retention of P-selectin-targeted microbubbles in inflamed tissue due to their direct attachment to the endothelial surface. Targeting to the endothelial cell adhesion molecule results in about 4-5 fold greater retention of microbubbles than strategies that rely on attachment to activated leukocytes (9). Endothelial inflammatory responses have been evaluated with renal ultrasound and P-selectin-targeted microbubbles following ischemia-reperfusion injury of the kidney (9). The main limitation for molecular imaging of inflammation with microbubbles targeted against P-selectin or any other specific adhesion molecule is that leukocyte retention still occurs and contributes to a small portion of the contrast signal. To counter this problem, shell modifications such as augmentation of the protective PEG coat are being made to decrease microbubble-leukocyte interactions. There are also limitations for targeting strategies that employ the use of antibodies or antibody fragments, the most important of which include cost and immunogenicity. The feasibility of targeting by conjugating oligopeptide ligands to the shell surface has been demonstrated. Preliminary studies with microbubbles bearing oligopeptides containing the RGD motif recognized by the glycoprotein IIb/IIIa receptor on platelets suggest that this agent can be used for the contrast enhancement of thrombi (23). Imaging endothelial inflammatory changes in a similar manner, such as using small glycoprotein ligands for selectins, may be possible.

In summary, a variety of strategies of have been used to create microbubble ultrasound contrast agents targeted to regions of inflammation. These strategies are schematically depicted in Figure 3 and rely on either chemical alteration of the microbubble shell which enhances microbubble-leukocyte avidity, or conjugation of specific ligands to the microbubble surface that bind cell surface molecules expressed in the inflammatory response on leukocytes, endothelial cells, and platelets. Future efforts will likely be directed towards creating new imaging methods to specifically detect the signal from microbubbles retained within inflamed vessels, and for characterizing the potential clinical uses of these agents in specific disease processes.

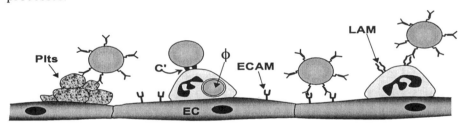

Figure 3. Schematic depicting potential mechanisms used to target microbubble contrast agents to inflammation. Strategies involve conjugation of ligands to the shell surface that recognize leukocytes adhesion molecules (LAM), endothelial cell adhesion molecules (ECAM), platelet (Plt) integrins, or an alteration of the microbubble shell to amplify complement (C') mediated attachment to activated leukocytes and subsequent phagocytosis (φ).

MAGNETIC RESONANCE IMAGING OF INFLAMMATION

The basis for magnetic resonance imaging (MR) imaging is the detection of radiofrequency signals generated by magnetic alignment and relaxation of the hydrogen nuclei in water. Non-contrast-enhanced magnetic resonance imaging has been used for more than a decade to indirectly assess the spatial extent of acute and chronic inflammatory disorders. This method relies on the detection of regional differences in signal on T2-weighted imaging caused by tissue edema. Limitations of this application are that the degree of edema is not predictably related to the severity of the inflammatory response, and that acute changes in the degree of inflammation in response to therapy cannot be quantified. Accordingly, newer methods are under investigation.

MR imaging with paramagnetic contrast agents has been used to assess the presence and spatial extent of active inflammation. Paramagnetic agents produce a contrast effect by locally altering proton relaxation in a magnetic field, with most effecting predominantly T2 shortening. Gadolinium-diethylenetriamine pentaacetic acid (Gd-DTPA) is the most widely used agent and is readily diffusible, owing to its small size and hydrophilic properties. Gd-DTPA signal enhancement on MR imaging is greater in regions of inflammation due to both increased capillary permeability and to interstitial edema that occurs in response to histamine, serotonin, bradykinin, and many of the pro-inflammatory cytokines. Interstitial edema expands the non-vascular extracellular compartment where Gd-DTPA can reside and delays diffusion of the tracer back into the vascular compartment. The delay in vascular reuptake provides a means to specifically detect inflammation by delayed imaging after contrast administration. The hyperemic response associated with acute inflammation may further increase Gd-DTPA contrast enhancement by augmenting the microvascular blood volume. Although Gd-DTPA-enhanced MR imaging has been used in experimental studies to detect and follow inflammatory conditions such as viral myocarditis, its clinical utility is hampered by some of the same limitations as non-contrast-enhanced MR.

MR with paramagnetic contrast agents containing iron oxide have also been used to image inflammatory processes. Superparamagnetic iron oxide (SPIO) particles are large (>50 nm) so that they remain within the vascular compartment and are rapidly taken up by the reticuloendothelial system. Their smaller counterparts, ultrasmall particles of iron oxide (USPIO) have a mean diameter of around 18 nm and, hence, are not recognized as readily by the reticuloendothelial system and can exit the vascular compartment. Although it is likely that selective accumulation of USPIO in inflamed tissue is in part related to increased endothelial permeability, histology of atherosclerotic plaques has revealed macrophage uptake of these particles (24). These findings suggest that USPIO signal in regions of inflammation, which can be detected days after intravenous administration of the agent, depends on phagocytic cell recognition. In animal models of hyperlipidemia, MR signal from accumulated USPIO has provided a means to detect inflamed atherosclerotic aortic plaques with high spatial resolution (24).

MR contrast agents with greater specificity for pathologic molecular processes have been developed using antibody targeting of paramagnetic contrast agents. One strategy has relied on the direct coupling of Gd-DTPA to monoclonal antibodies against cell surface integrins. A second strategy that has similarities to the microbubble targeting technique relies on the conjugation of monoclonal antibodies to the surface of 300-350 nm liposomes that contain gadolinium-lipid complexes.

Potential advantages of the liposome approach include greater binding affinity for the particles and greater signal afforded for any single binding event.   One of the initial applications of antibody-targeted paramagnetic contrast agents has been for the detection of $\alpha_v\beta_3$ integrin expressed in tumor neovessels (25).   Successful characterization of tumor phenotype with MR imaging suggests that similar approaches may be capable of detecting endothelial expression of adhesion molecules that are more central to leukocyte recruitment.

RADIONUCLIDE IMAGING OF INFLAMMATION

Radionuclide imaging techniques have been providing information on the presence and spatial distribution of inflammation longer than any other non-invasive imaging technique. Accumulation of radiopharmaceuticals at sites of inflammation has been accomplished by many different strategies. Some early methods have relied on the injection of ^{67}Gallium that exits the intravascular space in regions of inflammation and binds to leukocyte-associated lactoferrin and bacterial siderophores. More specific leukocyte targeting has been accomplished by ex vivo labeling of leukocytes with ^{99m}Technetium (^{99m}Tc) or ^{111}Indium (^{111}In). The routine use of all of these agents in the clinical arena has been limited by several drawbacks including long study duration, non-specific uptake in non-inflamed organs, high blood pool activity, and the expense and safety concerns associated with radiopharmaceuticals.   Ex-vivo labeling techniques are also hampered by the cumbersome leukocyte tagging protocols and unstable conjugation. These limitations have provided the impetus to develop non-radionuclide inflammation imaging techniques as well as new radionuclide contrast agents.

One promising new radionuclide imaging strategy involves isotope labeling of oligopeptides or small proteins that bind to leukocyte cell surface receptors in vivo. Examples of this strategy include the use of [99m]Tc- or [123]Iodine-labeled analogues of cytokines or chemoattractants, such as IL-1, IL-2, IL-8, platelet factor-4, and fMLP (26, 27). An example of uptake of a ^{99m}Tc-labeled agent targeted to the leukotriene-B$_4$ receptor expressed by activated neutrophils in a myocardial region injured by ischemia and reperfusion is shown in Figure 4.

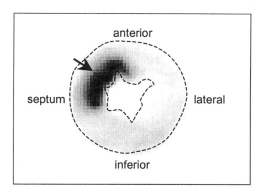

Figure 4. Short-axis images through the mid-left ventricle (cavity devoid of signal in the center) illustrating the spatial extent of enhancement of inflammation by radionuclide imaging with technetium-labeled agent targeted to the leukotriene-B4 receptor on leukocytes in a dog following ischemia and reperfusion of the left anterior descending coronary artery.

Although the signal enhancement from these agents in inflamed tissue is favorable, their application in humans is currently limited due concerns regarding systemic inflammatory responses, neutropenia, and high levels of non-specific uptake in the liver, spleen, kidneys, and bladder. Alternate methods for in vivo leukocyte-targeting that have much less potential for pro-inflammatory effects have been developed using radionuclide-labeled monoclonal antibodies or Fab' fragments against CD-15 and CD-66 (27). Although these agents appear safe, there still appears to be somewhat limited by non-specific uptake.

Experience with radionuclide targeting for endothelial adhesion molecules is currently still very preliminary. Monoclonal antibodies against E-selectin or oligopeptides that mimic the E-selectin glycoprotein ligand have labeled with technetium and tested in animal models of arthritis (28). Scintigraphic imaging has demonstrated uptake of these agents specifically within inflamed joints. However, spatial resolution with these and other radionuclide imaging techniques is still quite limited.

DRUG AND GENE DELIVERY BY ULTRASOUND CONTRAST AGENTS

Drugs can be attached to or incorporated into a targeted particle so that the drug (a biopolymer, enzyme, large or small molecule) may be then targeted to the areas of interest. Microbubble agents offer a key potential advantage over the classical drug delivery schemes, because the drug can be activated or released by an externally applied ultrasound field. The microbubbles with the drug are allowed to circulate through the target area or are concentrated in the target area via a selective ligand-receptor interaction. Then, a focused ultrasound field is applied, and rapidly vibrating bubbles are supposed to release the drug and, hopefully, facilitate drug passage into the tissue (in a manner similar to sonophoresis).

Incorporating the drug payload in the microbubble

There are several ways of outfitting a microbubble with a drug (depending on the nature of both). Because the inside core of a microbubble is occupied with gas, it is not possible to incorporate a drug inside that space. The drug is therefore placed within the shell or attached to the shell directly or indirectly. If a bubble is coated with a lipid monolayer shell, a hydrophobic drug can simply be added as a shell component (29). This results in a rather limited load of a drug per unit of bubble surface and low overall drug concentration. To improve the drug load, a thicker shell can be created (e.g., containing oil, which would also dissolve the drug component (30). However, a drug might be hydrophilic so it cannot be simply incorporated into the shell. In that case, it can be attached to the shell, for instance via a nonspecific adsorption technique (as suggested for protein-based PESDA microbubbles, which bind antisense oligonucleotides (31). Charge interaction is used widely for plasmid DNA attachment. In that case, a positively charged lipid component is added to the microbubble shell (usually, the same material as used in lipofection reagents), and negatively charged plasmid is easily and firmly bound to the surface of microbubbles upon mixing (32). The term "sonoporation" was suggested to describe ultrasound-assisted transfection.

The most promising design is the combination approach: a drug is incorporated into the liposomes, and the liposomes are attached to the microbubble surface (31). In the latter example, a hydrophilic drug may be entrapped inside the aqueous space of the liposomes, and released into the surrounding media due to the rapid movement of the microbubble surface during the application of the ultrasound field.

Targeted ultrasound-assisted drug delivery requires a high level of drug at the target, with minimal toxic effect of the drug towards normal non-target tissues. If the drug is nontoxic and inexpensive, it would not make sense to use expensive microbubble preparation and ultrasound activation to achieve the same effect as could be reached by simply increasing the drug dose. If the drug is toxic and only a small percentage of the administered dose is delivered into the target tissue, the improvement of target-to-nonspecific ratio may justify the use of a drug delivery system. Targeted delivery is most appropriate if the drug substance is costly, nontoxic and inactive in the absence of ultrasound activation, so that it is metabolized in the non-target tissues, and only capable of exercising its function after sonic activation. An example of the latter approach is plasmid DNA delivery with microbubbles and ultrasound-mediated transfection for the purpose of gene therapy.

Microvascular effects and potentiation of ultrasound action in the presence of microbubbles

Ultrasound has long been considered one of the safest diagnostic imaging modalities. Indeed, as compared with X-ray, which uses external ionizing radiation, or nuclear medicine, which requires radiotracer sources of ionizing radiation injected in the organism, sound waves seem to be quite harmless. However, strict limitations were applied in the design and implementation of ultrasound imaging equipment. The ultrasound energy emitted by the transducer should never exceed the suggested safety limits. If the presence of microbubbles modifies the interaction of ultrasound with tissues, changes the level of ultrasound energy absorption in the tissue, or creates some other effects that may be used for drug targeting/delivery purposes or tissue ablation, different energy levels may be necessary and appropriate. There are now a number of experimental studies that confirm the potentiating effect of microbubbles on the interaction of ultrasound and biological tissues.

The action of high-intensity sound waves, such as used in lithotripsy procedures to break kidney stones, is known to be potentiated in the presence of microbubbles (even first-generation air-filled microspheres such as Albunex). The action of ultrasound pulses with several MPa of peak pressure (that typically exceeds what is normally used for diagnostic imaging by several-fold) in the presence of microbubbles results in tissue hemorrhages. One of the hypotheses suggests that the microbubbles act as nuclei for ultrasound-induced inertial cavitation. Rapid cavitation events that take place during the microbubble collapse during lithotripsy may result in the localized generation of high temperature, ultraviolet and even soft X-ray radiation. Such extreme phenomena occur only at high intensities of ultrasound energy, which exceed by orders of magnitude what is normally used for diagnostic imaging. However, even the intermediate intensities of ultrasound energy may in certain conditions cause formation of some transient petechial hemorrhages in the insonified tissue in the presence of microbubbles. The proposed mechanism for these events is the rupture of microvessels by rapidly expanding and contracting microbubbles.

Local delivery by targeted destruction of microbubbles

The action of insonified microbubbles on cells in suspension or on monolayers of attached cells in culture varies from hemolysis of red blood cells to sonoporation and ultrasound-mediated transfection (32, 34). These results suggest that delivery of drugs or plasmid DNA to the layer of endothelial cell lining of the vasculature will be possible. In order to transfer drugs out of the vasculature into the bulk of the tissue, ultrasound-microbubble-mediated microvessel rupture, shown both with red blood cells and submicron polymer microspheres, could be useful (35). These microspheres were injected in the bloodstream of experimental animals at the same time as the microbubbles and transported into the bulk of the tissue, tens of micrometers from the vessel wall. It is assumed that the formation of microvessel ruptures may open a conduit for the materials from the bloodstream directly into the tissue. Microvessel ruptures might be helpful not only for drug delivery but also for the induction of therapeutic angiogenesis, because only a small percentage of capillaries need to be ruptured to achieve delivery to all of the tissue mass.

CONCLUSION

Sites of inflammation can be targeted by using endothelial, leukocyte and platelet surface molecules. Promising in vivo results have demonstrated feasibility for ultrasound imaging purposes. Incorporating drugs or DNA into ultrasound microbubbles may allow targeted therapy of the vascular endothelium and, in the future, tissue cells in the inflamed area.

The authors apologize for not being able to cite all relevant work because of space constraints. Parts of this work were supported by NIH HL 64381 and HL 03810.

REFERENCES

1. Boerman, O. C., Dams, E. T., Oyen, W. J., Corstens, F. H., and Storm, G. (2001). Radiopharmaceuticals for scintigraphic imaging of infection and inflammation. *Inflamm.Res.* **50**, 55-64.
2. Springer, T. A. (1994). Traffic signals for lymphocyte recirculation and leukocyte emigration: the multistep paradigm. *Cell* **76**, 301-314.
3. Jung, U. and Ley, K. (1997). Regulation of E-selectin, P-selectin and ICAM-1 expression in mouse cremaster muscle vasculature. *Microcirculation* **4**, 311-319.
4. Fries, J. W. U., Williams, A. J., Atkins, R. C., Newman, W., Lipscomb, M. F., and Collins, T. (1993). Expression of VCAM-1 and E-selectin in an *in vivo* model of endothelial activation. *Am.J.Pathol.* **143**, 725-737.
5. Bendas, G., Krause, A., Schmidt, R., Vogel, J., and Rothe, U. (1998). Selectins as new targets for immunoliposome-mediated drug delivery. A potential way of anti-inflammatory therapy. *Pharmaceutica Acta Helvetiae* **73**, 19-26.
6. Mayrovitz, H. N. (1992). Leukocyte rolling: A prominent feature of venules in intact skin of anesthetized hairless mice. *Am.J.Physiol.* **262**, H157-H161.
7. Johnson-Tidey, R. R., McGregor, J. L., Taylor, P. R., and Poston, R. N. (1994). Increase in the adhesion molecule P-selectin in endothelium overlying atherosclerotic plaques: Coexpression with intercellular adhesion molecule-1. *Am.J.Pathol.* **144**, 952-961.
8. Hickey, M. J., Kanwar, S., McCafferty, D. M., Granger, D. N., Eppihimer, M. J., and Kubes, P. (1999). Varying roles of E-selectin and P-selectin in different microvascular beds in response to antigen. *J.Immunol.* **162**, 1137-1143.
9. Lindner, J. R., Song, J., Christiansen, J., Klibanov, A., Xu, F., and Ley, K. (2001). Ultrasound assessment of inflammation and renal tissue injury with microbubbles targeted to P-selectin. *Circulation* **104**, 2107-2112.
10. Bevilacqua, M. P., Stengelin, S., Gimbrone, M. A., Jr., and Seed, B. (1989). Endothelial leukocyte adhesion molecule-1: An inducible receptor for neutrophils related to complement regulatory proteins and lectins. *Science* **243**, 1160-1165.
11. Keelan, E. T., Licence, S. T., Peters, A. M., Binns, R. M., and Haskard, D. O. (1994). Characterization of E-selectin expression in vivo with use of a radiolabeled monoclonal antibody. *Am.J.Physiol.* **266**, H278-H290.
12. Stahn, R., Grittner, C., Zeisig, R., Karsten, U., Felix, S. B., and Wenzel, K. (2001). Sialyl Lewis(x)-liposomes as vehicles for site-directed, E-selectin-mediated drug transfer into activated endothelial cells. *Cellular & Molecular Life Sciences* **58**, 141-147.
13. Roebuck, K. A. and Finnegan, A. (1999). Regulation of intercellular adhesion molecule-1 (CD54) gene expression. *J.Leukocyte Biol.* **66**, 876-888.
14. Sipkins, D. A., Gijbels, K., Tropper, F. D., Bednarski, M., Li, K. C., and Steinman, L. (2000). ICAM-1 expression in autoimmune encephalitis visualized using magnetic resonance imaging. *Journal of Neuroimmunology* **104**, 1-9.
15. Demos, S. M., Alkan-Onyuksel, H., Kane, B. J., Ramani, K., Nagaraj, A., Greene, R., Klegerman, M., and McPherson, D. D. (1999). In vivo targeting of acoustically reflective liposomes for intravascular and transvascular ultrasonic enhancement. *Journal of the American College of Cardiology* **33**, 867-875.
16. Salmi, M., Alanen, K., Grenman, S., Briskin, M., Butcher, E. C., and Jalkanen, S. (2001). Immune cell trafficking in uterus and early life is dominated by the mucosal addressin MAdCAM-1 in humans. *Gastroenterology* **121**, 853-864.
17. Nakashima, Y., Raines, E. W., Plump, A. S., Breslow, J. L., and Ross, R. (1998). Upregulation of VCAM-1 and ICAM-1 at atherosclerosis-prone sites on the

endothelium in the apoE-deficient mouse. *Arteriosclerosis Thrombosis & Vascular Biology* **18**, 842-851.

18. Lindner, J. R., Coggins, M. P., Kaul, S., Klibanov, A. L., Brandenburger, G. H., Ley, K. (2000) Microbubble persistence in the microcirculation during ischemia-reperfusion and inflammation: integrin- and complement-mediated adherence to activated leukocytes. *Circulation* **101**, 668-675.

19. Lindner, J. R., Ismail S., Spotnitz, W. D., Skyba, D. M., Jayaweera, A. R., Kaul, S. (1998) Albumin microbubble persistence during myocardial contrast echocardiography is associated with microvascular endothelial glycocalyx damage. *Circulation* **98**, 2187-2194.

20. Lindner, J. R., Song, J., Xu, F., Klibanov, A. L., Singbartl, K., Ley, K., Kaul, S. (2000) Noninvasive ultrasound imaging of inflammation using microbubbles targeted to activated leukocytes. *Circulation* **102**, 2745-2750.

21. Lindner, J. R., Dayton, P. A., Coggins, M. P., Ley, K., Song, J., Ferrara, K., Kaul, S. (2000) Non-invasive imaging of inflammation by ultrasound detection of phagocytosed microbubbles. *Circulation* **102**,531-538.

22. Villanueva, F. S., Jankowski, R. J., Klibanov, S., Klibanov, S., Pina, M. L., Alber, S. M., Watkins, S. C., Brandenburger, G. H., Wagner, W. R. (1998) Microbubbles targeted to intercellular adhesion molecule-I bind to activated coronary endothelial cells. *Circulation* **98**, 1-5.

23. Unger, E. C., McCreery, T. P., Sweitzer, R. H., Shen, D., Wu, G. (1998) In vitro studies of a new thrombus-specific ultrasound contrast agent. *Am. J. Cardiol.* **81**,58G-61G.

24. Ruehm, S. G., Corot, C., Vogt, P., Kolb, S., Debatin, J. F. (2001) Magnetic resonance imaging of atherosclerotic plaque with ultrasmall superparamagnetic particles of iron oxide in hyperlipidemic rabbits. *Circulation* **103**,415-422.

25. Sipkins, D. A., Cheresh, D. A., Kazemi, M. R., Nevin, L. M., Bednarski, M. D., Li, K. C. P. (1998) Detection of tumor angiogenesis in vivo by $\alpha_v\beta_3$-targeted magnetic resonance imaging. *Nature Med.* **4**,623-626.

26. Corstens, F. H. M., van der Meer, J. W. M. (1999) Nuclear medicine's role in infection and inflammation. *Lancet* **354**,765-770.

27. Weiner, R. E., Thakur, M. L. (1999) Imaging infection/inflammations. *Q. J. Nucl. Med.***43**, 2-8.

28. Zinn, K. R., Chaudhuri, T. R., Smyth, S. C., Wu, Q., Hong-Gang, L., Fleck, M., Mountz, J. D., Mountz, J. M. (1999) Specific targeting of activated endothelium in rat adjuvant arthritis with a ^{99m}Tc-radiolabeled E-selectin-binding peptide. *Arthritis Rheum.***42**, 641-649.

29. Unger, E.C., McCreery, T., Sweitzer, R., Vielhauer, G., Wu, G., Shen, D., and Yellowhair, D. (1998). MRX 501: a novel ultrasound contrast agent with therapeutic properties. *Acad Radiol* **5** Suppl 1, S247-S249.

30. Unger, E.C., McCreery, T.P., Sweitzer, R.H., Caldwell, V.E., and Wu, Y. (1998). Acoustically active lipospheres containing paclitaxel: a new therapeutic ultrasound contrast agent. *Invest Radiol* **33**, 886-892.

31. Porter, T.R., Iversen, P.L., Li, S., and Xie, F. (1996). Interaction of diagnostic ultrasound with synthetic oligonucleotide-labeled perfluorocarbon-exposed sonicated dextrose albumin microbubbles. *J Ultrasound Med* **15**, 577-584.

32. Unger, E.C., Hersh, E., Vannan, M., and McCreery, T. (2001). Gene delivery using ultrasound contrast agents. *Echocardiography* **18**, 355-361.

33. Schneider, M., Yan, F., and Hiver, A. (2001). Delivery of biologically active substance to target sites in the body of patients. US Patent 6258378.

34. Miller, D.L, and Quddus, J. (2000). Sonoporation of monolayer cells by diagnostic ultrasound activation of contrast-agent gas bodies. *Ultrasound Med Biol* **26**, 661-667.

35. Price, R.J., Skyba, D.M., Kaul, S., and Skalak, T.C. (1998). Delivery of colloidal particles and red blood cells to tissue through microvessel ruptures created by targeted microbubble destruction with ultrasound. *Circulation* 98, 1264-1267.

GLOSSARY

E-selectin: carbohydrate-binding inflammatory adhesion molecule with restricted expression exclusive to endothelial cells

Flow cytometry: detection of expression of cell surface molecules by laser-induced fluorescence

Gamma imaging: Method of imaging using a gamma camera detecting gamma rays emitted by a radioisotope.

Glycocalyx: glycoprotein and carbohydrate-based layer lining endothelial and other cells

ICAM-1: Intercellular Adhesion Molecule-1 is an inflammatory adhesion molecule expressed by endothelial cells and most other cell types under conditions of inflammation

IL-1: Interleukin-1 is an inflammatory cytokine produced by macrophages and other cells

Integrin: a class of more than 30 heterodimeric cell surface molecules involved in cell adhesion to extracellular matrix molecules and to other cells

L-selectin: carbohydrate-binding inflammatory adhesion molecule expressed by most leukocytes

Leukocyte rolling: Movement of white blood cells driven by blood flow. The velocity of leukocyte rolling is controlled by the breakage of molecular bonds between the leukocytes and endothelial cells

LFA-1: lymphocyte function-associated antigen-1, an integrin expressed on most leukocytes

Liposome: lipid-shelled droplets of fluid, suitable for drug or gene delivery

LPS: lipopolysaccharide is a pro-inflammatory product of gram-negative bacteria that is recognized by a specific receptor and can cause severe inflammation

Mac-1: an integrin related to LFA-1 expressed on monocyte-macrophages and granulocytes

MAdCAM-1: Mucosal Addressin Adhesion Molecule-1 is expressed on endothelial cells of specialized venules in secondary lymphatic organs of the intestinal tract and is responsible for lymphocyte adhesion

Microbubbles: lipid-, protein- or polymer-shelled gas bubbles used to generate ultrasound contrast in blood for anatomic and perfusion measurements

MR: magnetic resonance imaging creates images based on the detection of radiofrequency signals from alignment and relaxation of hydrogen nuclei in water

Myocardial infarction: Injury to the heart muscle due to limited or no blood perfusion

P-selectin: carbohydrate-binding inflammatory adhesion molecule expressed by inflamed endothelial cells and activated platelets

RGD: arginine-glycine-aspartic acid, a tripeptide recognition sequence for some integrins

Rheology: science investigating the streaming properties of fluids including blood

Stroke: Injury to the brain due to limited or no blood perfusion

TNF-α: Tumor necrosis factor-α is an inflammatory cytokine produced by macrophages and other cells

VCAM-1: Vascular Cell Adhesion Molecule-1 is an inflammatory adhesion molecule expressed on endothelial cells, smooth muscle cells, and other cells

Vulnerable plaque: atherosclerotic lesions that are prone to rupture, induce acute thrombosis and heart attacks or strokes

9

INTRAVASCULAR RE-TARGETING OF VIRAL VECTORS

Paul N. Reynolds and Sergei M. Danilov
*Department of Thoracic Medicine, Royal Adelaide Hospital, Adelaide, South Australia 5000
and Department of Anesthesiology, University of Illinois in Chicago, Chicago IL USA.*

INTRODUCTION

In recent years, the concept of gene delivery has arisen as an alternative to more traditional drug delivery approaches. Although this concept was initially envisaged as a strategy to correct inherited genetic disorders, the approach has been substantially broadened to encompass the use of gene-based therapies for a variety of acquired diseases. In essence, the approach involves the delivery of nucleic acids (i.e. genes) into cells whereupon the host cell's machinery will be used for transcription and translation, leading to *in situ* production of a protein which in turn will have an impact on cell function.

There are several potential rationales for using a gene-based approach instead of administering the protein *per se*. Firstly, there is the possibility that life-long correction of genetic diseases can be achieved by this method; for example, there is now evidence that this has been achieved in X-linked severe combined immunodeficiency (SCID) in contrast to limited achievements in other inherited disorders.

Short of permanent correction, gene-based approaches may achieve localized, sustained release of the gene product thereby potentially avoiding systemic toxicity and reducing dosage frequency. In some cases, the therapeutic protein may be unsuitable for direct administration due to instability, cost, limitation in the production of pharmaceutical quantities, or may be of a nature that standard direct administration is not feasible (e.g. a membrane based receptor).

In the context of vascular disease, direct gene delivery to vessels has been proposed as a means to prevent post-angioplasty re-stenosis and early graft failure. Further, the delivery of genes for angiogenic growth factors has been shown to stimulate the growth of new vessels into ischemic areas. The recent discovery that primary pulmonary hypertension (PPH) is in many cases caused by an inherited mutation in bone morphogenetic protein type 2 receptors suggests a gene-based approach for this disease could be developed. Beyond specific vascular application, gene delivery to endothelium could provide a "factory" for secreted therapeutic factors for other diseases by way of direct access to the circulation. Thus, gene-based approaches to therapy are continuing to emerge as an attractive complement to standard approaches – a major issue however, remains the best method for actually delivering the genes to target cells.

In broad terms, gene delivery may be achieved either by *ex vivo* or *in vivo* approaches. *Ex vivo* strategies were the first attempted in human trials. These approaches involve removal of target cells from the body, followed by transduction with the relevant therapeutic gene, then re-implantation back into the patient. For obvious reasons, this sort of approach is best suited for hematological conditions (although the approach is being broadened). The isolation of circulating endothelial progenitor cells from the circulation could potentially allow for an *ex vivo* approach for gene delivery to areas of angiogenesis (e.g. wound healing, tumor vasculature).

However, for most disease states, direct *in vivo* administration of the gene is needed and in many cases this would ideally be achieved using intravascular administration of a gene delivery agent that would specifically home to target cells. Among the available gene delivery systems, viral vectors have typically had the greatest gene delivery efficacies. This is due in large part to the fact that non-viral systems are often compromised by endosomal entrapment and degradation of delivered DNA, whereas viruses have developed strategies to achieve endosomal escape, thereby allowing their DNA to be delivered to the cell nucleus for subsequent processing. A direct comparison of transfection efficiency of adenoviral (Ad) vectors compared to a non-viral approach using liposomes in the pulmonary arteries of rats showed that Ad was approximately 100-fold more efficient (1). However, the efficacy of native viral vectors is in large part determined by the natural distribution of viral receptors on potential target cells. Experience has shown that many target cells lack sufficient accessible receptors for optimal application of viral vectors. Even in clinical trials where local or regional administration has been attempted, such as via the airways by inhalation, into the pleural or peritoneal space or even via direct injection into tumor masses, the transduction efficiency has often been poor. On the other hand, certain non-target cells may express high levels of receptors and thus potentially be at risk of toxicity due to inadvertent transduction. Thus, there has been a great deal of attention in recent years devoted to the development of targeted, cell-specific, viral gene delivery vectors.

Targeted Viral Vectors

Although viral targeting strategies were first attempted with retroviral vectors, these approaches were somewhat hampered by alterations in intracellular trafficking when the virus entered the cell via a non-native route leading to substantial reductions in efficacy. Subsequently, there has been considerably more effort directed at retargeting adenoviral vectors; the principles established here are increasingly being applied to other agents.

Ad vectors have several positive attributes that favor their use as intra-vascular delivery agents. They can readily be produced to high titer, have the ability to infect both dividing and non-dividing cells, and are stable when administered into the bloodstream. However, the vast majority of Ad vector administered systemically is sequestered into the liver, a phenomenon due to a number of factors including the high level of expression of Ad receptors on hepatocytes, the fenestrated nature of the hepatic sinusoids, phagocytosis of Ad by Kupffer cells, and other less-well defined mechanisms which mediate hepatocyte uptake. Thus, for Ad vectors to be used via the vascular route for anything other than hepatic gene delivery, they must be modified to impart specific targeting properties.

Adenovirus infection pathway

Strategies for re-targeting of Ad vectors are based on an understanding of the native infection pathway. The adenovirus is a non-enveloped icosahedral particle with 12 fibers projecting outwardly from the vertices (Fig 1, below). Each fiber consists of a homotrimer of 62 kDa subunits, with each subunit being comprised of a tail, shaft, and knob domain. During the assembly phase of viral replication, fiber monomers trimerize in the cytoplasm, and the tail of the fiber binds to a viral penton base protein that is subsequently incorporated into the rest of the viral capsid within the cell nucleus. The knob region of the fiber is responsible for two critical functions: correct trimer formation and binding to the primary Ad cell-surface receptor (the coxsackie and adenovirus receptor, CAR (2, 3)). Thus, an understanding of the biology of the knob domain and CAR is an important basis from which to consider targeting strategies.

CAR is a member of the immunoglobulin superfamily of molecules, possessing two extracellular immunoglobulin-like domains (D1 and D2) (2). The intracellular region of the molecule does not appear to be critical for Ad infection as truncated receptors lacking this domain function as Ad receptors. A relative deficiency of CAR has been noted in several Ad-resistant cells, especially tumor cells. For example, analysis of CAR levels in primary ovarian cancer cells from malignant ascites has shown that these cells are variably low in CAR expression and that this correlates to poor transducibility with Ad vectors (4). Recently, some evidence has been presented suggesting that the relative paucity of CAR on tumors may actually have functional significance asR may have some role as a tumor suppressor. Okegawa et al (5) found a correlation between low CAR state and high rate of tumor growth. New evidence indicates that CAR may have a role in cell-cell adhesion (6). Interestingly, it has also been shown that CAR expression in cultured endothelial cells increases as the cells become confluent and that this correlates to increased infectiousness with Ad vectors (7).

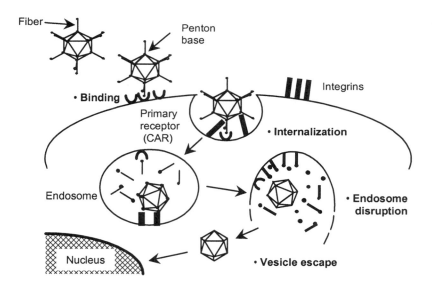

Figure 1. The pathway of adenovirus infection

The regions of the Ad knob responsible for interacting with CAR have been determined. Through a combination of sequence comparison and extensive mutation analysis, regions predicted to be exposed on the side of the knob domain were found to be critical for binding to CAR (8). These regions are loop structures that link together the eight B strands of the knob, which are arranged in two sheets; the V sheet faces the virion and the R sheet faces outward. The crystal structure of the complex formed between the CAR D1 domain and Ad12 knob has also been determined.

Following attachment, viral entry requires a second step involving an interaction between Arg-Gly-Asp (RGD) motifs in the Ad penton base and cell surface integrins (typically $\alpha_v\beta_3$ or $\alpha_v\beta_5$ but others may be used) which then leads to endocytosis of the virion (9). A lack of integrins on the cell surface contributes to poor Ad transducibility for certain cells; for cells that express high amounts of CAR, a lack of integrins is not a major impediment to transduction. In general, CAR-deficiency seems more widespread and tends to be the dominant rate-limiting factor.

In the endosome, the virus undergoes stepwise disassembly and endosomal lysis (a process mediated by the penton base and low endosomal pH) followed by transport of the viral DNA to the cell nucleus. This step is critical for efficient gene delivery and the ability of Ad to effect endosomal escape is one of the key factors in its efficiency as a vector. Based on the foregoing, strategies to modify the interaction between the knob domain and CAR, plus or minus the penton RGD- integrin interaction have formed the basis for the majority of Ad retargeting approaches.

Conjugate-based re-targeting strategies

Strategies to retarget Ad vectors can be broadly classified into either "adapter" approaches or direct genetic modification. So far, adapter approaches have achieved better results in terms of cell-specific gene delivery. These strategies involve the use of bi-specific molecules that have affinity both for the Ad capsid (typically the knob domain, thus neutralizing knob-CAR interaction) and a specific cell-surface marker (i.e. a receptor). A number of bi-specific molecules have been constructed by chemically cross-linking the Fab fragment of an anti-knob antibody to either natural ligands (such as folate, basic fibroblast growth factor (10), epidermal growth factor, or secretin) or anti-receptors antibodies (e.g., anti-EGFR, -ErbB2, -Tag72(4)). Using this approach, targeting efficacy has been demonstrated in several *in vitro* systems, often to tumor cell lines, but also to endothelial cells in the case of bFGF (Fig 2, below) (10). There has been much less success in translating this approach to the stringent *in vivo* situation of systemic vascular delivery.

To determine the feasibility of specifically retargeting Ad vectors upon systemic administration, we recently developed a strategy to target Ad to pulmonary vascular endothelium (11). This approach served both as a proof of principle for the more general application of targeted Ad as well as having potential utility for the investigation and treatment of pulmonary vascular disease. To achieve the retargeting of Ad to pulmonary vascular endothelium, it was necessary to select a suitable target molecule on the surface of the cells.

Angiotensin converting enzyme (ACE) is a 170 kD membrane-anchored ectoenzyme primarily responsible for the conversion of angiotensin I to angiotensin II. ACE is present throughout the pulmonary capillary circulation at significantly higher levels the in the circulation elsewhere (12). This property (combined with the large size of the pulmonary vascular bed) makes this enzyme a suitable target for pulmonary endothelial targeting. The utility of this approach had previously been established in the context of protein delivery through the use of an anti-ACE monoclonal antibody mAb 9B9 (see also Chapter 7). This antibody has been shown to have excellent pulmonary endothelial targeting properties in many species ranging from rats to humans. We have also recently described an expanded repertoire of anti-ACE antibodies with targeting potential in primates (13).

Conjugates formed between mAb 9B9 and candidate therapeutic proteins, such as superoxide dismutase (SOD) or catalase, have been derived and the pulmonary localization of these agents after systemic administration confirmed. Thus, we developed a conjugate (Fab-9B9) between mAb 9B9 and the Fab fragment of the anti-Ad knob antibody 1D6.14. The conjugate was constructed by cross-linking using SPDP followed by separation of unlinked components by size exclusion chromatography. The functionality of the conjugate molecule was then tested *in vitro* using western blots and ELISA to confirm binding to recombinant Ad5 knob and purified ACE respectively.

Because the principle aim was to develop a strategy with *in vivo* utility, we then assessed the *in vivo* pulmonary localization of Fab-9B9 versus parent mAb 9B9. The molecules were labeled with radioactive iodine and injected into the tail veins of rats. Animals were sacrificed two hours later and the biodistribution of labeled molecules was determined by gamma counting. The conjugate had a similar biodistribution profile to the parent mAb 9B9 with 9 and 11% of injected dose/gram of tissue detected in the lungs respectively. These studies indicated that a bispecific molecule had been created which had the specificities of the parent components, as well as the desired pulmonary localizing properties.

We next sought to determine whether Ad-mediated gene delivery could indeed be achieved via ACE targeting; we employed an *in vitro* model system using Chinese Hamster Ovary cells that have been stably transfected to express human ACE at levels similar to those seen in the pulmonary endothelium *in vivo*. The rationale for using this system is that endothelial cells tend to rapidly lose their ACE expression when placed in culture. To achieve targeted gene delivery, Ad vector was combined with conjugate and simply incubated at room temperature for 30 minutes. The Ad/conjugate mix was then applied to cell monolayers for one hour to allow infection, then the cells were washed, fresh tissue culture medium was applied, then after 24 hours incubation transgene expression was assessed. A number of studies were conducted, first to determine the optimal Ad: conjugate ratio, then to confirm specificity of infection by using ACE-positive and ACE negative cells, and blocking with either an excess of free mAb 9B9 or free ACE. In summary, these studies showed that enhanced CAR-independent gene delivery could be achieved to ACE-positive cells.

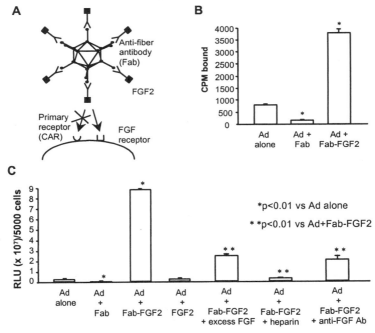

Figure 2. Conjugate-based retargeting to FGF receptors on endothelial cells. A. Retargeting schema. B. 3H labeled Ad vector alone or after incubation with Fab or Fab-FGF2 was bound to human umbilical vein endothelial cells (HUVECs) at 4°C for 1 hour. Following washing, cell bound radioactivity (CPM) was measured in a scintillation counter. Enhanced binding of virus to cells in the presence of conjugate is shown. C. Anti-knob Fab alone or Fab-FGF2 was incubated with 10^8 particles of an Ad vector carrying the luciferase reporter gene (AdCMVLuc). Thirty minutes later the complexes were added to 24-well plates containing HUVECs. After incubation for 24 hours at 37°C, cells were lysed and extracts assayed for luciferase activity. Specificity of FGF2 retargeting was confirmed by blocking with heparin, excess FGF or anti-FGF antiserum. Free FGF2 alone had no stimulatory effect on Ad mediated luciferase expression. CPM = radioactivity counts per minute, RLU = relative light units, a measure of luciferase activity (Adapted from Reynolds et al, ref 10).

Our primary objective was to evaluate whether cell-specific retargeting of Ad could be achieved after systemic vascular administration *in vivo*, thus we proceeded to animal studies. Rats were injected via the tail vein with either Ad alone (AdCMVLuc, carrying the luciferase reporter gene) or in combination with Fab-9B9. The animals were sacrificed three days later and the luciferase expression per mg protein in various organs was determined. We found that the use of the Fab-9B9 targeting conjugate significantly increased pulmonary transgene expression by a mean of 22.7-fold. In conjunction with this, expression in the liver was reduced by 83% compared to untargeted Ad. Expression in the spleen was reduced by 54%. Examination of other organs revealed no significant changes from the low levels seen with untargeted Ad. Thus, these findings were in keeping with our hypothesis that Ad vectors could be specifically retargeted. To further confirm the specificity of the approach, we conducted studies comparing Fab-9B9 to an irrelevant conjugate, and performed *in vivo* blocking of retargeting by co-injecting an excess of free 9B9.

Although these studies indicated evidence for retargeting to the appropriate organ, we wished to confirm transduction specificity of the correct target cells (i.e., pulmonary endothelial cells). For these studies, we used an alternative reporter system, using an Ad vector carrying the gene for carcinoembryonic antigen (CEA), followed by immunohistochemistry. These studies indeed confirmed that the targeting system achieved gene expression in endothelium that we confirmed to the level of electron microscopy and immuno-gold analysis for CEA. Thus, the use of an ACE-targeting approach was the first illustration that some measure of specific retargeting of Ad vectors could be achieved after systemic vascular administration.

Nevertheless, the approach has at least two clear shortcomings at this stage. Although transgene expression in non-target organs, especially the liver, was significantly reduced; in absolute terms, the levels were still much higher than would be desired. While this may in part reflect some differences between the synthetic capabilities of hepatocytes versus endothelial cells for the reporter proteins used, there is still an undesirably high level of hepatocyte transduction taking place. In theory, this could either be due to a degree of instability of the Ad-conjugate bond *in vivo*, residual transduction mediated directly via the RGD motif in the penton base, or via less well-defined mechanisms such as interactions with cell-surface heparan sulfates. Another shortcoming was revealed when we assessed vector particle localization. Using real-time PCR analysis of rat organs harvested ninety minutes after vector injection, we did find an increase in pulmonary localization of vector consistent with the transgene expression results. We did not, however, see a significant reduction in vector particle levels in the liver despite reductions in hepatocyte transgene expression. The most likely explanation for this is that a substantial fraction (as much as 90%) of an injected dose of Ad vector is actually phagocytosed by the Kupffer cells that line the hepatic sinusoids (14). This vector fraction is then steadily degraded over 24 hours and does not lead to transgene expression. Clearly then, more efficient transductional targeting approaches are required that can avoid both residual hepatocyte and Kupffer cell uptake.

In terms of antibody approaches, anti-PECAM antibodies may have some utility for general vascular targeting and have been shown to enhance non-viral transduction to pulmonary vasculature. Anti-ICAM or anti-E-selectin antibodies could potentially be used to target to areas of inflammation. Other, more refined conjugate-based approaches are emerging based on the use of recombinant targeting molecules. These molecules may incorporate either an anti-Ad single chain antibody (15) or monomeric or trimeric recombinant CAR (16) to achieve binding to Ad. The Ad-binding component can then be linked genetically to a receptor-binding component that may be either another single chain antibody (thus forming a diabody), a natural ligand (such as EGF), or a peptide. This approach has technical advantages over antibody cross-linking in that there is greater control of the structure of the final product. Nevertheless, no recombinant targeting molecule has yet been produced which has efficacy *in vivo* either in a loco-regional or systemic delivery context.

Genetic retargeting strategies

An alternative approach to conjugate-based retargeting is the direct genetic incorporation of targeting ligands into the Ad capsid itself. Work in this area has run in parallel to the conjugate approaches, but so far has had more limited success. Nevertheless, the approach is attractive as it potentially avoids the complexities of the "two-component" system and may ultimately be more readily extended to human clinical trials. Genetic retargeting approaches have to a large extent been limited by the structural constraints of Ad capsid proteins; only a modest number of ligands have been inserted without causing disruption of the viability of the virus. Conversely, certain small peptide ligands have successfully been inserted, but have then been found to lose their targeting properties when placed in the virion. Because of the central role of the knob domain in mediating primary viral attachment, genetic modifications have focused on this region – either the c-terminus or an extended loop region known as the HI loop.

In general, these approaches have achieved a measure of success in producing "infectivity-enhanced" vectors rather than more specific vectors, because CAR-recognition has been retained. Such infectivity enhancement has been achieved by introducing an integrin-binding RGD motif either at the c-terminus or HI-loop of the fiber knob (17, 18). Enhancement has also been achieved by introducing a poly-lysine sequence at the c-terminus for binding to heparan sulfates (18). In the context of vascular gene delivery, either of these approaches has been shown to increase transduction of endothelial or vascular smooth muscle cells in culture, sometimes by over two orders of magnitude. Further, the poly-lysine approach was shown to increase transduction of smooth muscle *in vivo* in a porcine iliac artery balloon injury model. We investigated the effect of inserting an RGD motif into the HI-loop on the biodistribution of transgene expression when Ad is injected systemically into mice (19). As for unmodified virus, liver transgene expression predominated consistent with the fact that the RGD-modified Ad still retains recognition for CAR. However, there were some significant differences noted with relative increases in expression seen in the lungs and kidney compared to unmodified vector. This suggests that the ligand in the HI-loop is accessible for interaction with cells in the context of systemic administration and that this site might be useful for the insertion of more specific ligands.

To achieve truly specific targeting by genetic means, however, the recognition of the native binding to CAR must be abolished. Roelvink et al. have defined a number of amino acids located on the side of the knob domain that are critical for CAR recognition (8). Further, they determined a series of point mutations that could abolish CAR recognition without disrupting the tertiary structure of the knob domain. In theory, this makes it possible to superimpose targeting specificity on a tropism-ablated background. Recently, Nicklin et al. were the first to construct an Ad vector combining a cell-specific targeting motif with CAR tropism-ablation (20). Firstly, they had identified a novel peptide with endothelial binding properties using the technique of *in vitro* phage panning against cultured endothelial cells. This peptide had then been shown to have targeting utility for Ad vectors when it was incorporated into a recombinant targeting adapter with an anti-Ad single chain antibody (15). In this context, transduction of endothelial cells was improved whereas transduction of non-endothelial cells was reduced. The peptide was then inserted into the HI-loop of an Ad knob that had been modified to ablate CAR recognition. Reduced transduction of CAR-positive non-endothelial cells was seen in conjunction with enhanced transduction of endothelial cells. These studies established several important principles and represent the first successful combination of native –tropism ablation with a cell-specific ligand. However, this vector has not yet been evaluated *in vivo*.

Limited evaluation of the effect of CAR-recognition ablation on the systemic transgene expression profile of Ad vectors has been undertaken. A consistent finding in the studies to date has been that ablation of CAR recognition alone has minimal if any impact on the level of hepatocyte transduction, vector particle localization to the liver, or hepatic toxicity after systemic vascular administration (21). This came as something of a disappointment as it had been widely assumed that a large contributing factor to the hepatic sequestration of Ad vectors was the high level of CAR expression on hepatocytes. Recently, Wickham et al. has combined CAR-recognition ablation with deletion of the RGD motif in the penton base to ablate integrin recognition (22). This "doubly-ablated" vector does appear to lead to much less liver transgene expression, although we have developed similar doubly ablated constructs that do not show this reduction (unpublished data). Whether this is due to subtle differences in the construction strategy is yet to be determined. Recent evidence that Ad transduction can be achieved via binding to heparan sulfates could also possibly be a factor.

Although combinations of ligand insertion with CAR-recognition ablation show promise, at least *in vitro*, the insertion of ligands will still be restricted by the structural constraints of the knob domain. Thus, other, more radical modifications of Ad vectors are being undertaken, although these are at an earlier phase of development. Viruses have now been generated in which the entire knob domain has been replaced by an artificial trimerization motif and shaft (23). These vectors have shown some promise *in vitro* using model ligands to achieve "proof of principle", but their transduction efficiency is significantly reduced compared to unmodified vectors. There is a suggestion that the Ad fiber may have other important functions in addition to primary attachment that is being compromised by these approaches, but further studies are required. Other Ad capsid proteins are also being evaluated for their capacity to accept targeting ligands, including the hexon and pIX proteins. Along with efforts to re-engineer the virus, considerable attention has been given in recent years to the discovery of new targeting ligands for endothelial-specific binding, particularly through phage-panning approaches. A large effort is currently underway to use phage panning *in vivo* in humans to define unique vascular "addresses" for specific vascular beds.

Combined transductional and transcriptional targeting

While improvements in transductional targeting strategies are being pursued, the difficulties being faced have raised the idea that optimal achievement of cell-specific transgene expression will require a multifaceted approach. In addition to transductional targeting, transgene expression may also be targeted at the transcriptional level, through the use of cell-specific promoters. The use of cell-specific promoters in Ad vectors has not proven to be a trivial endeavor because many promoters have been shown to lose their specificity when placed in the context of the Ad genome. Nevertheless, an expanding cohort of promoters that do retain specificity in this setting is now emerging and strategies such as flanking promoters with insulator sequences has been shown to help. Therefore, we evaluated candidate endothelial specific promoters for their strength and specificity in Ad vectors. Ads were constructed containing either the promoter for vascular endothelial growth factor receptor type 1 (flt-1), von-Willebrand factor, or ICAM-2 (24). When tested *in vitro* using a panel of endothelial and non-endothelial cells, the flt-1 promoter had the clear advantage in terms of strength and specificity. Furthermore, when injected *in vivo* into mice via the tail vein, the flt promoter was seen to have much less activity in the liver than the commonly used strong, non-specific CMV promoter. Thus the flt promoter appeared to be an ideal candidate to improve targeting specificity for the vasculature *in vivo*.

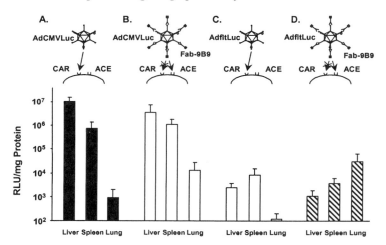

Figure 3. Combined transductional and transcriptional targeting improves the specificity of transgene expression in vivo. Step-wise improvement in transgene expression in pulmonary endothelium is shown. Rats were injected via the tail vein with vectors carrying the luciferase reporter gene, then organs were harvested and luciferase activity determined three days later. A. Untargeted vector, AdCMVLuc, showing dominant transgene expression in liver and spleen. B. Addition of Fab-9B9 for targeting to ACE leads to enhanced pulmonary gene expression and reduction in liver expression (note log scale). C. AdfltLuc, containing an endothelial specific promoter results in dramatic reduction in expression in all organs. D. AdfltLuc + Fab-9B9 restores transgene expression levels in lungs, but still further reduces expression in non-target liver and spleen, thereby dramatically improving selectivity ratio. RLU = relative light units (Adapted from Reynolds et al, ref 25).

To assess the specificity gains that could be achieved using combined transductional and transcriptional targeting, we used Ad vectors containing the flt-1 promoter (AdfltLuc) in combination with the ACE-targeting approach using Fab-9B9 (Fig 3, previous page) (25). Use of the Fab-9B9 with an Ad vector containing the CMV promoter resulted in an increase in pulmonary transgene expression as seen earlier with a modest reduction in liver expression compared to untargeted vector. Use of AdfltLuc alone resulted in marked reduction in transgene expression, especially in liver and spleen. When we combined AdfltLuc with Fab-9B9, the levels of transgene expression in the lungs were restored to those seen using the AdCMVLuc/Fab-9B9 combination, however, expression in liver and spleen was further reduced. The combined effect resulted in a net 300,000-fold improvement in the lung/liver ratio of transgene expression compared to untargeted vector. Further studies comparing tail vein injection of vector complex with injection into the left ventricle indicated that the targeting was not dependant on the first pass effect of vector passage through the pulmonary circulation.

These results indicated that a synergistic improvement in specificity could be achieved with the combined approach. This implies that whatever improvements may be achieved with further refinements of transductional and transcriptional targeting approaches, a combined approach should be considered because of the complementary advantages that can be achieved. To date, no other combined approach has shown utility *in vivo*, but this will likely change as new transductional targeting ligands are developed. Similarly, other promoters are already showing *in vivo* promise for endothelial specificity such as the promoter for preproendothelin.

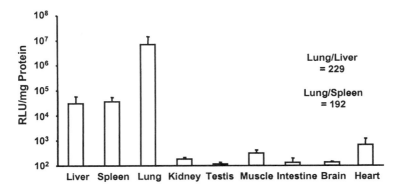

Figure 4. Targeting specificity enhanced at high vector dose: Rats were injected with a high dose of Ad vector in combination with Fab-9B9 and transgene expression determined on day 3. RLU = relative light units. (Adapted from Reynolds et al, ref 25).

Our previous studies using Fab-9B9 had indicated that a substantial amount of vector complex was still localizing to the liver and presumably being phagocytosed by Kupffer cells. Others have clearly shown that Kupffer cell uptake is a saturable phenomenon, which in the context of an untargeted Ad, leads to a sudden increase in hepatocyte transduction above a threshold dose (26). We evaluated this phenomenon in our system by evaluating the effect of a high dose of vector complex (3×10^{11} particles). In this setting, we found a substantial improvement in the lung/liver and lung/spleen ratios of expression (up to 200) compared to the lower doses of 5×10^{10} particles used in the initial experiments (Fig 4 above).

These data provide some evidence that the Kupffer cell threshold effect is operating in the context of the targeted system and that avoidance of Kupffer cell uptake could further improve the efficiency of the gene delivery system. Pre-administration of Kupffer cell inhibitors, such as gadolinium, has been shown to improve hepatocyte transduction with non-targeted vectors. Strategies to coat Ad vectors with agents to avoid Kupffer cell uptake, such as polyethylene glycol (PEG) and other polymers, are currently being explored in an effort to develop "stealth" particles that can avoid RES uptake (as has been achieved for liposomes). If these approaches are successful, they may allow for a substantial reduction in the dose of vector required, thereby reducing the direct pro-inflammatory effects of the vector.

Other viral vectors

Although this discussion has focused mainly on the targeting of Ad vectors, there are now increasing efforts to retarget other viruses. There is, however, little *in vivo* data as yet. In the context of intravascular gene delivery, Gordon et al have recently developed a highly novel approach for systemic targeting of retroviruses. Rather than target to a cellular receptor, they have targeted to areas of exposed collagen as is seen in vascular injury and tumor vasculature (27). This leads to a local accumulation of vector at the target site, but actual cellular entry is achieved via the natural retroviral entry mechanisms. In this way, transduction efficiency was preserved in contrast to the direct targeting approaches where differences in intracellular trafficking had lead to reductions in efficiency.

Targeting efforts have also been applied to adeno-associated virus (AAV) vectors, both through the use of bi-specific conjugates (28) and through direct genetic modification of capsid proteins (29). Nicklin et al. recently showed that an endothelium –specific peptide could be inserted into the AAV capsid thus allowing for the retention of targeting specificity for endothelium *in vitro* (30). *In vivo* efficacy has not yet been shown. As an evolution of the use of bacteriophage for ligand definition, there is now a growing interest in using this agent as a targeted vector *per se*. Further studies are required to determine the *in vivo* efficacy of this approach.

CONCLUSION

In conclusion, the systemic targeting of viral vectors is gradually becoming a practical reality, although much work remains to be done to optimize efficiency and avoid RES sequestration. At this time, tropism-modified, "infectivity-enhanced" agents are already poised to enter human clinical trials for locoregional disease. Further developments in this area should see the use of targeted agents via the systemic route.

ACKNOWLEDGEMENTS

Data concerning the pulmonary vascular targeting strategies discussed herein was generated in the Division of Human Gene Therapy, University of Alabama at Birmingham, Birmingham, Alabama, directed by David T. Curiel. Supported by grants from the American Heart Association, National Institutes of Health, National Health and Medical Research Council of Australia and a grant from Allen and Hanbrurys and the Thoracic Society of Australia and New Zealand.

REFERENCES

1. Rodman DM, San H, Simari R, Stephan D, Tanner F, Yang Z, Nabel GJ, Nabel EG: In vivo gene delivery to the pulmonary circulation in rats: transgene distribution and vascular inflammatory response. *Am J Respir Cell Mol Biol* 1997; 16:640-649.
2. Bergelson JM, Cunningham JA, Droguett G, Kurt-Jones EA, Krithivas A, Hong JS, Horwitz MS, Crowell RL, Finberg RW: Isolation of a common receptor for Coxsackie B viruses and adenoviruses 2 and 5. *Science* 1997; 275:1320-1323
3. Tomko RP, Xu R, Philipson L: HCAR and MCAR: the human and mouse cellular receptors for subgroup C adenoviruses and group B coxsackieviruses. *Proc Natl Acad Sci USA* 1997; 94:3352-3356
4. Kelly FJ, Miller CR, Buchsbaum DJ, Gomez-Navarro J, Barnes MN, Alvarez RD, Curiel DT: Selectivity of TAG-72-targeted adenovirus gene transfer to primary ovarian carcinoma cells versus autologous mesothelial cells in vitro. *Clin Cancer Res* 2000; 6:4323-4333.

5.   Okegawa T, Li Y, Pong RC, Bergelson JM, Zhou J, Hsieh JT: The dual impact of coxsackie and adenovirus receptor expression on human prostate cancer gene therapy. *Cancer Res* 2000; 60:5031-5036.

6.   Cohen CJ, Shieh JT, Pickles RJ, Okegawa T, Hsieh JT, Bergelson JM: The coxsackievirus and adenovirus receptor is a transmembrane component of the tight junction. *Proc Natl Acad Sci U S A* 2001; 98:15191-15196.

7.   Carson SD, Hobbs JT, Tracy SM, Chapman NM: Expression of the coxsackievirus and adenovirus receptor in cultured human umbilical vein endothelial cells: regulation in response to cell density. *J Virol* 1999; 73:7077-7079.

8.   Roelvink PW, Mi Lee G, Einfeld DA, Kovesdi I, Wickham TJ: Identification of a conserved receptor-binding site on the fiber proteins of CAR-recognizing adenoviridae. *Science* 1999; 286:1568-1571.

9.   Wickham TJ, Mathias P, Cheresh DA, Nemerow GR: Integrins alpha v beta 3 and alpha v beta 5 promote adenovirus internalization but not virus attachment. *Cell* 1993; 73:309-319.

10.   Reynolds PN, Miller CR, Goldman CK, Doukas J, Sosnowski BA, Rogers BE, Gomez-Navarro J, Pierce GF, Curiel DT, Douglas JT: Targeting adenoviral infection with basic fibroblast growth factor enhances gene delivery to vascular endothelial and smooth muscle cells. *Tumor Targeting* 1998; 3:156-168.

11.   Reynolds PN, Zinn KR, Gavrilyuk VD, Balyasnikova IV, Rogers BE, Buchsbaum DJ, Wang MH, Miletich DJ, Douglas JT, Danilov SM, Curiel DT: A targetable injectable adenoviral vector for selective gene delivery to pulmonary endothelium in vivo. *Mol Ther* 2000; 2:562-578.

12.   Danilov SM, Gavrilyuk VD, Franke FE, Pauls K, Harshaw DW, McDonald TD, Miletich DJ, Muzykantov VR: Pulmonary uptake and tissue selectivity of antibodies to surface endothelial antigens: key determinants of vascular immunotargeting. *Am. J. Physiol. (Lung Cell. Mol. Physiol.)* 2001; 280:L1335-L1347.

13.   Balyasnikova IV, Yeomans DC, McDonald TB, Danilov SM: Antibody-mediated lung endothelium targeting: in vivo model on primates. *Gene Ther* 2002; 9:282-290.

14.   Worgall S, Wolff G, Falckpedersen E, Crystal RG: Innate immune mechanisms dominate elimination of adenoviral vectors following in vivo administration. *Hum Gene Ther* 1997; 8:37-44.

15.   Nicklin SA, White SJ, Watkins SJ, Hawkins RE, Baker AH: Selective targeting of gene transfer to vascular endothelial cells by use of peptides isolated by phage display. *Circulation* 2000; 102:231-237.

16.   Kashentseva EA, Seki T, Curiel DT, Dmitriev IP: Adenovirus targeting to c-erbB-2 oncoprotein by single-chain antibody fused to trimeric form of adenovirus receptor ectodomain. *Cancer Res* 2002; 62:609-616.

17.   Dmitriev I, Krasnykh K, Miller CR, Wang M, Kashentseva E, Mikheeva G, Belousova N, Curiel DT: An adenovirus vector with genetically modified fibers demonstrates expanded tropism via utilization of a coxsackievirus and adenovirus receptor-independent cell entry mechanism. *J Virol* 1998; 72:9706-9713.

18.   Wickham TJ, Tzeng E, Shears LL, Roelvink PW, Li Y, Lee GM, Brough DE, Lizonova A, Kovesdi I: Increased in vitro and in vivo gene transfer by adenovirus vectors containing chimeric fiber proteins. *J Virol* 1997; 71:8221-8229.

19.   Reynolds PN, Dmitriev I, Curiel DT: Insertion of an RGD motif into the HI loop of adenovirus alters the transgene expression profile of the systemically administered vector. *Gene Ther* 1999; 6:1336-1339.

20   Nicklin SA, Von Seggern DJ, Work LM, Pek DC, Dominiczak AF, Nemerow GR, Baker AH: Ablating adenovirus type 5 fiber-CAR binding and HI loop insertion of the SIGYPLP peptide generate an endothelial cell-selective adenovirus. *Mol Ther* 2001; 4:534-542.

21. Alemany R, Curiel DT: CAR-binding ablation does not change biodistribution and toxicity of adenoviral vectors. *Gene Ther* 2001; 8:1347-1353.
22. Einfeld DA, Schroeder R, Roelvink PW, Lizonova A, King CR, Kovesdi I, Wickham TJ: Reducing the Native Tropism of Adenovirus Vectors Requires Removal of both CAR and Integrin Interactions. *J Virol* 2001; 75:11284-11291.
23. Krasnykh V, Belousova N, Korokhov N, Mikheeva G, Curiel DT: Genetic targeting of an adenovirus vector via replacement of the fiber protein with the phage T4 fibritin. *J Virol* 2001; 75:4176-4183.
24. Nicklin SA, Reynolds PN, Brosnan MJ, White SJ, Curiel DT, Dominiczak AF, Baker AH: Analysis of cell-specific promoters for viral gene therapy targeted at the vascular endothelium. *Hypertension* 2001; 38:65-70.
25. Reynolds PN, Nicklin SA, Kaliberova L, Boatman BG, Grizzle WE, Balyasnikova IV, Baker AH, Danilov SM, Curiel DT: Combined transductional and transcriptional targeting improves the specificity of transgene expression in vivo. *Nat Biotechnol* 2001; 19:838-842
26. Tao N, Gao GP, Parr M, Johnston J, Baradet T, Wilson JM, Barsoum J, Fawell SE: Sequestration of adenoviral vector by Kupffer cells leads to a nonlinear dose response of transduction in liver. *Mol Ther* 2001; 3:28-35.
27. Gordon EM, Chen ZH, Liu L, Whitley M, Wei D, Groshen S, Hinton DR, Anderson WF, Beart RW, Jr., Hall FL: Systemic administration of a matrix-targeted retroviral vector is efficacious for cancer gene therapy in mice. *Hum Gene Ther* 2001; 12:193-204.
28. Bartlett JS, Kleinschmidt J, Boucher RC, Samulski RJ: Targeted adeno-associated virus vector transduction of nonpermissive cells mediated by a bispecific F(ab'gamma)2 antibody. *Nat Biotechnol* 1999; 17:181-186.
29. Girod A, Ried M, Wobus C, Lahm H, Leike K, Kleinschmidt J, Deleage G, Hallek M: Genetic capsid modifications allow efficient re-targeting of adeno-associated virus type 2. *Nat Med* 1999; 5:1052-1056.
30. Nicklin SA, Buening H, Dishart KL, de Alwis M, Girod A, Hacker U, Thrasher AJ, Ali RR, Hallek M, Baker AH: Efficient and selective AAV2-mediated gene transfer directed to human vascular endothelial cells. *Mol Ther* 2001; 4:174-181.

GLOSSARY

AAV: Adeno-Associated Virus, a small non-pathogenic virus that may be used as a vector.

ACE: Angiotensin converting enzyme

CAR: Coxsackie and Adenoviral Receptor.

CEA: Carcino-Embryonic Antigen, used herein simply as a reporter to be detected by immunohistochemistry.

CMV promoter: Cytomegalovirus immediate early promoter, a DNA sequence having strong, non-specific promoter activity for driving the expression of delivered genes.

Flt-1: Also referred to as VEGFR 1, vascular endothelial growth factor receptor type one, an endothelial cell-specific receptor.

Flt-1 promoter: The natural promoter for flt-1

Knob domain: The distal tip of adenoviral fiber that binds to CAR

Luciferase gene: The gene for an enzyme that catalyses a reaction that emits light (e.g., as in firefly luciferase) that can be detected in a luminometer. It is a common, sensitive reporter gene assay used in gene delivery studies.

Penton base: The region of adenovirus at base of fiber that contains an Arg-Gly-Asp (RGD) motif that binds to integrins.

RLU: Relative Light Units, a measure of luciferase activity.

Vector: A vehicle to achieve gene delivery.

SECTION 3:

TUMOR TARGETING

10

POLYMER-DRUG CONJUGATES: TARGETING CANCER

Ruth Duncan
Centre for Polymer Therapeutics, Welsh School of Pharmacy, Cardiff University, King Edward VII Avenue, Cardiff CF10 3XF, UK

INTRODUCTION

Synthetic polymers are well known through their widespread use in biomedical materials, for example hip prostheses, contact lenses, vascular grafts and most recently as scaffolds for tissue engineering. Polymers are also routinely used as pharmaceutical excipients. Both these applications are far removed from the concept of "disease targeting." However, the last decade has seen the emergence of several novel classes of therapeutic that exploit the properties of natural or synthetic water soluble polymers to provide opportunities for improved chemotherapy. They include biologically active polymeric drugs, polymer-drug conjugates, block copolymer micelles, polymer-protein conjugates and polymer-based non-viral vectors are currently being designed for gene delivery.

This family of technologies has been termed "polymer therapeutics" (1). The phrase was coined to distinguish them from the polymer-based depot formulations used for local or systemic controlled drug delivery. Comprehensive reviews describing all classes of polymer therapeutic can be found elsewhere. This chapter describes polymer-anticancer drug conjugates and explains their ability to target tumors "passively" due to the hyperpermeability of tumor vasculature and "actively" as a result of ligand-directed receptor-mediated targeting (2, 3). Our work with N-(2-hydroxypropyl) methacrylamide (HPMA) copolymer-derived conjugates (the most extensively studied so far) will be used as the primary example. The current status of ongoing early phase clinical trials involving all polymer anticancer conjugates will be reviewed.

POLYMER-DRUG CONJUGATES

The original model for the idealized polymer-drug conjugate (Figure 1b) imagined a tripartite structure (4). A hydrophilic polymer backbone chosen to aid drug solubilization, a biodegradable polymer-drug linker designed to ensure stability in the circulation and subsequently facilitate enzymatic or hydrolytic intratumoral drug release, and the inclusion of a targeting ligand to promote tumor-specific delivery. In practice, tumor-specific ligands (including antibodies) have proved almost impossible to identify and consequently, with a single exception, all the polymer-anticancer conjugates thus far transferred into the clinic are more "simple" polymeric pro-drugs (Figure 1a) composed only of a polymer backbone conjugated to drug. It has become apparent that such conjugates still show significant tumor targeting of drug due to their pharmacokinetic profile and the pathophysiology of tumor vasculature.

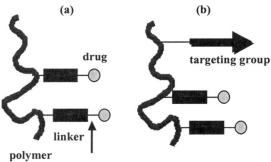

Figure 1. Polymer-anticancer conjugates designed for (a) passive targeting and (b) receptor-mediated targeting

Choice of Polymer, Drug and Linker

A wide variety of natural, synthetic and pseudo-synthetic polymers have been explored as carriers for anticancer agents as reviewed in (3). Used clinically, those conjugates have utilized one of the following polymeric carriers: N-(2-hydroxypropyl) methacrylamide (HPMA) copolymers, polyglutamate (PGA), polyethyleneglycol (PEG), or dextran. When selecting a carrier a number of polymer features must be considered to ensure suitability for human use. The polymer should be non-toxic and non-immunogenic. Preferably the polymer backbone should be biodegradable. If the backbone is not degradable (e.g. HPMA copolymers and PEG) molecular weight should be limited to < 40,000 Da to ensure eventual renal elimination.

To guarantee efficacy, the conjugate must have sufficient carrying capacity in relation to the potency of the anticancer drug to be carried (reviewed in 1, 3, and 5). Without exception the first clinically tested polymer-drug conjugates all contained commonly used, and relatively potent, anti-tumor agents. This was essential to obtain the necessary ethical permission for progression into humans. Combining drugs of known clinical profile (efficacy and toxicity) with polymeric carriers (HPMA copolymers and PGA never before administered to man) gave greater confidence that an early proof of concept could be obtained with minimal risk. The remarkable success of the first clinical trials, lack of polymer toxicity, and observation of antitumor activity in chemotherapy refractory patients (a rare event in Phase I anticancer trials) has now opened the door to design of second generation conjugates containing a wide variety of both established and experimental chemotherapy. Some examples of HPMA copolymer anticancer conjugates currently under investigation are listed in Table 1.

Table 1. Anticancer agents linked to HPMA copolymers

Class	Compound	Status	Ref
Anthracyclines	daunorubicin	preclinical	6
	doxorubicin	clinical	7
Natural Products	camptothecin	clinical	8
	paclitaxel	clinical	9
	emetine	preclinical	10
	aminoellipticine	preclinical	11
	geldanamycin	preclinical	12
Alkylating Agents	platinates	clinical	13
	melphalan	preclinical	14
	Bis(2-chloroethyl)amine	preclinical	15
Photoactivatable drugs	Cholorin e6	preclinical	16
Membrane Active Agents	melittin	preclinical	17

Choice of Polymer-Drug Linker

The fundamental aim of polymer-drug conjugation is to modify pharmacokinetics at the cellular level and promote increased tumor targeting of drug whilst minimizing exposure of sensitive normal tissues (reviewed in 1, 5). Polymer conjugation of a compound with a large volume of distribution restricts cellular uptake to the mechanisms of fluid-phase or receptor-mediated endocytosis (Figure 2). Unless rapidly taken up by the cells, the polymer conjugate is retained in the circulation immediately after IV injection is reflected by its small volume of distribution.

Once internalized, the conjugate is trafficked via the endosomal compartments (acid pH 6.5 - 5.5) to lysosomes where it is exposed to both acid pH (~ pH 5.0) and an array of lysosomal hydrolases. This route of cellular entry has been called lysosomotropic delivery. Experience has shown that drug conjugation alone does not necessarily bring therapeutic benefit unless the polymer-drug linker is carefully designed.

It is essential that the linker chosen does not degrade too rapidly. Polymer conjugation seems to be an attractive opportunity to simply solubilize, and thus improve the formulation of poorly water-soluble drugs (8). However, it is clear that rapid drug liberation in the bloodstream after I.V. injection brings no therapeutic benefit compared to the parent compound (18).

To ensure maximum tumor targeting, the polymer-drug linker should be completely stable in the circulation, but usually must be amenable to enzymatic or hydrolytic cleavage intratumorally. Unless the pharmacophore is membrane-active, e.g. melittin (17), a non-biodegradable or poorly labile linker will never yield an adequate local concentration of active drug within tumor cells. The rate and site of drug liberation must be carefully optimized to reflect the whole body pharmacokinetics of the conjugate, the precise mechanism of (and cell cycle-dependence of) drug action, and the potential mechanisms of inherent or acquired resistance.

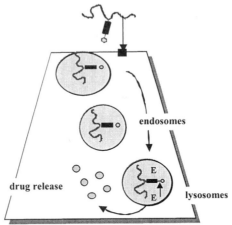

Figure 2. Lysosomotropic delivery of polymer-drug conjugates

Extensive studies involving HPMA copolymers bearing libraries model peptidyl linkers (reviewed in 1, 3, and 5) enabled design of sequences stable in the bloodstream but amenable to lysosomal activation. A tetrapeptide linker, Gly-Phe-Leu-Gly, cleaved by the lysosomal cysteine proteases was selected for doxorubicin conjugation (6, 7). This sequence has been used to synthesize many other conjugates. Fortuitously, more aggressive metastatic human tumors have higher levels of the cysteine proteases thus providing another element of "tumor selectivity".

pH-Responsive cis-aconityl and hydrazone linkers have also been explored for polymer-drug conjugation (reviewed in 3) with the aim of using lower intracellular pH to liberate drug from the carrier. However, the peptidyl linkages have remained a firm favorite (reviewed in 19) even though the chemistry of most antitumor agents makes it impossible to link them to polymer directly via an amide bond. A combination of the Gly-Phe-Leu-Gly linker and a terminal ester bond was used to synthesize an HPMA copolymer-paclitaxel conjugate (19). A simplified Gly-C_6-Gly sequence was used to bind camptothecin to HPMA copolymers - again the terminal bond being an ester (8). Most recently, a variety of platinum binding ligands including a pendant diamine, malonate, and simple carboxylate were used to generate a family of HPMA copolymer-platinates (13). Whereas the malonate and carboxylate released biologically active platinum species hydrolytically, the HPMA copolymer-Gly-Phe-Leu-Gly- ethylenediame-platinate required enzymatic activation.

TUMOR TARGETING

Globally ~10 million people are diagnosed with cancer each year and currently > 6 million die each year of their disease. In the USA and Europe, cancers are overtaking coronary disease to become the major cause of mortality. Current treatments routinely involve surgery, radiation therapy, immunotherapy, cytotoxic chemotherapy or use of hormones. Cure is however seen in only ~35% of cases and commonly used cytotoxic chemotherapy is generally poorly effective (< 5 % of cures). Potential efficacy is limited by lack of drug selectivity (tumor cells retain most of the characteristics of the parent normal cell), non-specific damage to healthy tissue, and multiple mechanisms of drug resistance. An obvious and urgent need exists for new and improved cancer therapy. Delivery of chemotherapy more selectively to tumor tissue would circumvent non-specific toxicity and the application of high enough local drug concentrations would in theory circumvent all resistance mechanisms. Clinical resistance is typically a < 5-10 fold decrease in drug sensitivity.

Tumor-specific (or tumor-enhanced) receptors offer, at least theoretically, the most elegant opportunity for targeted delivery. Antitumor antibodies have been consistently heralded as the "magic bullets" that could seek out and selectively destroy tumor cells whilst sparing healthy normal tissue. Despite the fact that neither antibodies nor immunoconjugates have yet been identified that provide significantly improved treatments for common solid tumors (e.g. breast, prostate, colon and lung) progress is being made. An anti-CD20 antibody Rituxan® is now available for the treatment of relapsed or refractory non-Hodgkin's lymphoma (NHL) and the anti-HER2 antibody

Herceptin® is effective in treating those 15% of breast cancer patients who are C-ERB B2+ve. The first immunoconjugate has recently entered routine clinical use. This is an anti-CD33 antibody conjugated to calicheamicin (Mylotarg®) and it is used for the treatment of relapsed acute myeloid leukemia (AML).

The three strategies are currently being used to target polymer-drug conjugates to tumors and these are illustrated in Figure 3.

(a)   passive tumor targeting due to leaky tumor   vasculature
e.g. HPMA copolymer- doxorubicin

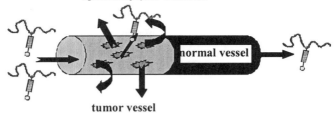

(b)   receptor-mediated tumor targeting

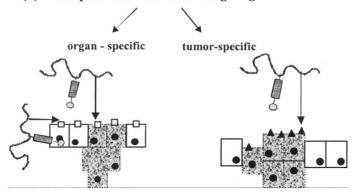

Figure 3. Strategies for tumor targeting with polymer-drug conjugates.
Panel (a) shows passive targeting due to enhanced permeability of angiogenic tumor vessels. Panel (b) shows the opportunities for receptor-mediated targeting. The tumor cells are shown by ▨ and the normal cells present on the tissue shown by ☐ . In certain cases, it is only possible to target a receptor present on both normal and tumor cells ● (e.g., HPMA copolymer-doxorubicin-galactose). But in other cases it is possible to identify a tumor-specific receptor not present on adjacent normal cells ▲. For example, HPMA copolymer-doxorubicin bearing also melanocyte stimulating hormone (MSH).

Passive Targeting due to the EPR Effect

Remarkably, and contra the original paradigm for polymer-drug conjugate design, passive targeting gives the most significant and reproducible tumor targeting so far discovered. This mechanism of targeting, the so-called the enhanced permeability and retention (EPR) effect (20), results from tumor vasculature hyperpermeability and subsequent intratumoral retention of the conjugate localized there due to lack of lymphatic drainage. Angiogenic tumor vessels are quite distinct from normal capillaries. They are poorly formed with thin walls, often just a basement membrane and endothelial cells. Gaps between endothelial cells lead to vascular "leakiness" allowing extravasation of circulating macromolecules into tumor tissue. Plasma half-life of the polymer conjugate, i.e. the plasma concentration, is the primary driving force leading to continued tumor accumulation. A variety of probes (including liposomes, nanoparticles, and microparticles) suggest that the capillary defects can be large, up to 1.2 μm in diameter, and HPMA copolymer molecular weight fractions (~10,000 to 800,000 Da) all showed equivalent ability to localize in s.c. B16F10 and sarcoma 180 tumor models (21) confirming wide tolerance limits for extravasation of hydrophilic polymers (< 30 nm diameter).

The magnitude of targeting achieved by the EPR effect is surprisingly high, up to ~20% dose/g (22). Interestingly, the extent of targeting seen (expressed as % dose/g tumor) is often highest in smaller tumors (22), perhaps as they are more actively involved in angiogensis. If this were true clinically, the smaller micrometastases that are so often hard to eradicate using conventional therapy would be best targets for polymer-drug therapy.

Due to EPR-mediated targeting, substantially elevated tumor-drug levels (a > 70 fold increase compared to free drug) have been reported following IV injection of doxorubicin (23) and platinum (13) conjugates (Figure 4 below). This magnitude of targeting would be easily sufficient to overcome all resistance mechanisms, providing that the chemotherapy is liberated from the conjugate in an active form and at an optimal rate once it arrives. Preclinical antitumor experiments have shown repeatedly shown that targeting by the EPR effect correlates with improved activity compared to free drug (for examples see 5,7,8).

There is still much to learn about the quantitative contribution of EPR-mediated targeting in the clinical setting. Few pharmacokinetic and imaging studies have been conducted in patients, but there is a growing body of evidence showing of selective targeting. In particular, highly vascularized tumors like Kaposi's sarcoma and head and neck cancer show good uptake. Clinical imaging using liposomal systems has indicated preferential localization in head and neck cancers > lung > breast. Interestingly, prior radiotherapy enhances EPR-mediated targeting in animal models (24) and this might prove an interesting clinical combination for future evaluation.

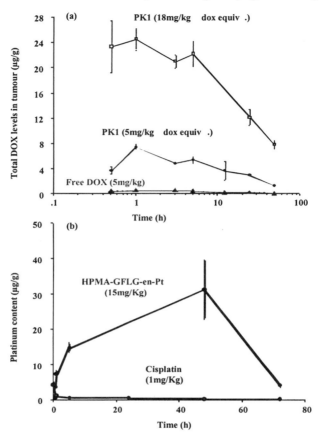

Figure 4. S.c. B16F10 tumor levels of (a) doxorubicin and HPMA copolymer-doxorubicin (called PK1) (from 23) and (b) cisplatin and HPMA copolymer-platinate (from 13) after I.V. injection at the doses stated.

Active Targeting

A vast array of putative tumor targeting residues has been investigated. Ligands bound to HPMA copolymer conjugates are typical representatives (Table 2). However, so far the only "targeted" conjugate to enter clinical testing is a HPMA copolymer-doxorubicin conjugate containing additionally galactosamine. This conjugate was designed (25) to target the asialoglycoprotein receptor present on normal hepatocytes and hepatocellular carcinoma with the hope of improving treatment of primary and secondary liver cancer. Targeting has been verified by clinical gamma camera imaging (26) but it is important to note that this conjugate produces organ-specific targeting. The conjugate localizes within normal hepatocytes as well as hepatoma, but it is likely that the overall high local concentrations of drug will also produce a bystander effect.

Table 2. Targeting ligands incorporated into HPMA copolymer conjugates

Ligand	Target	Ref
Saccharide		
Galactose	Liver hepatocyte asialoglycoprotein receptor	25
Peptides and Proteins		
MSH†	Melanoma	27
Transferrin	Tumor cells of high transferring receptor density	28
FGF†	Tumor cells of high FGF receptor density	29
EBV peptide†	CD21+ve lymphocytes	30
Antibodies or their Fragments		
Anti-Thy 1.2	Receptor +ve cells	31, 32
CD71mAb	Tumor cells of high transferring receptor density	33
B1mAb	BCL1 on leukemia and lymphoma	34
OV-TL	Ovarian carcinoma	35

†Abbreviations as follows. MSH: melanocyte stimulating hormone; FGF: fibroblast growth factor; EBV peptide: EDPGFFNVE an Epstein-Barr virus epitope

In principle, any ligand identified for tumor targeting is a candidate for polymer conjugation. The ability of polymers, including PEG and HPMA copolymers, to reduce the immunogenicity of bound proteins brings an additional incentive to use this combination. The fundamental question still remains. Is there a significant advantage of targeting ligands over and above the EPR-mediated targeting in the treatment of solid tumors? Few studies allow direct comparison of the two strategies as this relies upon the use of conjugates identical Mw and conformational characteristics (plasma half-life). Antibody polymer conjugates increase targeting simply due to their higher molecular weight and thus increased circulation time. So far the best indication we have of the importance of targeting is seen with the comparison of the antitumor activity of HPMA copolymer-doxorubicin and HPMA copolymer -doxorubicin-MSH-containing conjugate in an established s.c. B16F10 murine melanoma model (27). Free doxorubicin displayed is poorly active in this model (T/C = 148%), HPMA copolymer doxorubicin maximum activity of 175% whereas HPMA copolymer-doxorubicin has maximum activity of 324%.

CLINICAL STATUS: POLYMER-DRUG CONJUGATES

An increasing number of polymer-anticancer conjugates are making the transition into man (Table 3). Early results are very promising, especially as several of the polymeric carriers had never before been used in humans, and the optimum dosing schedule for such macromolecular pro-drugs is still unknown. Consistently throughout these trials antitumor activity has been seen in chemotherapy refractory patients. Results emerging from the first Phase I studies conducted to "good clinical practice (GCP)" guidelines are briefly described below. Three groups of compound have emerged: (i) Conjugates that have failed because of toxicity of the carrier (dextran-doxorubicin); (ii) Conjugates that have failed because of unacceptable toxicity of the conjugate (HPMA copolymer-paclitaxel and HPMA copolymer camptothecin) probably due inadequacy of the polymer-drug linkage; and (iii) Conjugates that have progressed into further Phase I/II trials.

The natural polymer conjugate, dextran-doxorubicin (36) was the first to be tested clinically. The conjugate had a molecular weight of ~ 70,000 Da and was administered using a three weekly dosing schedule. Dextran is already used as a plasma expander so it was hoped that conversion into a drug carrier would lead to minimal toxicity. This was not the case. The conjugate had a maximum tolerated dose (MTD) of 40 mg/m^2 doxorubicin-equivalent, significantly lower than the routine doxorubicin dose (60-80 mg/m^2). Severe hepatotoxicity occurred and was attributed to the uptake of the polysaccharide by the reticuloendothelial system in the liver.

The novel synthetic polymer conjugates have faired better. HPMA copolymer-doxorubicin (all HPMA copolymer conjugates have a molecular weight of ~ 30,000 Da) was also given once every three weeks and it displayed greatly reduced toxicity with a MTD of 320 mg/m^2 (doxorubicin-equivalent) (37). No polymer-related toxicity was observed and the dose limiting toxicity was typical of the anthracyclines (febrile neutropenia and mucositis). Cardiotoxicity (typical of anthracyclines) was absent despite individual cumulative doses of up to 1680 mg/m^2 doxorubicin-equivalent.

Responses were seen in four of the 36 patients enrolled in non-small cell lung cancer (NSCLC), colorectal cancer and anthracycline -resistant breast cancer. Antitumor activity was demonstrated in cancers considered resistant/refractory to conventional chemotherapy at low doses (80-180 mg/m^2 doxorubicin-equivalent) it was suggested that the EPR effect might also be important clinically. Recent Phase II trials reported no activity in a colorectal trial although there has been further activity seen in breast and lung cancer. Clinical pharmacokinetics of HPMA copolymer-doxorubicin had good correlation with pre-clinical studies; although gamma camera imaging using a ^{131}I-labelled analogue had poor resolution conjugate accumulation was seen in some tumors including head and neck cancer (37).

As the HPMA copolymer carrier was not toxic or immunogenic the evaluation of other HPMA copolymer anticancer conjugates was justified.

Twelve patients were entered into a Phase I study to evaluate HPMA copolymer-paclitaxel given by 1 h infusion every 3 weeks (9). The highest dose administered was 196 mg/m² (paclitaxel-equivalent). Unfortunately dose-escalation was discontinued prematurely due to concerns over neurotoxicity seen in emerging preclinical animal studies (9). Even so, antitumor activity was observed - a partial response in paclitaxel refractory breast cancer and disappearance of sigmoid cancer ascites.

The liver targeted conjugate HPMA copolymer-doxorubicin-galactosamine was evaluated in 31 patients with primary or secondary liver cancer. Of twenty-three patients with primary hepatocellular carcinoma, three achieved partial response (one continuing for 47 months) and a further eleven had stable disease as demonstrated on sequential CT scans (26). Superimposition of SPECT and CT scans following gamma camera imaging using an I-labeled analogue confirmed liver targeting. The majority of radioactivity was associated with normal liver (after 24h 16.9%) with lower accumulations within hepatic tumor (3.2 % of the dose) although this still represented substantially higher intratumoral drug levels than seen following IV administration of doxorubicin.

The HPMA copolymer-camptothecin (so called MAG-CPT) was less successful (38). Patients received an I.V. infusion over 30 min every 3 weeks or the alternative schedule of daily treatment (x 3) repeated every 4 weeks. The conjugate showed unpredictable toxicity that was severe and unpredictable. It included myelosuppression, GI toxicity and cystitis. At 240 mg/m² camptothecin-equivalent diarrhea was dose limiting. These problems were attributed to variable conversion of the inactive open ring form to the active closed ring form of the drug (37). Although no objective responses were seen a patient with renal cell carcinoma had tumor shrinkage.

Table 3. Polymer-drug conjugates in early clinical trials as anticancer agents

Polymer-drug	Status	Ref
Passive Targeting		
Dextran-doxorubicin	Phase I	36
HPMA copolymer-doxorubicin (FCE 28068)	Phase I/II	37
HPMA copolymer-paclitaxel (PNU166945)	Phase I	9
HPMA copolymer-camptothecin (MAG-CPT)	Phase I	38
PGA-paclitaxel (CT-2103)	Phase I/II	39, 40
Active Targeting		
HPMA copolymer-doxorubicin-galactosamine (FCE 28069)	Phase I/II	26

Two Phase I studies are currently ongoing with the PGA-paclitaxel conjugate CT-2103 (39, 40). The drug is linked through the 2' position via an ester bond to a poly-L-glutamate (PGA) polymer of ~ 80,000 Da molecular weight. This higher molecular weight carrier can be used as the polymer is biodegradable. One trial uses the conjugate as a single agent and the other involves a combination with cisplatin at a dose of 75 mg/m^2. In each case the drug was given every 3 weeks. The trials are continuing. At higher doses toxicities including neutropenia, sensorimotor neuropathy are emerging but a significant number of patients have displayed partial responses or stable disease (mesothelioma, renal cell carcinoma, NSCLC and when combined with cisplatin patients with paclitaxel-resistant ovarian showed responses.

Several other conjugates (including an HPMA copolymer - platinate (AP5280), a PEG-camptothecin, and a polysaccharide -camptothecin) have commenced Phase I trials and the results of these studies are awaited with interest.

CONCLUSIONS AND FUTURE CHALLENGES

Interdisciplinary collaboration between chemistry, biology, medicine, as well as academia and industry, has led to the first synthetic polymer-anticancer conjugate entering Phase I trial in 1994. Limited research and development during the 80's and 90's (compared to liposomes and immunoconjugates) was responsible for the relatively slow emergence of polymer-drug conjugates as a new class of targetable carriers. Exponential growth in this field, however, fuelled by the commercialization of polymer-protein conjugates and polymeric drugs, is rapidly redressing the balance.

Polymer therapeutics will undoubtedly contribute increasingly to drug targeting both of anticancer chemotherapy and treatments for other diseases. To the future it is important to profit from the lessons learned so far.

Clearly novel polymers like the HPMA copolymers and PGA can safely be transferred into humans. However, it is essential that all new polymeric carriers (and their conjugates) are always carefully studied pre-clinically to ensure acceptable biocompatibility.

The initial rationale for polymer-drug conjugation was improvement of pharmacokinetics *in vivo* and facilitate better drug targeting, so it is essential that the polymer-drug linker is optimized to match the known *in vivo* pharmacokinetics of the conjugate. Drug must be released at optimal rate at the therapeutic target, but not prematurely in the circulation, and neither slowly during renal elimination nor in any other normal tissues.

Due to conjugate cellular uptake by endocytosis routine *in vitro*, cytotoxicity screening of anticancer conjugates is not suitable for selection a "lead" for further evaluation. Although easy experiments to do, the vast body of data being generated in this way has very limited value. *In vitro* testing gives false positive results for conjugates that contain free drug (all do to some extent) and conjugates that are poorly stable, as these offload drugs rapidly into the culture medium.

Pleasingly, the pharmacokinetic studies reported in humans have shown good correlation with the pre-clinical animal studies and have indicated lack of dose dependency. Early animal pharmacokinetic studies *in vivo* are essential.

A number of studies in animal and humans have indicated that polymer conjugation can assist chemotherapy to overcome mechanisms of drug resistance. However, too little thought has been given to potential new resistance mechanisms specific to polymeric conjugates. For example, it is clear that cells which are able to limit or stop endocytic internalization of the conjugate would be completely protected. Also, levels of the activating enzymes would minimize activity.

The emerging clinical results illustrate clearly the key issues for future trials. The dose-schedule needs optimization to reflect the pharmacokinetics and therapeutic index of the conjugate. Too many trials have used only the classical dosing schedule used for the parent compound. The pharmacokinetic profile of free drug and conjugate is patently very different. Clinical protocols will in the future anticipate better the potential for unexpected toxicity with greater consideration of the known biodistribution of the conjugate. In particular, trial design will take account the fact that many polymer conjugates have shown clinical activity at doses lower than the MTD.

The polymer approach potentially provides a universal "platform" for tumor selective delivery of many different kinds of anti-tumor agent. Now that the concept has been validated using existing chemotherapy, future developments will enable the creation of conjugates containing novel drugs with new therapeutic targets, polymer-drug combinations, and increasing numbers of clinical trials investigating combinations of polymer conjugate with existing chemotherapy and radiotherapy.

REFERENCES

1   Duncan R., Dimitrijevic S. and Evagorou E.G. The role of polymer conjugates in the diagnosis and treatment of cancer. *S.T.P. Pharma Sciences* 1996; *6:237.*

2   Duncan, R. Polymer conjugates for tumor targeting and intracytoplasmic delivery. The EPR effect as a common gateway? *Pharm. Sci. and Tech. Today* 1999; *2(11):441.*

3   Brocchini, S. and Duncan, R. Pendent drugs, release from polymers. In *Encyclopaedia of Controlled Drug Delivery*, E. Mathiowitz, ed. John Wiley & Sons, New York, 1999.

4   Ringsdorf, H. Structure and properties of pharmacologically active polymers. *J. Pharm Sci. Polymer Symp.51;* 1975:135.

5   Duncan, R. Drug-polymer conjugates: potential for improved chemotherapy. *Anti-Cancer Drugs* 1992; *3:175.*

6   Duncan R., Kopeckova-Rejmanova P., Strohalm J., Hume I.C., Lloyd J.B., Kopecek J. Anticancer agents coupled to N-(2-hydroxypropyl) methacrylamide copolymers. 2. Evaluation of daunomycin conjugates in vivo against L1210 leukemia. *Brit J Cancer* 1988; *57:147.*

7   Duncan, R., Seymour, L.W, O'Hare, K.B., Flanagan, P.A., Wedge, S., Ulbrich, K., Strohalm, J., Subr, V., Spreafico, F., Grandi, M., Ripamonti, M., Farao M. and Suarato, A. Preclinical evaluation of polymer-bound doxorubicin. *J. Cont. Rel.* 1992; *19:331.*

8   V.R. Caiolfa, V.R., Zamal, M., Fiorini, A., Frigerio, E., D'Argy, R., Ghigleri, A., Farao, M., Angelucci, F. and Suarato, A. Polymer-bound camptothecin: Initial biodistribution and antitumor activity studies. *J. Cont. Rel.* 2000;*65:105.*

9   Meerum Terwogt, J.M., ten Bokkel Huinink, W.W., Schellens, J.H.M., Schot, M., Mandjes, I.A.M., Zurlo, M.G., Rocchetti, M., Rosing, H., Koopman, F.J. and Beijnen, J. Phase I clinical and pharmacokinetic study of PNU166945, a novel water soluble polymer-conjugated pro-drug of paclitaxel. *Anti-Cancer Drugs* 2001;*12:315.*

10   Dimitrijevic, S. and Duncan R. Synthesis and characterization of N-(2-hydroxypropyl)methacrylamide (HPMA) copolymer-ementine conjugates. *J. Bioact. Compat. Polymers* 1998;*3:165.*

11   Searle F., Gac-Breton S., Keane R., Dimitrijevic S., Brocchini S., Duncan R. N- (2-hydroxypropyl)methacrylamide   copolymer-6(3-aminopropyl)-ellipticineconjugates, synthesis, characterization and preliminary *in vitro* and *in vivo* studies, *Bioconj. Chem.* 2001;*2:711.*

12   Kasuya, Y., Lu, Z-R., Kopeková, P., Minko, T., Tabibi, S.E. and Kopecek, J. Synthesis and characterization of HPMA copolymer aminopropylgeldanamycin conjugates. *J. Cont. Rel.* 2001;*74(1-3):203.*

13   Gianasi, E., Wasil, M., Evagorou, E.G., Keddle, A., Wilson, G. and Duncan, R. HPMA copolymer platinates as novel antitumour agents: *in vitro* properties, pharmacokinetics and antitumour activity. *Eur. J. Cancer* 1999;*3:994.*

14   Duncan, R., Hume, I.C., Yardley, H.J., Flanagan, P.A., Ulbrich, K., Subr, V., Strohalm, J. Macromolecular pro-drugs for use in targeted cancer chemotherapy: Melphalan covalently coupled to N-(2-hydroxypropyl)methacrylamide copolymers. *J Controlled Rel* 1991;*16:121.*

15   Ringsdorf, H., Schmidt, B., Ulbrich, K. Bis (2-chloroethyl)amine bound to copolymers   of   N-(2-hydroxypropyl)methacrylamide   and   methacryloylated oligopeptides via biodegradable bonds. *Makromol Chem* 1987;*188:257.*

16   Krinick, N.L., Rihova, B., Ulbrich, K., Strohalm, J., Kopecek, J. Targetable photoactivatable drugs 2. Synthesis of N-(2-hydroxypropyl)methacrylamide copolymer anti-Thy 1. 2 antibody-chlorin e6 conjugates and a preliminary study of their photodynamic effect on mouse splenocytes in vitro. *Makromol Chem* 1990;*191:839.*

17   Musila, R. and Duncan, R. Synthesis and evaluation of HPMA copolymer-melittin as a potential anticancer agent. *J. Pharm. Pharmacol.* 2000;*52:51.*

18   Przybylski, M., Fell, E., Ringsdorf, H., Zaharko, D. Pharmacologically active

polymers. 17. Synthesis and characterization of polymeric derivatives of the antitumour agent methotrexate. *Makromol Chem* 1978;*179:1719*.

19   Soyez, H., Schacht, E., Vanderkerken, S: The crucial role of spacer groups in macromolecular pro-drug design. *Adv. Drug Delivery Rev.,* 1996;*21:81*.

20   Matsumura, Y. and Maeda, H. A new concept for macromolecular therapies in cancer chemotherapy: mechanism of tumoritropic accumulation of proteins and the antitumour agent SMANCS. *Cancer Res.* 1986;*6:6387*.

21   Seymour, L.W., Miyamoto, Y., Brereton, M., Styger, P.S., Maeda, H., Ulbrich, K. and Duncan. R. Influence of molecular size on passive tumor-accumulation of soluble macromolecular drug carriers. *Eur. J. Cancer*, 1995;*5:766*.

22   Sat, Y.N., Burger, A.M., Fiebig, H.H., Sausville, E.A. and Duncan, R. Comparison of vascular permeability and enzymatic activation of the polymeric pro-drug HPMA copolymer-doxorubicin (PK1) in human tumor xenografts. *American Association for Cancer Research 90th Annual Meeting, Philadelphia, USA* 1999.

23   Seymour, L.W., Ulbrich, K., Styger, P.S., Brereton, M., Subr, V., Strohalm, J. and Duncan, R. Tumoritropism and anticancer efficacy of polymer-based doxorubicin pro-drugs in the treatment of subcutaneous murine B16F10 melanoma. *Br. J. Cancer* 1994;*70:636*.

24   Ke S., Milas L., Charnsangavej C., Wallace S. and Li C. Potentiation of radioresponse by polymer-drug conjugates. *J. Cont. Rel.* 2001;*74(1-3):237*.

25   Duncan, R., Seymour, L.C.W., Scarlett, L., Lloyd, J.B., Rejmanova, P. and Kopecek, J. Fate of *N*-(2-Hydroxypropyl)methacrylamide copolymers with pendant galactosamine residues after intravenous administration to rats. *Biochimica et Biophysica Acta* 1986;*880:62*.

26   Seymour, L.W., Ferry, D.R., Anderson, D., Hesslewood, S., Julyan, P.J., Payner, R., Doran, J., Young, A.M., Burtles, S., Kerr, D.J, Hepatic drug targeting: Phase I evaluation of polymer bound doxorubicin. *J. Clin. Oncol.* 2002;*20:1668*.

27   O'Hare, K.B., Duncan, R., Strohalm, J., Ulbrich, K. and Kopeckova, P. Polymeric drug-carriers containing doxorubicin and melanocyte-stimulating hormone: *In vitro* and *in vivo* evaluation against murine melanoma. *J. Drug Targeting* 1993;*1:217*.

28   Flanagan, P.A., Duncan, R., Subr, V, Ulbrich, K. Kopeckova, P. and Kopecek, J. Evaluation of protein *N*-(2-hydroxypropyl)methacrylamide copolymer conjugates as targetable drug-carriers. 2. Body distribution of conjugates containing transferrin, anti-transferrin receptor antibody or anti-Thy 1.2 antibody and effectiveness of transferrin-containing daunomycin conjugates against mouse L1210 leukemia *in vivo*. *J. Cont. Rel.* 1992;*19:25*.

29   Sunassee, K.R. The evaluation of polymer-peptide and polymer-protein conjugates for targeted melanoma chemotherapy. *PhD Thesis University of Keele, UK* 1994.

30   Omelyanenko V., Kopeckova P. Prakash R.K., Ebert C.D. Kopecek J. Biorecognition of HPMA copolymer-adriamycin conjugates by lymphoctes mediated by synthetic receptor binding epitopes. *Pharm. Res.* 1999;*16:1010*.

31   Krinick, N.L., Rihova, B., Ulbrich, K., Strohalm, J. and Kopecek, J. Targetable photoactive drugs. 2. Synthesis of N-(2-hydroxypropyl)methacrylamide copolymer-anti-Thy 1.2 antibody-chlorin e6 conjugates and a preliminary study of their photodynamic effect on mouse splenocytes in vitro. *Makromol Chem* 1990;*191:839*.

32   Rihova, B., Jelinkova, M., Strohalm, J., St'astny, M., Hovorka, O., Plocova, D., Kovar, M., Draberova, L. and Ulbrich, K. Antiproliferative effect of a lectin- and anti-Thy-1.2 antibody-targeted HPMA copolymer-bound doxorubicin on primary and metastatic human colorectal carcinoma and on human colorectal carcinoma transfected with the mouse Thy-1.2 gene. *Bioconj. Chem.* 2000;*11(5):664*.

33   St'astny, M., Strohalm, J., Plocova D., Ulbrich, K. and Rihova, B. A possibility to overcome P-glycoprotein (PGP)-mediated multidrug resistance by antibody-targeted drugs conjugated to N-(2-hydroxypropyl)methacrylamide (HPMA) copolymer carrier. *Eur. J. Cancer* 1999;*35(3);459*.

34   Rihova, B., Strohalm, J., Kubackova, K., Jelinkova, M., Hovorka, O., Kovar, M., Plocova, D., Sirova, M., St'astny, M., Rozprimova, L. and Ulbrich, K. Acquired and specific immunological mechanisms co-responsible for efficacy of polymer-bound drugs. *J. Cont. Rel.* 2002;*78(1-3):97*.

35   Omelyanenko, V., Gentry, C., Kopeckova, P. and Kopecek, J. HPMA copolymer anticancer drug OV-TL16 antibody conjugates. II. Processing in epithelial ovarian carcinoma cells in vitro. *Int. J. Cancer* 1998;*75(4):600*.

36   Danauser-Reidl, S. Hausmann, E. Schick, H., Bender, R., Dietzfelbinger, H., Rastetter J. and Hanauske, A. Phase-I clinical and pharmacokinetic trial of dextran conjugated doxorubicin (AD-70, DOX-OXD). *Invest. New Drugs*, 1993;*11:187*.

37   Vasey, P., Twelves, C., Kaye, S., Wilson, P., Morrison, R., Duncan, R., Thomson, A., Hilditch, T., Murray, T., Burtles, S. and Cassidy, J. Phase I clinical and pharmacokinetic study of PKI (HPMA copolymer doxorubicin) first member of a new class of chemotheraputics agents: drug-polymer conjugates. *Clin. Cancer Res.* 1999;*5:83*.

38   Twelves, C. Clinical experience with MAG-CPT. *Proc. 5th Int Symp. Polymer Therap.: Laboratory to Clinic Cardiff, UK* 2002.

39   Bolton, M.G., Kudekla, A., Cassidy, J., Calvert, H. Phase I studies of PG-paclitaxel(CT-2103) as a single agent and in combination with cisplatin. *Proc. 5th Int Symp. Polymer Therap.: Laboratory to Clinic Cardiff, UK* 2002.

40   Sabbatini P., Aghajanian C., Hensley M., Pezzulli S., Oflaherty C., Soigner S. Lovegren M., Esch J., Funt S., Odujinrin O., Warner M., Bolton M.G. Spriggs D. Early findings in a Phase I/II study of PG-paclitaxel (CT-2103) in recurrent ovarian or primary peritoneal cancer. *Proc. 5th Int Symp. Polymer Therap.: Laboratory to Clinic Cardiff, UK* 2002.

GLOSSARY

Bystander effect: The passage of drug targeted to one cell, usually by diffusion, to the adjacent cells resulting in amplification of an antitumor effect.

EPR effect: The process by which enhanced permeability and retention effect tumor vascular hyper-permeability and lack of lymphatic drainage in tumor tissue allows passive targeting of macromolecular and liposomal anticancer agents to tumor tissue.

Fluid-phase endocytosis: Endocytic internalization of macromolecules present in the extracellular fluid without any membrane adsorption. Uptake is proportional to extracellular concentration.

Herceptin®: An anti C-ERB2 antibody used to treat receptor +ve breast cancer.

HPMA copolymer: Water soluble methacylamide-based polymers. Most extensively studied as targetable drug carriers.

Lysosomotropic delivery: Entry of drugs or macromolecular pro-drugs via the lysosomal compartment of the cell.

MTD: Maximum tolerated dose of an anticancer when given to humans.

Mylotarg®: An anti CF33 antibody conjugate containing the natural product anticancer agent calicheamicin used to treat acute myeloid leukemia.

Polymer-drug linker: The "biodegradable" spacer used to conjugate drug to a water soluble polymer. Its design ensures stability during transport and optimum release at the target.

Polymer therapeutics: Water soluble polymer drugs, polymeric drug carriers, polymer-protein conjugates, and polymeric non viral vectors for gene delivery.

Receptor-mediated endocytosis: Endocytic internalization of macromolecules in association with specific or non-specific cell surface receptors. Allows high efficiency uptake in receptor-positive cells.

Rituxan®: An anti-CD20 antibody used to treat non-Hodgkins lymphoma.

11

ENHANCED PERMEABILITY AND RETENTION (EPR) EFECT: BASIS FOR DRUG TARGETING TO TUMOR

Hiroshi Maeda
Department of Microbiology, Kumamoto University School of Medicine, Kumamoto 860-0811, Japan

INTRODUCTION

Tumor vascular permeability is becoming increasingly important in tumor biology because of its critical role in tumor growth and perhaps in metastasis, as well as in the selective delivery of anticancer agents, particularly macromolecular compounds, to tumors (see Refs. 1-5 for reviews). This issue of vascular permeability is significant primarily in tumorous tissues (and in inflammatory tissues). Macromolecular (or polymeric) drugs are of interest because they are in the class of substances manifesting enhanced extravasation in tumor tissue. The tumor-selective phenomenon has been characterized and termed the enhanced permeability and retention (EPR) effect of macromolecules and lipidic particles (2-4). One can best take advantage of this unique EPR effect for tumor-targeted delivery of drugs. Thus, polymeric drugs and microparticles, including micellar compounds or liposomes, can be delivered with greater selectivity to tumors because of the EPR effect.

Such selective targeting is not possible with low-molecular-weight substances, as described later in this chapter. Small molecules, as are many of the drugs being used today for cancer chemotherapy, do not discriminate tumor tissue from normal tissue: they reach most normal tissues and organs as well as tumor tissues by free diffusion-dependent equilibrium. For example, common drugs such as ordinary antibiotics spread throughout the body within a few minutes after intravenous or subcutaneous injection, and their plasma and tissue concentrations decrease rapidly. Such drugs are less toxic or cause fewer problems to the host when compared to anticancer agents, even though they are distributed throughout entire body tissues. In contrast, polyethylene glycol (PEG)-conjugated interferon-α (MW 52K) reaches the blood circulation more slowly when given by subcutaneous injection and exhibits a much longer plasma half-life (80 hrs vs. 8 hrs) compared with native interferon-α (MW about 20K) as discussed later.

Tumor tissues exhibit extensive extravasation of macromolecules including plasma proteins and liposomes (1-9); inflammatory tissues also show similar characteristics, although to a lesser extent. Unlike the situation with tumor tissues, the clearance of macromolecules and lipids from the interstitial space is much more rapid via the lymphatic system in normal and inflammatory tissues after extravasation from blood vessels. (2-4, 9-11) Clearance of macromolecules and lipids from tumor tissue is impaired, so that these substances remain in the tumor interstitium for a long time (2-5). For example, we found that SMANCS mixed in Lipiodol (SMANCS/Lipiodol) remained within a primary liver cancer site for more than 2 months (12, 13). During this period, the drug was released slowly (1, 4), and cytotoxic activity or antitumor effect occurred (13).

The EPR concept is now regarded as the "gold standard" to be considered in the design of new anticancer agents (3-7, 14-17). This chapter therefore describes the mechanism of the EPR effect in tumor tissues, the prolonged residence time of macromolecular drugs in plasma and delivery of these drugs to cancer sites. This chapter also describes the pathophysiology of tumor vessels with a focus on the EPR effect, as well as the vascular mediators involved.

VASCULAR PERMEABILITY OF SOLID TUMOR TISSUE AND THE ENHANCED PERMEABILITY AND RETENTION EFFECT FOR POLYMERIC DRUGS

The *"magic bullet"* concept proposed by Paul Ehrlich at the turn of 20th century prevailed for more than 100 years. This magic bullet concept was the basis of many efforts to discover cancer-selective therapeutic agents in the last half-century, with no good results. In the 1970s and later, many reports were published on so-called tumor-specific or tumor-associated antigens; the *missile drug* concept was developed using an antibody, usually a monoclonal antibody would be directed against a tumor-specific or tumor-associated antigen as a sensing device. Although this concept had shown much promise and many attempts to utilize antibodies for tumor-selective drug targeting were carried out, again, there was no luck, namely, no truly selective anticancer agent that was clinically satisfactory was discovered. Despite great expectations, a critical evaluation of targeting to tumors by using a monoclonal antibody against a tumor antigen showed no great difference compared with a non-monoclonal antibody (or ordinary immunoglobulin G, IgG) (8).

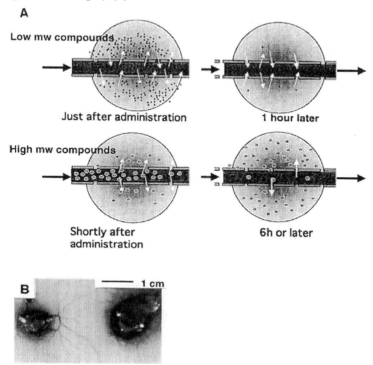

Figure 1. Schematic representation of the EPR effect of macromolecules in solid tumor (A), and the EPR effect demonstrated in mouse tumor (B). (A) Intratumor accumulation of low-molecular-weight compounds (upper panel) and high-molecular-weight compounds (lower panel) is represented in a time-dependent manner. Low-molecular-weight compounds rapidly disappear from the blood stream, and little tumor accumulation is observed after 1 hr. Large molecules, which remain for a longer time in circulation, gradually accumulate in tumor tissue (after 6 hr), and they are not washed out even as the plasma level becomes lower. Thus, selective targeting to tumor is possible. (B) Selective accumulation of albumin in tumor. Evans blue was injected intravenously which then bound to albumin. The dark blue stain of albumin in the tumor demonstrates the EPR effect (see (A) above and Figure 2). Note the unstained background of normal skin (from Refs. 2, 20 with permission). Tumor; S-180 sarcoma.

Three reasons may explain this unexpected outcome. First, any tumor consists of many heterogeneous cell populations, so a specific antibody cannot apply to the entire tumor cell population. Second, many putative tumor-specific antigens are also found in other normal organs and tissues; thus, the antibody conjugates can cause unpredictable side effects. The third reason concerns an intrinsic matter: the use of IgG. That is, when IgG was of murine origin, the so-called idiotypic anti-mouse IgG antibody, the human antibody against mouse IgG, would nullify the antibody's capacity in about 10-14 days. Thus, IgG of nonhuman origin may be inactivated rather quickly.

The cost of humanized IgG may discourage use rather unfavorably. In contrast to these immunological targeting characteristics, the EPR effect is universal in all solid tumors and is observed not only with various proteins including IgG and albumin but also with polymeric conjugates and lipidic microparticles, as discussed above as far as they are biocompatible (see Figure 1 above) (1-9).

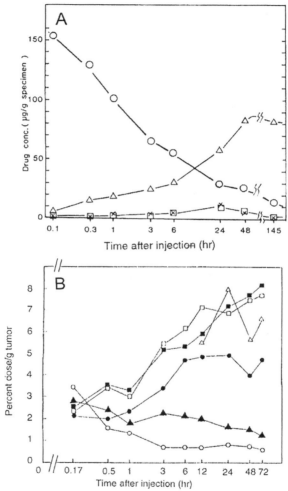

Figure 2. Tumor-selective accumulation of plasma proteins and other proteins and Evans blue-bound albumin in tumor (Ref. 2).

(A) Time course of drug uptake and drug concentration in tumor ($\triangle$) as compared with that in plasma ($\circ$) and normal tissue (muscle, skin) ($\times$, $\square$), quantified by using Evans blue-bound albumin and excised tissue or blood. Tumor; S-180 sarcoma

(B) Time course of dose retained in tumor for radiolabeled plasma proteins and other low-molecular-weight proteins. $\blacksquare$, bovine albumin (67K); $\square$, mouse albumin (67K); $\triangle$, human IgG (150K); $\bullet$, SMANCS (16K bound to albumin); $\blacktriangle$, ovomucoid (30K); $\circ$, neocarzinostatin (12K) (from Ref. 2 with permission).

Even though a few tumors, such as those found in pancreatic or prostate cancer, show hypovascularity, they become visible under angiography using X-ray if blood pressure is elevated by infusing angiotensin II and one can verify that they are well vascularized (18-20). It is noteworthy that delivery of macromolecules is highly enhanced when systemic blood pressure is increased (as described later). As discussed in this chapter, many polymeric drugs now show increasing promise for tumor-selective drug delivery on the basis of the more universal characteristic of tumor vasculature, namely, the EPR effect. Examples of the special characteristics of tumor vessels that are not usually observed in normal blood vessels are summarized in Table 1. In addition to vasculature architecture (21, 22), various vascular mediators, such as bradykinin, nitric oxide, and collagenase, are quite important for the EPR effect (9-11, 23-25).

Table 1. Unique characteristics of tumor blood vessels and various factors affecting the EPR effect in solid tumor

(1) Active angiogenesis and high vascular density in tumor tissue
(2) Extensive production of vascular mediators that facilitate extravasation, including:
    (a) bradykinin
    (b) nitric oxide
    (c) VPF/VEGF (vascular permeability factor/vascular endothelial growth factor)
    (d) prostaglandins
    (e) collagenases (same as matrix metalloproteases; MMPs)
    (f) peroxynitrite
(3) Defective vascular architecture: for example, lack of smooth muscle cells, lack of or reduced numbers of receptors for angiotensin II, large gap in endothelial cell-cell junctions, anomalous vascular conformation (e.g., branching or stretching)
(4) Impaired lymphatic clearance of macromolecules and lipids from interstitial tissue at tumor (resulting in their retention)

FACTORS AFFECTING TUMOR VACSCULAR PERMEABILITY

The EPR effect in cancerous tissue is the result of multiple causes, some of which are also known to affect inflammatory tissue (10, 11, 21-25). Tumor angiogenesis in a solid tumor that results in higher vascular density is also well known (see for example, Ref. 26). A more important point is that a great difference exists in the anatomical architecture of tumor vessels compared with vessels in normal tissue (21, 22): a lack of smooth muscle cells surrounding the endothelial cells. This difference helps to explain the impaired response to vasoconstricting mediators (e.g., angiotensin II). As a result of all these factors, tumor blood vessels are quite leaky (see Figure 1 above).

We first demonstrated the EPR effect by using plasma proteins such as albumin, transferrin, and IgG, which are by far the most biocompatible macromolecules. Also used were various synthetic polymers including SMANCS, HPMA [hydroxypropylmethacrylate] copolymer (1-7, 14-17), PEG and polyvinyl alcohol [PVA] -conjugates (see reviews in Ref. 9, 15), many lipidic particles, and liposomal or micellar particles of PEG-poly-(L-Asp) (5, 12, 13, 27).

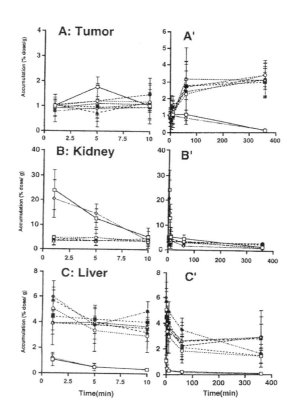

Figure 3. Accumulation of ^{125}I-labeled HPMA copolymers in tumor (A, A'), kidney (B, B'), and liver (C, C'). Please note time frames in A, B, C and A', B', C' are greatly different. A, B, C are only for initial short time. Symbols used for copolymers of different molecular singes are □, 4.5K; ◇, 16.5K; ○, 40K; △, 80K; ■, 150K; ◆ 300K; ●, 600K; and ▲, 800K. Note the lack of substantial accumulation in kidney, or a gradual washout in liver. Only tumor showed increased accumulation of macromolecules with molecular size more than 40K (from Ref. 7 with permission)

For these EPR characteristics to be exhibited, the molecular size of the drug is critical for tumor targeting. A systematic study using HPMA copolymer or natural proteins showed that a molecular size greater than 40 kDa is needed for the EPR effect (2-4, 7, 14-17), although the maximum size is not so clear (Figure 3 above). For instance, liposomes and microsphere lipids, and even bacteria (*Bifidobacillus*) (28), injected intravenously showed greater retention in tumor and much less accumulation in normal tissues and organs (5-9, 12, 13, 25, 27, 28, 31) (Figure 3).

HALF-LIFE OF DRUGS IN PLASMA AND MOLECULAR SIZE

For the EPR effect, as important as the highly facilitated extravasation from blood vessels in the tumor is the long plasma residence time ($t_{1/2}$). More than 6 hours of circulation time seems to be needed for the EPR effect to be exhibited clearly (1, 2, 4, and 7) (Figures 1-3). The residence times of macromolecules in plasma appear to be quite different among various mammalian species: we found that the $t_{1/2}$ of neocarzinostatin (12 kDa) in mice is < 2 min but that this time in humans is approximately 2 hr. We also found that the $t_{1/2}$ changes with polymer conjugation of drugs: the $t_{1/2}$ for neocarzinostatin conjugated with poly(styrene-co-maleic acid) half-butyl ester copolymer (SMA), known as SMANCS becomes about 19 min in mice, i.e., a 10-fold increase. Native superoxide dismutase (SOD) (30kDa) had a $t_{1/2}$ of about 3 min in mice, whereas SMA and other polymer conjugates had a $t_{1/2}$ of 25 min or longer. The $t_{1/2}$ of native human interferon-α in human plasma was about 8 hr, which became 80 hr after PEG conjugation of interferon-α (Tables 2 and 3). These data are summarized in Tables 2 and 3, and more detailed data will be found in references 1-4, 7, and 15.

It should be noted that the intratumor concentration of SMANCS, albumin, HPMA-Dox, or other macromolecules becomes several folds higher than the plasma concentration several hours after intravenous injection, indicating that clearance is slower than uptake velocity. Figure 4 below shows the relationship between molecular size, tumor uptake and urinary clearance of HPMA copolymers: renal clearance and tumor uptake has a reverse relationship. The intratumor concentration of macromolecules was found to parallel the AUC (area under the concentration curve) (7).

Furthermore, the concentration of macromolecules in the tumor can be as much as 30 times higher than that in normal tissue. The accumulation increases progressively with time in the tumor, whereas clearance from the tumor does not (2-4) (Figure 3A vs. 3A'). In contrast, the initial uptake of macromolecules in normal tissue can be high after intravenous injection, although their clearance from this tissue continues and concentration of these substances reaches a very low level (Figure 3B', and 3C', for kidney and liver) compared with that in a tumor (7) (Figure 3A'). Thus, the release velocity of the active component or principle from polymeric conjugates or liposomal drugs should be very slow so that the active component is retained in the conjugates. Subsequently the active component should be released slowly and at an adequate level, one that results in an effective therapeutic concentration.

For example, we found that SMANCS in Lipiodol is cleared very slowly from tumor (clearance takes several weeks), whereas it is delivered to and deposited in tumor very quickly. The activity of SMANCS was detected at 20~30 μg/g tumor tissue even 2~3 months after arterial injection (1 mg/ml) (13), and this remaining activity was more than 100 times the minimal inhibitory concentration against tumor cells in culture.

Table 2. Pharmacokinetic parameters of native and polymer-conjugated interferons in human, monkey, rat, and mouse (from Ref. 15 with permission).

Types of Conjugates of Interferon [b]	Approximate Molecular Mass (kDa)	$t_{1/2}$* (hr)			
		Human, s. c.[a]	Monkey, i. v.[a]	Rat, i. v.[a]	Mouse, i. v.[a]
Native IFN-α	18	8	—	—	4
Native IFN-β-1a	22.3	—	3.2	1.5	0.92
FMS $_7$-IFN-α-2[b]	21.4	—	—	—	34
PEG-IFN-β-1a	42.27	—	9.5	10.1	9.96
PEG-IFN-α-2b	30	54	—	—	—
PEG-IFN-α-2a	52	80	—	—	—

- $t_{1/2}$: plasma half-life ; [a] Routes of administration. [b] FMS $_7$-IFN-α-2, seven moieties of 2-sulfo-9-fluorenylmethoxycarbonyl conjugate with interferon-α-2 ; PEG-IFN-β-1a , 20-kDa straight-chain PEG conjugate with interferon-β-1a ; PEG- IFN-α-2b , 12-kDa straight-chain PEG conjugate with interferon-α-2b ; PEG-IFN-α-2a , 40-kDa branched-chain PEG conjugate with interferon-α-2a.

Tumor uptake ($\cdot$)

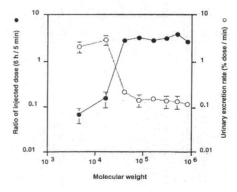

Figure 4. Relationship between tumor uptake and renal clearance of polymers (HPMA) of various molecular sizes. AUC (area under the concentration curve) is parallel to the tumor uptake of polymers and mirror image to the renal clearance (from Ref. 7 with permission).

Table 3. Plasma clearance times of various proteins and their polymer conjugates or modified proteins (from Ref. 4 with permission).

Protein	Type of polymer or modification	Molecular mass (kDa)	$t_{1/2}$	$t_{1/10}$	Test animal
Neocarzinostatin (NCS)	None	12	1.8 m	15 m	Mouse
SMANCS	SMA[a]	16	19 m	5 hr	Mouse
Ribonuclease	None	13.7	5 m	30 m	Mouse
Ribonuclease dimer		27	18 m	5 hr	Mouse
Soybean trypsin inhibitor (SBTI [b])	None	20	<2.0m	3 m	Rabbit
Dextran-SBTI	dextran	127	20 m	>80m	Rabbit
Ovomucoid	DTPA /NH$_2$ / ^{51}Cr [c]	29	5 m	34 m	Mouse
Cu $^{2+}$, Zn $^{2+}$ superoxide–dismutase (SOD)	None	30	4 m	30 m	Rat
SMA-SOD	SMA conjugate [a]	40	>300m	>10hr	Rat
Bilirbin oxidase	None	50	<1.0m	1.8 m	Rat
PEG [d]-bilirubin oxidase	PEG	70	5 m	48 hr	Rat
Serum albumin, mouse	None	68	3- 4d [e]	—	Mouse
Serum albumin, mouse	Evans Blue dye	—	2 hr	30 hr	Mouse
Serum albumin, human	Formaldehyde/ ^{125}I	—	25 m	4 hr	Rat
L-Asparaginase	None	65×(2-8)	1.5-3.4hr	—	Rat
PEG-L-Asparaginase	PEG	—	56 hr	11 d	Mouse
Immunoglobin G, mouse	DTPA	150	60 hr	—	Rat
α_2-Macroglobulinf [f]	Iodination/ ^{125}I	180×4	140 hr	22 d	Mouse
α_2-Macroglobulinf [f] -plasmin complex	Iodination/ ^{125}I	180×2	2.5 m	20 m	Mouse

*m, min; d, day. [a] binds to albumin. [b] SBTI, Kunitz type. [c] DTPA, diethylenetriaminepentaacetic acid. [d] PEG, polyethylene glycol. [e] Human albumin in human, 19 days. [f] Human

AUGMENTATION OF THE EPR EFFECT AND CLINICAL APPLICATION

Angiotensin II-Induced Hypertension

As discussed briefly above, the architecture of blood vessels in tumors is quite different from that in normal tissue (21, 22). The response of tumor vessels to vascular mediators, i.e. vasoconstriction by angiotensin II, is impaired, which is consistent with the finding of differences in tumorous vessels and reflects the anatomical defect observed under the electron microscope. For instance, a slow intravenous infusion of angiotensin II with a macromolecular drug such as SMANCS, causes elevation of the systemic blood pressure, e.g., from 100 mmHg to 160 mmHg in rats. If this blood pressure is maintained at 160 mmHg for about 15-20 min, then one can attain 50-100 % increase of drug delivery to tumor, as evidenced by assay of SMANCS (aqueous formulation) or radiolabeled albumin (29). This angiotensin II-induced systemic hypertension opens the vascular endothelial junction in a passive fashion, thus facilitating transvascular leakage in tumor tissue. In contrast, the vascular mediator causes vessels in normal tissues and organs to constrict, and endothelial junctions to contract tighter as smooth muscle cells surrounding the vessels constrict (vasoconstriction) (9, 11, 18-20, and 29).

Consequently, less delivery of drug to normal tissues and organs results under vasoconstriction, and accordingly, a smaller side effect. This facilitated targeting of drug to cancer site is much more pronounced with macromolecular drugs than with low-molecular-weight drugs such as mitomycin C or doxorubicin. This is because these small molecules leak out from the tumor interstitium and back into the blood plasma very quickly, i.e., within 5-10 min. Indeed, we observed that, with induced hypertension, the toxicity of SMANCS such as bone marrow cellularity and toxicity to the kidney and the intestine can be suppressed to a significant extent (29, 30). Delivery of the polymeric drug SMANCS into tumor tissue reached a much higher level than drug delivery to normal tissue (29). This effect can also be demonstrated by delivery of SMANCS/Lipiodol administered arterially (via the hepatic artery) under angiotensin II-induced hypertensive conditions: deposition of the drug in the peripheral area of metastatic liver cancer was observed clearly even after 1 week (see Figure 5).

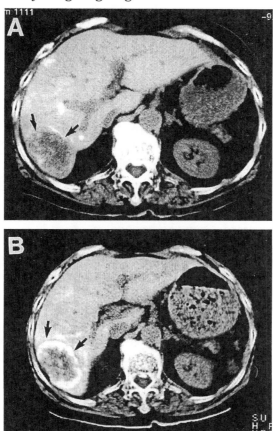

Figure 5. Enhanced drug delivery under angiotensin II-induced hypertension as demonstrated by computed topography. In this case, a patient with liver cancer received an arterial injection of SMANCS/Lipiodol under normotension (A) or under angiotensin II-induced hypertension (160 mmHg for 15 min) (B). The interval between A and B was 1 week. Each time, about 3 ml of SMANCS/Lipiodol was injected. The arrows indicate the tumor area. Note the more intense high-density (light) area at tumor periphery in B when injected under angiotension-induced hypertension, which demonstrates enhanced deposition of SMANCS/Lipiodol (cf. A. see details in text) (personal communication; A. Nagakitsu et al.). This staining, defined type B in the liver, is a typical one for metastatic liver cancer having a low density area near the central area, and a high area at the tumor periphery where more prominent tumor growth occurs. This type B staining is different from that of hepatocellular carcinoma, which exhibits high density staining in entire tumor, (defined type A staining) (34).

Arterial Administration in Cancer Chemotherapy

Ever since my discovery of SMANCS, we have used SMANCS/Lipiodol (oily formulation) administered via the hepatic artery for hepatoma, or via the upstream of the corresponding tumor-feeding artery (see details in Refs. 4, 5, 12, 13, 25 and 31). This method has been approved for clinical use in Japan since 1993 and has been found to be very effective. The rationale behind this therapeutic maneuver (arterial administration) is related to the greatest tumor-targeting efficacy, which is attained by use of this method and is attributed to the first-pass effect in addition to the EPR effect. Namely, lipid formulation of SMANCS administered via the tumor-feeding artery results in drug concentrations in the tumor of more than 2000 times the concentrations in blood, with missile targeting accuracy (4, 5, 12, 13, 25 and 31) and of course, sustained drug retention and slow release from the lipid milieu at the tumor site. This slow release makes it possible to have a long interval, a month or longer, before the next administration of drug is needed.

In addition to the greater therapeutic efficacy with this technique, tumor imaging becomes much sharper and more sensitive. Tumors smaller than 5 mm in diameter can be readily identified (5, 12, 13, 25). Furthermore, the need for subsequent drug administrations and the approximate doses can be decided on a more quantitative basis by using the high-density stained area of tumor, related to the presence of iodine (Lipiodol). This method therefore allows the dose of the drug (e.g., SMANCS/Lipiodol) for the patient to be decided not by use of the maximum tolerable dose (mg of drug/square meter of body surface), as in conventional chemotherapy, but by use of measured tumor size. This method also offers very sensitive diagnostic and rational therapeutic information. That the dose of the drug to be administered depends on tumor size is a striking consequence of the application of this method. Such a new concept of dose determination not based on maximum tolerable dose but on tumor size, will be important as the technology of interventional radiology is being developed. More detailed comments and precautions in practical settings are found in reference (25).

Angiotensin I-Converting Enzyme (ACE) Inhibitor

This enzyme inhibitor is one of a class of antihypertensive agents that are widely used and very safe. Not only does it inhibits conversion of angiotensin I to II (thus blocking hypertension), but it also inhibits the degradation of bradykinin, which is one of the most potent vascular permeability inducers (i.e., EPR effect) generated at the tumor or inflammatory site (9, 10, 11, 25). Therefore, with the use of ACE inhibitors such as enalapril or temocapril that also inhibit degradation of bradykinin, one can ultimately activate endothelial nitric oxide synthase to yield nitric oxide (NO), while at the same time increasing the level of bradykinin. Thus, the EPR effect induced by both bradykinin and NO will be enhanced (9-11, 20, 23, 24). Such inhibitors increase delivery of macromolecular drugs to the tumor even under normotension. Enalapril and temocapril can therefore enhance the EPR effect (9, 11, 23 and S. Tanaka et al., unpublished data), similar to the results seen with angiotensin II-induced hypertension (20, 29).

Intracavitary Administration for Carcinomatosis

Another advantage of macromolecular drugs over drugs that are small molecules is therapeutic effectiveness after administration into a cavitary compartment, either the pleural or the peritoneal cavity. This method can easily be used when the physician is removing excessive ascitic or pleural fluid, in which cancer cells are floating (carcinomatosis). The intrapleural or intraperitoneal route is most useful because the polymeric drugs are retained in the cavitary compartment for more than several hours, whereas small molecules (e.g., doxorubicin) disappear within a few minutes (32, 33). The period of drug accessibility to floating cancer cells in the cavity is thus far superior with the macromolecular drugs than with the smaller molecular drugs (Figure 6 below). We have identified a rodent model as well as human cases of carcinomatosis, in which SMANCS treatment by this route is remarkably effective (32, 33).

Drug Resistance and Immunogenicity

Drug resistance is one of the major problems associated with cancer chemotherapy. Our group and others have demonstrated that SMANCS and HPMA doxorubicin copolymer are not subject to so-called p-glycoprotein-dependent efflux (see review Refs. 9, 14, 15, 25 and 35). Thus, polymeric drugs may hold some answers for the problem of drug resistance of tumors.

Of great concern is usually whether these polymers elicit an immunological reaction. The agents SMANCS, PEG-asparaginase, PEG-interferon-α, and HPMA, PVA, or gelatin conjugates are well tolerated by patients and animals. Necarzinostatin and many other protein drugs, when conjugated with biocompatible polymers, exhibit significantly suppressed immunogenicity compared with native proteins (1, 3, 4, and 15). Polyanions, however, cause an endotoxin-like reaction, as noted with large size pyran-copolymers [DIVEMA] of rather unrefined quality. Some, including SMANCS, activate components of the immune system such as macrophages, NK- and T-cell functions (36), and interferon induction (37).

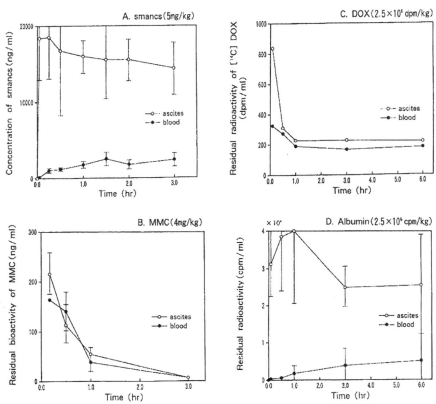

Figure 6. Compartmental retention of low- and high-molecular-weight substances in AH130 ascitic tumor-bearing rats. As shown in A and D, macromolecules (SMANCS and ^{14}C-labeled albumin, respectively) were retained in the peritoneal ascitic compartment at high levels for a long period without reaching equilibrium. (B) and (C), Mitomycin C (MMC) and ^{14}C-labeled doxorubicin (DOX), respectively, injected intraperitoneally disappeared from the peritoneal compartment rapidly; drug concentrations in blood and in the peritoneal compartment reached equilibrium in a short time (< 0.5 hr). These results mean that macromolecules do not traverse normal blood vessels readily and are ideal, because of a long retention time, for maintaining effective concentrations for the control of peritoneal and pleural carcinomatosis in human as well (from Ref. 33 with permission).

Table 4. Side effects of SMANCS/Lipiodol injected into the hepatic artery of patients with hepatocellular carcinoma [a]

Symptoms	Frequency (%) observed
Dermatological (exanthema)	0.36
Nausea	5.35 [b]
Vomiting	4.06 [b]
Anorexia	3.63 [b]
Abdominal pain (transitory)	5.53
Liver function	
GOT [c], increased	2.16 [b]
GPT, increased	2.12 [b]
Bilirubin (>1.5 mg/dl)	3.45 [b]
Hypotension	2.22
Blood counts	
WBCs, decreased	0.38
increased	0.83
PMNs, decreased	0.04
increased	0.28
Platelets, decreased	0.83 [b]
Renal function, impaired	0.71
BUN [c], increased	0.41
Anaphylaxis/shock	0.14
Rigor (transitory)	4.88
Chest pain (transitory)	0.20
Fever (low grade, 2-7 days)	27.80
CRP [c], increased	0.67
Ascites formation	1.35 [b]

[a] Based on 3956 patients . (From Yamanouchi Pharmaceutical Co. PMS material of 2000.)
[b] These results are frequently associated with impaired hepatic function (e.g. , due to liver cirrhosis), and most patients tend to show these effects as liver function deteriorates and disease progresses without the use of SMANCS .
[c] GOT , glutamic-oxaloacetic transaminase ; GPT , glutamic-pyruvic transaminase ; PMNs , polymorphonuclear neutrophils ; WBCs , white blood cells ; BUN , blood urea nitrogen ; CRP , C-reactive protein. Many details and precautions related to the arterial injection of SMANCS/Lipiodol may be found in Reference 25 (page 57).

CONCLUDING REMARKS

By the end of 2001, a number of polymeric drugs had already been approved by regulatory agencies. These drugs include SMANCS, PEG-asparaginase, PEG-adenosine deaminase, and PEG-interferon-α . SMANCS has been used in many thousands of patients, and the remarkable results with this agent warrant further development of this category of drugs, as Muggia pointed out (16). Side effects of SMANCS/Lipiodol given by the arterial route, when properly administered, are very few, as expected when compared with conventional cancer chemotherapy (Table 4). In our experience, the compliance of treated patients and their quality of life are far better with these drugs than with conventional chemotherapy. I hope that the development of similar drugs will gain greater appreciation.

REFERENCES

1   H. Maeda, T. Matsumoto, T. Konno, K. Iwai and M. Ueda: Tailor-making of protein drugs by polymer conjugation for tumor targeting: A brief review on smancs. J. Protein Chem. 3, 181-193 (1984).
2   Y. Matsumura and H. Maeda: A new concept for macromolecular therapeutics in cancer chemotherapy: Mechanism of tumoritopic accumulation of proteins and the antitumor agent smancs. Cancer Res. 46, 6387-6392 (1986).
3   H. Maeda and Y. Matsumura: Tumoritropic and lymphotropic principles of macromolecular drugs. Crit. Rev. Ther. Drug Carrier Syst. 6, 193-210 (1989).
4   H. Maeda: SMANCS and polymer-conjugated macromolecular drugs: Advantages in cancer chemotherapy. Adv. Drug Deliv. Rev. 6, 181-202 (1991).
5   K. Iwai, H. Maeda, and T. Konno: Use of oily contrast medium for selective drug targeting to tumor: Enhanced therapeutic effect and X-ray image. Cancer Res. 44, 2115-2121 (1984).
6   R. Duncan, I.C. Home, H.J. Yardley, P.A. Flanagan, K. Ulbrich, V. Subr and J. Strohalm: Macromolecular prodrugs for use in targeted cancer chemotherapy: melphalan covalently coupled to N-(2-hydroxypropyl) methacrylamide copolymer. J. Control. Release 16, 121-136 (1991)
7   Y. Noguchi, J. Wu, R. Duncan, J. Strohalm, K. Ulbrich, T. Akaike , and H. Maeda: Early phase tumor accumulation of macromolecules: A great difference in clearance rate between tumor and normal tissues. Jpn. J. Cancer Res. 89, 307-314 (1998).
8   E Marecos., R. Weissleder, and A. Bogdanov, Jr. : Antibody-mediated versus nontargeted delivery in a human small cell lung carcinoma model. Bioconjug.. Chem. 9,184-191 (1998)
9   H. Maeda: Enhanced permeability and retention (EPR) effect in tumor vasculature: The key role of tumor-selective macromolecular drug targeting. Adv. Enzyme Regul. 41, 189-207 (2001).
10 R. Kamata, T. Yamamoto, K. Matsumoto, and H. Maeda: A serratial protease causes vascular permeability reaction by activation of the Hageman factor-dependent pathway in guinea pig. Infect. Immun. 48, 747-753 (1985).
11 H. Maeda, J. Wu, T. Okamoto, K. Maruo, and T. Akaike: Kallikrein-kinin in infection and cancer. Immunopharmacology 43, 115-128 (1999).
12 T. Konno, H. Maeda, K. Iwai, S. Tashiro, S. Maki, T. Morinaga, M. Mochinaga, T. Hiraoka, and I. Yokoyma: Effect of arterial administration of high molecular-weight anticancer agent SMANCS with lipid lymphographic agent on hepatoma: A preliminary report. Eur. J. Cancer Clin. Oncol. 19, 1053-1065 (1983).
13 T. Konno, H. Maeda, K. Iwai, S. Maki, S. Tashiro, M. Uchida, and Y. Miyauchi: Selective targeting of anti-cancer drug and simultaneous image enhancement in solid tumors by arterially administered lipid contrast medium. Cancer 54, 2367-2374 (1984).
14 J. Kopecek, P. Kopecekova, T. Minko, and Z-R. Lu: HPAA copolymer anticancer drugs conjugates: Design, activity, and mechanism of action. Eur. J. Pharm. Biopharm. 50, 61-81 (2000).

15   T. Sawa, S.K. Sahoo, and H. Maeda: Water-soluble polymer therapeutics with special emphasis on cancer chemotherapy. *in* Polymers in Medicine and Biotechnology , Ashady ed, Washington D.C.: Am. Chem Soc. Monograph, *in press*, 2002

16   F.M. Muggia: Doxorubicin-polymer conjugates: Further demonstration of the concept of enhanced permeability and retention. Clin. Cancer Res. 5, 7-8 (1999).

17   L.W. Seymour, Y. Miyamoto, H. Maeda, M. Brereton, J. Strohalm, K. Ulbrich , and R. Duncan: Influence of molecular weight on passive tumor accumulation of a soluble macromolecular drug carrier. Eur. J. Cancer 31A, 766-770 (1995).

18   M. Suzuki, K. Hori, Z. Abe, S. Saito and H. Sato: A new approach to cancer chemotherapy: Selective enhancement of tumor blood flow with angiotensin II. J. Natl. Cancer Inst. 67, 663-669 (1981).

19   K. Hori, S. Saito, H. Takahashi, H. Sato, H. Maeda, and Y. Sato: Tumor-selective blood flow decrease induced by an angiotensin converting enzyme inhibitor, temocapril hydrochloride. Jpn. J. Cancer Res. 91, 261-269 (2000).

20   K. Hori, M. Suzuki, S. Tanda, S. Saito, M. Shinozaki , and Q-H. Zhang: Fluctuation in tumor blood flow under normotension and the effect of angiotensin-II induced hypertension. Jpn. J. Cancer Res. 82, 1309-1316 (1991).

21   S.A. Skinner, P.J. Tutton, and P.E. O'Brien: Microvascular architecture of experimental colon tumors in the rat : Cancer Res. 50, 2411-2417 (1990).

22   M. Suzuki, T. Takahashi, and T. Sato: Medial regression and its functional significance in tumor-supplying host arteries, Cancer 59, 444-450 (1987).

23   J. Wu, T. Akaike, and H. Maeda: Modulation of enhanced vascular permeability in tumors by a bradykinin antagonist, a cyclooxygenase inhibitor, and a nitric oxide scavenger. Cancer Res. 58, 159-165 (1998).

24   J. Wu, T. Akaike, K. Hayashida, T. Okamoto, A. Okuyama, and H. Maeda: Enhanced vascular permeability in solid tumor involving peroxynitrite and matrix metalloproteinases. Jpn. J. Cancer Res. 92, 439-451 (2001).

25   H. Maeda, T. Sawa, and T. Konno: Mechanism of tumor-targeted delivery of macromolecular drugs, including the EPR effect in solid tumor and clinical overview of the prototype polymeric drug SMANCS. J. Control. Release 74, 47-61 (2001).

26   J. Folkman: Angiogenesis in cancer, vasculature, rheumatoid and other disease. Nat. Med. 1, 27-31 (1995).

27   M. Yokoyama, T. Okano, Y. Sakurai, H. Ekimoto, C. Shibasaki, and K. Kataoka: Toxicity and antitumor activity against solid tumors of micelle-forming polymeric anticancer drug and its extremely long circulation in blood. Cancer Res. 51, 3229-3236 (1991).

28   N.T. Kimura, S. Taniguchi, K. Aoki, and T. Baba: Selective localization and growth of *Bifidbacterium bifidum* in mouse tumors following intravenous administration. Cancer Res. 40, 2061-2068 (1980).

29   C.J. Li, Y. Miyamoto, Y. Kojima, and H. Maeda: Augmentation of tumour delivery of macromolecular drugs with reduced bone marrow delivery by elevating blood pressure. Br. J. Cancer 67, 975-980 (1993).

30   C. J. Li, Y. Miyamoto, Y. Noguchi, M. Kimura and H. Maeda: Improved therapeutic effect of the macromolecular anticancer agent smancs combined with time -lagged administration of antidote tiopronin. J. Exp. Clin. Cancer Res. 13, 394-404 (1994).

31   K. Iwai, H. Maeda, T. Konno, Y. Matsumura, R. Yamashita, K. Yamasaki, S. Hirayama, and Y. Miyauchi : Tumor targeting by arterial administration of lipids: Rabbit model with VX2 carcinoma in the liver. Anticancer Res. 7, 321-327 (1987).

32   M. Kimura, T. Konno, Y. Miyamoto, T. Oda, and Y. Miyauchi: Intracavitary treatment of malignant ascetic carcinomatosis with oily anticancer agents in rats. Anticancer Res. 13, 1287-1292 (1993).

33   M. Kimura, T. Konno, Y. Miyauchi, Y. Kojima, and H. Maeda: Pharmacokinetic advantages of macromolecular anticancer agents against peritoneal and pleural carcinomatosis. Anticancer Res. 18, 2547-2550 (1998).

34   S. Maki, T. Konno, and H. Maeda: Image enhancement in computerized tomography
     for sensitive diagnosis of liver cancer and semiquantitation of tumor selective drug
     targeting with oily contrast medium. Cancer 56, 751-757 (1985).
35   Y. Miyamoto, T. Oda and H. Maeda: Comparison of the cytotoxic effect of the high
     and low-molecular weight anticancer agents on multidrug-resistant Chinese hamster
     ovary cells in vitro. Cancer Res. 50, 1571-1575 (1990).
36   E. Masuda and H. Maeda: Host-mediated antitumor activity induced by
     neocarzinostatin and its polymer-conjugated derivative SMANCS in tumor bearing
     mice. in Neocarzinostatin: the Past ,Present and Future of an Antitumor Anticancer
     Drug. ed. H. Maeda, K. Edo and N. Ishida, Springer-Verlag, Tokyo (1997).
37   F. Suzuki T. Munakata and H. Maeda: Interferon-γ induction by SMANCS:polymer
     conjugated derivative of neocarzinostatin. Anticancer Res. 8 97-104 (1988).

GLOSSARY

AUC: area under the concentration curve (in plasma) vs. time course, i.e.
plasma residence time. This is usually very large for polymer drugs.

EPR-effect: enhanced vascular permeability and retention effect observed in
biocompatible macromolecules or microparticles. This effect results in tumor
selective accumulation of such drugs.

SMANCS: poly [styrene maley (*n*-buthylate)] conjugated neocarzinostatin,
is the first polymeric drug, which is used in clinic in Japan.

12

LIGAND-DIRECTED DESTRUCTION OF TUMOR VASCULATURE

Sophia Ran[1], Michael Rosenblum[2] and Philip E. Thorpe[1]
[1]*The University of Texas Southwestern Medical Center at Dallas, 2201 Inwood Road, Dallas, TX 75390-8594 and* [2]*M.D. Anderson Cancer Center, 1515 Holcombe Boulevard, Box 44, Houston, TX 77030-4009*

INTRODUCTION

Vascular targeting agents (VTA) are designed to bind selectively to components of tumor vasculature and deliver an effector molecule that, directly or indirectly, causes occlusion of the tumor vessels. Blood flow to the tumor thus ceases, resulting in tumor cell death due to the cells' inability to obtain oxygen and nutrients (Fig. 1, below). This approach has several advantages. Firstly, the tumor endothelial cells are directly accessible to intravenously administrated therapeutic agents, permitting rapid localization of a high percentage of the injected dose. Secondly, since each capillary provides oxygen and nutrients for thousands of tumor cells, occlusion of the vessel has an amplified effect on tumor cells. Thirdly, the outgrowth of mutant endothelial cells lacking the target antigen is unlikely because they comprise a normal, genetically stable cell population. Finally, since tumor vessels share common morphological and biochemical properties, this strategy should be applicable to different tumor types.

VTA are composed of two main components: a targeting moiety and an effector moiety. The two components are linked using chemical cross-linkers or via peptide bonds. The function of the targeting moiety is to deliver an effector specifically to the tumor vasculature. The function of the effector moiety is to occlude the tumor vasculature. The effector could act by directly thrombosing tumor blood vessels, by inducing vascular injury that later leads to coagulation or by causing shape changes in the tumor endothelium that physically block the vessels. Typically antibodies directed against a specific marker of tumor endothelium are used as targeting moieties. Alternatively, a ligand that binds to high affinity receptors that are over-expressed on the tumor vessels can be used. Effector moieties include tissue factor (TF), a drug, a toxin or a radioisotope that induce thrombosis on the injured vasculature indirectly.

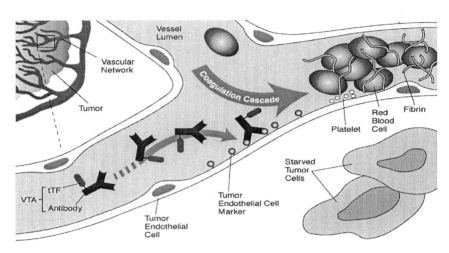

Figure 1. How vascular targeting agents that employ TF work. Tumors rely on a vascular network for oxygen and nutrients. Vascular targeting agents are designed to destroy this vasculature. Selectivity is attained by means of an antibody (or other ligand) that binds to antigens on the vascular endothelial cells of the tumor. The antibody delivers a molecule of truncated tissue factor (tTF) to the lipid surface of endothelial cells. Once the VTA binds to its target, tTF activates the extrinsic pathway of coagulation. The clotting cascade rapidly produces fibrin, and the ensuing clot occludes the vessel.

VTA are conceptually different from drugs that inhibit angiogenesis (Table 1, below). Inhibitors of angiogenesis prevent vascular endothelial cell division while having little or no effect on vasculature where division is not taking place (1). These drugs inhibit tumor growth in regions of neovascularization but do not prevent tumor growth along existing vascular tracts or tumor survival in regions of the tumor served by mature, non-proliferating vessels.

Angiogenesis inhibitors are most effective against tumors and metastases at their early growth stage, when extensive angiogenesis occurs. These inhibitors are less effective against large tumors having a more established vasculature. Giving the drug for prolonged periods is essential to prevent endothelial cell division as the tumor revascularizes zones of necrosis that occur naturally or that are created by earlier courses of the drug. Recent clinical trials have shown that anti-angiogenic drug treatment of patients with bulky advanced tumors results in stabilization of the disease but not usually of tumor shrinkage.

Table 1. Advantages and disadvantages of anti-angiogenesis and vascular targeting approaches

Anti-angiogenic drugs		Vascular targeting agents	
Advantages	Disadvantages	Advantages	Disadvantages
Low toxicity	Chronic treatment that requires a large amount of drug	Acute treatment that requires a small amount of drug	Dose-limiting toxicity may occur with some effectors
Effective at preventing growth of small tumors and metastases	Large tumors are less responsive	Large tumors responsive	Only a few markers are selectively and homogeneously expressed on tumor vasculature
		Regressions and complete eradication have been observed	
Applicable to wide range of tumor types	Tumor growth resumes upon termination of the treatment	Effect extends to vessels located up-and down-stream of thrombosed vasculature	Thrombosis may trigger compensatory angiogenesis as a secondary event

In contrast, VTA are designed to induce platelet activation and coagulation of blood in vessels where division is taking place and where it is not. Blood transporting vessels are occluded, in addition to capillary sprouts. This broadens the effect on the tumor because most vessels are affected and because blood flow is halted in tumor vessels upstream and downstream of the thrombosed vessels, even if they lack the target marker. The action of the VTA is therefore particularly suited to the treatment of large tumors, which are the least responsive to cytotoxic and anti-angiogenic drugs therapy. The downside, however, is that VTA are riskier to use than angiogenesis inhibitors because any mis-targeting or non-specific interaction with the normal vasculature could result in toxicity. The other potential problem with using thrombosis-inducing drugs is that thrombin and other final products of the coagulation cascade are inducers of angiogenesis (2). Tumor angiogenesis may occur as a compensatory response around a partially thrombosed tumor vascular network. This, in turn, may allow re-building of the angiogenic network and expansion of tumor growth. Ultimately, VTA might be used together with anti-angiogenic drugs to suppress the secondary angiogenic response and to take advantage of the complementary strengths of both approaches.

TISSUE FACTOR AS AN EFFECTOR MOIETY OF VTA

Tissue factor is the major initiator of the coagulation cascade. Cells typically in contact with plasma, including vascular endothelial cells, are devoid of tissue factor under normal circumstances, whereas fibroblasts, smooth muscle cells and epithelia that are outside the blood, have tissue factor incorporated into their plasma membranes (3). Blood coagulation is normally triggered at sites of injury when factor VIIa in the blood comes in contact with tissue factor expressed on the extravascular tissues. The tissue factor:VIIa complex then rapidly activates factors IX and X by limited proteolysis, which leads to formation of thrombin and the fibrin clot (3).

The recombinant, truncated form of tissue factor (tTF) lacks the cytosolic and transmembrane domains and has only one hundred-thousandth of the factor X-activating activity of native tissue factor despite its retained ability to bind factor VIIa (4). This is because the truncated tissue factor:VIIa complex is soluble and does not associate with plasma membranes. Membrane association is required for the coagulation cascade to proceed since membrane phospholipids (mainly phosphatidylserine) provide the organizational surface upon which the coagulation complexes assemble.

We reasoned that linking truncated TF to an antibody directed against antigens on tumor endothelium would enable it to bind to the surface of the endothelial cells. Such conjugates, termed "coaguligands", bring truncated TF into proximity to the lipid membrane, restoring its ability to interact with downstream coagulation factors. Binding of the antibody to the endothelial cell surface would, in effect, switch on the thrombogenic activity of the truncated TF and cause thrombosis of tumor vessels.

The use of tTF as the effector also offers other advantages: (a) it is fully functional as a coagulant in rodents, enabling a realistic evaluation of the construct in animal tumor models; (b) neither free tTF nor antibody-conjugated tTF is functional in the absence of acidic phospholipids, thereby preventing nonspecific blood coagulation; (c) even if the target marker of tumor vasculature were present on normal cells outside the bloodstream, toxicity should not result because TF is thrombogenic only when in contact with the blood.

PROOF OF CONCEPT IN A MOUSE MODEL

This approach was first validated in a mouse model (Figure 2, below) in which tumor vasculature was induced to express a unique tumor endothelial antigen (5). The murine neuroblastoma line, C1300, was transfected with the mouse interferon (IFN)-gamma gene and implanted subcutaneously into nude mice. The IFN-gamma secreted by the tumor cells induced local vascular expression of MHC class II antigen, normally absent from rodent blood vessels.

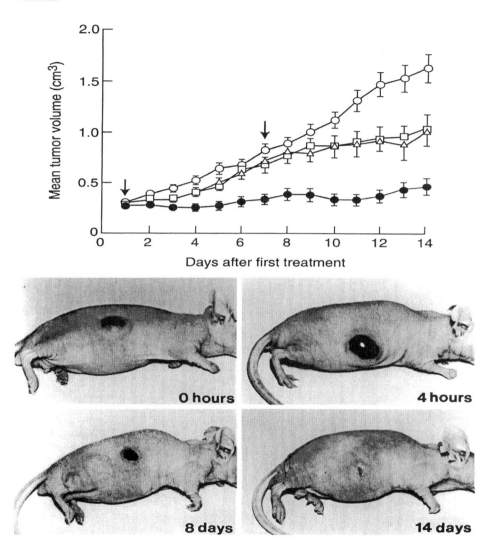

Figure 2. Tumors regressions induced by a coaguligand directed against an MHC class II antigen on tumor endothelial cells. (Top) Nu/nu mice bearing solid neuroblastoma tumors having MHC class II-expressing tumor endothelial cells were injected intravenously with a coaguligand directed against this antigen (•). Other groups received equivalent doses of unconjugated tTF (□) a control coaguligand of irrelevant specificity (Δ) or saline (○). Arrows indicate days of treatment. (Bottom) A representative mouse at selected times after treatment.

To target tumor vasculature, a bispecific antibody was constructed. One arm of the bispecific antibody recognized the MHC class II antigen and the other arm directed against a non-inhibitory epitope on truncated TF. The antibody was mixed with tTF before injection to create the coaguligand. When mice bearing large tumors (0.8 cm in diameter) were injected with anti-class II-coaguligand, thrombosis of tumor vasculature followed by dramatic tumor regressions was observed. Thirty-eight percent of treated animals showed complete tumor regressions (Fig. 2) and a further 24% showed more than 50% tumor shrinkage (5).

A histological study of the time course of events in the tumors confirmed that tumor necrosis was secondary to intravascular thrombosis. Within 30 minutes, vessels throughout the tumor were thrombosed, containing occlusive platelet aggregates, packed erythrocytes and fibrin. After 4 hours, tumor cells showed pyknotic changes that became progressively more marked. By 72 hours, the entire central region of the tumor had condensed into amorphous debris.

TARGETING COAGULIGANDS TO NATURALLY OCCURRING MARKERS OF TUMOR VESSELS

Targeting VCAM-1 on the vessels of Hodgkin's tumor in mice

VCAM-1 is moderately to strongly expressed on the vascular endothelium of tumors having marked leukocytic infiltrates, in particular Hodgkin's disease (6), non-small cell lung carcinoma, breast carcinoma and nasopharyngeal carcinoma. VCAM-1 is absent from vessels in normal tissues, apart from thyroid, testis and tonsil, and is present on activated macrophages and dendritic cells.

A mouse model of Hodgkin's disease was established by implanting L540Cy lymphoma cells subcutaneously into immunodeficient mice. This xenograft shows all hallmarks of the human disease, including the expression of inflammatory cytokines and up-regulation of VCAM-1 on tumor vasculature. The murine VCAM-1 is also present on postcapillary venules in the heart and lungs of the mice. The expression on these vessels is constitutive, rather than cytokine-induced, since identical VCAM-1 expression is found on heart and lung vessels in the control and tumor-bearing mice.

To deliver TF to Hodgkin's tumor vasculature, a VTA was constructed consisting of rat IgG against murine VCAM-1 chemically linked to tTF (7). Intravenous injection of 20 μg of anti-VCAM-1•tTF caused a profound thrombosis in 40-70% of the tumor blood vessels. Within four hours of injection of coaguligand, all VCAM-1-positive vessels were thrombosed, containing occlusive platelet aggregates, packed erythrocytes and fibrin. By 24 hours, the blood vessels were still occluded and tumor cells showed pyknotic changes. By 72 hours, advanced necrosis was evident throughout the tumor. Necrosis was even present in the central region where the vessels do not originally express VCAM-1.

Treatment with anti-VCAM-1•tTF coaguligand reduced the tumor growth rate in mice bearing established (0.3-0.4 cm in diameter) L540 tumors. The mean tumor size 21 days after treatment was 50% of that in control mice receiving antibody alone or coaguligand of irrelevant specificity. No toxicity was observed in the anti-tumor growth experiments.

Vasculature of the heart and lungs in all tumor-bearing animals was resistant to the thrombotic action of the coaguligand despite the localization of the conjugate to VCAM-1-positive vessels of both normal organs (7). These results demonstrate that binding of coaguligand to VCAM-1 on normal vasculature in heart and lung does not induce coagulation, and that tumor vasculature provides additional factors to support coaguligand action.

Targeting TF to fibronectin isoform containing extracellular B (ED-B) domain

A human single-chain Fv antibody L19 specific for the ED-B isoform of fibronectin (see below) was isolated using phage display libraries and combinatorial mutagenesis (8). When administrated to nude mice bearing syngeneic teratocarcinoma, 20% of the injected L19 antibody localized to the tumor (8). These results demonstrated that, although tumor vasculature represents a small fraction of the total tumor mass, high affinity antibodies to selectively expressed markers could accumulate in tumors *in vivo* in large amounts.

To generate a coaguligand, an L19 fragment was genetically fused with truncated TF and expressed as one entity in E. coli (9). The anti-ED-B fibronectin coaguligand was administered to mice bearing large syngeneic tumors. After one injection of 35 μg of the fusion protein, tumors were eradicated in thirty percent of the treated mice (9). The rest of the treated group showed a significant growth delay but tumors eventually grew back. Histologic examination revealed that 80% of the tumor vessels in the center of the tumor mass were thrombosed four hours after injection. Peripheral intratumoral vessels were unaffected despite the fact that they expressed

ED-B isoform. It is likely that this residual vasculature supported renewed angiogenesis and resumption of tumor growth.

This study is interesting from several points of view. First, it demonstrated that, contrary to prior belief, an abluminal marker could be efficiently targeted by tissue factor conjugates. Perhaps, leaky tumor vessels allow extravasation of factor VIIa into sub-endothelial spaces where it can bind to tTF anchored to the target molecule. Alternatively, perhaps ED-B domain is present in small but sufficient quantities on the luminal surface. Second, the anti-tumor effect of anti-ED-B coaguligand was much more impressive than that of the comparable anti-VCAM-1 construct. This suggests that the homogenous distribution and abundance of the drug-binding sites are of greater importance for successful treatment than location of a target. Third, the results of the study confirmed that circulating coaguligands, despite their highly potent effector moiety, are not toxic to normal organs, in accordance with previously published results from our laboratory (7). Last, the authors showed a clear dose-dependency of the therapeutic effect, suggesting that the efficacy can still be improved by better formulation, dosage, and scheduling of the treatment or by combination therapies.

SUPPORT OF COAGULIGAND ACTIVITY BY EXTERNALIZED PHOSPHATIDYLSERINE

The lack of thrombosis induced by anti-VCAM-1•tTF in VCAM-1-positive vessels in heart and lungs suggested that normal vessels lack an ancillary molecule that was needed to support the thrombotic action of the coaguligand. We postulated that the ancillary molecule might be phosphatidylserine (PS). PS exclusively resides on the inner leaflet of the plasma membrane in all normal, quiescent cells, including endothelial cells [10]. Externalization of PS on activated endothelium supports the coagulation cascade as it allows binding of coagulation factors to cell membrane and assemble into enzymatically-active complexes (10). Dependence on PS is supported by the fact that PS-neutralizing protein, annexin V, inhibits the coaguligand's activity *in vitro* in a dose-dependent manner (S. Ran, unpublished results). We reasoned that normal vessels might segregate PS to the cytosolic side of the plasma membrane, whereas tumor vessels might expose PS to the external luminal side.

To test this hypothesis, we determined the distribution of specific anti-PS monoclonal IgM in L540 tumor-bearing mice. Anti-PS antibody specifically bound to the majority of L540 tumor blood vessels but not to vessels in normal organs, including VCAM-1-positive vessels in the heart and lung (7). Similar results were obtained in mice bearing colon, lung and breast carcinomas. A mouse monoclonal IgM antibody against another acidic phospholipid, cardiolipin, did not localize to any organ, confirming the specificity of the detection by anti-PS IgM. We concluded that PS is exposed on the external surface of vascular endothelial cells in tumors but not in normal tissues. In the absence of PS surface exposure, anti-VCAM-1•tTF binds to VCAM-1-positive vessels in heart and lungs but cannot induce coagulation. In contrast, VCAM-1-expressing vessels in the tumor show coincident expression of surface PS. This enables endothelium-bound coaguligand to activate coagulation factors and to induce local formation of thrombi. It is plausible that lack of PS exposure on the ED-B-positive peripheral vessels might be a contributing factor to inactivity of the localized ED-B coaguligand in some tumor regions.

The requirement for coincident expression of the target molecule and PS on tumor endothelium contributes to the safety of coaguligands. Even if the marker of tumor vasculature were present on endothelial cells in normal tissues, PS is likely to be absent from the luminal surface of such cells. Normal vessels are known to maintain the fibrinolytic status through numerous mechanisms, including segregation of PS to the inner side of the membrane (10). It is currently unclear whether non-malignant pathological conditions (e.g., inflammation) could cause exposure of endothelial PS. If PS is externalized under these conditions, the target marker of tumor endothelium will have to be absent from endothelium in these lesions for it to be a safe and useful marker for coaguligand therapy.

CANDIDATE TARGETS EXPRESSED ON HUMAN TUMOR VESSELS

An ideal marker for targeting tumor vasculature would be a luminal protein that is expressed on a high proportion of tumor endothelium and absent from normal vessels. An abluminal marker can also be targeted (9), provided it is located on leaky and fenestrated vessels that allow direct contact with coagulation factors in the blood. Success of the targeting approach will ultimately depend on the extent of a marker's expression, its consistency and favorable distribution within the tumor vasculature. Of these criteria, a homogeneous expression of a marker on the majority of the tumor vessels is probably of the greatest importance. This is because it would allow a simultaneous vascular attack in all tumor regions, minimizing chances for angiogenic recovery and eliminating a need for repetitive, potentially toxic, treatments. A perfect marker would be also absent from sites of inflammation, tissue re-modeling and other pathological non-malignant conditions that might be found in cancer patients. Many tumor endothelial cell markers are expressed either on normal angiogenic endothelium or inflamed vessels.

Despite these concerns, a number of antibodies have been reported to recognize antigens that show preferential expression in tumor vascular endothelial cells. The most promising of these antigens are reviewed below.

Fibronectin isoform containing ED-B domain

An isoform of fibronectin containing ED-B domain is present in the stroma of fetal and neoplastic tissues and in vessels in sites of angiogenesis (11). The epitope is recognized by BC-1 antibody that was raised against transformed fibroblasts. BC-1 antibody stained 38% of human tumors tested, including breast, hepatocellular and colorectal cancers. In almost all the positive tumors, BC-1 staining was confined to the tumor interstitium surrounding tumor cell nests and to the vascular intima. ED-B fibronectin is also present at angiogenic (such as endometrium and ovary), inflammatory (synovium) and proliferative sites but otherwise is undetectable in normal adult tissues.

Administration of technetium 99m-labeled BC-1 antibody to patients with brain tumors resulted in high uptake at the tumor site. In contrast, the uptake in bone marrow, liver and spleen was very low, suggesting that the ED-B fibronectin is specifically associated with malignant vessels (12).

Prostate-specific membrane antigen (PSMA)

PSMA is a membrane enzyme with at least two different enzymatic activities: (a) N-acetylated α-linked L-amino dipeptidase (NAALDase); (b) a folate hydrolase. The expression of PSMA was originally thought to be exclusively restricted to the epithelial cell membrane of the prostate (13). It was initially considered only as a candidate for prostate-specific targeting therapies, since it is expressed on a high proportion of prostate cancers, and the expression is increased in metastatic disease. Follow-up studies showed that antibodies to PSMA also strongly reacted with the vascular endothelium in a wide range of carcinomas, including lung, colon and breast (14), but did not react with normal endothelium. The reason why tumor endothelium should express PSMA is currently unknown. PSMA is also expressed in epithelial cells of normal brain, kidney, and brush border of the intestine (14). However, these extravascular sites should not be accessible to intravenously administered anti-PSMA antibodies.

PSMA holds high promise as a target as it is one of the very few markers that are both selective for the tumor vasculature and homogeneously distributed within the vascular network. Clinical applications of PSMA targeting have been hindered by the lack of animal models with tumor vascular distribution of PSMA similar to that observed in human tumors, and by the absence of anti-mouse PSMA antibodies. Such antibodies have been recently generated.

VEGF and VEGF•Receptor complex

VEGF, also known as vascular permeability factor (VPF), is a dimeric glycoprotein (Mr 34000-42000) that is secreted by many tumor cells in response to hypoxia (15). The molecule is an endothelial cell-specific chemotactic factor mitogen that enhances vascular permeability, all of which are important in the neovascularization of solid tumors. Two endothelial cell surface receptors, VEGFR-1 (Flt-1) and VEGFR-2 (Flk-1 in mouse and KDR in human) are the mediators of the angiogenic responses of VEGF. Anti-VEGF antibodies intensely stain tumor endothelial cells as well as the tumor cells themselves. In contrast, endothelial cells in normal tissue do not stain. VEGF mRNA is localized to tumor cells and is absent from endothelial cells. By contrast, the mRNA for the VEGFR-1 and VEGFR-2 are mainly restricted to endothelium and are upregulated on tumor endothelium (16). These findings indicate that VEGF synthesized by the tumor cells is secreted and binds to VEGF receptors on adjacent endothelial cells. Thus, within the tumor microenvironment, the high concentration of both VEGF and its receptors leads to an accumulation of VEGF•Receptor complex on the tumor endothelium.

Our laboratory generated and characterized six monoclonal antibodies to VEGF, the VEGF-receptor complex, or both. Five of the monoclonal antibodies did not interfere with the binding of VEGF to its receptor, whereas one (2C3) blocked this interaction. The 2C3 antibody prevented binding of VEGF to VEGFR-2, blocked VEGF-induced permeability *in vivo* and significantly suppressed tumor growth in 3 different mouse models (17). The nonblocking antibodies recognized VEGF in association with Flk-1 in *in vitro* assays, stained blood vessels of human and rodent tumors, and localized to tumor endothelium *in vivo* (17).

Similar results have been shown for a single chain Fv antibody LL4 that reacts preferentially with receptor-bound VEGF (18). The tumor uptake of the LL4 antibody was 2 to 10 fold higher than the uptake in various normal organs with the exception of kidney. The high kidney uptake of LL4 occurs partly because kidneys tend to retain single chain antibodies and partly because normal mouse kidney expresses VEGF receptors. It may not be a problem in patients because the expression of VEGF in human tumors is higher than it is in kidneys (18).

Antibodies against VEGF•Receptor complex do not neutralize VEGF and, therefore, have no therapeutic effect by themselves. However, the specificity of their localization makes them good candidates to deliver cytotoxic or pro-thrombotic agents to the tumor vasculature.

VEGF receptors

VEGF receptors, which are highly expressed on tumor endothelium, have been used as targets for VEGF toxin conjugates. A construct containing VEGF and a truncated form of diphtheria toxin was selectively toxic to endothelial cells *in vitro* and inhibited tumor growth *in vivo* by inducing vascular injury followed by hemorrhagic necrosis of the tumor mass (19).

We have recently produced a construct consisting of $VEGF_{121}$ fused to a plant toxin, gelonin ($VEGF_{121}$/rGel). Studies have demonstrated that cells over-expressing the Flk-1/KDR receptor but not the Flt-1 receptor were specifically killed by this construct. Upon systemic administration to mice bearing MDA-MB-231 breast tumors, $VEGF_{121}$/rGel localized to the tumor endothelium but was undetectable on the endothelium of normal tissues. Histological analysis of the tumor sections derived from mice treated with $VEGF_{121}$/rGel revealed thrombotic occlusion of blood vessels and escape of erythrocytes into the tumor interstitium. Treatment of mice bearing human xenografts of breast, prostate, bladder and melanoma tumors resulted in 60% to 80% inhibition of tumor growth.

One of the concerns when targeting VEGF-based toxins is the expression of VEGF receptors at low levels on endothelium of normal tissues. However, injury to normal vascular endothelium was not detected in mice treated with $VEGF_{121}$/rGel or with VEGF- diphtheria toxin (19). It is plausible that the expression of VEGF receptors on the normal vasculature is below the threshold necessary to cause toxicity.

Endoglin

Endoglin is an essential component of the TGF-β receptor system on human endothelial cells, binding TGF-β1 and TGF-β3 with high affinity. Endoglin is upregulated on tumor endothelium in most human solid tumors, probably as a result of endothelial cell activation or proliferation (20).

An immunotoxin prepared by linking anti-endoglin antibody TEC-11 to ricin A-chain was 3000-fold more potent at killing subconfluent, dividing HUVEC than it was at killing confluent, non-dividing HUVEC (21). The greater sensitivity of dividing HUVEC to the drug can be attributed partly to the greater level of expression of endoglin on dividing HUVEC, and partly to a difference in the routing of the drug after it binds to cell surface (21). Whereas non-dividing HUVEC degrade the immunotoxin (presumably in lysosomes), dividing HUVEC appear to internalize the drug by a pathway that avoids degradation. This pathway favors A-chain translocation to the cytosol, where the A-chain exerts its toxic action.

Mice bearing human breast carcinoma MCF-7 (22) that were treated with the anti-endoglin immunotoxin showed complete and durable regressions of the tumors. No apparent toxicity was reported in these studies, indicating that quiescent endothelial cells in normal tissues were unharmed by the immunotoxin despite their expression of endoglin at low levels. In contrast, dividing endothelial cells in the tumor, which express higher levels of endoglin, were killed.

Endosialin

Endosialin is a membrane glycoprotein of 165 kDa which is made up of a 95 kDa core polypeptide and several highly sialyated O-linked oligosaccharides. It was originally identified as a selective tumor endothelial marker in human tumors by means of a monoclonal anti-endosialin antibody, FB5, raised against cultured human fetal fibroblasts (23). FB5 reacted with endothelial cells in about two-thirds of human tumors whereas normal blood vessels and other adult tissues lacked detectable endosialin. There was considerable variability between tumors in the number of FB5 positive vessels, ranging from a small subset of capillaries to virtually the entire capillary bed. FB5 also reacted with cultured fibroblasts and neuroblastoma cell lines but not with normal human endothelial cells even after activation with cytokines.

The selective expression of endosialin on human tumor vessels has been recently confirmed by serial analysis of gene expression (SAGE) (24). The gene expression profile of endothelial cells derived from normal and malignant tissues was compared. One of the most abundantly expressed markers specifically detected in tumor endothelial cells was termed TEM1 (tumor endothelial marker 1). The sequence of the TEM1 gene identified it as endosialin (25). *In situ* hybridization studies showed that mouse endosialin is selectively expressed in tumors.

$\alpha_v\beta_3$ integrin

The integrin $\alpha_v\beta_3$ is a marker of angiogenic vascular tissue (26). After induction of angiogenesis, endothelial cells enter the cell division cycle and express increased levels of $\alpha_v\beta_3$. Anti-$\alpha_v\beta_3$ antibody, LM609, antagonizes the binding of the endothelial cells via their $\alpha_v\beta_3$ integrins to extracellular matrix components. The cells fail to receive a survival signal from the extracellular matrix and undergo apoptosis (26).

The $\alpha_v\beta_3$ integrin is expressed on blood vessels in human wound granulation tissue but not in normal skin, and it shows a 4-fold increase in expression during angiogenesis on the chick chorioallantoic membrane (CAM) (27). Similar induction of the $\alpha_v\beta_3$ expression was observed on the neovasculature of human breast carcinoma melanoma and various epithelial cancers. The LM609 antibody inhibited tumor-induced and bFGF-induced angiogenesis (26). Likewise, the disruption of $\alpha_v\beta_3$ integrin – ligand interaction by peptides mimicking the binding site on the ligand (28) results in apoptosis of tumor vasculature and suppression of tumor growth. Simultaneous administration of integrin antagonist and anti-tumor-IL-2 fusion protein induced tumor regressions and eradicated hepatic metastases, whereas the individual therapies were only partially effective (29).

In addition to direct therapy, anti-integrin peptides have been used to deliver cytotoxic drugs to tumor endothelium (30). It has been shown that coupling of α_v integrin-binding peptide to the anti-cancer drug doxorubicin enhanced the efficacy of the drug against breast cancer xenografts and reduced its toxicity to normal organs (30).

Tumor Endothelium Specific (TES) antigen -23

TES-23 antibody was selected from hybridoma lines that were differentially screened on tumor and normal rat endothelial cells (31). The antibody recognizes an 80 kDa protein related to CD44 that is preferentially expressed on sprouting endothelial cells in tumors of rodent origin (31). Although TES-23 accumulated in tumors at high concentration, repeated injections of unconjugated antibody had no effect on tumor growth. By contrast, an immunoconjugate consisting of TES-23 and neocarzinostatin caused tumor-restricted hemorrhagic necrosis concomitant with a marked anti-tumor effect. No toxic side effects were observed in these studies. These results suggest that analogous markers on human tumor vessels may be exploited for selective destruction of the tumor vasculature.

APPROACHES TO IDENTIFYING NEW TUMOR ENDOTHELIAL ANTIGENS

Powerful new techniques for searching for tumor endothelial cell markers are being developed. Jacobson and colleagues (32) described a method for extracting endothelial cell luminal membrane proteins from solid tumors using perfusion with cationic colloidal silica. The silica binds to the luminal membrane of the endothelial cells. The tumor is then separated from the normal tissue, homogenized and the silica-coated membranes sedimented by density centrifugation. Two-dimensional gel electrophoresis is then used to compare the proteins extracted from tumor vessels with those from normal vessels. Proteins present only in tumor endothelium are then isolated and sequenced or are used to raise specific monoclonal antibodies. Preliminary results indicated that at least 20 new proteins (or ones differing in their glycosylation patterns) can be detected in the endothelium of lung tumors in rats.

Genes differentially expressed in malignant endothelia can be identified by SAGE technique (33). Messenger RNA of endothelial cells derived from malignant and normal tissues was compared to an extensive SAGE library of more than 193,000 expressed sequence tags (ESTs). This analysis revealed 46 tags that were 10-fold or more elevated in tumor endothelia. Twelve tags of this group identified known markers of angiogenesis and tissue remodeling. The remaining transcripts corresponded to uncharacterized genes, deposited in databases as ESTs. Nine of the transcripts from the latter group attracted the most attention because their gene structures predicted the presence of at least one transmembrane domain, suggesting that a putative marker is located on the surface of the cell membrane. These genes were termed TEM (tumor endothelial markers) and labeled 1 through 9. *In situ* hybridization confirmed the selective expression of most of the TEMs in the endothelium of several human primary and metastatic tumors (33). All TEMs with the exception of TEM8 were detected in the corpus luteum and in the granulation tissue of healing wounds. These results are consistent with the idea that a truly specific tumor endothelial marker may not exist because of similarity of stimuli driving both physiological and pathological angiogenesis.

A third technique having enormous promise has been developed by Pasqualini, Arap, Ruoslahti and colleagues (34). They used a method of *in vivo* selection of peptides displayed on the surface of filamentous phage particles. Millions of different peptide sequences were expressed by individual virions. A phage display library was injected intravenously into mice and the phages that homed to specific organs were recovered. After several rounds of amplification and *in vivo* selection, peptides with affinity for vascular receptors expressed in normal and malignant tissues were isolated (34). *In vivo* screening in tumor bearing mice yielded a panel of peptides with three major tripeptide motifs: RGD, NGR and GSL (35). The RGD peptides are selective binders of $\alpha_v\beta3$ and $\alpha_v\beta5$ integrins, known markers of angiogenesis. Peptides containing NGR motif bind to aminopeptidase N (CD13), a protein that is over-expressed on both tumor endothelial and perivascular cells (35). The exact nature of the receptors for GSL peptides is yet to be established. The tumor homing of these peptides was independent of tumor type, suggesting that their receptors were universally expressed on the angiogenic endothelium. Analogous techniques using phage antibody display libraries or aptameric libraries are currently being developed for identifying luminal markers on tumor endothelium in man.

CONCLUDING REMARKS

The main advantages of targeting tumor vessels versus targeting tumor cells themselves are the accessibility of tumor endothelial cells and their lower likelihood of developing treatment-induced resistance. The main advantage of vascular targeting over anti-angiogenic approaches is the ability of VTA to regress well-established tumors through destruction of the pre-existing vasculature. Large-size tumors are less responsive to angiogenesis inhibitors, probably because little angiogenesis takes place at this stage of tumor growth. By contrast, VTA seem to be more effective against large tumors than against small ones. It is plausible that more tumor vessels externalize PS as the tumor grows because of the increased stress conditions in the tumor environment. PS-positive vessels are able to support coagulation whereas PS-negative vessels, which are more prevalent in small tumors, do not.

The main challenge for vascular targeting is to identify a surface marker that is specifically and homogeneously expressed on the majority of tumor vessels. Most tumor endothelial markers are expressed at low levels in some normal tissues or are heterogeneously distributed within the tumor vasculature. Also, all known markers are upregulated on vessels in sites of inflammation, tissue remodeling or physiological angiogenesis, consistent with the concept that "tumors are wounds that do not heal". If a perfect marker were not found, it would be important to assure that cross-reactivity of VTA with normal and pathological non-malignant tissue can be tolerated. There are several reasons to believe that some cross-reactivity might be tolerated. Firstly, the level of expression of the marker in normal or inflamed endothelium may be below the threshold level for a destructive response. Secondly, specifically with regard to immunotoxins, the internalization route of an immunoconjugate may differ between dividing endothelial cells in tumors and quiescent endothelial cells in normal tissues, rendering the latter refractory to the toxic effects of the cytotoxic moiety. Thirdly, coaguligand-induced thrombosis requires co-incident expression of a target and PS. Tumor vessels express PS whereas quiescent normal endothelium does not; thus normal endothelium is resistant to coaguligand action, even if it expresses the target molecule (7). In animal models, treatment with TF or toxin conjugates caused little or no toxicity at the therapeutic dose, suggesting that such experimental therapies could be safely translated into clinical treatments.

REFERENCES

1. Folkman, J. and Shing, Y. Angiogenesis. J.Biol.Chem., *267*: 10931-10934, 1992.
2. Hillen, H. F. Thrombosis in cancer patients. Ann.of Oncol., *11 (SUPPL 3)*: 273-276, 2000.
3. Wilcox, J. N., Smith, K. M., Schwartz, S. M., and Gordon, D. Localization of tissue factor in the normal vessel wall and in the atherosclerotic plaque. Proc.Natl.Acad.Sci.USA, *86*: 2839-2843, 1989.
4. Ruf, W., Rehemtulla, A., and Edgington, T. S. Phospholipid-independent and -dependent interactions required for tissue factor receptor and cofactor function. J.Biol.Chem., *266*: 2158-2166, 1991.
5. Huang, X., Molema, G., King, S., Watkins, L., Edgington, T. S., and Thorpe, P. E. Tumor infarction in mice by antibody-directed targeting of tissue factor to tumor vasculature. Science, *275*: 547-550, 1997.
6. Ruco, L. P., Pomponi, D., Pigott, R., Stoppacciaro, A., Monardo, F., Uccini, S., Boaraschi, D., Tagliabue, A., Santoni, A., Dejana, E., Mantovani, A., and Baroni, C. D. Cytokine production (IL-a alpha, IL-1 beta, and TNF alpha) and endothelial cell activation (ELAM-1 and HLA-DR) in reactive lymphadenitis, hodgkin's disease, and in non-hodgkin's lymphomas. Am.J Pathol., *137(5)*: 1163-1171, 1990.
7. Ran, S., Gao, B., Duffy, S., Watkins, L., Rote, N. S., and Thorpe, P. E. Infarction of solid Hodgkin's tumors in mice by antibody-directed targeting of tissue factor to tumor vasculature. Cancer Res, *58(20)*: 4646-4653, 1998.
8. Viti, F., Tarli, L., Giovannoni, L., Zardi, L., and Neri, D. Increased binding affinity and valence of recombinant antibody fragments lead to improved targeting of tumoral angiogenesis. Cancer Res, *59* : 347-352, 1999.
9. Nilsson, F., Kosmehl, H., Zardi, L., and Neri, D. Targeted delivery of tissue factor to the ED-B domain of fibronectin, a marker of angiogenesis, mediates the infarction of solid tumors in mice. Cancer Res, *61(2)*: 711-716, 2001.
10. Williamson, P. and Schlegel, R. A. Back and forth: the regulation and function of transbilayer phospholipid movement in eukaryotic cells. Molec.Mem.Biol., *11*: 199-216, 1994.
11. Carnemolla, B., Balza, E., Siri, A., Zardi, L., Nicotra, M. R., Bigotti, A., and Natali, P. G. A tumor-associated fibronectin isoform generated by alternative splicing of messenger RNA precursors. J.Cell Biol., *108*: 1139-1148, 1989.
12. Karelina, TV. and Eisen, A. Z. Interstitial collagenase and the ED-B oncofetal domain of fibronectin are markers of angiogenesis in human skin tumors. Cancer Detect.Prev., *22(5)*: 438-444, 1998.
13. Israeli, R. S., Powell, C. T., Fair, W. R., and Heston, W. D. W. Molecular cloning of a complementary DNA encoding a prostate-specific membrane antigen. Cancer Res, *53*: 227-230, 1993.

14. Silver, D. A., Pellicer, I., Fair, W. R., Heston, W. D. W., and Cordon-Cardo, C. Prostate-specific membrane antigen expression in normal and malignant human tissues. Clin.Cancer Res., *3*: 81-85, 1997.

15. Shweiki, D., Itin, A., Neufeld, G., Gitay-Goren, H., and Keshet, E. Patterns of expression of vascular endothelial growth factor (VEGF) and VEGF receptors in mice suggest a role in hormonally regulated angiogenesis. J.Clin.Invest., *91*: 2235-2243, 1993.

16. Dvorak, H. F., Sioussat, T. M., Brown, L. F., Berse, B., Nagy, J. A., Sotrel, A., Manseau, E. J., Vandewater, L., and Senger, D. R. Distribution of vascular permeability factor (vascular endothelial growth factor) in tumors - concentration in tumor blood vessels. J.Exp.Med., *174*: 1275-1278, 1991.

17. Brekken, R. A., Overholser, J., Stastny, V. A., Waltenberger, J., Minna, J., and Thorpe, P. E. Selective inhibition of vascular endothelial growth factor (VEGF) receptor2 (KDR/Flk-1) activity by a monoclonal anti-VEGF antibody blocks tumor growth in mice. Cancer Res, *60*: 5117-5124, 2000.

18. Cooke, S. P., Boxer, G. M., Lawrence, L., Pedley, R. B., Spencer, D. I. R., Begent, R. H. J., and Chester, K. A. A strategy for antitumor vascular therapy by targeting the vascular endothelial growth factor:receptor complex. Cancer Res, *61*: 3653-3659, 2001.

19. Ramakrishnan, S., Olson, T. A., Bautch, V. L., and Mohanraj, D. Vascular endothelial growth factor-toxin conjugate specifically inhibits KDR/flk-1-positive endothelial cell proliferation in vitro and angiogenesis in vivo. Cancer Res., *56*: 1324-1330, 1996.

20. Fonsatti, E., Del Vecchio, L., Altomonte, M., Sigalotti, L., Nicotra, M. R., Coral, S., Natali, P. G., and Maio, M. Endoglin: an accessory component of the TGF-E-binding receptor-complex with diagnostic, prognostic, and bioimmunotherapeutic potential in human malignancies. J.Cell.Physiol., *188*: 1-7, 2001.

21. Burrows, F. J., Derbyshire, E. J., Tazzari, P. L., Amlot, P., Gazdar, A. F., King, S. W., Letarte, M., Vitetta, E. S., and Thorpe, P. E. Endoglin is an endothelial cell proliferation marker that is upregulated in tumor vasculature. Clin.Cancer Res., *1*: 1623-1634, 1995.

22. Seon, B. K., Matsuno, F., Haruta, Y., Kondo, M., and Barcos, M. Long-lasting complete inhibition of human solid tumors in SCID mice by targeting endothelial cells of tumor vasculature with antihuman endoglin immunotoxin. Clin.Cancer Res., *3*: 1031-1044, 1997.

23. Rettig, W. J., Garinchesa, P., Healey, J. H., Su, S. L., Jaffe, E. A., and Old, L. J. Identification of endosialin, a cell surface glycoprotein of vascular endothelial cells in human cancer. Proc Natl.Acad.Sci.USA, *89*: 10832-10836, 1992.

24. Carson-Walter, E. B., Watkins, D. N., Nanda, A., Vogelstein, B., Kinzler, K. W., and St.Croix, B. Cell surface tumor endothelial markers are conserved in mice and humans. Cancer Res, *61(18)*: 6649-6655, 2001.

25. Christian, S., Ahorn, H., Koehler, A., Eisenhaber, F., Rodi, H. P., Garin-Chesa, P., Park, J. E., Rettig, W. J., and Lenter, M. C. Molecular cloning and characterization of endosialin, a C-type lectin-like cell surface receptor of tumor endothelium. J Biol.Chem, *276(10)* : 7408-7414, 2001.

26. Brooks, P. C., Clark, R. A., and Cheresh, D. A. Requirement of vascular integrin alpha v beta 3 for angiogenesis. Science, *264*: 569-571, 1994.

27. Brooks, P. C., Montgomery, A. M. P., Rosenfeld, M., Reisfeld, R. A., Hu, T., Klier, G., and Cheresh, D. A. Integrin alpha v beta 3 antagonists promote tumor regression by inducing apoptosis of angiogenic blood vessels. Cell, *79*: 1157-1164, 1994.

28. Pasqualini, R., Koivunen, E., and Ruoslahti, E. Alpha v integrins as receptors for tumor targeting by circulating ligands. Nature Biotechnology, *15(6)*: 542-546, 1997.

29. Lode, H. N., Moehler, T., Xiang, R., Jonczyk, A., Gillies, S. D., Cheresh, D. A., and Reisfeld, R. A. Synergy between an antiangiogenic integrin alpha V antagonist and an antibody-cytokine fusion protein eradicates spontaneous tumor metastases. Proc.Natl.Acad.Sci.(USA), *96(4)*: 1591-1596, 1999.

30. Arap, W., Pasqualini, R., and Ruoslahti, E. Cancer treatment by targeted drug delivery to tumor vasculature in a mouse model. Science, *279*: 377-380, 1998.

31. Ohizumi, I., Tsunoda, S., Taniguchi, K., Saito, H., Esaki, K., Koizumi, K., Makimoto, H., Wakai, Y., Matsui, J., Tsutsumi, Y., Nakagawa, S., Utoguchi, N., Ohsugi, Y. , and Mayumi, T. Identification of tumor vascular antigens by monoclonal antibodies prepared from rat-tumor-derived endothelial cells. Int J Cancer, *77(4)*: 561-566, 1998.

32. Jacobson, B. S., Stolz, D. B., and Schnitzer, J. E. Identification of endothelial cell-surface proteins as targets for diagnosis and treatment of disease. Nature Med., *2*: 482-484, 1996.

33. St.Croix, B., Rago, C., Velculescu, V., Traverso, G., Romans, K. E., Montgomery, E. , Lal, A., Riggins, G. J., Lengauer, C., Vogelstein, B., and Kinzler, K. W. Genes expressed in human tumor endothelium. Science, *289(5482)*: 1197-1202, 2000.

34. Pasqualini, R. and Ruoslahti, E. Organ targeting *in vivo* using phage display peptide libraries. Nature, *380*: 364-366, 1996.

35. Ruoslahti, E. Targeting tumor vasculature with homing peptides from phage display. Semin Cancer Biol, *10(6)*: 435-442, 2000.

GLOSSARY

Coaguligand: VTA consisting of tTF and an antibody or other high affinity ligand directed against marker of tumor endothelium.

Effector moiety: a component of VTA that directly or indirectly causes formation of occlusive thrombi within the tumor vessels.

Immunotoxin: VTA consisting of antibody or other high affinity ligand directed against marker of tumor endothelium and cytotoxic agent (e.g. ricin A or gelonin).

PS: phosphatidylserine; a negatively charged phospholipid that exclusively resides in the inner leaflet of the plasma membrane under normal conditions. PS is an essential component of enzymatically active coagulation complexes.

Single-chain Fv antibody: a recombinant fragment of variable region of an antibody that retains the antigen binding capacity.

Targeting moiety: a component of VTA that is selected for its ability to specifically recognize and bind to a marker expressed on tumor vascular endothelial cells.

TEM: Tumor Endothelial Marker; a molecule that is predominantly expressed in tumor endothelial cells and that is absent from endothelial cells in normal organs.

TF: Tissue Factor; a protein expressed on the surface of activated endothelial cells and cells outside of the bloodstream that is chiefly responsible for induction of coagulation cascade.

tTF: truncated TF; a modified tissue factor protein that lacks the cytosolic and transmembrane domains and has only one hundred-thousandth of the activity of native TF.

VTA: Vascular Targeting Agent; a conjugate that is designed to deliver pro-thrombotic, cytotoxic or radiolabeled molecule specifically to the components of tumor vessels.

13

TUMOR NECROSIS TREATMENT AND IMAGING OF SOLID TUMORS

Alan L. Epstein, Leslie A. Khawli, and Peisheng Hu
Department of Pathology, Keck School of Medicine at the University of Southern California, Los Angeles, CA 90033.

INTRODUCTION

A novel approach to cancer imaging and therapy utilizing necrotic cells as targets for the selective binding of monoclonal antibodies has been developed in our laboratory. Tumor Necrosis Therapy (TNT) represents a radical departure from current methods that employ monoclonal antibodies (MAbs) to bind to tumor-associated cell surface antigens and require the use of different antibodies for each type of tumor. In contrast, TNT is based upon the hypothesis that MAbs against intracellular antigens that are found in all cells and are retained by dying cells show preferential localization in malignant tumors due to the presence of abnormally permeable, degenerating cells not found in normal tissues. It has long been recognized that rapidly dividing tumors contain a proportion of degenerating or dead cells, but, with attention focused upon attempts to kill the dividing cells, the degenerating component has largely been ignored. Calculations of tumor cell loss have revealed that, in contrast to normal tissues, 30-80% of the progeny of tumor cell divisions shortly undergo degeneration. In tumors, the imperfect vasculature and impaired phagocytic response permit the accumulation of degenerating cells, often with the formation of large areas of necrosis, long recognized by pathologists to be a typical feature of malignant tumors. Thus, the accumulation within tumors of a high proportion of dying cells constitutes a major distinction between malignant tumors and normal tissues, where sporadic cell death occurs at a relatively low rate and is accompanied by a rapid and orderly removal of necrotic elements from the tissue. Since degenerating cells have permeable cell surface membranes not observed in viable cells, TNT MAbs enter and bind to their intracellular antigens in necrotic areas of the tumor. Contrarily, TNT antibodies diffusing in viable regions of the tumor and normal tissues do not bind and are removed from the circulation by normal clearance mechanisms. Hence, TNT provides a novel approach for specifically targeting necrotic regions of tumors and can be used to deliver diagnostic and therapeutic reagents into the central core of tumors.

As shown in Table 1, TNT has a number of unique features that distinguishes it from other forms of MAb therapy. Because of these attributes, TNT has several advantages that allow it to be used to deliver radionuclides, immunostimulatory molecules, and vasopermeability agents to treat experimental and human tumors. Over the next several years, it is anticipated that, as this approach moves from the laboratory bench into the clinic, it will be applied to a number of treatment options in order to determine its best use in patients.

Table 1. Major Characteristics of Tumor Necrosis Therapy for the Treatment of Refractory Solid Tumors.

1.	Applicable to a wide range of human and animal cancers
2.	Does not bind to normal tissues
3.	Targets microregionally in central necrotic areas
4.	MAbs have a long retention time in tumor
5.	Suitable for the treatment of bulky tumors
6.	Can be used as a delivery vehicle for radionuclides, immune effector molecules, vasopermeability enhancing agents, diagnostic reagents, and toxic drugs

CHIMERIC TNT ANTIBODIES AND THEIR ANTIGENS

Monoclonal antibodies are ideal reagents that can be used in the effective therapy and diagnosis of cancer. In order for these promising reagents to reach their full potential, however, several obstacles need to be circumvented including their low tumor uptake, non-specific binding in normal tissues, and poor pharmacokinetic characteristics (1). Many different methods have been devised to link radiodiagnostic and therapeutic reagents to MAbs for clinical evaluation. For radioimaging, an ideal reagent (high signal to noise ratio) should clear rapidly so that the background is minimal and high contrast is achieved to enable rapid detection of primary and secondary tumor lesions. In contrast, radioimmunotherapy strives to achieve optimal tumor targeting as its primary objective in order to obtain adequate therapy. To accomplish this, it is necessary for MAbs not only to target tumor effectively but also to clear quickly from normal organs, thereby minimizing the exposure of radiosensitive tissues to circulating radionuclide.

Our laboratory has developed a novel method to target solid tumors using monoclonal antibodies (MAbs) that bind to degenerating cells located in necrotic regions of tumors (2). Designated TNT, this approach can be used to target cancers of diverse origin while avoiding the problems of antigenic modulation and shedding. Three chimeric TNT MAbs developed in our laboratory, chTNT-1, chTNT-2 and chTNT-3, target intranuclear antigens consisting of histone DNA complexes, heterochromatic DNA, and single-stranded DNA, respectively (3, 4). In this section, we have investigated these three related MAbs and evaluated the pharmacokinetic and biodistribution characteristics of each in tumor-bearing mice. Monoclonal antibodies chTNT-1 and chTNT-3 were produced in our laboratory as previously described (4). chTNT-2 was genetically engineered in our laboratory from murine hybridoma 244 (IgM, κ) using primers based on the murine μ- and κ-chain sequences (5).

Pharmacokinetic and biodistribution studies

Six-week-old female BALB/c mice were used to determine the pharmacokinetic clearance of all three chTNT MAbs. chTNT-2 showed the longest circulation time ($T_{1/2}$ = 178.7 hours) compared to chTNT-1 ($T_{1/2}$ = 30.4 hours) and chTNT-3 ($T_{1/2}$ = 134.2 hours). Affinity binding studies were also conducted in which ^{125}I labeled chTNT antibodies were incubated with fixed Raji cells and the bound radioactivity was used to calculate the affinity constant K_a by Schatchard analysis. The affinity constants of chTNT-1, -2, and –3 were 2.5 x 10^9 M^{-1}, 1.2 x 10^9 M^{-1}, and 1.4 x 10^9 M^{-1}, respectively.

To examine the tissue biodistribution of these MAbs, a 0.2 ml inoculum containing 10^7 cells of the MAD109 murine lung adenocarcinoma or the LS174T human colon carcinoma was used. The tumors were grown for 5-7 days at which time they reached approximately 1 cm in diameter. Within each group (*n*=5), individual mice were injected I.V. with a 0.1 ml inoculum containing 100 μCi/10 μg of ^{125}I-labeled MAb. As shown in Table 2, chTNT-1, -2, and –3 had different biodistribution characteristics *in vivo* and showed good uptake in the tumor models tested. For chTNT-2 and chTNT-3, the % injected dose/g tended to be higher than that for chTNT-1 in all organs. However, tumor-to-blood ratios for chTNT-1 were significantly higher (except for muscle and intestine) compared with those of chTNT-2 and chTNT-3. These results demonstrate the *in vivo* binding characteristics of each chTNT antibody in tumor-bearing mice.

Table 2. One-Day Tissue Biodistribution of ^{125}I-labeled chTNT-1, -2 and –3 MAbs in Tumor Bearing Mice.[a]

% Injected Dose/Gram (%ID/g)

Organs	chTNT-1[b]	chTNT-2[c]	chTNT-3[b]
Blood	5.91((0.40)	11.8(1.74)	10.2(1.03)
Lung	1.10(0.07)	4.73(0.18)	2.51(0.47)
Liver	0.85(0.02)	4.81(0.23)	2.91(0.90)
Spleen	0.79(0.01)	3.60(0.49)	4.48(0.98)
Stomach	0.48(0.04)	1.80(0.23)	1.66(0.36)
Kidney	0.87(0.03)	2.86(0.43)	1.64(0.28)
Tumor	2.78(0.20)	6.29(0.62)	4.53(0.88)

[a]Data are expressed as mean (SD), n = 5 animals per group
[b]LS174T human colon carcinoma-bearing nude mice
[c]MAD109 murine lung adenocarcinoma-bearing BALB/c mice.

HUMAN TNT ANTIBODY NHS76

Anti-tumor antibodies are being used in a variety of ways including use as direct cytotoxic agents and carrier molecules for potent therapeutic compounds. An important obstacle, however, has been the potential for the immunological rejection of these antibodies due to their non-human composition. To address this problem, humanized antibodies using Complementary Determining Regions (CDR) grafting techniques have been developed to diminish the immunoreactivity of chimeric antibodies (6). These humanized MAbs, while greatly reducing the risk of immunologic rejection, still have the potential to elicit a human anti-mouse antibody (HAMA) response due to the murine content of the CDR, especially when linked to other immune regulatory molecules that can increase their antigenicity. With the advent of technology to produce antibodies in mammalian systems in a stabile manner, completely human monoclonal antibodies are becoming more readily available. To accomplish this, investigators rely on phage display libraries (7), immunization in human antibody-producing XenoMouse strains (8), and fusion using human myeloma cell lines (9). These human antibodies are better suited for use in therapeutic applications because of their compatibility in humans. In collaboration with scientists at Cambridge Antibody Technology (CAT, Slough, UK), a human TNT-1 antibody, designated NHS76 (10), has been generated using phage display methods. The characterization of this fully human antibody is described below to demonstrate its potential to target solid tumors of man.

Generation of NHS76

The cDNA of the light and heavy variable regions of NHS76 was provided by Cambridge Antibody Technology, Ltd. It was derived from screening a large scFv library using nuclear extracts form the Raji Burkitt's lymphoma cell line using methods described by Vaughan *et al.* (11). The variable heavy and light chains were then linked to human IgG1 heavy chain and human kappa light chain constant regions, respectively, and the complete NHS76 antibody was expressed in the mouse NSO myeloma cell line using the glutamine synthetase gene amplification expression system (10). Using fixed Raji Burkitt's lymphoma cells, the immunoreactivity of NHS76 was compared to that of chTNT-1. The ^{125}I-labeled antibodies were incubated with paraformaldehyde fixed Raji cells and the amount of bound radioactivity was used to calculate the affinity constant (K_a) by Scatchard analysis. The determined K_a for chTNT-1 and NHS76 were found to be 1.74 x 10^9 M^{-1} and 1.65 x 10^9 M^{-1}, respectively. This indicates that the human antibody was found to have close to the same binding ability as chTNT-1 against the same antigen.

Pharmacokinetic and biodistribution studies

Pharmacokinetic evaluation demonstrated differences in the clearance profile of the NHS76 MAb as compared to chTNT-1. The whole body clearance of the NHS76 in BALB/c mice was much greater than that of the chTNT-1 (a half-life of 212.4h vs. 30.4h) ($P \leq 0.01$). This was an unexpected result since most human antibodies tend to have a more rapid half-life than murine and chimeric antibodies in mice. Despite this finding, the NHS76 was able to target tumor similarly if not better than chTNT-1.

Relative tumor uptake of the chTNT-1 and NHS76 was determined by tissue biodistribution studies in LS174T human colon adenocarcinoma tumor-bearing nude mice. For these studies, biodistribution was performed on days 1, 2, 3, 5, and 7 after I.V. injection of ^{125}I-labeled MAbs. Figure 1 illustrates the tissue biodistribution for 1 to 7 days as depicted by the % injected dose per gram of tissue and the tumor to normal organ ratios. It is evident that because of the slower body clearance of the NHS76, the 1-day biodistribution values have high circulating blood levels. As the blood levels drop, however, the amount of antibody remaining at the tumor normalizes to about 2.7 % injected dose per gram by 7 days. This is comparable to the 3-day tumor retention level for chTNT-1. In fact, comparing 3-day tumor % injected dose per gram levels (Figure 2 below) shows a slightly higher uptake

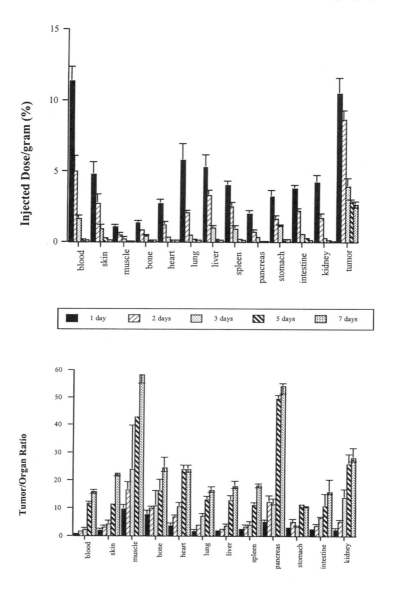

Figure 1.   Tissue biodistribution of ^{125}I-labeled NHS76 in LS174T human colon adenocarcinoma-bearing nude mice. **A)** Tissue uptake as measured by % injected dose of ^{125}I-labeled NHS76 per gram of tissue (mean ± SD). **B)** Tumor/normal organ ratios calculated from the cpm per gram of tumor/cpm per gram of organ (mean ± SD).

for the NHS76 (3.94 ± 0.96 vs. 2.74 ± 0.10) ($P \leq 0.01$). It appears that the high tumor uptake at day one mirrors that of the high blood levels. This can be expected since LS174T is a highly vascularized tumor and therefore, the circulating blood pool of MAb is detected by the sampling of tumor at day one. However, as time progresses and the circulating MAb disappears from the blood, the tumor uptake stabilizes at its true value of around 2.7 % injected dose per gram (Figure 2). The TNT target may also affect binding uptake since we have previously reported that chTNT-3 against DNA and RNA has over twice the tumor uptake of chTNT-1(12). Because of the unique nature of our targeting system, the TNT MAbs can be used as delivery vehicles for a variety of therapeutic modalities. Unlike cell-surface targeted MAbs which may require internalization for their cellular toxicity, the TNT MAbs are not involved in direct tumoricidal activity. Because of this, only the relative amount of uptake is important for TNT MAbs to be effective as delivery vehicles for therapeutic reagents.

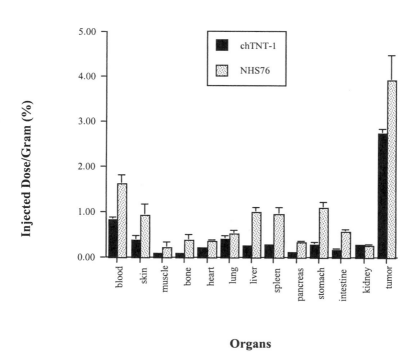

Figure 2. Three-day biodistribution of ^{125}I-labeled chTNT-1 and NHS76 in LS174T human colon adenocarcinoma-bearing nude mice. Tissue uptake as measured by % injected dose of ^{125}I-labeled antibody per gram of tissue (mean ± SD).

Tumor targeting studies

An imaging study was also performed to demonstrate the ability of NHS76 to localize to LS174T human colon adenocarcinoma xenografts. As depicted in Figure 3, imaging for 1, 3, and 5 days show strong signal at the tumor site indicating that the MAb is able to localize and remain within the tumor. Because of the apparent slower clearance of this human MAb, there is a greater amount of circulating radiolabeled MAb in the blood accounting for the relatively high background seen at the early time points. Tumor localization of the NHS76 was further examined with phosphor screen autoradiography. Using this macro-autoradiographic method on sections serially stained with H&E, we have previously demonstrated that the targeting of the TNT antibodies correlates to the necrotic regions of tumor xenografts (2, 13). NHS76 targets necrotic regions the LS174T tumor while normal tissues show little binding. By 7 days, there is still a strong signal in the tumor while the lung, liver and kidney show only background uptake.

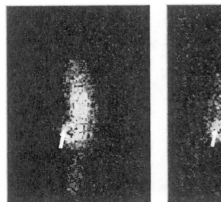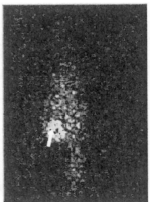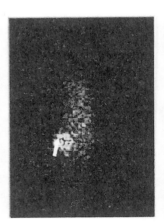

Figure 3. Images of LS174T human colon adenocarcinoma-bearing nude mice treated with ^{131}I-labeled NHS76 at 1, 3, and 5 days after injection. Arrows point to the tumor image.

This demonstration of the comparability of NHS76 to chTNT-1 indicates that the human MAb has potential to accomplish all of the therapeutic goals already demonstrated with the chimeric antibody. As a fully human, non-antigenic counterpart to the chTNT-1, it therefore appears to be a good candidate to be used in future clinical trials for the treatment of refractory solid tumors in man.

GENERATION OF TNT IMAGING AGENTS

Based upon the above results, our laboratory has attempted to develop a TNT imaging agent that could be used for the early diagnosis of cancer and/or the monitoring of cytoreductive therapies in common use. Intact monoclonal antibodies, although known to give the best quantitative uptake in tumors, are not ideal imaging agents due to their slow clearance from blood and tissues producing low signal-to-noise ratios (14). Although a number of monoclonal antibody fragments have been tested against tumor cell membrane antigens (15, 16), the novel nature of TNT monoclonal antibodies and their antigens mandated that a thorough analysis of TNT antibody derivatives would be required in order to identify the most useful reagent for immunoscintigraphy.

Fortunately, molecular biology provides the means to produce a series of antibody fragments from small single chain derivatives to F(ab')$_2$ (16, 17). The single chain Fv (scFv), is one of smallest forms of antibody which consists of variable light and heavy domains connected by a flexible peptide linker of approximately 15 amino acids (AA) generating one binding site. The ability of the scFv to bind to tumor lies in a fine balance between its ability to penetrate tumor tissues due to its small size (30 kDa) and its fast clearance from the body by the kidneys. To obtain better tumor binding, other variations of antibody structure have recently been described, including diabody and triabody molecules. Diabodies (60 kDa) consist of two single chain molecules joined by a very short linker (17) while triabodies are prepared without the linker thereby preventing dimer formation (18) and forcing trimerization (90 kDa).

For clinical studies, the selection of radionuclide is critical to the development of an imaging agent. ^{131}I is the most commonly used radionuclide for radioimmunotherapy but its use in cancer imaging is restricted by a long physical half-life (T½ = 8 days), a high energy photon which is only captured at 10% efficiency by imaging cameras, and dehalogenation issues. Use of ^{123}I has been restricted by its relatively high cost and short half-life (T½ = 13.2 hr). ^{99m}Tc has been used for radioimmunoscintigraphy, but because of its short half-life (T½ = 6 h), images must be obtained in a restricted time frame. Finally, ^{111}In and other radiometals require the use of chemical chelators to attach them to antibodies and have a high affinity for the liver in patients where metaloenzymes abound obscuring imaging in the abdomen.

In this section, we compare the imaging capabilities of chimeric TNT-3 derivatives including scFv, diabody, and triabody molecules and Fab and F(ab')$_2$ fragments previously generated by our laboratory (19), in order to identify candidate reagents for the immunoscintigraphy of solid tumors. For these studies, ^{125}I, ^{131}I, and ^{99m}Tc were used as radionuclides to determine optimal labeling methods. *In vivo* analyses were also performed after labeling to evaluate whole body half-life and tumor uptake.

Expression and characterization of the chTNT-3 fragments

All five chTNT-3 fragments were genetically engineered using the TNT-3 binding site and produced by PCR assembly. The Glutamine Synthetase Gene Amplification System was used to produce the chTNT-3 derivatives in mammalian cells enabling post-translational modifications to occur. While single chain reagents and their derivatives are in most cases produced in bacteria, in this case the recombinant antibody fragments were produced using the GS system in mammalian cells. Antibody fragments produced in mammalian systems are generally easier to purify since they are secreted into the supernatant and can be recovered under native conditions thereby bypassing denaturation and refolding steps often necessary when expression is performed in bacteria (20). In addition, the results of our studies showed that three cysteine residues are required to produce stable F(ab')$_2$ fragments and that different purification tags can be used with this variant to produce suitable reagents for *in vivo* studies. Those constructs containing one or two cysteines were found to be unstable and broke down to Fab fragments regardless of the purification tag used.

Affinity constants

In studies (21) which compared the relative affinity constants of scFv fragments with other antibody fragments, the constants for the bivalent forms (IgG and F(ab')$_2$) were 7- to 10-fold greater than those for the monovalent forms (Fab and scFv). As seen in other antibody models (22), all single chain-derived chTNT-3 fragments were found to have diminished avidity constants compared to chTNT-3 (Table 3). In addition, the immunoreactivity of all fragments was approximately 25% lower than the parent antibody probably attributable to changes in conformation during the assembly of newly constructed molecules producing a modification in the active site. We also found that the diabody showed a relatively higher affinity than the triabody. This finding is particularly important and in agreement with other studies, which demonstrated that multivalent fragments such as triabody and tetrabody did not show, as expected, an improvement in binding. This was due to the fact that their configurations that prevented them from utilizing all binding sites, and, in fact, reduced their valencies compared to the diabody.

Pharmacokinetic and biodistribution studies

The affinity binding characteristics and pharmacokinetic behavior (Table 3) of all the fragments were studied in parallel. These studies showed that they had rapid whole-body clearances in BALB/c mice compared to that of parental chTNT-3.

Table 3. Percentage Binding, Affinity Constants and Half-lives ($T_{1/2}$) of chTNT-3 Antibody and Fragments [a].

Antibody	# Of Binding Sites	Size (kDa)	% Binding	Affinity Constant (M^{-1})	$T_{1/2}(h)$ [b]
chTNT-3	2	150	89.0	1.43×10^9	134.2 (4.0)
ScFv	1	30	67.9	0.25×10^9	4.9(0.98)
Diabody	2	60	68.5	0.40×10^9	6.1(7.9)
Triabody	3	90	68.1	0.31×10^9	7.9(1.25)
Fab	1	55	65.8	0.48×10^9	6.3(0.77)
F(ab')$_2$	2	120	65.7	0.54×10^9	8.1(0.48)

[a] All of the antibody variants were labeled with ^{125}I. Standard Deviations of the Mean are given in Parentheses.
[b] $T_{1/2}$ as Determined by Whole-Body Clearance in BALB/c Mice (n=5).

The principle determinants of the rate with which radiopharmaceuticals are cleared from the circulation are their size and the presence of an intact Fc portion. Both factors determine whether they radiopharmaceuticals will be removed by filtration in the kidney or by the reticuloendothelial system. Consistent with these concepts, our results showed that the clearance rate is in accordance with the molecular size of each fragment, meaning that smaller fragments are cleared more rapidly than the larger ones. Despite their rapid elimination, all fragments did, however, retain their ability to localize to tumor, as depicted in the biodistribution studies shown in Table 4.

Table 4. Tumor Uptake (% Injected Dose/Gram) at Different Times after Administration of ^{125}I-Labeled and ^{99m}Tc-Labeled chTNT-3 Antibody and Fragments in MAD109 Murine Lung Carcinoma Tumor-Bearing BALB/c Mice (n=5).[a]

[125]I-Labeled chTNT-3 and Fragments

Time (h)	chTNT-3	ScFv	Diabody	Triabody	Fab	F(ab')$_2$
6	10.7(0.77)	4.59(0.48)	3.05(0.28)	4.62(0.47)	3.68(0.51)	6.13(0.47)
12	12.5(0.66)	1.50(0.37)	1.72(0.06)	2.26(0.33)	1.75(0.16)	5.30(0.35)
24	11.6(1.03)	1.41(0.12)	1.64(0.07)	2.10(0.23)	1.40(0.26)	5.01(0.41)

[99m]Tc-Labeled chTNT-3 and Fragments

Time (h)	chTNT-3	ScFv	Diabody	Triabody	Fab	F(ab')$_2$
24	3.45(0.09)	0.58(0.09)	0.57(0.09)	0.68(0.05)	0.54(0.04)	1.34(0.14)

[a] Standard Deviations of the Mean are Given in Parentheses

The biodistribution data also showed that at all time points after injection, tumor uptake of the ^{125}I-labeled fragments was lower than the parental antibody. These data suggest that tumor uptake appears to correlate with the molecular size (kDa) of each variant, since the more rapid clearance of smaller fragments decreased the amount of binding to the tumors. However, at 6h and 12h after injection, tumor-to-organ ratios for all the fragments were higher (except kidney and stomach) compared with those of parental chTNT-3. By 24h after injection, the difference was more pronounced, and the lowest tumor-to-organ ratios for kidney and stomach were only observed with scFv and Fab fragments. Our data appear to confirm those of other studies (23) and showed a slight improvement of diabodies over scFv, as well as a ratio of approximately 1:8 as compared to whole chTNT-3 at 24h post injection. Biodistribution of ^{99m}Tc-labeled preparations showed that tumor uptake had a lower %ID/g for smaller fragments compared to those of parental chTNT-3. A comparison of tumor uptake with [125]I- and ^{99m}Tc-labeled preparations (Table 4) suggests that labeling with technetium had a significant effect on tissue biodistribution. This is a common finding in mouse studies (23, 24) that show heterogeneity of antibody accumulation due to differences in the animal model used or differences in the techniques and radioisotopes used for labeling. Although absolute levels of ^{99m}Tc-labeled fragments in the tumor were lower compared with their corresponding ^{125}I-labeled fragments, the lower levels of background with ^{99m}Tc in all organs suggest the contrast would be greatly improved. In particular, tumor-to-blood ratios for ^{99m}Tc-labeled fragments were far better than their corresponding

[125]I-labeled fragments (except $F(ab')_2$) at equivalent time points after injection. Moreover, the biodistribution data with ^{99m}Tc labeling demonstrated that the highest tumor-to-organ ratios were observed with scFv and Fab fragments. In contrast, the highest tumor-to-organ ratios with ^{125}I labeling were observed with $F(ab')_2$, diabody and triabody.

Imaging studies

The ability to produce pure antibody fragments allowed evaluation of the imaging properties with ^{131}I-labeled chTNT-3 fragments (Fig. 4). These data are encouraging and consistent with previous publications using chTNT-3 and mutant chTNT-3 (24). Figure 4F demonstrates the capability of [131]I-$F(ab')_2$ to localize in tumor at 24h post injection and shows that total body activity cleared sufficiently to allow excellent visualization of the tumor. With the ^{131}I-diabody (Fig. 4C) and the ^{131}I-triabody (Fig. 4D), however, visualization of the tumor was not as clear at 24h because of the higher background noise.

Images with the ^{131}I-scFv (Fig. 4B) and the ^{131}I-Fab (Fig. 4E) showed a faint signal in the tumor and a very high signal visible in the bladder, which is consistent with the kidney being the major route of clearance of activity for these small molecular sized fragments. Thus, these pharmacokinetic and biodistribution data are consistent with our imaging results that show that smaller fragments have higher clearance rates and less time to bind to tumor. Furthermore, the predominant renal clearance of monovalent (scFv and Fab) fragments that impedes the accumulation of activity in tumor should result in poor discrimination of abdominal tumors. The observed immunoscintigraphic results showed a marked difference between the [131]I- and ^{99m}Tc-labeled fragments (Fig. 5). Thus, for ^{99m}Tc-scFv and ^{99m}Tc-Fab, better images were observed at 24h. These images agree well with our biodistribution results, which show higher tumor-to-organ ratios in most tissues at these time points. In addition, the better performance of ^{99m}Tc-labeled scFv and Fab compared with ^{131}I-labeled scFv and Fab might be attributable to differences in the experimental variables used in this study. For example, tumor uptake and tumor-to-organ ratios are known to be influenced by nonspecific factors such as the radionuclides used, the size of the tumor, and the dose administered. The different radionuclides (^{125}I, ^{131}I and ^{99m}Tc) used by our laboratory may have contributed to the difference in performance, since each labeling method might have influenced the amount of non-specific binding, resulting in different tumor-to-organ ratios. Tumor uptake is also increased as the dose (specific activity/quantity of antibody) is increased, although this is usually at the expense of higher background accumulation. The biodistribution data show that the better tumor-to-organ ratios of ^{99m}Tc-labeled scFv and Fab compared with ^{125}I-labeled scFv and Fab were mostly attributable to better clearance from the normal tissues and not to higher tumor uptake. These comparisons suggest that not all factors examined appear to have been responsible for the observed differences in the performance of scFv, diabody, triabody, Fab and F(ab')$_2$. Rather the performance observed here appears to be influenced by the type of radionuclide used. Additional studies are currently in progress to test different human tumor models as well as different labeling methodologies and radionuclides, such as ^{123}I and ^{111}In, in order to define the optimal parameters for tumor targeting.

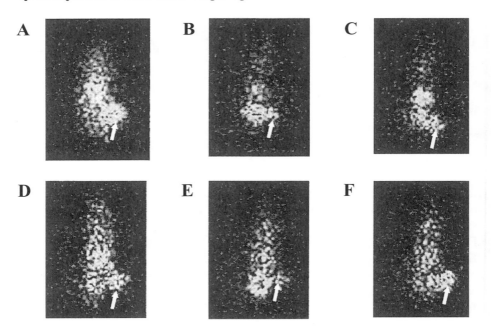

Figure 4. Images of MAD109 tumor-bearing BALB/c mice with ^{131}I-labeled chTNT-3 antibody and fragments at 24 hours after injection. (**A**) Whole chTNT-3 antibody. (**B**) Single Chain Fv (scFv). (**C**) Diabody. (**D**) Triabody. (**E**) Fab. (**F**) F(ab')$_2$. Arrows point to the tumor image.

In conclusion, because of their smaller size, recombinant antibody fragments of chTNT-3 were found to clear more rapidly than the intact molecule. The data show that all fragments can be labeled directly with ^{131}I or ^{99m}Tc while retaining their stability *in vitro* and *in vivo*. Tumor-imaging with ^{131}I labeling demonstrated the following order of efficacy: F(ab')$_2$ > triabody > diabody. In contrast, ^{99m}Tc labeling exhibits properties *in vivo* that make the scFv and Fab superior for imaging. On the basis of these results, different chTNT-3 fragments appear to be best suited to image solid tumors when radiolabeled with ^{99m}Tc or ^{131}I.

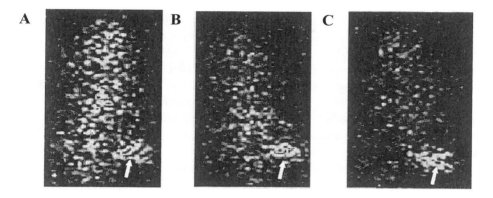

Figure 5. Images of MAD109 tumor-bearing BALB/c mice with ^{99m}Tc-labeled chTNT-3 antibody and fragments at 24 hours after injection. **(A)** Whole chTNT-3 antibody. **(B)** single chain Fv (scFv). **(C)** Fab. Arrows point to the tumor image.

STRATEGIES TO ENHANCE ANTIBODY AND DRUG TARGETING USING TNT

Chemical modification

Monoclonal antibodies are basic, positively charged proteins while mammalian cells are negatively charged due to outer membrane sialic acid residues. Therefore, electrostatic interactions between the two can create higher levels of background binding. In order to decrease background signal and enhance tumor uptake, our laboratory has determined that charge modification that decreases the isoelectric points (pI) of antibodies can significantly improve their pharmacokinetic performance (25).

Using this approach, we have developed a simple method of chemical modification with biotin for the chTNT MAbs. Biotin (vitamin H) is a naturally occurring compound and is a nontoxic and nonimmunogenic normal component of the body. Because biotin is commonly used with immunologic reagents, derivatives are available to simplify the chemistry. Changing the pharmacokinetic characteristics of intact MAbs can improve their clearance to rates similar to those of their F(ab')2 counterparts. Changing these characteristics is advantageous in radioimmunotherapy as well as biologic therapies in which the Fc portion of the antibody is desired for interaction with the immune response. By using a neutral molecule like biotin, the charge of the antibody can be better optimized for increased clearance without loss in tumor localization. Biotinylation blocks the ε-amino groups of lysine residues, thereby reducing the antibody's net positive charge. In this study, we have biotinylated three different TNT monoclonal antibodies to determine the optimal level of biotinylation that will yield the highest tumor to organ ratios without appreciable loss in tumor activity. As expected, biotinylation had the effect of decreasing pI in a concentration-related manner (Table 5). Consistent with our previous studies, this chemical modification had the effect of enhancing whole body antibody clearance of two out of the three antibodies, leading to decreased non-specific uptake of the reagent by normal tissues, as demonstrated by the markedly improved tumor/organ ratios (Table 6).

Table 5. Physicochemical Properties, Affinity Constants, Optimal Biotinylation Ratios and Half-lives ($T_{1/2}$) of Chimeric TNT MAbs.[a]

Antibody	Isoelectric Point (pI)	Affinity Constant (M^{-1})	Optimal Biotinylation Ratio (MAb/biotin)	$T_{1/2}$ (h)[b]
chTNT-1	>9.6	2.5×10^9	-	30.4(1.8)
chTNT-1/B	7.2-7.8	2.0×10^9	1:3	17.4(2.4)
chTNT-2	>9.6	1.2×10^9	-	178.7(7.2)
chTNT-2/B	8.2-9.6	1.2×10^9	1:5	175.1(3.0)
chTNT-3	>9.6	1.4×10^9	-	134.2(4.0)
chTNT-3/B	7.2-7.8	1.5×10^9	1:8	90.1(3.8)

[a] All of the antibody variants were labeled with ^{125}I. Standard Deviations of the Mean are Given in Parentheses.
[b] $T_{1/2}$ as Determined by Whole-Body Clearance in BALB/c Mice (n=5).

Unlike other chemical modification methods described thus far, biotinylation of the chimeric TNT MAbs did not increase their uptake in normal organs such as the spleen and liver. Rather, there was a dramatic drop in uptake by all organs with biotinylated chTNT-1 and chTNT-3 and by the majority of tissues with biotinylated chTNT-2. Furthermore, although the clearance of chTNT-2 was not affected by biotinylation, it too demonstrated an improvement in the non-specific uptake by normal tissues following chemical modification. Interestingly, despite the fact that chemically modified chTNT-1 and chTNT-2 displayed shortened circulation times *in vivo*, biodistribution analyses demonstrate that they had enhanced uptake in tumors compared to the native antibodies. Hence, this method can be used to improve both the diagnostic and therapeutic potential of MAbs by improving their signal to noise ratio and the absolute tumor accretion of MAb, respectively. Interestingly, chTNT-2 demonstrated no improvement in clearance regardless of charge modification with up to 10 biotin molecules per antibody. Indeed, this particular antibody was relatively insensitive to the alterations in isoelectric point through biotinylation. chTNT-2 has an unusually long circulation time for chimeric MAbs tested in mice and, unlike chTNT-1 and –3, this did not change after biotinylation. The reason for its resistance to the beneficial effect of biotinylation, which is demonstrated by the lack of change in pI and *in vivo* half-life, is at this time unknown.

Table 6. Tumor/Organ Ratios at One Day after Administration of ^{125}I-Labeled Parental and Biotinylated chTNT MAbs in LS174T Human Colon Carcinoma-Bearing Nude Mice (n=5).[a]

Organ	chTNT-1	chTNT-1/B	chTNT-2	chTNT-2/B	chTNT-3	chTNT-3/B
Blood	0.47(0.13)	1.28(0.18)	0.53(0.17)	0.73(0.20)	0.44(0.11)	0.96(0.32)
Muscle	7.51(0.56)	11.6(1.40)	10.1(1.82)	14.0(2.03)	6.76(1.05)	10.4(2.21)
Lung	2.52(0.64)	3.15(0.69)	1.32(0.46)	2.02(0.35)	1.80(0.38)	2.67(0.86)
Liver	3.27(0.53)	4.77(1.25)	1.30(0.37)	2.07(0.51)	1.55(0.37)	3.61(0.83)
Spleen	3.51(0.32)	4.33(0.99)	1.74(0.43)	3.51(0.53)	1.01(0.29)	2.35(0.78)
Stomach	5.79(1.01)	6.50(1.12)	3.49(0.90)	4.51(0.98)	2.73(0.58)	4.17(1.15)
Kidney	3.19(0.15)	4.27(1.30)	2.19(0.47)	2.90(0.31)	2.76(1.12)	3.98(0.57)

[a]Data are expressed as mean (SD), n = 5 animals per group.

As shown in Table 5, chTNT-1, -2, and -3 had different optimal biotinylation ratios that improved their performance *in vivo* (Table 6). For those TNT MAbs amenable to pI shifts, chemical modification with biotin should improve the therapeutic value of these reagents by reducing non-specific binding, increasing tumor uptake, and decreasing pharmacological half-life.

Vasopermeability enhancing agents

A second approach to improving the uptake of TNT MAbs in tumors is the use of vasopermeability enhancing agents as originally described by our laboratory (26-28). Physiological barriers to the delivery of therapeutic reagents to solid tumors are major obstacles to the clinical success of developing targeting therapies. For example, the limited clinical responses observed in radioimmunotherapy of solid tumors can be attributed in large part to low tumor localization of radiolabeled MAb. Although xenograft models in nude mice have shown levels of tumor uptake ranging from 1-20% ID/g, patient studies have demonstrated exceedingly low tumor uptake in the range of 0.01% ID/g of tissue. Thus, an extremely small fraction of antibody delivers radionuclide to tumor sites, while the majority of the injected dose disperses throughout the body, where it can cause dose-limiting myelosuppression. Recognizing that blood flow and vascular permeability are key parameters controlling the egress of therapeutic molecules into tumors, our laboratory developed a strategy to utilize MAbs to direct proteins with vasoactive properties to tumor sites in order to increase local vascular permeability without affecting normal tissues(26). A study of several candidate vasopermeability inducing agents eventually revealed that IL-2 had the desired properties (27).

IL-2 is a 15 kD protein secreted by activated T-cells that supports the proliferation and activation of lymphocytes and other immune cells. In clinical studies, IL-2 has shown success in the treatment of several human malignancies, in particular melanoma and renal cell carcinoma. It is well established, however, that systemic administration of IL-2 leads to increased permeability of blood vessels in the lungs and other organs, leading to a toxic side effect known as the capillary leak syndrome (29). To enhance antibody uptake in tumors, however, the undesirable property of IL-2 was harnessed to increase local tumor vascular permeability enabling more antibody to enter the tumor parenchyma. Surprisingly, the magnitude of enhancement was similar whether the IL-2 was delivered by an antibody directed against tumor-associated cell surface antigens, an extracellular matrix protein in the basement membranes of tumor vessels, or an intracellular antigen accessible in the necrotic regions of solid tumors (30). For this reason, we chose to develop a TNT based IL-2 fusion protein to serve as a universal targeting agent, depending on its ability to target degenerating cells within all solid tumors. In the current section, we describe a fusion protein consisting of chTNT-3 and human IL-2 (chTNT-3/IL-2), which can increase the specific tumor uptake of both MAbs and chemotherapeutic drugs in various experimental tumor models. Once these studies were completed, our strategy was to develop a fully human vasopermeability agent which consisted of the human TNT MAb NHS76 and Permeability Enhancing Peptide (PEP), a fragment of IL-2 that contains the vasopermeability activity of the intact molecule but is devoid of cytokine activity. Completion of these studies sets the foundation for testing this novel concept in man.

The recombinant chTNT-3/IL-2 fusion protein was expressed in mammalian cells using the Glutamine Synthetase Gene Expression System (28). The IL-2 cDNA was inserted downstream of the terminal codon of the chimeric heavy chain, following a short linker peptide to promote proper folding of the cytokine. The fusion protein was found to retain both the immunoreactivity of the parent antibody and the biologic activity of the IL-2 moiety.

The ability of chTNT-3/IL-2 to increase tumor uptake of both MAbs and drugs (IUdR) was examined in the ME-180 cervical carcinoma xenograft model. Radiolabeled IUdR has been evaluated in animal tumor models for the diagnosis and therapy of cancers and was used in our studies to determine whether chemotherapeutic drugs can also be enhanced in tumors in a specific manner. Under optimal conditions, however, pretreatment with chTNT-3/IL-2 resulted in a nearly 3-fold increase in tumor accretion of ^{125}IUdR (Table 7) with no effect on normal tissues. The necessity for tumor localization of IL-2 was evidenced by the absence of an effect when mice were pretreated with the control fusion protein chCLL-1/IL-2 directed against B-cell malignancies.

Table 7. Effects of Vasoconjugate Pretreatment on Chemotherapeutic Drug (^{125}IUdR) Uptake in ME-180 Human Cervical Carcinoma-bearing Nude Mice Following Pretreatment with chTNT-3/IL-2[a].

Pretreatment Time (h)	No Pretreatment	Pretreatment
1	1.53	4.54
3	1.31	3.44
6	1.37	3.49

[a]Data expressed as % injected dose/gram of tumor

The effects of pretreatment with chTNT-3/IL-2 on the specific tumor uptake of radiolabeled antibodies were examined in two additional tumor models. The MAb NR-LU-10 recognizes a membrane glycoprotein expressed in many carcinomas of epithelial origin. The tumor targeting ability of this MAb has been demonstrated previously in colon tumor-bearing mice by both biodistribution and imaging studies (31). Moreover, clinical studies have illustrated the potential of NR-LU-10 both for the diagnostic imaging and staging of patients with lung cancer and for the radioimmunotherapy of ovarian cancer (32). In the present study, the ability of pretreatment with chTNT-3/IL-2 to enhance the tumor uptake of NR-LU-10 was demonstrated in nude mice bearing the A427 human lung adenocarcinoma (Table 8).

Pretreatment with chTNT-3/IL-2 was also performed with the MAb CYT-351/LNCaP antibody/tumor model, which is reactive with the prostate-specific membrane antigen (33) and has been used for the immunoscintigraphy of patients with prostate cancer (34). As shown in Table 8, pretreatment with chTNT-3/IL-2 significantly increased the specific tumor uptake of CYT-351 in LNCaP prostate tumor-bearing mice. This pretreatment strategy can thus be applied to tumors of different histologic origins. The optimal dose of chTNT-3/IL-2 varied somewhat from one tumor model to the next, which might be attributable to different amounts of fusion protein accumulating at the tumor site.

Table 8. Tumor Uptake (% Injected Dose/Gram) at Five Days after Administration of ^{125}I-Labeled Antibody in human tumor-bearing nude mice following pretreatment with chTNT-3/IL-2.

Organ	^{125}I-Labeled NR-LU-10[a]		^{125}I-Labeled CYT-351[b]	
	No pretreatment	Pretreatment	No pretreatment	Pretreatment
Blood	2.32	1.68	7.75	6.25
Muscle	0.17	0.16	0.38	0.45
Heart	0.58	0.39	2.30	1.70
Lung	0.68	0.61	3.17	2.43
Liver	0.46	0.33	1.40	1.27
Spleen	0.49	0.32	1.40	0.93
Stomach	0.39	0.32	0.99	0.80
Kidney	0.64	0.36	1.78	1.16
Tumor	3.09	6.37	18.59	31.85

[a]A427 human lung adenocarcinoma-bearing nude mice
[b]LNCap human prostatic adenocarcinoma-bearing nude mice.

The findings described in this report provide evidence for the potential of this approach as a universal pretreatment to enhance the delivery of therapeutic molecules to solid tumors. In order to generate a clinically useful vasopermeability agent, the NHS76 human MAb described above was used to generate a fusion protein with a fragment of IL-2 (PEP) that contains 100% of the vasopermeability activity of the cytokine. Designated NHS76/PEP$_2$, this vasopermeability agent has been used as a pretreatment to enhance the uptake of antibodies and drugs in experimental tumor models (35). Using methods described above, biodistribution, imaging, and vasopermeability assays *in vivo* were performed to evaluate the tumor-targeting and vasopermeability characteristics of the fusion protein. As shown above in Figure 6, this newly generated vasopermeability agent enhances antibody uptake in tumor in a similar manner as chTNT-3/IL-2 as shown by immunoscintigraphy.

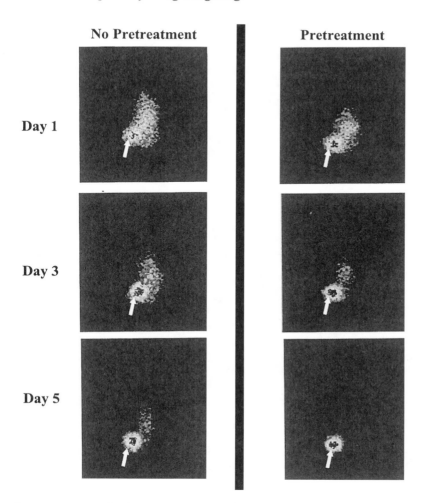

Figure 6. 1, 3, and 5 day images of LS174T human colon carcinoma in nude mice treated with I-131 labeled B72.3 murine monoclonal antibody with and without pretreatment with NHS76/PEP₂. Arrows point to the tumor image.

Pretreatment and chemotherapy

To demonstrate the therapeutic potential of targeted vasopermeability, a series of experiments was performed using single agent chemotherapeutic drugs to treat solid tumors of mouse and man. In these studies, groups of mice were treated with chemotherapeutic drugs using doses that were identified to have little therapeutic value. Half of these groups, however, were pretreated with NHS76/PEP₂ in order to demonstrate that increased vasopermeability at the tumor site could translate into better drug uptake and therapy.

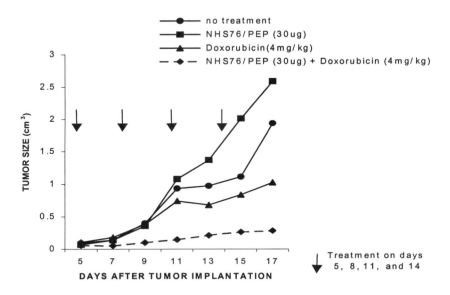

Figure 7. Chemotherapy of LS174T human colon adenocarcinoma xenograft in nude mice with and without NHS76/PEP$_2$ pretreatment.

As exemplified in Figure 7 above, one such study is presented which clearly demonstrates the value of NHS76/PEP$_2$ pretreatment in altering tumor growth. In general, those tumors which were sensitive to specific drugs exhibited the most profound effects, but tumors which are normally resistant to a specific drug, such as the MAD109 murine lung carcinoma (36, 37) treated with Taxol or Vinblastine (data not shown), now could be responsive. These results demonstrate the efficacy of vasopermeability enhancement to improve the therapeutic value of chemotherapeutic drugs and lay the foundation for using NHS76/PEP$_2$, a completely human fusion protein, for the therapy of patients with cancer and related diseases.

ACKNOWLEDGEMENTS

The authors wish to acknowledge the excellent technical assistance of Aoyun Yun for performing the molecular biology procedures and Jingzhong Pang for conducting the animal experiments. These studies were supported in part by grant 2 RO1 CA47334 from the National Cancer Institute, Bethesda, MD and Peregrine Pharmaceuticals, Inc., Tustin, CA.

REFERENCES

1. Kemshead J, Hopkins K. Uses and limitations of monoclonal antibodies in the treatment of malignant disease: A review. Diagnostic Oncology 1993;2:219-224.
2. Epstein AL, Chen F-M, Taylor CR. A Novel Method for the Detection of Necrotic Lesions in Human Cancers. Cancer Research 1988;48:5842-5848.
3. Miller GK, Naeve GS, Gaffar SA, Epstein AL. Immunologic and biochemical analysis of TNT-1 and TNT-2 monoclonal antibody binding to histones. Hybridoma 1993;12:689-698.
4. Hornick JL, Hu P, Khawli LA, Biela BH, Yun A, Sharifi J, et al. chTNT-3/B, a new chemically modified chimeric monoclonal antibody directed against DNA for the tumor necrosis treatment of solid tumors. Cancer Biotherapy and Radiopharmaceuticals 1998;13(4):255-268.
5. Jones ST, Bendig MM. Rapid PCR-cloning of full-length mouse immunoglobulin variable regions. Bio/Technology 1991;9:88-89.
6. Winter G, Harris WJ. Humanized antibodies (review). Trends in Pharmacolog. Sci. 1993;14:139-143.
7. Marks JD, Hoogenboom HR, Bonnert TP, McCafferty J, Griffiths AD, Winter G. Bypassing immunization. Human antibodies from V-gene libraries displayed on phage. J. Mol. Biol. 1991;222:581-597.
8. Yang XD, Jia XC, Corvalan JR, Wang P, Davis CG. Eradication of established tumors by a fully human monoclonal antibody to the epidermal growth factor receptor without concomitant chemotherapy. Cancer Res 1998;59:1236-1243.
9. Karpas A, Dremucheva A, Czepulkowski BH. A human myeloma cel line suitable for the generation of human monoclonal antibodies. Proc Natl Acad Sci U S A 2001;98:1799-1804.
10. Sharifi J, Khawli LA, Hu P, King S, Epstein AE. Characterization of a Phage Display-Derived Human Monoclonal Antibody (NHS76) Counterpart to Chimeric TNT-1 Directed Against Necrotic Regions of Solid Tumors. Hybridoma and Hybridomics 2001;20(5):305-312.
11. Vaughan TJ, Williams AJ, Pritchard K, Osbourn JK, Pope AR, Earnshaw JC, et al. Human antibodies with subnanomolar affinities isolated from a large non-immunized phage display library. Nature Biotechnology 1996;14:309-314.
12. Hornick JL, Sharifi J, Khawli LA, Hu P, Biela BH, Mizokami MM, et al. A new chemically modified chimeric TNT-3 monoclonal antibody directed against DNA for the radioimmunotherapy of solid tumors. Cancer Biotherapy & Radiopharmaceuticals 1998;13(4):255-268.
13. Chen F-M, Epstein AL, Li Z, Taylor CR. A comparative autoradiographic study demonstrating differential intratumor localization of monoclonal antibodies to cell surface (Lym-1) and intracellular (TNT-1) antigens. Journal of Nuclear Medicine 1990;31:1059-1066.
14. Larsen SM. Radiolabeled monoclonal anti-tumor antibodies in diagnosis and therapy. J. Nucl. Med. 1985;26:538-550.
15. Yokota T, Milenic DE, Whitlow M, Schlom J. Rapid tumor penetration of single-chain Fv and comparison with other immunoglobulin forms. Cancer Research 1992;52:3402-3410.

16. Hudson PJ, Kortt AA. High avidity scFv multimers, diabodies and triabodies. J. Immunological Methods 1999;231:177-189.

17. Holliger P, Prospero T, Winter G. Diabodies: Small bivalent and bispecific antibody fragments. Proc Natl Acad Sci U S A 1993;90:6444-6448.

18. Whitlow M, Filpula D, Rollence ML, Feng S-L, Woods JF. Multivalent Fvs: characterization of single chain Fv oligomers and preparation of bispecific Fv. Protein Engineering 1994;7:1017-1026.

19. Khawli LA, Biela BH, Hu P, Epstein AL. Stable, genetically engineered F(ab')2 fragments of chimeric TNT-3 expressed in mammalian cells. Hybidoma and Hybridomics 2002;21(1):11-18.

20. Verma R, Boleti E, George AJT. Antibody engineering: Comparison of bacterial, yeast, insect, and mammalian expression systems. J. Immunol. Methods 1998;216:165-181.

21. Milenic DE, Yokota T, Filpula DR, Finkelman MAJ, Dodd SW, Wood JF, et al. Construction, binding properties, metabolism, and tumor targeting of a single-chain Fv derived from the pancarcinoma monoclonal antibody CC49. Cancer Research 1991;51:6363-6371.

22. Adams GP, Schier R. Generating improved single-chain Fv molecules for tumor targeting. J. Immunol. Methods 1999;231:249-260.

23. Kang N, Hamilton S, Odili J, Wilson G, Kupsch J. In vivo targeting of malignant melanoma by 125iodine- and 99mTc-labeled single-chain Fv fragments against high molecular weight melanoma-associated antigens. Clin. Cancer Res. 2000;6:4921-4931.

24. Hornick JL, Sharifi J, Khawli LA, Hu P, Bai WG, Alauddin MM, et al. Single Amino Acid Substitution in the Fc Region of Chimeric TNT-3 Antibody Accelerates Clearance and Improves Immunoscintigraphy of Solid Tumors. Journal of Nuclear Medicine 2000;41:355-362.

25. Khawli LA, Glasky MS, Alauddin MM, Epstein AL. Improved tumor localization and radioimaging with chemically modified monoclonal antibodies. Cancer Biotherapy & Radiopharmaceuticals 1996;11:203-215.

26. LeBerthon B, Khawli LA, Alauddin M, Miller GK, Charak BS, Mazumder A, et al. Enhanced tumor uptake of macromolecules induced by a novel vasoactive interleukin 2 immunoconjugate. Cancer Research 1991;51:2694-2698.

27. Khawli LA, Miller GK, Epstein AL. Effect of seven new vasoactive immunoconjugates on the enhancement of monoclonal antibody uptake in tumors. Cancer 1994;73:824-831.

28. Hornick JL, Khawli LA, Hu P, Sharifi J, Khanna C, Epstein AL. Pretreatment with a Monoclonal Antibody/Interleukin-2 Fusion Protein Directed against DNA Enhances the Delivery of Therapeutic Molecules to Solid Tumors. Clinical Cancer Research 1999;5:51-60.

29. Rosenstein M, Ettinghausen SE, Rosenberg SA. Extravasation of intravascular fluid mediated by the systemic administration of recombinant interleukin 2. Immunology 1986;137:1735-1742.

30. Epstein AL, Khawli LA, Hornick JL, Taylor CR. Identification of a Monoclonal Antibody, TV-1, Directed against the Basement Membrane of Tumor Vessels, and Its Use to Enhance the Delivery of Macromolecules to Tumors after Conjugation with Interleukin-2. Cancer Res. 1995;55:2673-2680.

31. Goldrosen MH, Biddle WC, Pancook J, Bakshi S, Vanderheyden J-L, Fritzberg AR, et al. Biodistribution, pharmacokinetic, and imaging studies with [186]Re-labeled NR-LU-10 whole antibody in LS174T colonic tumor-bearing mice. Cancer Research 1990;50:7973-7978.

32.   Breitz HB, Sullivan K, Nelp WB. Imaging lung cancer with radiolabeled antibodies. Seminars in Nuclear Medicine 1993;23:127-132.
33.   Lopes AD, Davis WL, Rosenstraus MJ, Uveges AJ, Gilman SC. Immunohistochemical and pharmacokinetic characterization of the site-specific immunoconjugate CYT-356 derived from antiprostate monoclonal antibody 7E11-C5. Cancer Research 1990;50:6423-6429.
34.   Chengazi VU, Feneley MR, Ellison D, Stalteri M, Granowski A, Granowska M, et al. Imaging prostate cancer with technetium-99m-7E11-C5.3 (CYT-351). Journal of Nuclear Medicine 1997;38:675-682.
35.   Epstein AL, Mizokami MM, Hu P, Khawli LA. Permeability enhancing peptide (PEP): A protein fragment of IL-2 responsible for vasopermeability and useful in the generation of agents to increase the effectiveness of chemotherapy. Nature Biotechnology in press.
36.   Marks TA, Woodman RJ, Geran RI, Billups LH, Madison RM. Characterization and Responsiveness of the Madison 109 Lung Carcinoma to Various Antitumor Agents. Cancer Treatment Reports 1977;61(8):1459-1470.
37.   Rose WC. Evaluation of Madison 109 Lung Carcinoma as a Model for Screening Antitumor Drugs. Cancer Treatment Reports 1981;65(3-4):299-312.

GLOSSARY

Biodistribution: Uptake of radiolabeled antibodies in normal organs and tumor at different time points. Measurements are calculated as % injected dose/gram and tumor/normal organ ratios. Used as a method to determine the targeting abilities of monoclonal antibodies.

Chemical Modification: Attachment of small organic molecules, such as biotin, to antibodies used to decrease non-specific binding of the antibodies. This chemical method decreases the isoelectric point (charge) of the antibody thereby decreasing its circulation half-life *in vivo* and improving its uptake in tumors.

Chemokines: Small peptides elaborated at the site of injury to recruit and arm the immune system. These chemoattractants facilitate leukocyte migration, positioning, and degranulation and have a positive or negative influence on angiogenesis. Examples of these potent immune modulators include RANTES, IP-10, MCP-1, Mig, and LEC.

Chimeric MAb: Genetically engineered monoclonal antibodies consisting of murine variable heavy and light chains (binding sites) and human constant regions. Chimeric MAbs are approximately 35% mouse and 65% human in origin.

Cytokines: Cell activators of the immune system. Among others, includes the interleukins, tumor necrosis factor, and the interferons.

Fusion Proteins: Genetically engineered proteins consisting of monoclonal antibodies linked with immune modulatory proteins such as cytokines and chemokines.

NHS76/PEP$_2$:   Vasopermeability enhancing agent used to increase the permeability of vessels in tumors before the administration of chemotherapeutic drugs or monoclonal antibodies. Consists of a human TNT antibody (NHS76) and a fragment of interleukin-2 (PEP dimer) containing the vasopermeability activity of the cytokine.

Pharmacokinetics: Whole body clearance of radiolabeled antibodies in mice using a dosimeter.

Tumor Necrosis Treatment: A method for targeting tumors by directing antibodies to abundant, internal antigens (chromatin) accessible in dead and dying cells present in tumors.

Vasoconjugate Enhancing Agent: A fusion protein consisting of a tumor targeting monoclonal antibody linked to a vasopermeability inducing peptide or protein.   Administered as a pretreatment to increase the vascular permeability of tumor vessels before the administration of drugs or radiolabeled monoclonal antibodies.   Enhances uptake of diagnostic and therapeutic drugs/antibodies in tumors.

Vasopermeability: A condition where vessels become leaky due to relaxation of the interdigitating cell membranes of endothelial cells, allowing the efflux of fluids into surrounding tissue.

14

TARGETED APOPTOSIS: ANTIBODIES LINKED TO RNA DAMAGING AGENTS

Susanna M. Rybak [1], Michaela Arndt[2], Juergen Krauss[2], Dianne L. Newton[2], Bang K. Vu[2], and Zhongyu Zhu[2]

[1] *Developmental Therapeutics Program, Division of Cancer Treatment and Diagnosis, National Cancer Institute at Frederick, Frederick, MD 21702;* [2] *SAIC Frederick, National Cancer Institute at Frederick, Frederick, MD 21702*

INTRODUCTION

Generally, the new strategy in cancer drug discovery and development is to define and validate the most promising cancer related molecular targets to which new drugs can be designed. For small molecule drugs, the focus is on interfering with molecular targets that contribute to deregulated cell growth and signaling pathways, predominantly within the cancer cell. Antigens aberrantly expressed on the cancer cell surface also afford possible valid molecular targets. Thus antibodies against tumor related antigens are a class of drugs that fit the new paradigm for cancer drug development and treatment.

In this review we illustrate the potential success of this approach since early studies have led to approval of monoclonal antibodies for cancer therapy. Pharmaceutical companies are now pursuing strategies to increase the number and duration of responses to naked antibody treatment. Combination therapy will almost certainly be the case for most molecular target based approaches to cancer treatment since the pathogenesis of the cancer cell is due to multiple abnormalities. Therefore, the best antibody based therapeutics will likely be composed of antibodies that activate cellular processes, directly leading to cancer cell death, coupled with agents that accomplish the same result by different mechanisms. One novel combination is described within this review. The RNA damaging action of RNAses independently leads to apoptosis and cell death. This effect is enhanced thousands of times when RNAses are linked to antibodies. Moreover, the effectiveness of the antibody is enhanced as well. These targeted RNA-damaging drugs build on the promising immunotoxin technology platform because preclinical studies show that RNAses cause fewer problems related to immunogenicity and host toxicity. For all these reasons, the combination of antibody and RNAse should be attractive to the clinical and pharmaceutical communities. Consequently, future generations of designed antibody fragments are needed as molecular RNase targeting agents.

Antibodies

The invention of the hybridoma technology by Köhler and Milstein (1), which enabled the generation and production of antibodies with predefined specificities (monoclonal antibodies), revolutionized the role of antibodies as diagnostic and therapeutic tools in oncology. As a consequence, several monoclonal antibodies have been evaluated in clinical trials as cancer therapeutics since the early 1980's. Clinical outcomes, however, were generally poor. The main factors responsible for these initial shortcomings were related to the immunogenicity of the murine protein, to modulation of targeted antigens, and to the poor ability of these antibodies to sufficiently mediate antibody-dependent effector functions in humans (2).

Antibodies (immunoglobulins) are composed of two types of polypeptide chains of different molecular weights, designated as light chains (L) and heavy chains (H). Two heavy chains and light chains associate to a monomeric "Y" shaped IgG, IgD, or IgE antibody molecule. IgM antibodies are comprised of five monomers connected by a joining peptide. IgA as a secretory immunoglobulin exists both in a monomeric and dimeric form. Structural data have shown the antibody molecule to consist of several similar subunits (domains). Dependent on the immunoglobulin class, heavy chains are comprised of three or four domains with little sequence variability (constant domains) and one constant light chain. Antibody effector functions [e.g., complement activation and antibody dependent cellular cytotoxicity (ADCC)] are mediated by properties of the individual heavy chain constant domains. The N-terminal domains of the light chain (V_L) and heavy chain (V_H) are highly variable in sequence (variable domains), accounting for the diversity of the antibody repertoire. The antigen binding site is formed by three complementarity determining regions (CDR1-3) within each V_H and V_L domain. These structural features are illustrated in Figure 1.

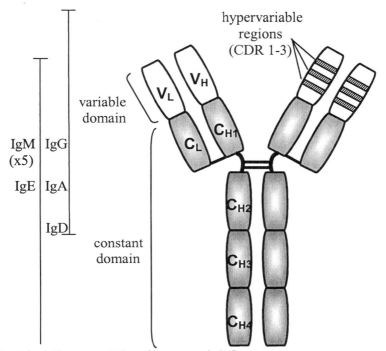

Figure 1. Schematic representation of a monomeric IgG.
The hypervariable regions (CDR1-3) within the variable domains of the heavy chain (V_H) and the light chain (V_L), respectively, represent the antigen binding site. Effector functions are mediated by the constant domain of the molecule.
C_L = constant light chain domain; C_H1-C_H4 = constant heavy chain domains; IgM, IgE, IgG, IgA, IgD = immunoglobulin isotypes

RNA as a Drug Target

RNA has an appeal as a molecular target because it is more structurally diverse than DNA. RNA plays key roles in many biological processes such as protein synthesis and regulation of gene expression [for review, see (3) and references therein]. Similar to proteins, RNA folds into complex tertiary structures thereby creating highly specific binding sites for molecular recognition. Structural information of many protein enzymes has aided in mechanism-based design of drugs and now similar strategies are beginning to emerge for the rational design of drugs that target RNA. Moreover, unlike DNA, in which resistance to drugs can develop, there are no RNA repair mechanisms, thus enhancing the impact of therapeutics directed at RNA. Furthermore, RNA is more accessible than nuclear DNA. Recent reviews show an increased interest in the development of RNA-based therapeutics with the RNA damaging enzymes, RNAses (4-6).

RNA Damaging Agents as Therapeutics

The appeal of RNA as a drug target has stimulated the investigation of possible therapeutic applications for more than forty years (5). In 1955, bovine pancreatic RNAse A was reported to impede tumor growth after injection into tumor bearing mice. This led to the use of the bovine pancreatic RNAse A in human clinical trials for the treatment of leukemia and encephalitis. In 1958, patients were given daily s.c. injections of 0.5-1 mg of RNAse A for the treatment of chronic myelogenous leukemia. These patients showed decreases in spleen size and general improvement. In another study reported in 1976, RNAse A was administered to 246 patients with tick-borne encephalitis, and the results obtained were compared to 261 patients treated with antiencephalitic gamma globulin. Administration of 30 mg of RNAse A every 4 hours for 5 to 6 days provided high levels of the enzyme in the blood with no adverse reactions and a clinical outcome superior to that obtained with gamma globulin.

In more recent clinical trials, another member of the RNAse A superfamily, onconase, is being evaluated for the treatment of a variety of solid tumors. Onconase is an amphibian RNAse isolated from *Rana pipiens* oocytes by following cytotoxic activity against cancer cells *in vitro* and *in vivo* (5). It is the only unconjugated RNAse currently in clinical trials. Phase I and Phase I/II studies of onconase as a single agent have been recently completed (7) and have progressed to Phase III studies. In addition, onconase has been shown to enhance the cytotoxic activity of some chemotherapeutic agents *in vitro* and *in vivo* even in the presence of the mdr1 form of multidrug resistance (5). There have been no problems associated with repeated weekly administration of onconase even though it is an amphibian protein (7). The small size (12 kDa), the very basic nature, as well as its high degree of homology to human serum RNAses may render it relatively non-immunogenic to humans. Furthermore, onconase is rapidly cleared from the circulation. In BALB/c mice, onconase exhibits a $t_{1/2\alpha}$ of 2.3 min.

The cytotoxic activity of onconase depends on its ability to enter cells through an as yet unidentified receptor and degrade RNA (5). Binding is saturable, correlates with cytotoxicity, and routing to the cytoplasm occurs through the Golgi apparatus. Recent studies show that onconase damages cellular tRNA causing a caspase-dependent apoptosis (8). In a recent study by Iordanov et al. (9), onconase was found to be a potent activator of the stress-activated protein kinase cascade, SAPK1 (JNK1 and JNK2) and SAPK2 (p38 MAP kinase), and did not activate the nuclear factor-kappa B (NF-kB). Unlike DNA damage and apoptosis, onconase induced apoptosis through tRNA damage is not affected by the absence of a functional p53 protein (8), yet another advantage to targeting RNA.

Recombinant Cytotoxic RNAses

Other members of the RNAse A superfamily have been shown to have antitumor activity [reviewed in (4-6)]. Bovine seminal RNAse (BS-RNAse), a dimeric member of this family, has shown both *in vitro* and *in vivo* to be selectively cytotoxic for malignant cells [reviewed in (10)]. Monomeric derivatives of BS-RNAse, although active enzymes, are not cytotoxic. BS-RNAse binds to specific sites on the extracellular matrix and blocks protein synthesis by degrading rRNA. Recently BS-RNAse has been reported to deplete multi-drug resistant tumor cells from *ex vivo* expanded blood-derived CD34+ hematopoietic progenitor cells (11). Until recently there have been no reports of a human RNAse with cytotoxic activity against tumor cells. Following inhibition of mouse oocyte maturation, Sakakibara et al. (12) isolated a uniquely processed form of EDN from the urine of pregnant women. A genetically engineered version of this EDN, (-4)EDN, containing amino acid residues, SLHV, -4 to -1 of its signal peptide region was found to be selectively cytotoxic towards Kaposi's sarcoma cells, KS Y-1 in *vitro* (13). Native EDN is predominantly expressed without this peptide, even though the predicted cleavage site based on signal peptidase recognition sites should occur between the -5 and -4 sites in the signal peptide sequence (5). Recent studies show that, in contrast to EDN, (-4)EDN displays saturable binding to KS Y-1 cells. Furthermore, binding of (-4)EDN is inhibited by onconase, suggesting that (-4)EDN may be binding to the same or similar cell-surface sites as onconase, causing an alteration in cellular routing or processing that results in cytotoxicity. The physiological significance of this uniquely modified version of EDN remains unknown (S.M.R., unpublished results).

The nature of the N-terminus is crucial to the cytotoxicity of RNAses (5). Dimeric BS-RNAse expressed as a (Met-1) fusion protein retains full enzymatic activity but decreased cytotoxic activity. X-ray crystallography studies of onconase reveal that the N-terminal <Glu residue forms part of the active enzyme site. In fact, all native cytotoxic amphibian RNAses contain an N-terminal <Glu amino acid residue that is necessary for activity. Expression of these RNAses with Met as the first amino acid results in enzymes with both reduced catalytic and cytotoxic activities. Amphibian RNAses with full activities result from either reconstituting <Glu as the first amino acid or modifying the N-terminus to restore the active site interaction.

Recently, a recombinant cytotoxic amphibian RNAse, *rap*LR1, lacking the post-translational modification of the amino terminus was cloned from a cDNA library using poly[A]RNA purified from *Rana pipiens* liver (5). An open reading frame encoding a 127 amino acid protein was identified. A characteristic signal peptide sequence was identified in amino acid residues 1-23, followed by an amino acid sequence in residues 24-127 that was highly conserved but not identical when compared to onconase. Four amino acid differences between *rap*LR1 and onconase were identified: 11 Leu < - >Ile, 20 Asn <- >Asp, 85 Thr < - >Lys, and 103 His < - >Ser. With the exception of the change at amino acid 11, the changes are between polar and charged amino acid residues. These changes result in *rap*LR1 being fully active without the N-terminal <Glu amino acid residue (IC_{50} was 0.8 µg/mL for both native onconase and *rap*LR1). Furthermore, this simplifies the expression of the recombinant protein, since expression of onconase without the restored <Glu is >100 fold less active than native onconase [IC_{50} >100 µg/mL]

Designing New Antibody Forms to Target RNAses

The successful expression of functional antigen binding domains in *E.coli* (14, 15) provided the basis for the rapid development of a new generation of antibody-based molecules with therapeutic impact. Antibody fragments have the full binding specificity and affinity of the parental antibody molecule and can be generated as monovalent, bivalent or multivalent fragments. The Fv fragment consisting only of the variable domains of the heavy and light chain (V_H and V_L) is the smallest antibody fragment carrying the whole antigen-binding site. The association between the non-covalently linked V_H and V_L is not very strong and the domains tend to dissociate from each other. To stabilize the association of the two domains, a synthetic flexible linker peptide (15-20 residues) has been introduced connecting both variable domains to a single chain variable fragment (sFv) (16). Another approach to enhance the stability of Fv fragments can be achieved by introducing artificial intermolecular disulfide bonds in the framework regions of V_H and V_L (17). The disulfide-stabilized Fv (dsFv) molecules are more stable than sFvs or chemically cross-linked Fv fragments.

The sFv fragment is the obvious format for generating multivalent antibody fragments. Dimeric antibody fragments can be produced from sFv's containing an additional carboxy-terminal cysteine residue by chemical coupling, (sFv')₂ (18). Other approaches to construct bivalent sFv molecules are the genetic fusion of the sFv with proteins that naturally form dimeric structures, such as the human IgG₁ CH3 domains (minibody), or amphipatic helices (miniantibody). In a similar way, streptavidin can be fused to the C-terminus of the sFv to allow spontaneous tetramerization. A more elegant approach to increase the antigen-binding sites of a sFv fragment is to shorten

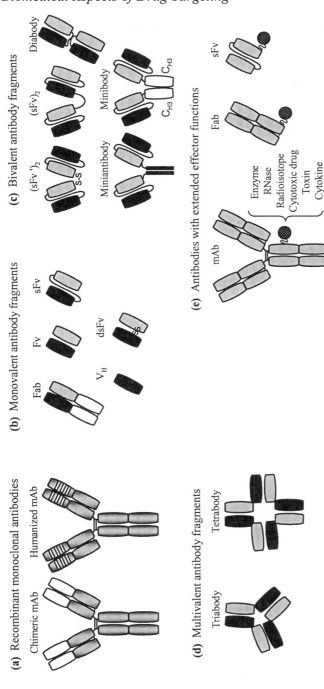

Figure 2. Schematic representation of recombinant antibody formats (panels a-e)

(a) Recombinant monoclonal antibodies. Fusion of murine variable regions to human constant domains results in a chimeric antibody. In a humanized antibody, the hypervariable regions of a murine monoclonal antibody are grafted onto the framework of a human antibody. (b) Monovalent antibody fragments. Fab fragments composed of the light chain ($V_L + C_L$) and the two N-terminal domains of the heavy chain ($V_H + C_H1$); Fv fragments are heterodimers consisting of the non-covalent association of the V_H and V_L domains. Some single variable heavy chain domains (V_H) retain full antigen binding properties. Fv fragments can be stabilized by the covalent linkage of the variable domains with a short linker peptide (single chain antibody, sFv) or by the introduction of intermolecular disulfide bonds within the variable domain framework regions (disulfide stabilized Fv, dsFv). (c) Bivalent and (d) multivalent antibody fragments. Two sFv fragments can be connected by C-terminal cysteine residues (sFv')$_2$, linker peptides (sFv)$_2$, dimerizing peptides or proteins (miniantibody) or constant region C_H3 domains (minibody). Bivalent diabodies, trivalent triabodies and tetravalent tetrabodies can be generated by variation of the linker lengths of sFv's. (e) Antibodies with extended effector functions. Recombinant monoclonal antibodies and derivatives acquire novel effector functions by linkage to various cytotoxic agents.

the length of the linker peptide connecting the variable domains. Reducing the linker length to three to twelve residues prevents pairing between domains of the same polypeptide chain and forces the pairing between complementary domains of a second sFv molecule to form a bivalent diabody (19). When further shortening the linker below three residues, the variable domains can associate to trivalent triabodies or tetravalent tetrabodies (20). Due to the lack of symmetry in the three-dimensional structure of the non-covalently associated variable domains, the orientation of the domains (V_H-V_L versus V_L-V_H) influences the trivalent or tetravalent transition. Different antibody forms are illustrated in Figure 2 above.

Targeted Apoptosis

Human RNAses, such as EDN, angiogenin or pancreatic RNAse A, are not cytotoxic to normal or tumor cells. Cell-type-specific cytotoxicity can be acquired by chemically conjugating or recombinantly fusing these RNAses to internalizing cell-binding ligands (5, 21). These targeted RNAses are reminiscent of the naturally occurring targeted bacterial enzymes, the colicins E3 and E6, that are comprised of both targeting and effector domains. The effector domains are RNAses that cleave the small rRNA in susceptible bacteria.

Both chemical and recombinant fusion proteins have been made between RNAses and antitransferrin antibody proteins or the genes encoding these proteins [(5, 21) and references therein]. Several different architectures have been used in the construction of the fusion proteins. In one variation, the 5′ end of the angiogenin gene was fused to the 3′ end of the CH2 domain of a chimeric antihuman-transferrin receptor antibody without a spacer peptide. The fusion took place in a manner that left the hinge region unaffected and dimerization of the heavy chain possible. The design of this construct allowed the formation of F(ab′)$_2$ antibody-angiogenin fusion proteins. Expression of the fusion protein occurred in myeloma cells that had been engineered to secrete an antitransferrin receptor chimeric light-chain. This fusion protein killed human leukemia cells with an IC$_{50}$ of 50 pM, however, the low level of secretion of the fusion protein into the culture media precluded purification of the antitransferrin receptor-targeted RNAse to homogeneity. The potency of this fusion protein most likely reflects the bivalent structure of the protein, which could have increased the avidity of binding. Additionally, angiogenin may have dimerized, which may have enhanced the translocation.

Another RNAse fusion protein, H17-BS-RNAse, was also designed using BS-RNAse to allow RNAse dimerization (5, 21). As discussed above,

BS-RNAse dimerizes naturally by the formation of two intersubunit disulfide bonds and an exchanged amino terminus. In this construct, the 5′ end of the RNAse was fused directly without a spacer to the 3′ end of the H17 sFv, an antibody that targets the human tumor-associated antigen placental alkaline phosphatase. Although designed to be a dimeric fusion protein, most of the correctly folded protein was monomeric, most likely due to the complexity of refolding and reconfiguring of the dimeric fusion. Toxicity of this fusion protein was in the nM range. Various modifications, such as the addition of the KDEL sequence to the C-terminus of BS-RNAse or the insertion of the diphtheria toxin disulfide loop between the sFv and the RNAse to increase translocation with and without the KDEL sequence, were made to improve the cytotoxicity of this molecule. This resulted in a 4-fold and 10-fold improvement in activity, respectively.

Single chain antibody constructs using the same chimeric antitransferrin receptor antibody used for the $F(ab')_2$ antibody-angiogenin fusion protein described above and three different human RNAses, EDN, pancreatic RNAse, or angiogenin, have also been prepared (5, 21). Both the nature of the linker connecting the V_L and V_H domains of the sFv [best linker was $(GGGGS)_3$] and the presence of a spacer peptide separating the RNAse and sFv [FB, residues 48-60 of staphylococcal protein A] proved to be important for the function of the antibody and the RNAse portion of the molecule. In all constructs, binding of the sFv was weaker than that of the parental IgG, most likely due to the valency, i.e. univalent vs. bivalent. In some of the fusion proteins, the activity of the RNAse was also impaired, ranging from 2-5 fold or 9-40 fold less than free enzyme for the angiogenin and EDN fusion proteins respectively. For the pancreatic RNAse fusion proteins, however, either the same or two times greater potency than that of the free enzyme was observed. Cytotoxicity varied when the same sFv fusion architecture was used but the human RNAse was changed. The EDN-sFv fusion protein proved to be more potent to a variety of human carcinoma cell lines tested in vitro with IC_{50}s ranging from 1-17 nM.

Other human RNAse fusion proteins have been constructed with growth factors or cytokines such as EGF, FGF, or IL2 as the targeting agent (21). These fusion proteins are fully humanized since both domains are built from human proteins. Possible drawbacks to using these types of specific cell binding ligands, in addition to receptor expression on normal tissues, are competitive inhibition by endogenous circulating ligand and the expression of natural biological activity of the ligand at concentrations too low to kill the cell but suitable for receptor binding and activation.

With one exception, RNAse chemical conjugates are less cytotoxic than RNAse fusion proteins (21). A comparison of chemical conjugates targeted to the human transferrin receptor shows that the chemical conjugates are 2-4 logs less potent than the recombinant RNAse-sFv fusion proteins. This decrease in activity may be due to the heterogeneous nature of the chemical conjugates. The inability to control sites of derivatization, and thus linkage, could lead to the inadvertent modification of key residues involved in the catalytic activity of the enzyme. Indeed enzymatic activity of the RNAse when chemically coupled is generally less than that of the free enzyme.

Yet the most potent targeted RNAse to date is composed of antibodies against the CD22 B-cell antigen chemically coupled to the natural amphibian RNAse, onconase (22), or the recombinant amphibian RNAse, *rap*LR1 (23) ($IC_{50}s$ range from 10-100 pM). Onconase and *rap*LR1 cytotoxicity are increased 10,000 ($IC_{50}s$, 500,000 and 50 pM for onconase and LL2-onconase, respectively) and 25,000-fold ($IC_{50}s$, 1,500,000 and 60 pM for *rap*LR1 and LL2-*rap*LR1, respectively) when chemically conjugated to antibodies against the CD22 receptor. The increase in cytotoxicity is due to specifically binding the CD22 antigen as free antibody against the CD22 receptor abrogates the cytotoxicity and protein synthesis is not inhibited in cells that do not express the CD22 antigen.

Targeted Apoptosis *In Vivo*

RNAses should overcome some of the limitations experienced in using plant or bacterial toxins as the effector proteins. These include immune responses against the toxins and toxin associated adverse effects, such as the dose limiting toxicity, vascular leak syndrome (VLS), characterized by: weight gain, edema, serum albumin decrease and pulmonary edema [reviewed in (24)]. Targeted RNAses are not immunogenic in animal studies nor does naked RNAse cause immunological problems in humans (5, 21).

While the potency and specificity of anti-CD22 RNAses is comparable to anti-CD22 immunotoxins made with plant and bacterial toxins, the anti-CD22 RNAse immunofusion proteins cause less non-specific toxic side effects in mice (22). Animals can tolerate 300 mg/kg and 500 mg/kg of LL2-onconase (22) and LL2-*rap*LR1 (23), respectively. This compares very favorably to the toxicity profiles for anti-CD22 *Pseudomonas* exotoxin derivatives [$LD_{50}s$ 1-6 mg/kg], anti-CD22 deglycosylated ricin A-chain immunotoxins [$LD_{50}s$ 12-80 mg/kg], and anti-CD22 ribosomal inactivating proteins [$LD_{50}s$ 0.5-1.75 mg/kg] (reviewed in (25)).

The *in vivo* activity of RNAse conjugates was first studied in a system in which the tumor cell burden was minimal as well as accessible to the conjugate. Cells were administered i.p. to mice; one day later i.p.

administration of the antibody plus RNAse or antibody-RNAse conjugate at 100 µg/day for 5 consecutive days began. Both LL2-onconase and LL2-*rap*LR1 were more effective than the mixture of RNAse and antibody in increasing the life span (ILS) of animals [ILS, 100-200% (22, 23)]. Intravenous injection of Daudi cells resulted in widely disseminated neoplasia with a more rapid onset of death compared with mice inoculated in the peritoneal cavity with the same number of tumor cells. Compression of the spinal cord causing hind limb paresis is predictive of survival time and is used as the end point (MPT). In this model, treatment is also I.V. and begins six days after tumor cell injection (100 µg/day for 5 consecutive days). Again, the covalently linked conjugates, LL2-onconase or LL2-*rap*LR1 significantly increased the lifespan of Daudi tumor-bearing mice 102-135% over that of the vehicle control or the mixture of antibody and RNAse. These studies show that significant increases in survival can be obtained with a dose of 25 mg/kg or less than 8% of the LD_{50}. Experiments in progress now demonstrate that significant responses can be obtained with doses as low as 0.25-2.5 mg/kg (D. L. N., unpublished observations).

Rationale for Clinical Use of Different Antibody Forms

The efficacy of tumor targeting by antibody-based molecules *in vivo* is dependent not only on the targeted tumor antigen but also on the tumor characteristics, e.g. tumor type (hematological malignancies or solid tumors), tumor mass, accessibility and density of the target antigen. The efficacy is also dependent on characteristics of the antibody molecule itself, e.g. size, charge, affinity and avidity. The comparison of pharmacokinetics and biodistribution of whole immunglobulins, enzymatically prepared fragments thereof, and engineered antibody fragments, indicates a correlation between size, tumor penetration and systemic clearance. The nominal molecular weight cut-off for the ultrafiltration in the kidney of uncharged proteins is approximately 60-70 kDa. Antibody fragments lacking the constant domain such as sFv (30 kDa), (sFv')$_2$ (55 kDa), Fab' (55 kDa) and diabodies (60 kDa) are cleared from the circulation within a few hours (26, 27), whereas intact chimeric and humanized IgG molecules (150 kDa) persist in the circulation for several days (28, 29). The passage of molecules across the glomerular filtration barrier decreases progressively with increasing molecular size. In contrast to conventional F(ab')$_2$ and Fab' distribution, intact IgG molecules barely exceed the perivascular regions of the tumor even at 24 h after administration, and the intratumoral diffusion distances of IgGs in solid tumor tissue is only about one millimeter in two days (30). In general, small antibody molecules are retained at relatively low levels but with much higher specificity at the tumor site (26).

Affinity describes the interaction of an antibody with its antigen and plays an important role in tumor-targeting properties. High affinity sFv antibody variants ($1x 10^{-9}$ M) were shown to have a prolonged tumor retention compared to mutants of lower affinity ($3x 10^{-7}$ M) (31, 32). Contrary to the theory that high affinity antibodies are preferable for successful tumor targeting *in vivo*, there is evidence of an existing physical penetration barrier for antibody-based molecules with extremely high affinities. Weinstein and colleagues (33) described the theory that a strong binding of high affinity monoclonal antibodies was confined mainly to the periphery of the tumor, thereby preventing deeper tumor penetration. This theory was experimentally validated for antibody fragments with extremely high affinities (10^{-11} M) (34), thus questioning their favorable value as therapeutics when rapid and uniform tumor penetration is required.

Naturally occurring antibodies differ from recombinant antibody fragments in their valencies of antigen binding. The multi-valency of natural antibodies contributes to an increased functional affinity due to simultaneous binding to the targeted antigen epitopes, the avidity effect. As a consequence, multivalency has a significant influence on the dissociation kinetics, which is of particular importance under non-equilibrium conditions of antibody-antigen interactions. Multivalent recombinant antibody fragments with increased avidity were shown to enhance tumor targeting much better than their monovalent counterparts (26, 35), providing a promising role for these constructs as novel therapeutic agents with improved biodistribution characteristics and pharmacokinetics. Through rational protein modeling and genetic engineering, antibody fragments can be designed to meet the requirements for optimal antibody-based therapeutic molecules.

CONCLUSIONS

Antibodies are now in the main stream of drug development. One of these is an anti-CD22 antibody that can evoke objective responses in patients with non-Hodgkin's lymphoma. Since the CD22 antigen rapidly internalizes, antibodies against it are well-suited to deliver molecular bombs to cancer cells. RNAses that damage RNA have tremendous potential as candidate bombs. They are well tolerated in humans and have potent anti-tumor effects when targeted by an antibody to CD22 expressing lymphoma cells. Other antibody-RNAse combinations are also effective against different types of cancer cells. The future lies with designing and engineering new variations of antibody-RNAse molecules with improved biodistribution and tumor penetration characteristics as well as optimal pharmacokinetics. Since preclinical studies show that RNAses cause fewer problems related to immunogenicity and host toxicity, the combination of antibody and RNAse should be attractive to the clinical and pharmaceutical communities.

ACKNOWLEDGEMENTS

This project has been funded in whole or in part with federal funds from the National Cancer Institute, National Institutes of Health, under Contract No. NO1-CO-56000. The content of this publication does not necessarily reflect the views or policies of the Department of Health and Human Services, nor does mention of trade names, commercial products, or organizations imply endorsement by the U.S. Government. The publisher or recipient acknowledges right of the U.S. Government to retain a nonexclusive, royalty-free license in and to any copyright covering the article. We appreciate the continued support of Dr. Edward A. Sausville and the Developmental Therapeutics Program.

REFERENCES

1.   Köhler, G. and Milstein, C. Continuous culture of fused cells secreting antibody of predefined specifity, Nature. *256:* 495-497, 1975.
2.   Gavilondo, J. V. and Larrick, J. W. Antibody engineering at the millennium, Biotechniques. *29:* 128-145, 2000.
3.   Caprara, M. and Nilsen, T. RNA: versatility in form and function, Nature Structural Biology. *7:* 831-833, 2000.
4.   Schein, C. H. From housekeeper to microsurgeon: The diagnostic and therapeutic potential of ribonucleases, Nature Biotechnol. *15:* 529-536, 1997.
5.   Rybak, S. M. and Newton, D. L. Natural and engineered cytotoxic ribonucleases: Therapeutic Potential, Exp. Cell Res. *253:* 325-335, 1999.
6.   Leland, P. A. and Raines, R. T. Cancer Chemotherapy - ribonucleases to the rescue, Chem. Biol. *8:* 405-413, 2001.
7.   Mikulski, S. M., Grossman, A. M., Carter, P. W., Shogen, K., and Costanzi, J. J. Phase 1 human clinical trial of ONCONASE (P-30 protein) administered intravenously on a weekly schedule in cancer patients with solid tumors, Int. J. Oncol. *3:* 57-64, 1993.
8.   Iordanov, M. S., Ryabinina, O. P., Wong, J., Dinh, T.-H., Newton, D. L., Rybak, S. M., and Magun, B. E. Molecular determinants of programmed cell death induced by the cytotoxic ribonuclease onconase: Evidence for cytotoxic mechanisms different from inhibition of protein synthesis, Cancer Res. *60:* 1983-1994, 2000.
9.   Iordanov, M., Wong, J., Newton, D., Rybak, S., Bright, R., Flavell, R., davis, R., and Magun, B. Differential requirement for the stress-activated protein kinase/c-Jun NH_2-terminal kinase in RNA damage-induced apoptosis in primary and in immortalized fibroblasts, Molec Cell Biol Res Com. *4:* 122-128, 2000.
10.   D'Alessio, G. New and cryptic biological messages from RNases, Trends in Cell Biol. *3:* 106-109, 1993.
11.   Cinatl, J. J., Cinatl, J., Kotchetkov, R., Motousek, J., Woodcock, B., Koehl, U., Vogel, J., Kornhuber, H., and Schwabe, D. Bovine seminal ribonuclease exerts

selective cytotoxicity toward neuroblastoma cells both sensitive and resistant to chemotherapeutic drugs, Anticancer res. *20:* 853-859, 2000.

12. Sakakibara, R., Hashida, K., Tominaga, N., Sakai, K., Ishiguro, M., Imamura, S., Ohmatsu, F., and Sato, E. A putative mouse oocyte maturation inhibitory protein from urine of pregnant women: N-terminal sequence homology with human nonsecretory ribonuclease, Chem. Pharm. Bull. *39:* 146-149, 1991.

13. Newton, D. L. and Rybak, S. M. Unique recombinant human ribonuclease and inhibition of kaposi's sarcoma cell growth, J Natl. Cancer Inst. *90:* 1787-1791, 1998.

14. Better, M., Chang, C. P., Robinson, R. R., and Horwitz, A. H. Escherichia coli secretion of an active chimeric antibody fragment, Science. *240:* 1041-3., 1988.

15. Skerra, A. and Pluckthun, A. Assembly of a functional immunoglobulin Fv fragment in Escherichia coli, Science. *240:* 1038-41., 1988.

16. Huston, J. S., Levinson, D., Mudgett-Hunter, M., Tai, M. S., Novotny, J., Margolies, M. N., Ridge, R. J., Bruccoleri, R. E., Haber, E., Crea, R., and Oppermann, H. Protein engineering of antibody binding sites: recovery of specific activity in an anti-digoxin single-chain Fv analogue produced in Escherichia coli, Proc Natl Acad Sci U S A. *85:* 5879-5883, 1988.

17. Glockshuber, R., Malia, M., Pfitzinger, I., and Plückthun, A. A comparison of strategies to stabilize immunoglobulin Fv fragments, Biochemistry. *29:* 1362-1367, 1990.

18. Adams, G. P., McCartney, J. E., Tai, M. S., Oppermann, H., Huston, J. S., Stafford, W. F. d., Bookman, M. A., Fand, I., Houston, L. L., and Weiner, L. M. Highly specific in vivo tumor targeting by monovalent and divalent forms of 741F8 anti-c-erbB-2 single-chain Fv, Cancer Res. *53:* 4026-4034, 1993.

19. Holliger, P., Prospero, T., and Winter, G. "Diabodies": small bivalent and bispecific antibody fragments, Proc Natl Acad Sci U S A. *90:* 6444-8., 1993.

20. Kortt, A. A., Lah, M., Oddie, G. W., Gruen, C. L., Burns, J. E., Pearce, L. A., Atwell, J. L., McCoy, A. J., Howlett, G. J., Metzger, D. W., Webster, R. G., and Hudson, P. J. Single-chain Fv fragments of anti-neuraminidase antibody NC10 containing five- and ten-residue linkers form dimers and with zero- residue linker a trimer, Protein Eng. *10:* 423-33., 1997.

21. Rybak, S. M. and Newton, D. L. Immunoenzymes. *In:* S. M. Chamow and A. Ashkenazi (eds.), Antibody Fusion Proteins, pp. 53-110. New York, NY: John Wiley & Sons, 1999.

22. Newton, D. L., Hansen, H. J., Mikulski, S. M., Goldenberg, D. M., and Rybak, S. M. Potent and specific antitumor activity of an anti-CD22-targeted cytotoxic ribonuclease: potential for the treatment of non-Hodgkin lymphoma, Blood. *97:* 528-535, 2001.

23. Hursey, M., Newton, D. L., Hansen, H., Ruby, D., Goldenberg, D. M., and Rybak, S. M. Specifically targeting the CD22 receptor of human B-cell lymphomas with RNA damaging agents: a new generation of therapeutics, Leukemia and Lymphoma 1-7, 2001.

24. Baluna, R. and Vitetta, E. S. Vascular leak syndrome: a side effect of immunotherapy, Immunopharmacol. *37:* 117-132, 1997.

25. Newton, D. L. and Rybak, S. M. Antibody targeted therapeutics for lymphoma: new focus on the CD22 antigen and RNA, Expert Opin Biol Ther. *1:* 995-1003, 2001.

26. Adams, G. P., Schier, R., McCall, A. M., Crawford, R. S., Wolf, E. J., Weiner, L. M., and Marks, J. D. Prolonged in vivo tumour retention of a human diabody targeting the extracellular domain of human HER2/neu, Br J Cancer. *77:* 1405-12, 1998.

27. Milenic, D. E., Yokota, T., Filpula, D. R., Finkelman, M. A., Dodd, S. W., Wood, J. F., Whitlow, M., Snoy, P., and Schlom, J. Construction, binding properties, metabolism, and tumor targeting of a single-chain Fv derived from the pancarcinoma monoclonal antibody CC49, Cancer Res. *51:* 6363-71, 1991.

28. Berinstein, N. L., Grillo-Lopez, A. J., White, C. A., Bence-Bruckler, I., Maloney, D., Czuczman, M., Green, D., Rosenberg, J., McLaughlin, P., and Shen, D. Association of serum Rituximab (IDEC-C2B8) concentration and anti-tumor response in the treatment of recurrent low-grade or follicular non- Hodgkin's lymphoma, Ann Oncol. *9:* 995-1001., 1998.

29. Cobleigh, M. A., Vogel, C. L., Tripathy, D., Robert, N. J., Scholl, S., Fehrenbacher, L., Wolter, J. M., Paton, V., Shak, S., Lieberman, G., and Slamon, D. J. Multinational study of the efficacy and safety of humanized anti-HER2 monoclonal antibody in women who have HER2-overexpressing metastatic breast cancer that has progressed after chemotherapy for metastatic disease, J Clin Oncol. *17:* 2639-48., 1999.

30. Clauss, M. A. and Jain, R. K. Interstitial transport of rabbit and sheep antibodies in normal and neoplastic tissues, Cancer Res. *50:* 3487-92, 1990.

31. Adams, G. P., Schier, R., McCall, A., Wolf, E. J., Marks, J. D., and Weiner, L. M. Tumor targeting properties of anti-c-erb-2 single-chain Fv molecules over a wide range of affinities for the same epitope, Tumor Targeting. *2:* 154, 1996.

32. Adams, G. P., Schier, R., Marshall, K., Wolf, E. J., McCall, A. M., Marks, J. D., and Weiner, L. M. Increased affinity leads to improved selective tumor delivery of single-chain Fv antibodies, Cancer Res. *58:* 485-90, 1998.

33. Weinstein, J. N., Eger, R. R., Covell, D. G., Black, C. D., Mulshine, J., Carrasquillo, J. A., Larson, S. M., and Keenan, A. M. The pharmacology of monoclonal antibodies, Ann N Y Acad Sci. *507:* 199-210, 1987.

34. Adams, G. P., Schier, R., McCall, A. M., Simmons, H. H., Horak, E. M., Alpaugh, R. K., Marks, J. D., and Weiner, L. M. High affinity restricts the localization and tumor penetration of single-chain fv antibody molecules, Cancer Res. *61:* 4750-5., 2001.

35. Nielsen, U. B., Adams, G. P., Weiner, L. M., and Marks, J. D. Targeting of bivalent anti-ErbB2 diabody antibody fragments to tumor cells is independent of the intrinsic antibody affinity [In Process Citation], Cancer Res. *60:* 6434-40, 2000.

GLOSSARY

Antibody: Proteins produced in a host in response to the presence of foreign molecules in the body called antigens.

Apoptosis: A type of cell death that can be induced in cancer cells by some types of drugs.

CD22: CD, cluster of differentiation, is cell surface antigens expressed on leukocytes. Antibodies that recognize CD markers can carry drugs to cells that express those markers and kill them. CD22 is present on B-lymphocytes in non-Hodgkin's lymphoma patients.

CDRs: complementarity determining regions: The sections of an antibody variable region that recognize the antigen.

EDN: Eosinophile derived neurotoxin: A human RNAse

Onconase: An amphibian cytotoxic RNAse in clinical trials as an anticancer drug.

rapLR1:   A recombinant cytotoxic RNAse that makes antibodies more effective in killing cancer cells by inducing apoptosis.

RNA: Ribonucleic acid: A polymeric structure in all living cells used in translating genetic information into proteins.

RNAse: Any number of enzymes that degrade RNA; in this chapter refers to members of the pancreatic type superfamily.

sFv: A type of antibody molecule produced by genetic engineering that only contains the V_L and V_H domains joined by a linker.

sFv fusion protein: A protein genetically engineered to contain an antibody domain fused to another protein e.g., RNAse. The specificity of the antibody for the antigen on tumor cells can increase the specificity of the RNAse to kill those cells.

Variable domains: Antibody domains of the variable light (V_L) or heavy (V_H) antibody chains. These vary in different antibodies and contain the CDRs with which they make up the antibody-combining site.

15

IMMUNOTOXINS AND ANTIBODY-DRUG CONJUGATES FOR CANCER TREATMENT

Victor S. Goldmacher, Walter A. Blättler, John M. Lambert, and Ravi V. J. Chari
ImmunoGen, Inc., Cambridge, MA 02139

INTRODUCTION

A large number of cytotoxic compounds are currently used as chemotherapeutic drugs to treat various malignancies. In general, the therapeutic efficacy of these drugs is limited by their narrow therapeutic window[i] primarily due to their lack of selectivity in killing cells that results in systemic toxicity at therapeutic doses.

An ideal anti-cancer drug should not be toxic in the compartment of its systemic delivery (such as blood compartment), but become toxic in the tumor compartment. This is the mode of action of the natural humoral immune response. Antibodies have no toxicity prior to reaching their targets. However, once antibodies are bound to the cell surface of the target cell, the antibody-dependent cellular cytotoxic response (ADCC) and complement-mediated cell lysis are activated.

The therapeutic efficacy of cytotoxic anti-cancer drugs can be improved by increasing their selectivity. One way of achieving this is to target such drugs to tumors with the help of antibodies, an idea first proposed by Paul Ehrlich about one hundred years ago. The practical application of this proposal became possible in the last twenty years with the advent of monoclonal antibodies, and identification of a number of tumor-associated antigens[ii]. A large number of conjugates of antibodies with a variety of cytotoxic agents were made and examined for their activity *in vitro* and *in vivo*. The first antibody-cytotoxic drug conjugates that were made lacked any selective potency *in vitro*, but a few of them demonstrated significant anti-tumor activity in mouse human xenograft tumor models. These conjugates were succeeded by immunotoxins, which were made with protein toxins, proved to be potent and selective in killing cultured cancer cell lines *in vitro*, as well as demonstrating anti-tumor activity towards xenograft tumors in immunodeficient mice. However, all early antibody-drug and antibody-protein toxin conjugates failed in clinical trials. These experiences revealed that cytotoxic potency and selectivity *in vitro* and in mouse xenograft tumor models, while perhaps necessary attributes, were not sufficient requirements for an immunoconjugate to be effective in patients. It became increasingly clear that *in vivo* properties of the early immunoconjugates in humans, such as their pharmacokinetics, tissue distribution, and the degree of their immunogenicity were unfavorable, and, at least in part, likely to be responsible for their lack of efficacy as anti-cancer drugs.

This chapter is not intended to be an exhaustive review of the vast literature devoted to the various types of conjugates of antibodies with toxic agents, a Herculean task. Instead, it provides our (inevitably subjective) critical analysis of the experiences accumulated with conjugates of monoclonal antibodies with various cytotoxic agents, hopefully serving as a guide towards the development of better anti-cancer drugs. Three types of targeting molecule-cytotoxic agent conjugates are beyond the scope of this chapter: protein hormone-toxin chemical conjugates or protein hormone-toxin fusion proteins, antibody-radionuclides, and small targeting molecule-small toxic molecule conjugates.

CONJUGATES OF MONOCLONAL ANTIBODIES WITH CLINICAL ANTI-CANCER DRUGS

Historically, the first cytotoxic agents conjugated with monoclonal antibodies were clinically used anti-cancer drugs and their derivatives (1). In the last twenty years, a large number of conjugates have been prepared with a variety of cytotoxic organic compounds such as doxorubicin, mitomycin c, daunomycin, methotrexate, *Vinca* alkaloids, *N*-acetyl-melphalan and chlorambucil (reviewed in (1, 2)) and taxol (3). These chemotherapeutic drugs, in non-conjugated form, are moderately to weakly cytotoxic to cultured cell lines with IC_{50} values in the range of 10^{-8} to 10^{-6} M (4). The drugs were linked to antibody molecules directly *via* covalent bonds not readily cleaved in cells, typically at a molar drug: antibody ratio of 4 to 8. When tested on cultured cells, virtually all these conjugates were found to be less potent than the non-conjugated drugs. Also, no cytotoxic selectivity could be demonstrated towards antigen-expressing cells.

These early results led quickly to the assumption that in order to kill cells, drugs need to be released from conjugates, most likely after their internalization. A variety of linkers designed to be cleavable inside the cells have been tested. These include: (a) acid-cleavable linkers based on *cis*-aconitic acid, acid-labile hydrazides, or acid-labile thiocarbamates, that could, in principle, be cleaved in acidified compartments of cells such as endosomes and lysosomes; (b) peptide linkers that could potentially be cleaved by lysosomal peptidases; (c) linkers containing an ester bond, that could potentially be hydrolyzed by intracellular esterases (reviewed in (2, 5)); (d) disulfide bond-containing linkers (6, 7) that could be cleaved by either intracellular thiols, or by protein disulfide isomerase. Conjugates of clinical anti-cancer drugs made with these linkers were found to be, at best, no more potent *in vitro*, than the non-conjugated drugs. Convincing selectivity in cell killing was rarely demonstrated.

Many of these antibody-drug conjugates utilizing cleavable linkers were evaluated for their anti-tumor activity in human tumor xenograft models in immunodeficient mice. Some of these conjugates displayed preferential accumulation at the tumor, and in spite of the somewhat disappointing *in vitro* results regarding selectivity of cell killing, showed a greater therapeutic efficacy *in vivo* than either the unconjugated drugs, or non-targeted antibody conjugates (2). In particular, several conjugates with doxorubicin, one of the most cytotoxic anti-cancer drugs in clinical use[iii] appeared very effective in these animal models, producing prolonged complete remissions in mice (7-9).

These encouraging *in vivo* data prompted clinical trials of the conjugates, but the results of these trials have been disappointing (reviewed in (2)). For example, the BR96-doxorubicin conjugate that displayed impressive anti-tumor activity in human xenograft tumor models in mice showed only marginal responses in cancer patients and exhibited a high degree of systemic toxicity (10). New clinical trials of this conjugate in combination with other chemotherapeutic drugs are ongoing, despite the unfavorable toxicity profile.

In an attempt to improve the potency of antibody-drug conjugates, the drug to antibody ratio was increased by linking a large number of drug molecules either directly to the antibody or with the help of a macromolecular carrier such as dextran, poly-glytamic acid, poly-lysine or serum albumin (5). These polymer conjugates, however, displayed diminished affinity and/or unfavorable pharmacokinetics (fast clearance from the circulation) in animal models and were not an improvement on direct antibody-drug conjugates having 4-8 drugs/antibody.

There may be several explanations why those of the early drug immunoconjugates that have shown anti-tumor activity in human xenograft models in mice had, at best, only marginal efficacy in clinical trials with cancer patients. One of the possible reasons for this discrepancy could be the design of the *in vivo* tumor models. In some studies, treatments of mice with a cytotoxic conjugate started almost immediately after inoculating the tumor cells into the animals (8), or the tumor cells were treated with the conjugates even before being injected into the animals (11). In other studies, it may be that the tumor xenografts were only marginally viable and so even a modest cytotoxic effect might have been sufficient to eradicate these tumors. A major reason might be the limitations of the mouse model to properly mimic the pharmacodynamics of conjugate distribution in the human body. It has been estimated, from quantifying the delivery of radiolabeled antibodies to both tumor xenografts in mice and to tumors in patients, that one can deliver in the range of 0.3% to 30% of the injected dose per gram of tumor in mice, but only up to 0.1% or less (depending on the tumor type) of the injected dose per gram of tumor in humans (12). We conclude that targeting the anti-cancer drugs via antibodies failed because the drugs were not potent enough to be effective at the concentrations that can be achieved at tumor sites in humans.

CONJUGATES OF MONOCLONAL ANTIBODIES WITH PROTEIN TOXINS (IMMUNOTOXINS)

In a search for cytotoxic agents of higher potency that could be targeted by antibodies, the attention of researchers shifted from conventional cancer drugs towards protein toxins of plant, fungal and bacterial origin. Two-chain toxins that consist of a binding subunit (or B-chain) linked to a toxic subunit (A-chain) are extremely cytotoxic. For example, ricin, a ribosome-inactivating protein isolated from castor beans, kills cells at concentrations lower than 10^{-11} M (13). Isolated A-chains of protein toxins and single-chain ribosome-inactivating proteins that functionally resemble ricin A-chain are only weakly cytotoxic for intact cells (in the concentration range of 10^{-7} to 10^{-6} M), but are very potent in killing cells once they get inside. For example, a single molecule of the A-subunit of diphtheria toxin injected into a cell can kill the cell (14). Protein toxins lack any selectivity in killing cells, and did not demonstrate any therapeutic window when tested in clinical trials (15). However, the remarkable cytotoxic potency of these toxins raised hopes that their conjugates with antibodies (collectively denoted immunotoxins) would be both highly effective and as selective as anti-tumor drugs.

The first generation immunotoxins were made with the toxic subunits (A-chains) of the two-chain toxins, such as ricin and diphtheria toxin, or with single-chain ribosome-inactivating proteins, such as gelonin or pokeweed antiviral protein (16-18). The nature of the linker between the antibody and the toxin proved to be a key parameter determining the cytotoxicity of such antibody-single-chain immunotoxins. It was assumed *a priori* that an ideal linker should be stable outside the cell but readily dissociate once the toxin is delivered inside the cell. Immunotoxins with various linkers were tested for their cytotoxicity, and it became clear that only cleavable linkers such as acid-labile, photolabile, and disulfide bond-containing linkers produced cytotoxic conjugates (16, 19). The most potent immunotoxins proved to be those constructed with a linker containing a disulfide bond. The mechanism of cell-induced reduction of these disulfide bonds has not been elucidated. The disulfide linker may possibly be cleaved by thiol/disulfide exchange with a low-molecular-weight thiol (such as glutathione, the most abundant thiol in the cytoplasm), or by protein disulfide isomerase (20), an enzyme capable of reducing disulfide bonds in proteins including intra-chain bonds in protein toxins (21). The enzyme is found in several intracellular locations, as well as at the cell surface (22, 23).

With a few exceptions, the antibody-single-chain immunotoxins turned out to be only moderately or weakly cytotoxic for cultured cell lines, killing cells in the concentration range of 10^{-9} to 10^{-7} M after a 24 h exposure[iv] (18). These observations were consistent with the cell biological properties of the A-chains and single-chain toxins. While two-chain protein toxins such as ricin and diphtheria toxin are capable of penetrating cell membranes, neither their isolated A-chains, nor the single-chain ribosome-inactivating proteins have this ability. As a result, only a tiny fraction (0.1% to 0.01%) of endocytosed antibody-single chain toxin conjugate molecules gains access to the cytoplasm and are able to reach their target (18).

Some antigens appear to be permanently anchored to the cell surface and do not mediate endocytosis of antibodies at all. Conjugates of single-chain-toxins with antibodies targeted towards such antigens are not any more cytotoxic towards the antigen-expressing cells than towards the antigen-negative cells (18). Thus, endocytosis is an obligatory step for activity of the single-chain-toxin immunotoxins.

The exceptions to the generalization that the single-chain immunotoxins were only moderately or weakly cytotoxic were those immunotoxins that were able to overcome the low efficiency of transfer of the cell-killing protein across a membrane (perhaps the endosomal membrane) into the cytoplasm. These were immunotoxins that targeted antigens, such as transferrin receptor or epidermal growth factor receptor, that are capable of achieving a higher internal quantity of receptor-bound antibody than the quantity found on the cell surface (18). These antigens thus enable the accumulation of large amounts of immunotoxin via endocytosis. A second group of cell surface antigens mediate endocytosis only to achieve an internal amount that is lower than the amount of antibody bound to the surface of the cell. However, immunotoxins targeting antigens of this type can also be very potent if they are present on the cell surface at very high density (5×10^5 or higher) (19).

Immunotoxins were also made with intact two-chain toxins on the premise that the binding subunit of these toxins also contains structural elements that facilitate the penetration of their toxic subunit across cellular membranes. The cytotoxic potency of such immunotoxins would be expected to be greatly enhanced compared to those made with A-chains or single-chain-toxins. To overcome the non-specific binding capacity of the binding subunit while preserving the ability of the toxin to efficiently translocate its A-chain across a cellular membrane into the cytoplasm, the binding site was either chemically blocked (as in ricin (25)), or specific deletions were made in the toxin's amino acid sequence (as in diphtheria toxin or pseudomonas exotoxin). Such chemically or genetically modified toxins were chemically conjugated or genetically fused to an antibody or an antibody fragment (26). Some of the resulting immunotoxins were remarkably potent and selective *in vitro*. For example, antibody conjugates of blocked ricin killed antigen-expressing cells in the 10^{-11} M range of concentrations[iv] while being about 1,000-fold less toxic towards antigen-negative cells (25).

Immunotoxins made with single-chain toxins (27), modified two-chain toxins (28), or with genetically engineered toxins (29), showed anti-tumor activity in xenograft models of human tumors in immunodeficient mice. In such *in vivo* models, efficacy was at least as high as could be achieved with conventional chemotherapeutic agents; several logs of cell killing could be demonstrated.

The results of efficacy studies with immunotoxins observed in *in vivo* models, together with the great selectivity shown by these agents *in vitro*, spurred the clinical evaluation of immunotoxins. Early clinical results demonstrated that immunotoxins could be administered safely with tolerable and reversible toxicity (30). However, more than 15 years of clinical studies with a variety of immunotoxins have yielded few clinically significant responses to date (17, 30). Novel clinical strategies, such as the use of immunotoxins to treat minimal residual disease, have also proved to be disappointing (31).

Again, as already discussed with regard to conjugates of clinically used cytotoxic drugs, the question arises of why immunotoxins showed such poor anti-tumor activity in humans despite promising data *in vitro*, and in animal xenograft models. One must again recognize the limitations of animal tumor models to mimic human disease, as well as the pharmacodynamic limitations of antibody distribution in the body where only 0.1% or less of the injected dose per gram of tumor actually arrives at the tumor site in humans compared to 0.3% to 30% in mice (12). This delivery limitation is very likely exacerbated by the unfavorable pharmacokinetics of immunotoxins. Unlike non-conjugated antibodies, most of the injected dose of these conjugates disappears from the circulation within several hours of the intravenous injection, probably *via* uptake by the reticulo-endothelial system.

Another factor limiting the efficacy of immunotoxins in the clinic is their immunogenicity. Both the toxin and the antibody moieties of immunotoxins were found to induce a humoral immune response in patients (17). Even patients with severely compromised immune systems (e.g., B-cell lymphoma patients following ablative chemotherapy) were able to generate an immune response to an immunotoxin (31). However in the case of immunotoxins that target B-cells, continuous infusion regimens can greatly delay, but not eliminate, the onset of neutralizing antibodies (31). As soon as patients produced antibodies against immunotoxins the therapeutic efficacy of immunotoxins was most likely abolished. Furthermore, there may be a risk that immune complexes will accumulate in the kidneys and cause nephrotoxicity, although it was not seen in one trial where an immune response was reported. (31). Thus, the clinical use of immunotoxins (unlike *in vivo* models utilizing immunodeficient mice) is limited to a single course of treatment before neutralizing antibodies appear, severely limiting the likelihood of clinical benefit. Immunotoxins made with humanized antibodies would not be a solution to this problem since their toxin moieties would still induce immune responses.

While immunotoxins in clinical trials have not lived up to the expectations generated by the *in vitro* and *in vivo* animal model data in general, very few of the patients treated with some of these agents did achieve partial responses and complete remissions (see for example (32, 33)). Indeed, one immunotoxin, an anti-CD22 variable fragment fused to a truncated pseudomonas exotoxin, was found highly efficacious in clinical trials of patients with chemotherapy-resistant hairy-cell leukemia (34). These isolated clinical successes suggest that some immunotoxins were just on the brink of having a clinically meaningful rate of anti-tumor activity in humans, and that, with further improvements, antibody-targeted cytotoxic agents could become effective anti-cancer drugs. If the systemic toxicity of immunotoxins could be reduced, and therefore higher doses administered, clinical efficacy might be increased. The major side effects at the maximum tolerated doses (MTD) included hepatotoxicity related to accumulation of immunotoxins in the liver (33, 35, 36), and capillary leak syndrome (37) resulting from damage to the vascular system. Recent studies suggest that the toxicity of the conjugates towards endothelial cells may be linked to a specific structural motif in toxins (38), raising hopes that this toxicity and the resulting capillary leak syndrome might be reduced by modifying the underlying amino acid sequences.

NOVEL CYTOTOXIC DRUGS FOR ANTIBODY-DRUG CONJUGATE PREPARATION (TUMOR-ACTIVATED PRO-DRUGS)

The experiences with early antibody-drug conjugates and immunotoxins suggest that the cytotoxic agents used in these conjugates have not been optimal. Immunoconjugates of conventional anti-cancer drugs did not have sufficient cytotoxic potency, while immunoconjugates of protein toxins retained some of the inherent properties of the toxins, including their fast clearance typical for foreign proteins and systemic toxicity which contributed to a narrow therapeutic window. Further, their high immunogenicity limited the number of courses of treatment.

These observations led us (and others) to the conclusion that for targeted drug delivery, we needed to search for novel cytotoxic agents that would combine the best properties of these two classes of agents. The cytotoxin should have a high cytotoxic potency approaching that of a protein toxin but should be non-immunogenic when conjugated to humanized (or human) antibodies, as expected for drugs of low molecular weight. Ideally, by conjugating such an agent to an antibody *via* a stable bond, the highly cytotoxic drug would be converted into an inactive pro-drug that would be stable in circulation *in vivo* and, thus, have low systemic toxicity even with high doses administered into the blood compartment.

Upon reaching a tumor cell the pro-drug would be activated by release of the fully active drug inside the cell. We named these conjugates tumor-activated pro-drugs (TAPs). The high potency of the drug would lead to the accumulation of a therapeutic (cytotoxic) dose of the drug at the tumor, despite the low percentage of the injected dose that ends up being retained in the tumor. The ideal immunoconjugates would have favorable pharmacokinetic properties, approaching those of unconjugated humanized (or human) IgG antibodies, so as to allow the maximum circulation time for optimum delivery of immunoconjugates from the blood compartment to the tumor.

To date, at least four types of highly cytotoxic drugs (Fig. 1) have been conjugated to monoclonal antibodies, calicheamicins, maytansinoids, DC1, and novel derivatives of taxol. These drugs are more potent than conventional cancer drugs and approach the potency of the protein toxins abrin, ricin and pseudomonas exotoxin in their *in vitro* cytotoxicity.

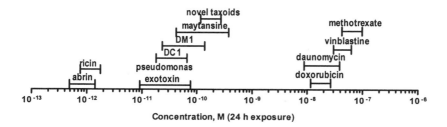

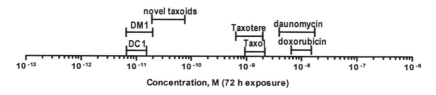

Figure 1. Comparison of the potency of various cytotoxic drugs for cultured human cells. The data are presented as the composite ranges of IC_{50} values for several representative cancer cell lines. The IC_{50} values were obtained in clonogenic assays after an exposure of cells to a drug.

Calicheamicin Immunoconjugates

The highly cytotoxic calicheamicins[v] were isolated from the broth extract of *Micromonospora echinospora ssp. Calichensis*. Calicheamicin γ_1^I, the most potent of the calicheamicins, is an enediyne compound that binds to the minor groove of DNA, ultimately resulting in DNA cleavage and cell death. Two immunoconjugates have been made with derivatives of calicheamicin, Mylotarg (40) and 138H11-Camθ (41).

Mylotarg consists of a humanized anti-CD33 antibody and the semisynthetic calicheamicin γ_1^I derivative, *N*-acetyl gamma calicheamicin dimethyl hydrazide. As a result, the conjugate contains two readily cleavable chemical bonds: an acid-cleavable hydrazide bond and a disulfide bond that can be cleaved through disulfide exchange with a sulfhydryl compound. Due to the hydrazide linker, the conjugate is not sufficiently stable in aqueous solutions and consequently the drug product is provided in a lyophilized form.

Mylotarg targets the CD33 antigen expressed on the surface of leukemic blasts in more than 80% of patients with acute myeloid leukemia (AML). Mylotarg proved to be highly potent and antigen-selective *in vitro* and showed anti-tumor effects in xenograft tumor models of myeloid leukemia in athymic mice (40). The promising pre-clinical data propelled the immunoconjugates into clinical trials, where it demonstrated a significant response rate in patients with CD33-positive acute myeloid leukemia (42). The conjugate was retained in the circulation for a long time (the calicheamicin elimination half-life being about 39 h), and did not induce an immune response in the vast majority of patients. Mylotarg is the first drug of this type to be approved for clinical use by the U.S. Food and Drug Administration (FDA). Its approval is for AML patients in first relapse who are 60 years of age or older and who are not considered candidates for cytotoxic chemotherapy.

The 138H11-Camθ conjugate, in which the anti-γ-glutamyl transferase antibody, 138H11, is coupled to calicheamicin θ_1^I *via* a disulfide bond-containing linker (41), appears to have high antigen-specific cytotoxicity in cultured renal cell carcinoma (RCC) cells. The conjugate is also active in a human RCC xenograft model in mice, although the *in vivo* results are difficult to interpret since the treatment of mice with the conjugate started almost immediately (on the next day) after the injection of the tumor.

Maytansinoid Immunoconjugates (4, 43)

Maytansine is a natural product originally isolated from the Ethiopian shrub *Maytenus serrata*. Maytansine inhibits tubulin polymerization resulting in a mitotic block and cell death. Thus, the mechanism of action of maytansine appears to be similar to that of vincristine and vinblastine. Maytansine, however, is about 200 to 1,000-fold more cytotoxic *in vitro* than these *Vinca* alkaloids. Human clinical trials of maytansine were disappointing: this drug did not display a therapeutic window (44).

We set out to enhance the target specificity of maytansine and to diminish its systemic toxicity by converting it to a prodrug that would be inactive in circulation, but selectively delivered to and cleaved inside a tumor cell to give active drug. In order to achieve this goal we sought to link maytansine, *via* disulfide bond, to monoclonal antibodies directed towards tumor-associated antigens. Since maytansine does not possess a suitable functional group that would allow linkage to antibodies, we synthesized a novel maytansinoid, DM1, bearing a sulfhydryl-containing substituent. The site of modification of maytansine was carefully chosen so as to maintain its cytotoxic potency. In fact, the new maytansinoid derivative was 3- to 10-fold more cytotoxic than maytansine itself (4).

Antibody-DM1 conjugates were prepared by disulfide exchange between the thiol moiety of DM1 and an antibody that had been modified to introduce a reactive disulfide group. Typically, an average of about four DM1 molecules was linked per antibody molecule. DM1 has been linked to several antibodies including (a) the TA.1 antibody directed against the *neu*/HER2/*erbB*-2 antigen expressed on breast tumors (4), (b) the C242 antibody directed against CanAg, (c) an antigen expressed on colorectal and pancreatic tumors (43), (d) the humanized N901 antibody which recognizes the CD56 antigen expressed on small cell lung cancer, (e) the J591 antibody that binds to prostate-specific membrane antigen, and (f) trastuzumab (Herceptin), another anti-*neu*/HER2/*erbB*-2 antibody.

In vitro evaluation of these conjugates indicated that linkage of about four DM1 molecules to these antibodies did not damage their binding affinities. These conjugates were highly cytotoxic for antigen-expressing cultured cell lines in an antigen-specific manner. For example, C242-DM1 killed antigen-positive colon cancer COLO 205 cells, with an IC_{50} of 3×10^{-11} M, while antigen-negative melanoma A-375 cells were only affected at a 1,000-fold higher concentration. Non-conjugated maytansinoid was equally cytotoxic for both cell lines with IC_{50} values in the range of 3×10^{-11} M. Thus, linkage of DM1 to an antibody converts it into an inactive prodrug that is rendered fully active only upon its association with a target antigen-expressing cell.

There was no measurable loss of the *in vitro* cytotoxic potency or antigen-specificity of these conjugates upon extended storage for more than 1 year in aqueous buffers at 4°C at near neutral pH. These results confirmed that the disulfide bonds in the linker were stable for the duration of this storage. *In vivo* evaluation of the stability of these conjugates in the circulation of mice and monkeys showed that the linker disulfide bond was remarkably stable under these conditions as well. The circulation half-life of the intact conjugates was about two days, much longer than that of immunotoxins.

Several of the DM1 conjugates mentioned earlier have been evaluated for their *in vivo* anti-tumor efficacy. The DM1 conjugates of C242, huN901, J591, and trastuzumab all displayed exceptional anti-tumor activity in human tumor xenograft models in immunodeficient mice. These conjugates completely eradicated the tumors in mice at doses below the MTD. For example, Tables 1 and 2 show the efficacy results obtained with the immunoconjugates C242-DM1 and huN901-DM1. As a reference, standard anti-cancer drugs used for these types of cancer showed only modest efficacy, i.e., tumor growth delays but no tumor regression, when used at their MTD (Table 1, 2), doses at which mice show clinical signs of toxicity effects.

Table 1. Comparison of the Anti-Tumor Efficacy of C242-DM1 and Standard Anti-Cancer Drugs (HT-29 Subcutaneous Xenograft Model)

Drug	Dose	Tumor growth-delay, days
CPT-11	60 mg/kg x 3, q3d	13
5-FU	15 mg/kg x 5, qd	6
Doxorubicin	3 mg/kg x 2, qd	7
Vincristine	0.4 mg/kg x 3, q2d	10
Maytansine	0.3 mg/kg x 5, qd	6
C242-DM1	0.3 mg/kg x 5, qd	complete remission (followed for 45 days)

Table 2. Comparison of the Anti-Tumor Efficacy of huN901-DM1 and Standard Anti-Cancer Drugs (SW2 Subcutaneous Xenograft Model)

Drug	Dose	Tumor growth-delay, Days
Cisplatin	4 mg/kg x 3, qd	12
Etoposide	15 mg/kg x 3, qd	13
Cisplatin + Etoposide	2 mg/kg x 3, qd 15 mg/kg x 3, qd	14
huN901	14.4 mg/kg x 5, qd	0
huN901 + Maytansine	14.4 mg/kg x 5, qd 0.3 mg.kg x 5, qd	2
huN901-DM1	0.3 mg/kg x 5, qd	cured (followed for 140 days)

The humanized version of C242-DM1, cantuzumab mertansine (huC242-DM1, code name SB-408075) is now undergoing phase I clinical evaluation in patients with colorectal, pancreatic, and non-small cell lung cancer. A phase I study administering a single intravenous (I.V.) dose of cantuzumab mertansine every three weeks resulted in a MTD of 235 mg/m^2. The dose-limiting toxicity was found to be reversible elevations (grade 3) in serum transaminases that occurred in two out of three patients treated at 295 mg/m^2. The MTD was 115 mg/m^2 upon weekly administration with similar reversible dose-limiting toxicities seen at 138 mg/m^2/week. Human anti-humanized antibody or anti-DM1 antibody was not detected in these studies. Several encouraging indications of biologic activity were seen in these studies with patients that had received many prior courses of chemotherapy and were (now) refractory to such treatment. Human clinical trials of huN901-DM1 (code name BB-10901) in small cell lung cancer patients have also commenced recently.

Bis-indolyl-*seco*-CBI derivative (DC1) conjugates (45)

CC-1065 is a structurally novel anti-tumor antibiotic isolated from microbial fermentation of *Streptomyces zelensis*. Its mode of action is binding with high affinity to the minor groove of DNA, followed by alkylation of adenine bases. CC-1065 is at least 1,000-fold more cytotoxic for cultured cell lines than most other DNA-interacting agents, such as the anti-cancer drugs doxorubicin and cis-platin.

Adozelesin is a structurally simpler synthetic analog of CC-1065, which retains the high potency of the parental compound. Adozelesin was evaluated in human clinical trials but showed high systemic toxicity and no therapeutic window. The high cytotoxic potency of adozelesin (Fig. 1) makes it a promising candidate for use in targeted delivery in the form of an antibody-drug conjugate.

In order to enable the linkage of DC1 to antibodies *via* disulfide bonds, we designed new disulfide-containing analogs of adozelesin, bis-indolyl-*seco*-CBI compounds, also known as DC1 derivatives. The alkylating cyclopropa-pyrroloindole (CPI) portion of adozelesin was replaced by the cyclopropa-benzindole (CBI) unit in these compounds. The terminal benzofuran moiety in adozelesin was replaced by an indole group bearing a sulfhydryl-containing side chain at the C-5 position. This functionality did not alter the cytotoxic potency of the drug toward cell lines. A methyldisulfide derivative of DC1 had an IC_{50} value of 2×10^{-11} M, which was similar to that reported for adozelesin.

In our first conjugate, DC1 was linked to the anti-B4 antibody, which binds to the CD19 antigen expressed in B cell lymphoma. We prepared an anti-B4-DC1 containing about 4 molecules of DC1 linked per antibody molecule, and examined its *in vitro* and *in vivo* properties.

In vitro, anti-B4-DC1 was evaluated for its cytotoxicity towards the antigen-positive human lymphoma cell line Namalwa and towards antigen-negative MOLT 4 cells (45). Anti-B4-DC1 was extremely cytotoxic for the target Namalwa cells with an IC_{50} value of 5×10^{-11} M, after a 72 h exposure to the drug. The killing curve was very steep, with greater than 99.999% of cells killed at a conjugate concentration of 1×10^{-9} M. Anti-B4-DC1 was at least 1,000-fold less cytotoxic to the non-target MOLT 4 cells ($IC_{50} > 5 \times 10^{-8}$ M), demonstrating the target specificity of the cytotoxic effect.

The anti-tumor activity of Anti-B4-DC1 was evaluated in an aggressive, metastatic model of human B cell lymphoma. Anti-B4-DC1 showed remarkable anti-tumor efficacy in this model (Fig. 2), resulting in a median increase in life span of 265%. The surviving animals (30% of the treated group) were sacrificed on day 100 and showed no evidence of disease upon necropsy. In comparison, the standard chemotherapeutic drugs, doxorubicin, vincristine, etoposide or cyclophosphamide, some of which are currently part of the standard treatment protocol of lymphoma, had only a modest effect (median increase in life span ranging from 22 to 91%).

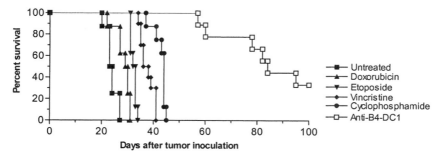

Figure 2. Anti-tumor activity of anti-B4-DC1 and of conventional chemotherapeutic drugs (a representative experiment). SCID mice were inoculated I.V. with 4×10^6 Namalwa cells. Animals were left either untreated (control) or were treated starting on day seven after tumor inoculation with one of the following agents: anti-B4-DC1 at a DC1 dose of 80 µg/kg/day x 5 every day (I.V.), or with one of the other drugs as described in (45).

Taxoid Conjugates

Paclitaxel (Taxol) and its semi-synthetic analogue docetaxel (Taxotere) are two of the most effective agents in the treatment of a variety of cancers. The taxoids target microtubules, but, unlike *Vinca* alkaloids or maytansine, taxoids inhibit the de-polymerization of tubulin polymers and stabilize microtubules, resulting in cell death.

Like other commonly used anti-cancer drugs, paclitaxel (Fig. 1) and docetaxel display moderate cytotoxic potency *in vitro*, and thus, are not sufficiently potent for use as antibody conjugates. Two independent research groups have reported the synthesis of new taxoids that are 50- to 100-fold more cytotoxic than the parental taxoids (46). The increased potency of these novel taxoids did not result in a greater therapeutic window, and thus did not make them more attractive as therapeutic drugs. The higher cytotoxicity of these taxoids made them attractive as candidate drugs for targeted delivery in the form of antibody conjugates.

To enable the linkage of taxoids to antibodies *via* disulfide bonds, we first had to modify them further to introduce a sulfhydryl-containing group. We synthesized a number of such compounds, and found a disulfide-containing taxoid derivative that was as cytotoxic as its precursor compound, and about 100-fold more cytotoxic than paclitaxel towards tumor cell lines *in vitro*. We are currently working on the conjugation of this promising new taxoid with monoclonal antibodies and the preclinical evaluation of the resulting conjugates.

CONCLUSION: EVOLUTION OF ANTIBODY-CYTO-TOXIC DRUG CONJUGATES

The discovery of the monoclonal antibody technology in 1975 fueled most if not all development work in the field of targeted delivery of cytotoxic agents to tumors. The development started with conjugates of antibodies with low molecular weight drugs and was then broadened to include conjugates with protein toxins. The latest development has returned to low molecular weight drugs, although to novel agents with much higher cytotoxic potency. The new conjugates combine the best qualities of the previous types of agents. It is this new generation of targeted cytotoxic drug delivery agents that may yet realize the old idea of Ehrlich, that effective treatments for cancer can be constructed from antibodies; "magic bullets" homing in on the cancer cell to deliver a lethal payload. The first agent of this type, Mylotarg, has been approved as an anti-cancer drug. We are confident that other approvals will follow, and that this approach will finally yield effective drugs for those types of cancers that used to be incurable.

---

[i] Therapeutic window is loosely defined as the interval of drug doses between the minimal dose that is producing a therapeutic effect and the maximal tolerated dose.

[ii] Tumor-associated antigens are those that are either over-expressed on cancer cells or expressed on only a limited number of cell lineages, including cancer cells.

[iii] The IC_{50} of doxorubicin for of cultured human cancer cell lines is about 30 to 50 nM after a 24 h exposure when measured in clonogenic assays.

[iv] The cytotoxicities of immunotoxins discussed here were measured in direct cytotoxicity assays such as clonogenic assays. A number of reports claimed high cytotoxic potencies (typically in the 10^{-10} M to 10^{-11} M range) for immunotoxins made with single-chain toxins or A-chains. These values were obtained by using indirect cytotoxicity assays, most commonly by measuring inhibition of incorporation of radiolabeled DNA or protein synthesis precursors. When we compared the IC_{50} values for single-chain toxin immunotoxins obtained by the indirect methods with those obtained by the benchmark clonogenic assay, we found that the indirect methods grossly overestimated cytotoxicities of immunotoxins. For a critical review of cytotoxicity assays see (24).

[v] These compounds have apparent IC_{50} values about 1 nM after a 1-day exposure, and below 1 pM after a 3-day exposure when measured by indirect cytotoxicity assays (39). To our knowledge, no direct measurements of cytotoxicities for these compounds (such as by clonogenic assays) have been reported.

REFERENCES

1. Pietersz, G. A., Krauer, K., and McKenzie, I. F. The use of monoclonal antibody immunoconjugates in cancer therapy. Adv Exp Med Biol, *353:* 169-179, 1994.
2. Chari, R. V. Targeted delivery of chemotherapeutics: tumor-activated prodrug therapy. Adv Drug Deliv Rev, *31:* 89-104, 1998.
3. Guillemard, V. and Saragovi, H. U. Taxane-antibody conjugates afford potent cytotoxicity, enhanced solubility, and tumor target selectivity. Cancer Res, *61:* 694-699, 2001.
4. Chari, R. V., Martell, B. A., Gross, J. L., Cook, S. B., Shah, S. A., Blättler, W. A., McKenzie, S. J., and Goldmacher, V. S. Immunoconjugates containing novel maytansinoids: promising anticancer drugs. Cancer Res, *52:* 127-131, 1992.
5. Pietersz, G. A. The linkage of cytotoxic drugs to monoclonal antibodies for the treatment of cancer. Bioconjug Chem, *1:* 89-95, 1990.
6. Trail, P. A., Willner, D., Knipe, J., Henderson, A. J., Lasch, S. J., Zoeckler, M. E., TrailSmith, M. D., Doyle, T. W., King, H. D., Casazza, A. M., Braslawsky, G. R., Brown, J., Hofstead, S. J., Greenfield, R. S., Firestone, R. A., Mosure, K., Kadow, K. F., Yang, M. B., Hellstrom, K. E., and Hellstrom, I. Effect of linker variation on the stability, potency, and efficacy of carcinoma-reactive BR64-doxorubicin immunoconjugates. Cancer Res, *57:* 100-105, 1997.
7. Zhu, Z., Kralovec, J., Ghose, T., and Mammen, M. Inhibition of Epstein-Barr-virus-transformed human chronic lymphocytic leukaemic B cells with monoclonal-antibody-adriamycin (doxorubicin) conjugates. Cancer Immunol Immunother, *40:* 257-267, 1995.
8. Sivam, G. P., Martin, P. J., Reisfeld, R. A., and Mueller, B. M. Therapeutic efficacy of a doxorubicin immunoconjugate in a preclinical model of spontaneous metastatic human melanoma. Cancer Res, *55:* 2352-2356, 1995.
9. Trail, P. A., Willner, D., Lasch, S. J., Henderson, A. J., Hofstead, S., Casazza, A. M., Firestone, R. A., Hellstrom, I., and Hellstrom, K. E. Cure of xenografted human carcinomas by BR96-doxorubicin immunoconjugates. Science, *261:* 212-215, 1993.
10. Tolcher, A. W. BR96-doxorubicin: been there, done that! J Clin Oncol, *18:* 4000, 2000.
11. Arnon, R. and Sela, M. In vitro and in vivo efficacy of conjugates of daunomycin with anti-tumor antibodies. Immunol Rev, *62:* 5-27, 1982.
12. Sedlacek, H.-H., Seemann, G., Hoffmann, D., Czech, J., Lorenz, P., C., K., and Bosslet, K. Antibodies as carriers of cytotoxicity, pp. 74-76. Basel; New York: Karger, 1992.
13. Lord, J. M., Roberts, L. M., and Robertus, J. D. Ricin: structure, mode of action, and some current applications. Faseb J, *8:* 201-208, 1994.
14. Yamaizumi, M., Mekada, E., Uchida, T., and Okada, Y. One molecule of diphtheria toxin fragment A introduced into a cell can kill the cell. Cell, *15:* 245-250, 1978.
15. Fodstad, O., Kvalheim, G., Godal, A., Lotsberg, J., Aamdal, S., Host, H., and Pihl, A. Phase I study of the plant protein ricin. Cancer Res, *44:* 862-865, 1984.
16. Frankel, A. E. Immunotoxins, Boston, Norwell: Kluwer Academic Publishers; 1988.
17. Ghetie, V. and Vitetta, E. Immunotoxins in the therapy of cancer: from bench to clinic. Pharmacol Ther, *63:* 209-234, 1994.
18. Goldmacher, V. S., Scott, C. F., Lambert, J. M., McIntyre, G. D., Blättler, W. A., Collnhson, A. R., Stewart, J. K., Chong, L. D., Cook, S., Slayter, H. S., and et al. Cytotoxicity of gelonin and its conjugates with antibodies is determined by the extent of their endocytosis. J Cell Physiol, *141:* 222-234, 1989.
19. Blakey, D. C., J., W. E., M., W. P., and E., T. P. Antibody toxin conjugates: a perspective. *In:* H. Waldmann (ed.), Monoclonal antibody therapy, Vol. 45, pp. 50-90. Basel: Karger, 1988.

20. Mandel, R., Ryser, H. J., Ghani, F., Wu, M., and Peak, D. Inhibition of a reductive function of the plasma membrane by bacitracin and antibodies against protein disulfide-isomerase. Proc Natl Acad Sci U S A, *90:* 4112-4116, 1993.

21. Barbieri, L., Battelli, M. G., and Stirpe, F. Reduction of ricin and other plant toxins by thiol:protein disulfide oxidoreductases. Arch Biochem Biophys, *216:* 380-383, 1982.

22. Varandani, P. T., Raveed, D., and Nafz, M. A. Insulin degradation. XXIII. Distribution of glutathione-insulin transhydrogenase in isolated rat hepatocytes as studied by immuno-ferritin and electron microscopy. Biochim Biophys Acta, *538:* 343-353, 1978.

23. Yoshimori, T., Semba, T., Takemoto, H., Akagi, S., Yamamoto, A., and Tashiro, Y. Protein disulfide-isomerase in rat exocrine pancreatic cells is exported from the endoplasmic reticulum despite possessing the retention signal. J Biol Chem, *265:* 15984-15990, 1990.

24. Sellers, J. R., Cook, S., and Goldmacher, V. S. A cytotoxicity assay utilizing a fluorescent dye that determines accurate surviving fractions of cells. J Immunol Methods, *172:* 255-264, 1994.

25. Lambert, J. M., Goldmacher, V. S., Collinson, A. R., Nadler, L. M., and Blättler, W. A. An immunotoxin prepared with blocked ricin: a natural plant toxin adapted for therapeutic use. Cancer Res, *51:* 6236-6242, 1991.

26. Kreitman, R. J. Immunotoxins. Expert Opin Pharmacother, *1:* 1117-1129, 2000.

27. Scott, C. F., Jr., Goldmacher, V. S., Lambert, J. M., Jackson, J. V., and McIntyre, G. D. An immunotoxin composed of a monoclonal antitransferrin receptor antibody linked by a disulfide bond to the ribosome-inactivating protein gelonin: potent in vitro and in vivo effects against human tumors. J Natl Cancer Inst, *79:* 1163-1172, 1987.

28. Shah, S. A., Halloran, P. M., Ferris, C. A., Levine, B. A., Bourret, L. A., Goldmacher, V. S., and Blättler, W. A. Anti-B4-blocked ricin immunotoxin shows therapeutic efficacy in four different SCID mouse tumor models. Cancer Res, *53:* 1360-1367, 1993.

29. Brinkmann, U., Pai, L. H., FitzGerald, D. J., Willingham, M., and Pastan, I. B3(Fv)-PE38KDEL, a single-chain immunotoxin that causes complete regression of a human carcinoma in mice. Proc Natl Acad Sci U S A, *88:* 8616-8620, 1991.

30. Grossbard, M. L., Press, O. W., Appelbaum, F. R., Bernstein, I. D., and Nadler, L. M. Monoclonal antibody-based therapies of leukemia and lymphoma. Blood, *80:* 863-878, 1992.

31. Grossbard, M. L., Multani, P. S., Freedman, A. S., O'Day, S., Gribben, J. G., Rhuda, C., Neuberg, D., and Nadler, L. M. A Phase II study of adjuvant therapy with anti-B4-blocked ricin after autologous bone marrow transplantation for patients with relapsed B-cell non-Hodgkin's lymphoma. Clin Cancer Res, *5:* 2392-2398, 1999.

32. Senderowicz, A. M., Vitetta, E., Headlee, D., Ghetie, V., Uhr, J. W., Figg, W. D., Lush, R. M., Stetler-Stevenson, M., Kershaw, G., Kingma, D. W., Jaffe, E. S., and Sausville, E. A. Complete sustained response of a refractory, post-transplantation, large B-cell lymphoma to an anti-CD22 immunotoxin. Ann Intern Med, *126:* 882-885, 1997.

33. Lynch, T. J., Jr., Lambert, J. M., Coral, F., Shefner, J., Wen, P., Blättler, W. A., Collinson, A. R., Ariniello, P. D., Braman, G., Cook, S., Esseltine, D., Elias, A., Skarin, A., and Ritz, J. Immunotoxin therapy of small-cell lung cancer: a phase I study of N901-blocked ricin. J Clin Oncol, *15:* 723-734, 1997.

34. Kreitman, R. J., Wilson, W. H., Bergeron, K., Raggio, M., Stetler-Stevenson, M., FitzGerald, D. J., and Pastan, I. Efficacy of the anti-CD22 recombinant immunotoxin BL22 in chemotherapy-resistant hairy-cell leukemia. N Engl J Med, *345:* 241-247, 2001.

35.   Ghetie, M. A., Ghetie, V., and Vitetta, E. S. Immunotoxins for the treatment of B-cell lymphomas. Mol Med, *3:* 420-427, 1997.
36.   Frankel, A. E., Kreitman, R. J., and Sausville, E. A. Targeted toxins. Clin Cancer Res, *6:* 326-334, 2000.
37.   Baluna, R. and Vitetta, E. S. Vascular leak syndrome: a side effect of immunotherapy. Immunopharmacology, *37:* 117-132, 1997.
38.   Baluna, R., Rizo, J., Gordon, B. E., Ghetie, V., and Vitetta, E. S. Evidence for a structural motif in toxins and interleukin-2 that may be responsible for binding to endothelial cells and initiating vascular leak syndrome. Proc Natl Acad Sci U S A, *96:* 3957-3962, 1999.
39.   Nicolaou, K. C., Stabila, P., Esmaeli-Azad, B., Wrasidlo, W., and Hiatt, A. Cell-specific regulation of apoptosis by designed enediynes. Proc Natl Acad Sci U S A, *90:* 3142-3146, 1993.
40.   Hamann, P. R., Hinman, L. M., Hollander, I., Beyer, C. F., Lindh, D., Holcomb, R., Hallett, W., Tsou, H. R., Upeslacis, J., Shochat, D., Mountain, A., Flowers, D. A., and Bernstein, I. Gemtuzumab Ozogamicin, A Potent and Selective Anti-CD33 Antibody-Calicheamicin Conjugate for Treatment of Acute Myeloid Leukemia. Bioconjug Chem, *13:* 47-58, 2002.
41.   Knoll, K., Wrasidlo, W., Scherberich, J. E., Gaedicke, G., and Fischer, P. Targeted therapy of experimental renal cell carcinoma with a novel conjugate of monoclonal antibody 138H11 and calicheamicin thetaI1. Cancer Res, *60:* 6089-6094, 2000.
42.   Dowell, J. A., Korth-Bradley, J., Liu, H., King, S. P., and Berger, M. S. Pharmacokinetics of gemtuzumab ozogamicin, an antibody-targeted chemotherapy agent for the treatment of patients with acute myeloid leukemia in first relapse. J Clin Pharmacol, *41:* 1206-1214, 2001.
43.   Liu, C., Tadayoni, B. M., Bourret, L. A., Mattocks, K. M., Derr, S. M., Widdison, W. C., Kedersha, N. L., Ariniello, P. D., Goldmacher, V. S., Lambert, J. M., Blättler, W. A., and Chari, R. V. Eradication of large colon tumor xenografts by targeted delivery of maytansinoids. Proc Natl Acad Sci U S A, *93:* 8618-8623, 1996.
44.   Issell, B. F. and Crooke, S. T. Maytansine. Cancer Treat Rev, *5:* 199-207, 1978.
45.   Chari, R. V., Jackel, K. A., Bourret, L. A., Derr, S. M., Tadayoni, B. M., Mattocks, K. M., Shah, S. A., Liu, C., Blättler, W. A., and Goldmacher, V. S. Enhancement of the selectivity and antitumor efficacy of a CC-1065 analogue through immunoconjugate formation. Cancer Res, *55:* 4079-4084, 1995.
46.   Ojima, I., Slater, J. C., Kuduk, S. D., Takeuchi, C. S., Gimi, R. H., Sun, C. M., Park, Y. H., Pera, P., Veith, J. M., and Bernacki, R. J. Syntheses and structure-activity relationships of taxoids derived from 14 beta-hydroxy-10-deacetylbaccatin III. J Med Chem, *40:* 267-278, 1997.

GLOSSARY

Calicheamicin: A highly cytotoxic antibiotic isolated from fermentation of *Micromonospora echinospora ssp. Calichensis.* It binds to the minor groove of DNA and induces double strand breaks.

DC1: A disulfide-containing analogue of adozelesin. DC1 is a bis-indolyl-*seco*-CBI compound. It kills cells by binding to the minor groove of DNA, followed by alkylation of adenine bases.

DM1: A derivative of maytansine that has a disulfide-containing group. DM1 is 3- to 10-fold more cytotoxic than maytansine.

Immunotoxins: Conjugates of monoclonal antibodies with highly cytotoxic protein toxins. Antibodies typically used for constructing immunotoxins are those targeted towards cell surface antigens.

Maytansine: A highly cytotoxic microtubular inhibitor isolated from the Ethiopian shrub *Maytenus serrata*.

Mylotarg: A conjugate of calicheamicin with a humanized anti-CD33 antibody. Mylotarg is approved by the FDA for treatment of certain kinds of leukemia.

Protein toxins: Cytotoxic proteins. There are several classes of protein toxins. Two classes have been widely used for construction of immunotoxins, both inhibit protein synthesis: (a) ribosome-inactivating proteins of plant origin, such as ricin, abrin, gelonin, and (b) a number of others, and bacterial toxins such as pseudomonas exotoxin and diphtheria toxin.

Tumor-activated pro-drugs (TAPs): Highly cytotoxic drugs converted into inactive pro-drugs by linking them *via* stable bonds to monoclonal antibodies directed against tumor-associated antigens. An ideal TAP is stable in circulation *in vivo* and thus, non-toxic. The pro-drug is specifically activated upon reaching a tumor cell, followed by release of fully active drug inside the cell.

SECTION 4:

TARGETING TO THE BRAIN

16

BLOOD-BRAIN BARRIER TRANSPORT AND DRUG TARGETING TO THE BRAIN

Ken-ichi Hosoya[1, 4], Sumio Ohtsuki[2-4], and Tetsuya Terasaki[2-4*]
*Faculty of Pharmaceutical Sciences, Toyama Medical and Pharmaceutical University, Sugitani, Toyama, 930-0194, Japan. [2]Department of Molecular Biopharmacy and Genetics, Graduate School of Pharmaceutical Sciences, and [3]New Industry Creation Hatchery Center, Tohoku University, Aoba, Aramaki, Aoba-ku, Sendai 980-8578, Japan. [4]CREST of Japan Science and Technology Corporation (JST). *Corresponding author*

INTRODUCTION

The transport of drugs to the central nervous system (CNS) from the circulating blood requires them to cross either the blood-brain barrier (BBB) or blood-cerebrospinal fluid barrier (BCSFB) (Fig. 1). The BBB, which is formed by complex tight-junctions of brain capillary endothelial cells, separates the circulating blood from the interstitial fluid in the brain. Although the BCSFB is also formed by the complex tight-junctions of the choroid plexus epithelial cells and separates the blood from the cerebrospinal fluid (CSF), the area of BBB is about 5,000-times greater than that of the BCSFB. There is an ependymal layer between the brain parenchymal cells and CSF, but this does not act as a barrier to prevent diffusion of drugs from the CSF to the CNS. Nevertheless, the diffusion rate of drugs between CSF and brain parenchymal cells is very slow. Although the cellular volume of the brain capillaries is only 0.1~0.2% of the entire brain, the total length of the brain capillaries is about 600 km and the total surface area is about 9~12 m^2 in humans. As the brain capillaries are ramified, like the network in the cerebrum at intervals of about 40 μm, small molecules such as nutrients immediately diffuse into the brain parenchymal cells following their passage across the BBB. In general, the BBB is a main route for drug transport from the blood to the CNS. In other words, a high drug concentration in the CSF is not necessary if the drug is able to cross the BBB very efficiently. The pericytes and astrocytes surrounding the brain endothelium (Fig. 1) provide paracrine interactions between the brain capillary endothelium and its neighboring cells. The in vivo BBB has a tight endothelium with an electrical

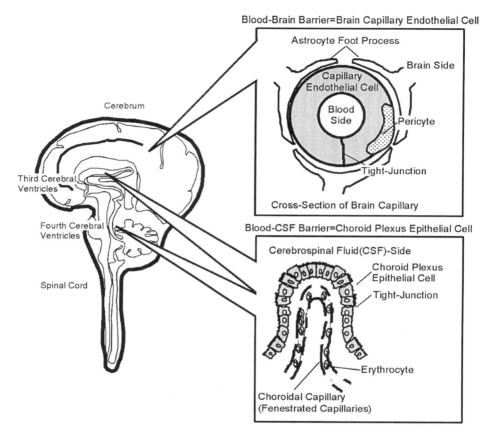

Figure 1. Schematic diagram of the blood-brain barrier (BBB) and blood-cerebrospinal fluid barrier (BCSFB).

resistance of ~8,000 $\Omega\cdot cm^2$. Therefore, circulating molecules gain access to brain parenchymal cells mainly via transcellular transport, but rarely viaparacellular transport. The transport mechanism for transcellular transport at the BBB basically involves three different processes: (i) passive diffusion (lipid-mediated transport), (ii) carrier-mediated transport for facilitated or active transport, and (iii) receptor mediated- or absorptive mediated-transcytosis (Fig. 2). One possible approach to achieve drug delivery to the CNS is to take advantage of the blood-to-brain influx transport process by designing drug molecules that are not substrates for the brain-to-blood efflux transport process.

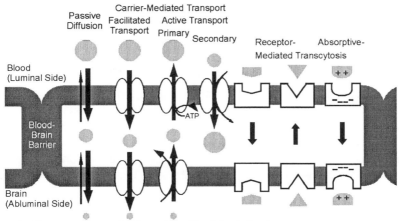

Figure 2. The transport mechanism of the blood-brain barrier.

In this chapter, we shall focus on the membrane transport processes that are currently known to allow small and macromolecular drugs to cross the BBB and their use in drug targeting to the CNS.

PHARMACOKINETIC CONSIDERATIONS

When designing CNS-active drugs, it is important to consider the pharmacokinetics of these drugs after administration. The pharmacological CNS effect of drugs reflects their brain interstitial fluid concentration ($C_{brain, ISF}$). Equation [1] represents the relationship between the $C_{brain, ISF}$ and other parameters, such as the free drug concentration of the circulating blood ($C_{blood, free}$), BBB influx and efflux permeability clearance ($PS_{inf, BBB}$, $PS_{eff, BBB}$, respectively).

$$\int_0^\infty C_{brain, ISF} dt = \frac{PS_{inf, BBB}}{PS_{eff, BBB}} \times \int_0^\infty C_{blood, free} dt \qquad \text{------[1]}$$

When a drug is administered intravenously and is not metabolized in the brain, Equation [2] can be obtained:

$$AUC_{brain, ISF} = \frac{PS_{inf, BBB}}{PS_{eff, BBB}} \times f_b \times \frac{D}{CL_{tot}} \qquad \text{------[2]}$$

where $AUC_{brain, ISF}$, f_b, D, and CL_{tot} represent the area under the drug concentration-time curve in the brain interstitial fluid (ISF), free fraction of drug in the blood, dose, and total body clearance, respectively, when the $AUC_{brain, ISF}$ is the integrated value of the $C_{brain, ISF}$ from time 0 to infinite time. According to Equation [2], there are several ways to achieve higher drug concentrations in the brain interstitial fluid. One is to increase the $PS_{inf, BBB}$ or

f_b value and the other is to reduce the $PS_{eff, BBB}$ or CL_{tot} value. Even the $C_{blood, free}$ value is relatively high for some drugs, and the $C_{brain, ISF}$ value is low when the ratio of $PS_{inf, BBB}/PS_{eff, BBB}$ is much less than 1. Therefore, the pharmacological CNS effect cannot be directly related to the $C_{blood, free}$ and dissociation constant (K_d) for receptors in the brain parenchymal cells and the inhibition constant (K_i) for enzymes in the brain if the drug is an efficient substrate for the BBB efflux transport system. Although making drugs more lipophilic may lead to an increased BBB permeability, this benefit may be offset by an increase in the CL_{tot} and a reduction in f_b. Therefore, it is necessary to design and select optimal drug candidates by considering their pharmacokinetic parameters and Equation [2] (Fig. 3).

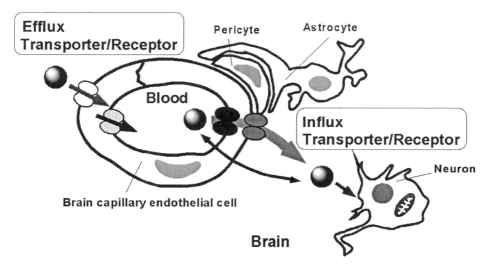

Figure 3. The relationship between blood-to-brain influx and brain-to-blood efflux transport and drug transport to the brain parenchymal cells.

MECHANISM OF DRUG TRANSPORT AT THE BBB

Passive diffusion

Blood-to-brain influx transport of a number of drugs and other compounds increases in parallel with their lipophilicity. For example, hydrophilic compounds such as sucrose and D-mannitol cannot be easily transported from the blood to the brain while lipophilic compounds, such as progesterone and testosterone can be transported relatively easily. Drug transport from the blood to the brain across the BBB (permeability surface area product, PS) has been measured using the brain uptake index (BUI) method (1). The lipophilicity was determined by measuring the partition coefficient (PC) between n-octanol and water. The PS values of various compounds are correlated with the PC divided by the square root of the molecular weight $(PC/MW^{1/2})$. Linear regression analysis gives following Equation [3]:

$$\log (PS) = -0.70 + 0.45 \log(PC/MW^{1/2}) \qquad ------[3]$$

According to this correlation, a drug with a molecular weight of 400 Da and a PC of 1 has an estimated PS of 0.05 mL/(min·g brain). This means that 5% of the drug is taken up by the brain following a single passage through the brain at a cerebrum blood flow rate of 1 mL/(min·g brain). Although the ratio of the transport of an administered drug to the brain is dependent on the CL_{tot}, some drugs are relatively lipophilic and, as a guide, a PC of 1 to 1000 is thought to be promising for delivery to the CNS and producing pharmacological effects in the CNS.

Carrier-mediated transport

There are two types of carrier-mediated transport at the BBB: facilitated and active. Facilitated carrier-mediated transport is a saturable, stereoselective, bi-directional and energy-independent process while active carrier-mediated transport is saturable, stereoselective, and either directly or indirectly dependent on energy expenditure in the cell. These mechanisms are referred to as primary and secondary active carrier-mediated transport, respectively (Fig. 2).

The PS values of D-glucose and several amino acids using the BUI method (2) are greater than those calculated from Equation [3] and their PC values since the carrier-mediated transport process involves blood-to-brain influx transport rather than passive diffusion. The blood-to-brain influx transporters at the BBB act as a support system for the brain since the BBB supplies nutrients and other essential molecules to the brain (Table 1) (3). D-Glucose, which is the main energy source for the brain, is transported from the circulating blood to the brain via an Na^+-independent glucose transporter, GLUT1 (SLC2A1), at the BBB. GLUT1 is a facilitated transporter of hexose and is localized on the luminal (blood) and abluminal (brain) side of the BBB (4). It also transports L-dehydroascorbic acid, an oxidized form of L-ascorbic acid (vitamin C), to supply the brain with L-ascorbic acid (5). The L-serinyl-β- D-glucoside analogues of Met[5]enkephalin have been shown to have greater BBB permeability than the parent peptides. This suggests that GLUT1 is responsible for transporting glycosylated peptides. However, chemotherapeutic agents coupled with D-glucose (D-glucose-chlorambucil derivatives) have been shown to inhibit GLUT1- mediated transport and so these derivatives are not transported. The substrate specificity of GLUT1 seems to be very strict and the choice of a carrier for drug delivery to the CNS needs to be considered very carefully.

Table 1. Representative transporters and transport processes at the blood-brain barrier (BBB)

Transporters and transport processes	Substrates	Energy-dependence	Molecular [a] Identification
Blood-to-brain influx transport			
GLUT1	D-Glucose/ L-dehydroascorbic acid	No	Yes
LAT1/4F2hc (system L)	Large neutral amino acids	No	Yes
CAT1(system y^+)	Cationic amino acids	No	Yes
EAAT1,2,3	Anionic amino acids	Na^+	Yes
MCT1	L-Lactate/monocarboxylates	H^+	Yes
OCTN2	Carnitine/organic cation	Na^+	Yes
CNT2	Nucleosides	Na^+	Yes
System β	β-Amino acids	Na^+/Cl^-	No
System ASC/B^{0+}	L-Ala/L-Ser/L-Cys and others	Na^+	No
System T	Thyroid hormons	?	No
Choline transport	Choline	?	No
Brain-to-blood efflux transport			
oatp2	Digoxin/organic anions	GSH	Yes
P-Glycoprtein (*mdr1a*)	Cyclosporin A and others	ATP	Yes
BGT1/GAT2	γ-Aminobutyric acid	Na^+/Cl^-	Yes
ATA2 (System A)	Small neutral amino acids	Na^+	Yes
MRP1	Leukotriene C_4 and others	ATP	Yes
PAH efflux transport	PAH	?	No
AZT efflux transport	AZT	?	No

(a), Molecular identification and localization have been recognized at the BBB.
References: 21, 23, 24, 32, 33, and 34

L-Lactate, pyruvic acid and ketone bodies are used as a major source of fuel in the brain during the early neonatal period. The monocarboxylic acid transporter 1 (MCT1) (SLC16A1) is responsible for the transport of these monocarboxylic acids coupled with H^+ and is located both on the luminal and abluminal side of the BBB. Although MCT1 is an H^+-dependent secondary active transporter, it allows both bi-directional blood-to-brain and brain-to-blood transport of L-lactate. Monocarboxylic acids, such as nicotinic acid and benzoic acid, appear to be substrates and are transported from the blood to the brain. Nonsteroidal anti-inflammatory drugs, which have a carboxyl moiety, like salicylic acid and ibuprofen, are recognized by MCT1 (6).

Neurotransmitters such as dopamine, norepinephrine, and epinephrine are synthesized from L-tyrosine. On the other hand, serotonin and histamine are synthesized from L-tryptophan and L-histidine, respectively, in the brain, particularly in neurons. L-Glutamic acid and γ-aminobutyric acid (GABA), an excitatory and a suppressive neurotransmitter, respectively, are synthesized directly from L-glutamine and L-glutamic acid, respectively. L-Tyrosine, L-tryptophan, and L-histidine, precursors of neurotransmitters, are transported from the blood to the brain via an Na^+-independent neutral amino acid transporter (system L; L-leucine-preferring) at the BBB. System L also transports L-leucine, L-isoleucine, L-valine, L-methionine, L-threonine, and L-phenylalanine to allow protein synthesis in the brain. Several amino acid mimetic-drugs are transported across the BBB by system L. Drug treatment of Parkinson's disease uses L-dopa as a prodrug of dopamine and is a good example of drug delivery to the CNS via a transport carrier at the BBB. L-Dopa is transported across the BBB and is readily biotransformed in the brain to dopamine. The alkylating agent melphalan (phenylalanine mustard), the antiepileptic drug gabapentin, and the muscle relaxant baclofen are substrates of system L and are transported to the brain. System L at the BBB is saturated by endogenous amino acids under normal conditions since the Michaelis-Menten constant (K_m) for system L is smaller than the plasma concentration of neutral amino acids. Although these drugs are thought to be continuously transported from the blood to the brain, a high-protein diet reduces the concentration of these drugs in the brain due to competitive inhibition at the BBB. In 1998, researchers succeeded in cloning system L and it has been found to be consist of LAT1 (SLC7A6) and the heavy chain of the 4F2 cell-surface antigen (4F2hc) (7). Although LAT2 (SLC7A8) has also been cloned, LAT1 is selectively expressed and functions at the BBB (8).

Nitric oxide (NO) may play a role as a neurotransmitter or neuromodulator in the brain. L-Arginine, which is a precursor of NO, and L-lysine are transported via an Na^+-independent basic amino acid transporter, system y^+ at the BBB. The CAT1 (SLC7A1) gene is 40-fold more highly expressed than other subtypes at the BBB compared with the whole brain (9), suggesting that CAT1 acts as system y^+ at the BBB.

Receptor- and absorptive-mediated transcytosis

Bioactive peptides do not undergo transport across the BBB by passive diffusion due to their high molecular weight and low lipophilicity.

However, the BBB possesses a receptor-mediated transcytosis process for some physiologically active peptides that are not synthesized in the brain. Insulin is transported from the circulating blood to the brain via insulin receptors at the BBB. Insulin binds to insulin receptors on the luminal side of the BBB and undergoes endocytosis, followed by exocytosis, on the abluminal side of the BBB. Thus, insulin is transported to the brain by transcytosis (Fig. 2). The K_d for insulin receptors at the BBB is 1.2 nM and the insulin concentration in blood is 150~300 pM. Thus, these receptors are not saturated with endogenous insulin. The difficulty in using native insulin as a transport vector is associated with hypoglycemia. Transferrin, the plasma protein that carries iron, binds to the transferrin receptors at the BBB. Although the K_d value is 5.6 nM, the transferrin concentration in blood is 25 μM, 5,000-fold greater than the K_d value. Thus these receptors are completely saturated with endogenous transferrin. Using these receptors for drug delivery to the CNS is a promising approach mentioned in the latter section of this chapter. Other bioactive peptides such as vasopressin, luteinizing hormone-releasing hormone (LHRH), delta sleep-inducing peptide, leucine-enkephalin, and interleukin-1α. are transported from the circulating blood to the brain, although it is not known if these peptide transport processes involve receptor-mediated transcytosis.

Cationic peptides are transported from the circulating blood to the brain via an absorptive-mediated transcytosis process at the BBB (Fig. 2). This process is triggered by an electrostatic interaction between the positively charged moiety of the peptide and the negatively charged plasma membrane surface of the BBB. The potent dynophin-like analgesic peptide, E-2078, and a potent adrenocorticotropic hormone (ACTH) analog, ebiratide, are transported from the circulating blood to the brain across the BBB (10, 11).

Brain-to-blood efflux transport

The BBB plays a role in acting not only as a structural barrier to regulate the passive diffusion of hydrophilic compounds but also as an efflux pump involved in the brain-to-blood efflux of xenobiotics and neurotransmitter metabolites in the brain as a detoxifying system (3) (Table 1). Lipophilic compounds, such as the immunosuppressive drug cyclosporin A, and anti-cancer drugs like vincristine and doxorubicin have relatively lower BBB permeabilities than those calculated from Equation [3] and their lipophilicities. The most well-known efflux pump at the BBB is P-glycoprotein (P-gp), which has two ATP binding cassettes and consists of 1,280 amino acids of 170 kDa. P-gp is localized on the luminal side of the BBB (12) and encodes *mdr1a* in rodents (13). On the other hand, research shows that P-gp (MDR1; ABCB1) is localized to the astrocyte foot process, rather than the capillary endothelium, in humans (14). There is a suggestion that P-gp may vary from one species to another as far as its localization at the BBB is concerned. This is a key issue for developing CNS-acting drugs in humans. Moreover, it is important to characterize non-P-gp efflux transporters at a molecular level and assess their contribution in vivo. P-gp is a primary active transporter of relatively lipophilic compounds, such as the anti-cancer drug vinblastine, cyclosporin A, and the cardiac glycoside digoxin, by direct consumption of ATP. When vinblastine, cyclosporin A, and digoxin were intravenously administered to *mdr1a* knock-out mice, their respective concentrations in brain were 22-, 66-, and 17-fold greater than those in normal mice (13, 15). This evidence indicates that P-gp plays a pivotal role in reducing the brain concentration of these drugs. However, inhibition of P-gp activity at the BBB is a promising way of obtaining higher concentrations of drugs that are P-gp substrates in the brain. PSC 833, an agent developed as a P-gp modulating drug and a cyclosporin A analog, reduces the pharmacological effects, inhibits P-gp activity at the BBB and increases the concentration of P-gp substrate drugs in the brain (16).

There are several other types of brain-to-blood efflux transport systems at the BBB apart from P-gp. Although homovanillic acid is produced as a metabolite from dopamine by monoamine oxidase and catechol-*O*-methyltransferase in the brain, it is hydrophilic and finally excreted in urine via the kidney. It is not yet known how homovanillic acid is transported from brain to blood across the BBB. Development of the Brain Efflux Index (BEI) method has made it possible to determine the brain-to-blood efflux transport of several compounds in vivo (17). Moreover, conditionally immortalized rat (TR-BBB) and mouse (TM-BBB) brain endothelial cell lines have been developed to study transport mechanisms in cellular and molecular levels at the BBB (18, 19). The combined use of the BEI method and conditionally immortalized brain endothelial cell lines has been used to investigate the brain-to-blood efflux transport of excitatory neurotransmitters such as L-glutamic acid and L-aspartic acid (20), inhibitory neurotransmitters such as GABA (21), and neuroactive steroids such as dehydroepiandrosterone sulfate (22) and estron-3-sulfate (23). Moreover, betaine/GABA transporter 1 (BGT-1 in rat; SLC6A12 in human; GAT2 in mouse) has been defined as a transporter responsible for GABA efflux at the BBB (24). System A, a transporter of small neutral amino acids, such as L-proline, glycine, and L-alanine, has been suggested to be localized on the abluminal side of the BBB by Betz and Goldstein (25). Using the BEI method and TR-BBB, ATA2 (SLC38A4) has been demonstrated to be responsible for the brain-to-blood efflux transport of L-proline (26). The anti-HIV viral drug, 3'-azido-3'-deoxythymidine (AZT), exhibits limited distribution into the brain. Although the efflux transporter has not yet been identified, AZT undergoes brain-to-blood efflux transport rather than limited blood-to-brain transport (27). It is necessary to take more AZT to obtain the expected anti-HIV effect in the brain since the AZT concentration in the brain is lower than that in the blood. Another approach is to administer a combination with the inhibitors of efflux transport, such as probenecid. To develop CNS-acting drugs, we need to consider not only the reaction with the blood-to-brain influx transporter but also the possibility of avoiding the brain-to-blood efflux transporter as indicated by Equation [2] (Fig. 3). Therefore, a complete understanding of the brain-to-blood efflux transport process is important in order to achieve higher concentrations in the brain interstitial fluid and to obtain the desired pharmacological CNS effects.

CHEMICAL MODIFICATION FOR BRAIN DELIVERY

The concept of a chemical delivery system (CDS) was proposed by Bodor in the early 1980s. The thinking behind drug targeting to the brain using CDS is as follows: (i) the lipophilic compound enters the brain across the BBB and is converted to a lipid-insoluble molecule in the brain, (ii) it will then not be released from the brain, i.e. it is locked-in, (iii) drug conjugation accelerates elimination even although the same conversions occur elsewhere in the body. The several CDSs, such as: (i) AZT-CDS, an anti-viral drug, (ii) ganciclovir-CDS, an anti-cancer drug, (iii) lomustine (CCNU)-CDS, antibiotics, (iv) benzylpenicillin-CDS, and (v) bioactive peptides-CDS, have been developed and used to improve drug delivery to the CNS (28).

Vector-mediated delivery systems for proteins and genes

Macromolecular drugs, such as brain-derived neurotrophic peptides and antisense oligonucleotides, could be very useful for the treatment of CNS diseases. Although these do not easily cross the BBB, vector-mediated drug delivery to the CNS using chimeric peptide technology is a promising way of improving the CNS targeting of peptide-based pharmaceutics, antisense therapeutics including peptide nucleic acids, and incorporating DNA within pegylated immunoliposomes (29). The strategy is based on the observation that conjugation of these macromolecular drugs with receptor-specific monoclonal antibodies to the receptors expressed at the BBB is facilitated by chemical linkers, avidin-biotin technology, polyethylene glycol linkers or liposomes. Therefore, this drug delivery system undergoes receptor-mediated transcytosis from the blood to the brain across the BBB in vivo. Monoclonal antibodies, OX-26 and Mab83-14, have been generated for transferrin and insulin receptors at the BBB, respectively. OX-26 specifically binds to transferrin receptors and undergoes receptor-mediated transcytosis (Fig. 2) at the BBB, even if the receptors are saturated by endogenous transferring. This is possible because the epitope of the receptors is different from the binding site of transferrin. Using this chimeric peptide technology, several agents have been developed and investigated by Pardridge and his group. Some examples are brain derived neurotrophic factor for treating brain ischemia, epidermal growth factor peptide radiopharmaceuticals for the diagnosis of brain cancer, amyloid β peptide radiopharmaceuticals for the diagnosis of Alzheimer's disease, and DNA and peptide nucleic acid for gene therapy in the brain (29). Very recently, they have succeeded in achieving the brain-specific expression of an exogenous gene after intravenous administration using both pegylated immunoliposomes gene targeting technology and a brain-specific promoter such as glial fibrillary acidic protein. It is an advantage to use a non-viral vector (30). Vector-mediated drug delivery system using the chimeric peptide technology could be useful for noninvasive drug delivery to the CNS.

CONCLUSION

The classical approach for drug delivery to the CNS involves the addition of a lipophilic moiety to the drug. The advantage of this approach is that it is very easy to convert drugs to prodrugs, but it is not a specific targeting system for the CNS. Lipophilic drugs have unfavorable plasma pharmacokinetics and some of them are substrates for P-gp. In the development of CNS drugs, over 98% of potential candidates drop out during the development stage. It is important to design CNS-acting drugs that are able to react with the blood-to-brain influx transporter to obtain a better rate of influx transport. The drugs must also avoid brain-to-blood efflux so as not to reduce drug concentrations in the brain. The latest technological advances have allowed more sophisticated drug delivery systems for the CNS, involving peptides and cDNA by taking advantage of BBB transport functions. The Human Genome Project has now been completed and all the human genes have been identified. There are at least 533 and 1,543 gene-related transporters and receptors, respectively (31). We will be able to elucidate the nature of BBB transport functions and identify the genes involved over the next 5 to 10 years. Moreover, the mechanisms of CNS diseases such as amyotrophic lateral sclerosis, Alzheimer's, Huntington's, and Parkinson's diseases will be identified at the molecular level in the near future. We will soon be able to examine the relationship between CNS diseases and BBB transport functions. This will give us access to higher quality information to develop better CNS drugs and design more rational drug delivery systems to target the CNS.

ACKNOWLEDGEMENTS

The authors gratefully acknowledge the support of a Grant-in-Aid for Scientific Research from the Ministry of Education, Science, Sports, and Culture, Japan, and thank M. Tomi and S. Hori for valuable discussions.

REFERENCES

1. Oldendolf, W.H. Measurement of brain uptake of radiolabeled substances using a tritiated water internal standard. *Brain. Res.* 1970; *24: 372.*
2. Oldendolf, W.H. Brain uptake of radiolabeled amino acids, amines and hexose after arterial injection. *Am. J. Physiol.* 1971; *221: 1629.*
3. Terasaki, T., and Hosoya, K. The blood-brain barrier efflux transporters as a detoxifying system for the brain. *Adv. Drug Deliv. Rev.* 1999; *36: 195.*
4. Pardridge, W.M., Boado, R.J., Farrell, and C.R. Brain-type glucose transporter (GLUT-1) is selectively localized to the blood-brain barrier. *J. Biol. Chem.* 1990; *265: 18035.*
5. Augus, D.B., Gambhir, S.S., Pardridge, W.M., Spielholz, C., Baselga, J., Vera, J.C., and Golde, D.W. Vitamin C crosses the blood-brain barrier in the oxidized form through the glucose transporters. *J. Clin. Invest.* 1997; *100: 2842.*
6. Tamai, I., Takanaga, H., Maeda, H., Sai, Y., Ogihara, T., Higashida, H., and Tsuji, A. Participation of proton-cotransporter, MCT1, in the intestinal transport of monocarboxylic acids. *Biochem. Biophys. Res. Commun.* 1995; *214: 482.*
7. Kanai, Y., Segawa, H., Miyamoto, K., Uchino, H., Takeda, E., and Endou, H. Expression cloning and characterization of a transporter for large neutral amino acids activated by the heavy chain of 4F2 antigen (CD98). *J. Biol. Chem.* 1998; *273: 23629.*
8. Boado, R.J., Li, J.Y., Nagaya, M., Zhang, C., and Pardridge, W.M. Selective expression of the large neutral amino acid transporter at the blood-brain barrier. *Proc. Natl. Acad. Sci. USA* 1999; *96: 12079.*
9. Smith, Q.R. Transport of glutamate and other amino acids at the blood-brain barrier. *J. Nutr.* 2000; *130; 1016S.*
10. Shimura, T., Tabata, S., Ohnishi, T., Terasaki, T., and Tsuji, A. Transport mechanism of a new behaviorally highly potent adrenocorticotropic hormone (ACTH) analog, ebiratide, through the blood-brain barrier. *J. Pharmacol. Exp. Ther.* 1991; *258: 459.*
11. Terasaki, T., Hirai, K., Sato, H., Kang, Y.S., and Tsuji, A. Absorptive-mediated endocytosis of a dynorphin-like analgesic peptide, E-2078 into the blood-brain barrier. *J. Pharmacol. Exp. Ther.* 1989; *251:351.*
12. Tsuji, A., Terasaki, T., Takabatake, Y., Tenda, Y., Tamai, I., Yamashima, T., Moritani, S., Tsuruo, T., and Yamashita, J. P-Glycoprotein as the drug efflux pump in primary cultured bovine brain capillary endothelial cells. *Lif, Sci.* 1992; *51: 1427.*
13. Schinkel, A.H., Smit, J.J.M., van Tellingen, O., Beijnen, J.H., Wagenaar, E., van Deemter, L., Mol, C.A.A.M., van der Valk, M.A., Robanus-Maandag, E.C., te Riele, H.P.J., Berns, A.J.M., and Borst, P. Disruption of the mouse *mdr*1a P-glycoprotein gene leads to a deficiency in the blood-brain barrier and to increased sensitivity to drugs. *Cell* 1994; *77: 491.*
14. Golden, P.L., and Pardridge, W.M. P-Glycoprotein on astrocyte foot processes of unfixed isolated human brain capillaries. *Brain Res.* 1999; *819:143.*
15. Schinkel, A.H. P-Glycoprotein, a gatekeeper in the blood-brain barrier. *Adv. Drug Deliv. Rev.* 1999; *36: 179.*
16. Kusuhara, H., Suzuki, H., Terasaki, T., Kakee, A., Lemaire, M., and Sugiyama, Y. P-Glycoprotein mediates the efflux of quinidine across the blood-brain barrier. *J. Pharmacol. Exp. Ther.* 1997; *283: 574.*

17. Kakee, A., Terasaki, T., and Sugiyama, Y. Brain efflux index as a novel method of analyzing efflux transport at the blood-brain barrier. *J. Pharmacol. Exp. Ther.* 1996; *277: 1550.*

18. Hosoya, K., Takashima, T., Tetsuka, K., Nagura, T., Ohtsuki, S., Takanaga, H., Ueda, M., Yanai, N., Obinata, M., and Terasaki, T. mRNA expression and transport characterization of conditionally immortalized rat brain capillary endothelial cell lines; a new in vitro BBB model for drug targeting. *J. Drug Target.* 2000a; *8: 357.*

19. Hosoya, K., Tetsuka, K., Nagase, K., Tomi, M., Saeki, S., Ohtsuki, S., Takanaga, H., Yanai, N., Obinata, M., Kikuchi, A., Okano,T., and Terasaki, T. Conditionally immortalized brain capillary endothelial cell lines established from transgenic mouse harboring temperature-sensitive SV 40 large T-antigen gene. *AAPS Pharmsci.* 2000b; *2:article 27*, (http://www.pharmsci.org/).

20. Hosoya, K., Sugawara, M., Asaba, H., and Terasaki, T. Blood-brain barrier produces significant efflux of L-aspartic acid but not D-aspartic acid: in vivo evidence using the brain efflux index method. *J. Neurochem.* 1999; *73: 1206.*

21. Kakee, A., Takanaga, H., Terasaki, T., Naito, M., Tsuruo, T., and Sugiyama Y. Efflux of a suppressive neurotransmitter, GABA, across the blood-brain barrier. *J. Neurochem.* 2001; *79: 110.*

22. Asaba, H., Hosoya, K., Takanaga, H., Ohtsuki, S., Tamura, E., Takizawa, T., and Terasaki, T. Blood-brain barrier is involved in the efflux transport of a neuroactive steroid, dehydroepiandrosterone sulfate, via organic anion transporting polypeptide 2. *J. Neurochem.* 2000; *75:1907.*

23. Hosoya, K., Asaba, H., and Terasaki, T. Brain-to-blood efflux transport of estrone-3-sulfate at the blood-brain barrier in rats. *Life Sci.* 2000c; *67: 2699.*

24. Takanaga, H., Ohtsuki, S., Hosoya, K., and Terasaki, T. GAT2/BGT-1 as a system responsible for the transport of γ-aminobutyric acid at the mouse blood-brain barrier. *J. Cereb. Blood Flow Metab.* 2001; *21: 1232.*

25. Betz, A.L., and Goldstein, G.W. Polarity of the blood-brain barrier: neutral amino acid transport into isolated brain capillaries. *Science 1978; 202: 225.*

26. Takanaga, H., Tokuda, N., Ohtsuki, S., Hosoya, K., and Terasaki, T. ATA2 is predominantly expressed as system A at the blood-brain barrier and acts as brain-to-blood efflux transport for L-proline. *Mol. Pharmacol.* 2002, *in press.*

27. Takasawa, K., Terasaki, T., Suzuki, H., and Sugiyama, Y. In vivo evidence for carrier-mediated efflux transport of 3'-azido-3'-deoxythymidine and 2',3'-dideoxyinosine across the blood-brain barrier via a probenecid-sensitive transport system. *J. Pharmacol. Exp. Ther.* 1997; *281: 369.*

28. Bodor, N., and Buchwald, P. Recent advances in the brain targeting of neuropharmaceuticals by chemical delivery systems. *Adv. Drug Deliv. Rev.* 1999; *36: 229.*

29. Pardridge, W.M. Vector-mediated drug delivery to the brain. *Adv. Drug Deliv. Rev.* 1999; *36: 299.*

30. Shi, N., Zhang, Y., Zhu, C., Boado, R.J., and Pardridge, W.M. Brain-specific expression of an exogenous gene after i.v. administration. *Proc. Natl. Acad. Sci. USA* 2001; *98: 12754.*

31. Venter, J.C., Adams, M.D., Myers, E.W., et al. The sequence of the human genome. *Science* 2001; *291: 1304.*

32. Terasaki, T., and Hosoya, K. Conditionally immortalized cell lines as a new in vitro model for the study of barrier functions. *Biol. Pharm. Bull.* 2001; *24: 111.*

33. Kakee, A., Terasaki, T., and Sugiyama, Y. Selective brain to blood efflux transport of para-aminohippuric acid across the blood-brain barrier: In vivo evidence by use of the Brain Efflux Index method. *J. Pharmcol. Exp. Ther.* 1997; *283: 1018.*

34. Komura, J., Tamai, I., Senmaru, M., Terasaki, T., Sai, Y., and Tsuji, A. Sodium and chloride ion-dependent transport of beta-alanine across the blood-brain barrier. *J. Neurochem.* 1996; *67: 330.*

GLOSSARY

BBB: Blood-brain barrier, which is formed by complex tight junctions of brain capillary endothelial cells and separates the circulating blood from the interstitial fluid in the brain.

BCSFB: Blood-cerebrospinal fluid barrier, which is formed by the complex tight junctions of the choroid plexus epithelial cells and separates the blood from the cerebrospinal fluid.

BEI: Brain Efflux Index, a method to determine brain-to-blood transport rate across the BBB in vivo.

GLUT1: Glucose transporter 1, a facilitated transporter of hexose. GLUT1 also transports L-dehydroascorbic acid.

MCT1: Monocarboxylic acid transporter 1, an H^+ dependent secondary active transporter of monocarboxylic acid.

mdr1a: Multidrug resistance protein 1a, a mouse subtype of P-gp, which is localized at luminal side of brain capillary endothelial cells and mediates the efflux transport to the circulating blood.

P-gp: P-glycoprotein (ABCB1), a member of the ATP binding cassette (ABC) transporter superfamily, which has two ATP binding cassettes and consists of 1,280 amino acids of 170 kDa. P-gp is a primary active transporter of relative lipophilic compounds.

17

LDL-RECEPTOR MEDIATED DRUG TARGETING TO MALIGNANT TUMORS IN THE BRAIN

Ranajoy Sarkar[1], David S. Halpern[2], Steven K. Jacobs[3] and D. Robert Lu[1]

[1]College of Pharmacy, University of Georgia, Athens, GA 30602, [2]Isotron, Inc. Alpharetta, GA 30022, [3]New York Medical College, New Windsor, NY 12553

INTRODUCTION

Malignant tumors are composed of abnormal cells that usually grow very aggressively. It is extremely difficult to treat many of these malignant tumors with conventional methods, including surgical resection, radiation therapy, chemotherapy and combinations of these modalities. To enhance the efficacy of tumor treatment with chemotherapy, targeted drug delivery resulting in high concentrations of therapeutic compounds in tumor cells and relatively low concentrations in neighboring normal cells has been attractive and many approaches for drug targeting have been extensively evaluated.

Rapidly dividing cells, such as those found within malignant tumors, have a high cholesterol requirement because cholesterol is utilized to construct the cell membranes. Cells can obtain cholesterol either by taking up plasma LDL (low-density lipoprotein) via receptor-mediated endocytosis or by de novo synthesis. The majority of cholesterol, however, is obtained from the receptor-mediated route. It is known that, for many malignant tumor cells, the expression of the LDL-receptor is upregulated on cell surfaces in order to acquire more cholesterol carried by LDL in blood circulation. The elevated LDL-receptor expression on tumor cells provides a rationale for targeted drug delivery to malignant tumors using drug-loaded LDL in blood circulation containing either cholesterol-based antitumor compounds or non-cholesterol-based antitumor compounds.

LIPOPROTEINS AND CHOLESTERYL ESTERS

Lipids (including cholesteryl esters) are carried from one part of the body to another by various lipoproteins as the primary transport form. Most of these lipids function as structural components of membranes (such as phospholipids and cholesterol) or as storage units of chemical energy (primarily triglycerides). These lipids are in general not soluble in aqueous solution and therefore need to be transported in blood through a suitable vehicle (i.e., lipoproteins). Lipoproteins also transport minor but important lipids such as steroid hormones, carotenoids, and tocopherols.

Structures and Functions of Lipoproteins

Lipoproteins are macromolecular complexes and generally have a spherical shape. Their structures consist of a hydrophobic core and a polar shell. Water-insoluble lipids are stored within the core and the polar shell allows the lipoprotein particles to float in blood circulation. Figure 1 shows the simplified structure of LDL. The lipid core is made up mostly of triglycerides and cholesteryl esters in varying proportions, depending on the type of lipoprotein. A group of polar molecules forms the outer polar shell, which mainly contains phospholipids, such as phosphatidylcholine and sphingomyelin, and specific proteins, referred to as apolipoproteins. Unesterified cholesterol molecules can also be present in the polar shell. Apolipoproteins are partially exposed at the surface. There are many types of apolipoproteins that recognize and bind specifically to enzymes or receptor proteins on cell membranes and are responsible for directing the lipoproteins to their sites of function and metabolism.

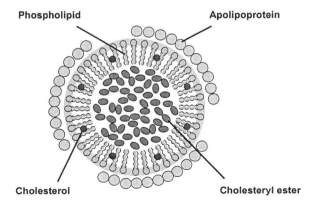

Figure 1. Structure of Low-Density Lipoprotein (LDL)

Table 1 lists those apolipoproteins that have been identified so far. The functions of the apolipoproteins are diversified. Apo A-I, apo A-IV, apo

C-I, apo C-II, and apo C-III function as activation or inhibition modulators for extracellular enzymatic reactions involved in lipid homeostasis. Apo B, apo E, apo J and apo A-I, on the other hand, recognize the cell surface receptors that mediate lipid uptake and work as receptor-specific ligands (1). The specific functions of many other apolipoproteins including apo C-IV, apo D, apo F, apo G and apo H remain unclear.

Table 1. Types of Apolipoproteins and their classifications and functions

Apolipoprotein	Lipoprotein	Function
A-I	LDL, HDL	LCAT activation
A-II	LDL, HDL	LCAT inhibition, hepatic lipase activation
B-100	VLDL, LDL	Cholesterol clearance
C-I	VLDL, HDL	Possibly LCAT activation
C-II	VLDL, HDL	LPL activation
C-III	VLDL, HDL	LPL inhibition, possibly LCAT activation
D	HDL	Unknown
E	HDL	Cholesterol clearance

LDL = Low Density Lipoprotein; HDL = High Density Lipoprotein;
VLDL= Very Low Density; LCAT = Lecithin:cholesterol acyltransferase;
LPL = Lipoprotein lipase

Various lipoproteins can be isolated according to their densities through ultracentrifugation with a salt gradient. Based on the separation, the plasma lipoproteins are divided into five major classes. Since they continuously undergo a metabolic course, lipoprotein particles have variable properties in chemical composition, apolipoprotein percentage, hydrated density and other physicochemical characteristics.

Table 2. Physicochemical properties of lipoproteins

Features	HDL	LDL	IDL	VLDL	Chylomicrons
Molecular weight (x 10^5)	1.9-3.9	20-25	35-45	50-100	10000-100000
Mass (kD)	175-360	2300	5-10000	10-80000	400000
Diameter (Å)	50-120	180-250	250-350	300-800	750-12000
Density (g/cm^3)	1.063-1.21	1.019-1.063	1.006-1.019	0.95-1.006	<0.95
Protein	40-55%	20-25%	15-20%	5-10%	1.5-2.5%
Total Lipids	45-60%	75-80%	80-85%	90-95%	97-99%
Cholesterol	3-4%	7-10%	8%	5-10%	1-3%
Cholesteryl esters	12%	35-40%	30%	10-15%	3-5%
Phospholipids	20-35%	15-20%	22%	15-20%	7-9%
Triglycerides	3-5%	7-10%	22%	50-65%	84-89%

The five major classes of lipoproteins have different physicochemical properties and functions (Table 2). Chylomicrons act as carriers to bring exogenous (dietary) triacylglycerols and cholesterol from the absorption site (intestines) to the tissues and liver. Very low density lipoprotein (VLDL), intermediate density lipoprotein (IDL) and low density lipoprotein (LDL) are a group of related lipid carriers responsible for transporting triacylglycerols and cholesterol from the liver to various tissues. LDL is the most important lipid carrier among this group and transports more than 60% of the plasma cholesterol (primarily as cholesteryl esters) in humans. High density lipoprotein (HDL) carries endogenous cholesterol from the tissues back to the liver.

Structure and Functions of Cholesteryl Esters

As shown in Figure 1, the majority of the molecules in the core of lipoproteins are the esterified form of cholesterol. Cholesterol is one of the major structural components of cell membranes and sub-cellular organelle membranes. Cholesterol molecules in plasma and various tissues exist either in the unesterified form in which the polar hydroxyl group is exposed or in the esterified form in which the hydroxyl group is esterified with long chain fatty acids. About 90% of the total cholesterol in animal tissue is present as unesterified cholesterol located within cell membranes, myelin and the polar shell of plasma lipoprotein particles. However, in plasma, about two-thirds of the cholesterol molecules are esters located in the lipid core of lipoproteins. The high proportion of cholesteryl esters, as opposed to unesterified cholesterol, in plasma results in high transport efficiency by lipoproteins. The cholesteryl esters are also in a chemical form that does not interact unnecessarily with plasma membranes. In addition, cholesteryl esters in the adrenal cortex and gonad cells provide the lipid storage as a reservoir of cholesterol in a physiologically inactive form.

The general chemical composition of cholesteryl esters can be seen in Figure 2. The structure can be divided into two major parts: cholesterol and fatty chains both of which are linked by an ester bond. This simple but versatile composition presents us with an opportunity to develop the mimics of native cholesteryl esters linked with drug molecules which can be carried by lipoproteins, especially LDL, for targeted drug delivery. The details of such a targeting strategy are described in the following sections.

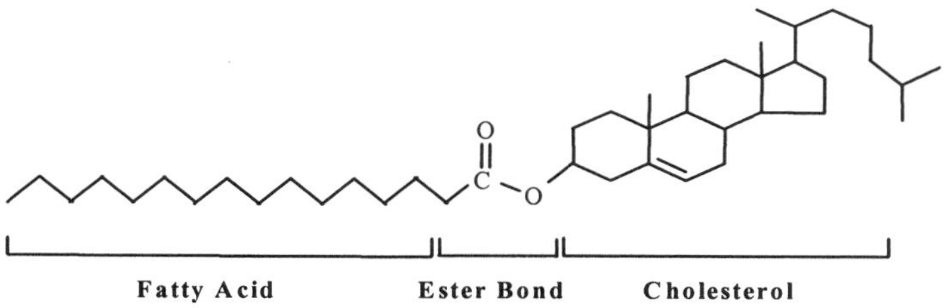

Figure 2. The general chemical composition of cholesteryl esters

All animal cells require cholesterol for cell growth and maintenance. The primary function of cholesterol is to stabilize the constituents of the cell bilaminar membrane. As such, it is well known that the requirement for cholesterol is much greater in cells that are rapidly dividing or growing than in those cells in a resting state. Consequently, the cholesterol requirement of tumor cells is greater since they divide rapidly. This presents a therapeutic rationale for cholesterol-based drug targeting. It should be emphasized that although there is a large amount of cholesterol molecules in the body, only a small portion of these molecules is present in blood and they are primarily in the form of cholesteryl esters. The mimics of cholesteryl esters conjugated with antitumor compounds can be administered systemically to compete with the native cholesteryl esters for targeted drug delivery to tumor cells.

TRANSPORT OF CHOLESTERYL ESTERS BY LIPOPROTEINS

Cholesteryl esters are synthesized with enzymatic assistance from Acyl CoA:cholesterol acyl transferase. The absorbed dietary cholesterol is thus esterified with fatty acids within intestinal and other cells. Chylomicrons are formed by intestinal mucosa and secreted from the intestinal cells into lymph and subsequently into the blood. The function of chylomicrons is to deliver dietary cholesterol to the liver as well as dietary triacylglycerols to muscle and adipose tissue. During the passage through the capillaries of adipose and other tissues, the apo C-II protein on the chylomicron surface activates lipoprotein lipase (LPL) and the component triacylglycerols of the chylomicron are progressively hydrolyzed. Consequently, the size of chylomicrons is reduced and they become cholesterol-enriched chylomicron-remnants containing a relatively high proportion of cholesteryl esters. The apo E protein on the surface enables them to bind to specific receptors on liver cells. During the interaction, these remnants are absorbed by liver cells through receptor-mediated endocytosis and are degraded within the cells.

VLDL is assembled in liver cells. During the process, microsomal triglyceride transfer protein in the lumen of endoplasmic reticulum within the liver facilitates the transfer of lipids to apolipoprotein B-100 by complexing with protein disulfide isomerase. This complexation step is essential for the assembly of triglyceride–rich lipoproteins. There are several apolipoproteins associated with VLDL including apo B-100, apo C-I, apo C-II, and apo C-III. VLDL is further metabolized and the triglyceride content is hydrolyzed. The VLDL becomes smaller with higher density and a higher proportion of cholesterol esters. As a result, VLDL is gradually transformed into IDL.

IDL contains a larger portion of apo E protein that enables it to bind to the LDL receptors on liver cells for internalization and degradation. However, only half of the IDL is taken up by liver cells. The other half experiences further metabolic processing and loses more triglycerides to eventually become LDL.

The lipid core of the LDL particle is mainly composed of cholesteryl esters. There are about 1500 cholesteryl ester molecules per LDL particle, surrounded by 500 cholesterol molecules and 800 phospholipid molecules as the polar shell. With the capacity of carrying large amounts of cholesteryl esters, LDL is the major vehicle to transport cholesteryl esters to peripheral cells. LDL contains one major apolipoprotein, apo B-100, which is associated with the surface monolayer of LDL. Apo B-100 allows LDL to bind the LDL receptors on the peripheral cell surfaces and to be internalized by these cells through a receptor mediated endocytosis.

In contrast to LDL, the function of HDL is to deliver excess cholesterol from various tissue cells back to the liver or to cells in demand of cholesterol. HDL is a smaller particle but contains a higher proportion of proteins. It is secreted by the liver and intestines as nascent HDL. Apo A-I protein on the nascent HDL activates the enzyme, lecithin:cholesterol acyl transferase (LCAT), to catalyze the esterification of cholesterol by transfer of an acyl group from lecithin to cholesterol. HDL receptors, named scavenger B1, exist on the surface of many different cells, including liver cells and the cells in demand of cholesterol. Through the recognition and binding of Apo A-I protein to the HDL receptors, cholesteryl esters in the HDL core are transferred to these cells without the internalization of HDL itself. After delivering its cholesterol content HDL again returns to the circulation to scavenge more cholesterol. The mediation process for the cholesteryl ester transfer from HDL to VLDL and LDL is provided by cholesteryl ester transfer protein (CETP).

LDL RECEPTORS AND TUMOR TARGETING

LDL receptors are transmembrane glycoproteins are present on cell surfaces and recognize and internalize LDL to obtain cholesterol from blood (2). This receptor family includes LDL-receptor (LDL-R), VLDL-receptor (VLDL-R), apolipoprotein E receptor 2, LDL-R Related Protein (LRP) and megalin. These receptors share several common structural and functional features. All members of this family show cell surface expression. They all have an extracellular binding domain that helps in recognition and binding of apo E-containing lipoproteins. LRP and gp330 also bind several other extracellular ligands. While most signaling receptors have a single large intracellular domain, the members of the LDL-R family are characterized by large extracellular and comparatively shorter intracellular domains. For LDL-R, the N-terminal domain is on the exterior side of the membrane and interacts with apo B-100 protein or other apolipoproteins on LDL. The C-terminal domain is on the cytosolic side of the membrane to interact with adapter proteins mediating the formation of the clathrin coat.

The LDL-R Family Members and Subtypes

LDL-R regulates the plasma cholesterol by mediating uptake and catabolism of plasma LDL. In normal tissues, the majority of the LDL-R is expressed on hepatic tissue and adrenal cortex. Several regions of the CNS including the blood-brain barrier (BBB) also express the LDL-R. Many types of tumor cells were found to have elevated LDL-R expression.

The presence of certain structural features like a particular complement- type and EGF precursor homology repeats of the LDL-R play a major role in the binding of apo E and apo B. It was found that complement-type repeats 3-7 and EGF precursor repeat A were both essential for the optimal binding of apo B while only complement-type repeat 5 was needed to bind apo E. The main function of the LDL-R is to bind and internalize those lipoproteins containing apo B-100 and apo E from the plasma.

In terms of structure, the very low density lipoprotein receptor differs from LDL-R only in the presence of an extra complement-type repeat in the ligand-binding domain present at the N- terminal. The VLDL-R has broad ligand binding ability. The majority of the VLDL-R is expressed in extrahepatic tissues such as the heart, muscle and adipose tissue. The VLDL-R may function in the uptake of triglyceride-rich, apo E containing lipoproteins in tissues where fatty acid metabolism occurs.

Cellular Uptake of LDL through LDL Receptor

Rapidly growing cells need a large amount of cholesterol. 90% of the cholesterol required by cells is acquired from receptor-mediated endocytosis while the remaining 10% is obtained by de novo synthesis. The endocytotic process begins by the formation of coated pits initiated by the binding of dephosphorylated adaptor protein to the plasma membrane. The coated pits are named because they are covered by the protein clathrin. Receptors from other regions of the plasma membrane move to the newly formed coated regions for internalization. Ligands containing apo B-100 and apo E are recognized and bound by the LDL-R to form a complex that is internalized into the coated pits.

After internalization of the LDL, the coated pits are pinched off and within a very short time, they shed their clathrin coating. The released clathrin can participate in the formation of new coated pits. The LDL particle that has been internalized is then transferred to endocytotic vesicles or endosomes. Due to the acidic pH within the endosomes, the LDL dissociates from its receptor. This is followed by the fusion of the endosomes with lysosomes that contain hydrolases. The protein component of the LDL, apo B-100, is broken down to free amino acids while the cholesteryl ester component is cleaved by lysosomal lipase. The free cholesterol is released and incorporated into the cell membrane. Excess cholesterol is re-esterified by the action of enzyme ACAT and the cholesteryl ester formed is stored for later use.

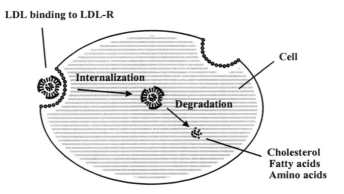

Figure 3. LDL receptor-mediated endocytosis of LDL particles

Elevated LDL Receptor Expression on Tumor Cells

Evidence has demonstrated an elevated LDL receptor activity on brain tumors. The human malignant glioma cell line (U-251 MG) was found to internalize and degrade LDL. The study by Murakami et al. indicated the presence of LDL receptors on the membrane of U-251 MG, which were responsible for the transport of cholesterol into the cell by receptor mediated endocytosis (3). A recent study was conducted by Maletinska et al. on seven human glioma cell lines to determine the levels of LDL receptors on the cell surface (4). It was found that all the cell lines had elevated LDL receptor expression. For example, the SF-767 glioma cells had 300,000 LDL receptors per cell with a very high binding affinity. Other glioma cells also showed high LDL receptor levels (128,000-950,000 LDL receptors per cell) with variable binding affinity.

Gueddari et al. studied the A-549 human lung adenocarcinoma cell line and found an over-expression of LDL receptors as compared to normal human fibroblasts (5). Yen et al. studied the Daudi Burkitt's Lymphoma cells and determined that the level of LDL receptors in these cells were much higher than normal peripheral blood lymphocytes and a majority of these receptors were not subject to downregulation (6). Chen et al. concluded from a study on human prostate cancer cells that over-expression of LDL receptors by cancer cells was important for obtaining essential fatty acids via the LDL receptor pathway (7). This led to an increased production of prostaglandins which in turn stimulated cell growth. Seven murine tumors were studied *in vivo* by determining the uptake of radio-labeled LDL (8). The high relative uptake of the radio-labeled LDL by the murine tumor cells *in vivo* corresponded to an elevated LDL receptor activity.

Vitols et al. studied 59 patients with acute leukemia and suggested a correlation between hypocholesterolemia in such patients and elevated LDL receptor activity in malignant cells (9.) They also proposed utilization of this pathway for targeted delivery of LDL-associated anti-cancer drugs to malignant cells. In another study, a patient diagnosed with adrenal tumor was found to suffer from severe hypocholesterolemia. To investigate whether there was any relation between a low cholesterol level and the tumor, Nakagawa et al. established a cell culture line of the adrenal tumor and found that these cells had twice the LDL receptor activity in these cells when compared to Hep G2 cells (10). This elevated LDL receptor activity resulted in low cholesterol levels in the patient. Furthermore, it was found that these receptors were not susceptible to downregulation.

LDL Transport across Blood Brain Barrier

Cholesterol in the brain can be derived either from the de novo synthesis or from the plasma by transport across the BBB. The presence of LDL receptors on the brain capillaries has been demonstrated. These LDL receptors are responsible for the transcytosis of LDL from the plasma across the BBB by a receptor-mediated mechanism.

Meresse et al. demonstrated the presence of LDL receptors on endothelial cells of brain capillaries. When radiolabeled LDL postmortem was injected into bovine brain circulation, it was found to bind to a specific LDL receptor (11). This LDL receptor was similar in characteristic to the LDL receptor on human fibroblasts. Lucarelli et al. suggested that LDL receptors on brain microvessels may be responsible for transport of lipids across the BBB (12). Dehouck et al. further demonstrated that the LDL receptors on the BBB capillary endothelial cells were responsible for the delivery of essential lipids to brain cells (13). LDL particles were specifically transcytosed across the BBB and this transcytotic process ceased when the receptor was blocked using a monoclonal antibody.

CHOLESTEROL-BASED DRUG TARGETING THROUGH LDL RECEPTORS

As indicated above, cholesterol is the essential component of cell membranes and is in high demand by rapidly dividing malignant tumor cells. Many types of tumor cells have elevated LDL receptor expression in order to acquire more cholesterol compared to corresponding normal cells. This phenomenon forms the basis of a cholesterol-based drug targeting approach through the synthesis of antitumor compounds that mimic native cholesteryl esters (14). As these compounds share similar chemical and physical characteristics with native cholesteryl esters, they can interact well with LDL. They may transfer effectively into LDL in the physiological environment, thus utilizing the elevated LDL receptor expression on tumor cells for targeted drug delivery. The cholesterol-based drug targeting to tumor cells is schematically illustrated in Figure 4.

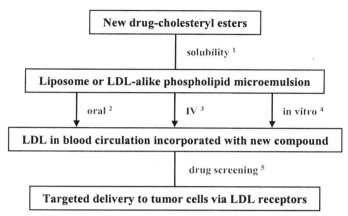

Figure 4. Schematic description of the cholesterol-based drug targeting approach. [1]These drug-cholesteryl esters are in general water-insoluble and thus require the pharmaceutical formulations. [2-4]The formulations containing drug-cholesteryl esters are administered in oral or IV route or incubated *in vitro* with freshly-isolated LDL for drug loading before the IV administration. [5]A series of such drug-cholesteryl esters are screened, *in vitro* or *in vivo*, to maximize the targeting capability.

To observe the therapeutic potential of the cholesterol-based drug targeting approach and to examine the interactions of such compounds with LDL and malignant tumor cells, our laboratory recently synthesized a series of compounds mimicking native cholesteryl esters for targeted drug delivery to tumor cells. One of these compounds, cholesteryl 1,12-dicarba-closo-dodecaboranel-carboxylate (BCH, see Figure 5), is a carborane ester of cholesterol designed for use in boron neutron capture therapy (BNCT).

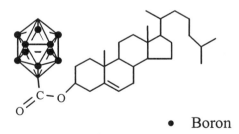

• Boron

Figure 5. The chemical structure of a carborane ester of cholesterol (BCH). The second carbon atom on the carborane allows the further addition of functional groups to generate a large number of similar compounds for drug screening.

The chemical reactions for making such a compound involve several steps as briefly described in Figure 6 (15). The resulting compound contains 10 boron atoms to maximize the amount of boron per molecule. The compound also possesses two carbon atoms on the boron cage allowing the formation of a cholesteryl ester bond on one carbon atom and further chemical modifications on the second carbon atom to generate a series of cholesteryl esters of carborane. Feakes et al. also reported the synthesis of boron-containing cholesterol derivatives for incorporation in liposomes (16).

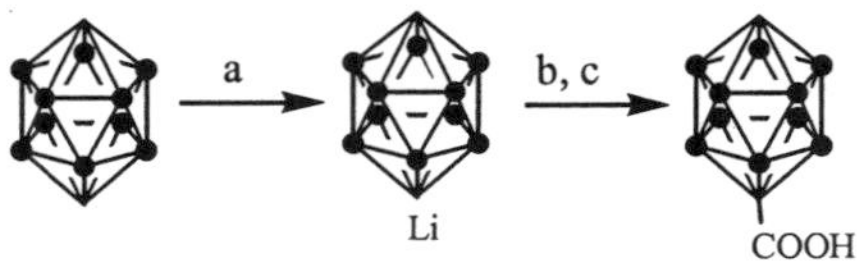

Scheme 1. (a) *n*-BuLi in ether at room temperature (RT); (b) Dry ice at −78 °C; (c) HCl.

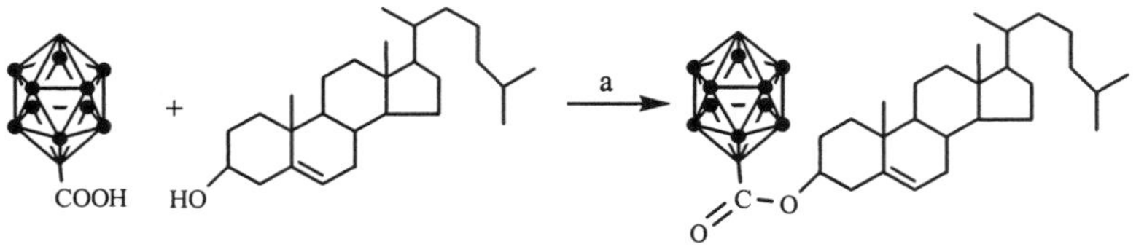

Scheme 2. (a) DCC and DMPA.

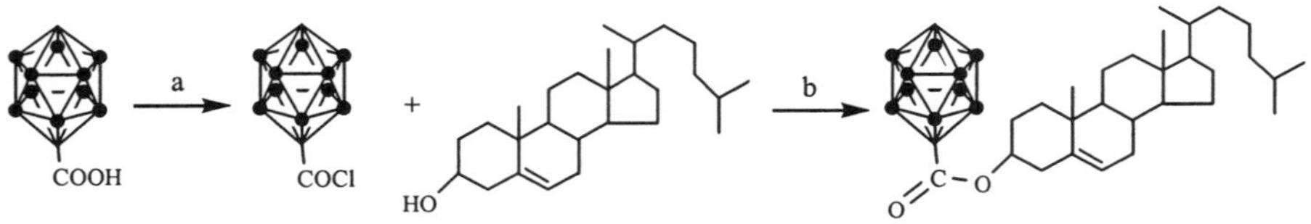

Scheme 3. (a) Reflux in $SOCl_2$; (b) DMAP in CH_2Cl_2 at RT.

Figure 6. Chemical synthesis of a carborane ester of cholesterol (BCH).

BNCT is an experimental therapy that has been used to treat glioma, melanoma and other malignant tumors. The basis for BNCT is a nuclear reaction which occurs when a stable isotope of boron, ^{10}B, is irradiated by a beam of low energy neutrons to yield high energy and short-range tumor-destroying α particles and ^{7}Li nuclei. For BNCT to be successful, the boron must preferentially localize in the tumor cells as compared to surrounding normal cells (17). Therefore, utilizing the cholesterol-based drug targeting approach by linking cholesterol to boron compounds to make the mimics of cholesteryl esters may result in a higher concentration of boron in tumor cells and thus enhance the efficacy for BNCT treatment. BCH is extremely hydrophobic and thus we have formulated the compound in liposomes and VLDL-resembling phospholipid-submicron emulsions for cell culture studies (18). In addition to solubilizing BCH, these formulations may also serve as suitable carriers to interact with LDL in the physiological environment. The formulations can be administered as indicated in Figure 4. Experiments involving tumor-bearing animal model may also supply direct information for the *in vivo* tumor-uptake of boron compounds formulated in these formulations (19).

Experiments were carried out in our laboratory to examine the cellular uptake of BCH from both liposomal formulation and VLDL-resembling phospholipid-submicron emulsion. Based on the studies using 9L rat glioma cell lines, sufficient levels of boron in the cells (about 50 μg boron/g of cells) were achieved with these BCH formulations. Maletinska et al. showed that seven human glioblastoma multiforme cell lines, including SF-767 and SF-763, had very high numbers of LDL receptors per cell (4). With the available information regarding the elevated LDL receptor expression on human tumor cells, further experiments were carried out in our laboratory using two human glioma cell lines (SF-767 and SF-763). The results indicated that extensive BCH uptake occurred in these human glioma cells. Although the concentration of BCH in the cell culture medium was low due to the limit of BCH formulation, the boron uptake reached 264 μg boron/g cells for the SF-767 cells, about 10 times higher than the required boron level ($\geq$ 20-25 μg boron per g cells) for successful BNCT. For SF-763 cells, the boron uptake reached 283.3 μg boron/g cells, about 11 times higher than the required boron level.

In addition to the requirement for the cells to obtain an adequate amount of boron, it is also essential for boron to remain in the cells for a sufficient time period so that the neutron radiation may be effectively applied. *In vitro* cell incubation experiments were carried out on SF-767 and SF-763 human glioma cells. The results showed that a majority of the BCH taken up in the human glioma cells was retained in the cells after the subsequent 24-hour incubation without the presence of BCH.

With the understanding of how LDL and LDL receptors work, better cholesterol-based compounds will be generated which can be used for the targeted delivery of anti-tumor agents. Clarifying the functions of LDL receptors within the blood-brain barrier may also aid in the development of other cholesterol-based therapeutical compounds for effective drug delivery across the blood-brain barrier.

NON-CHOLESTEROL-BASED DRUG TARGETING THROUGH LDL RECEPTORS

Non-cholesterol-based pharmaceutical compounds may also be incorporated into LDL for targeted delivery. The necessary requirement is that these compounds be hydrophobic in order to facilitate the loading. The incorporation is usually carried out *in vitro*. In general, human LDL is isolated from fresh serum by differential density ultracentrifugation. The incorporation of LDL with hydrophobic compounds is performed according to well-investigated protocols. The success of the incorporation requires the effective loading and a process to avoid the denaturation of apolipoproteins. The latter is a critical step because even a minor change in structure or conformation of apo B protein results in the rapid clearance of the modified LDL by the reticuloendothelial system. Studies have been conducted on drug-loading LDL in cell culture, as well as within preclinical and clinical experiments.

Lundberg successfully incorporated a steroid mustard carbamate, which is a lipophilic anti-cancer drug, into the core of reconstituted LDL and then evaluated its biological activity (20). The incorporation was first carried out using detergents. However, a newer method using enzymatic hydrolysis provided a milder process. The structure, as well as the cellular uptake, was found to be similar to those of native LDL. The cytotoxic activity of these compounds were tested using cultured human fibroblasts or neuroblastoma cells and it was found that the drug delivered to the cells via the LDL pathway was able to kill 100% of the cells. It was also found that inhibitors of LDL uptake blocked the cytotoxic activity of drug-lipoprotein complex indicating that the drug-LDL complex followed the same pathway as native LDL.

Lestavel-Delattre proposed that drugs from the 2-(aminomethyl) acrylophenones (AMA) class could be specifically targeted to cancer cells using LDL as the drug carrier (21). This class of drugs shows *in vitro* anti-leukemic activity but is ineffective *in vivo* since they are actively bound by blood proteins. When an AMA compound was loaded into LDL, the loading was about 100-300 drug molecules per LDL particle. The drug-LDL complex formed was highly electronegative. The drug-LDL complex was bound, internalized, and degraded through the LDL receptor of neoplastic A-549 cells but to a slightly smaller extent compared to native LDL. The drug-receptor interaction was demonstrated to induce *in vitro* cytotoxicity as evidenced by growth inhibition of the A-549 cells.

In vitro studies were conducted by Kerr et al. on human squamous lung tumor cells to assess the effectiveness of daunomycin-LDL receptor complex (22). The efficiency of the complex was compared with daunomycin itself and it was found that both were equally cytotoxic *in vitro*. Samadi-Baboli et al loaded eliptinium oleate (OL-NME) into LDL, about 400 molecules per LDL particle (23). Their results indicated that the complex enhanced the anti-tumor activity against B 16 melanoma model.

The success of anti-tumor treatment using photodynamic agents is dependent on the localization of the agent within tumor cells. The agents are required to be specifically delivered to tumor tissue followed by their activation after exposure to light. This approach is similar in certain extent to BNCT as described above. The selectivity of photodynamic agents for the tumors can be enhanced when LDL is used as the carrier. It was found that Haematoporphyrin (Hp), a photodynamic agent, was non-covalently bound with LDL (24). When administered, this Hp-LDL complex showed killing potential on tumor cells upon being internalized by the cells. Pharmacokinetic studies of a photodynamic agent, Zinc-phthalocyanate (Zn-Pc) were conducted by Reddi et al. using LDL as drug delivery system (25). These studies were carried out in mice bearing a transplanted MS-2 fibrosarcoma. It was found that the LDL approach resulted in a higher Zn-Pc uptake by the tumor as well as improved selectivity.

The potential of boron neutron capture therapy for the treatment of brain tumors has been extensively investigated. The treatment is based on the principle of interaction of boron atoms localized in brain tumors with thermal neutron generated from an external source. The efficiency of this method can be further enhanced when the selectivity of the boron compound is increased so that it is preferentially taken up by the brain tumor cells. Laster et al., at University of California, San Fransisco, prepared a boronated analogue of LDL containing almost 12,000 boron atoms per LDL (26). *In vitro* experiments were carried out using cell culture lines to investigate the biological efficacy when carborane carboxylic acid esters of fatty alcohols were used to boronate LDL. The boronated-LDL was incubated with hamster V-79 and CHO cells. On being irradiated with thermal neutron beams from the Brookhaven Medical Research Reactor, it was found that the boron was distributed intracellularly through a receptor-mediated process. Boron concentration achieved inside the cells was found to reach 10 times the concentration required for BNCT.

De Smidt incorporated the oleoyl derivatives of two anti-cancer drugs, methotrexate and floxuridine, into LDL particles (27). Three incorporation methods were used, namely the dry film method, the transfer protein method and the delipidation-reconstitution method. It was found that the drug loading was the highest with the delipidation-reconstitution method, resulting in about 50-70 dioleoyl-FdUrd molecules per LDL particle. *In vitro* studies were carried out using hepatocellular carcinoma cell line Hep G2 and it was found that the drug-LDL complex competed effectively with native LDL for binding to LDL receptors. *In vivo* studies in rats showed that the half-life of the drug-LDL complex was prolonged when compared to the free drug. Vitols et al. incorporated a water insoluble mitoclomine derivative (WB 4291) into LDL (28). The drug loading was about 1500 drug molecules per

LDL particle. The drug-LDL complex was tested *in vivo* in Balb-C mice with experimental leukemia. After intraperitoneal administration the median survival time was prolonged two to five-fold. Versluis et al. prepared a liposomal formulation containing apo E and found that it behaved similar to native LDL *in vivo* (29). When cultured with B 16 melanoma cell lines the apo E containing liposome was bound 15 times more by the LDL receptor than native LDL. A lipophilic derivative of Daunorubicin was incorporated into this liposomal formulation and when tested in B 16 tumor-bearing mice it was found that the tissue distribution of the complex was comparable to that of native LDL.

A clinical study was conducted at Karolinska Hospital in Sweden (30). Eleven adult patients diagnosed with acute myelogenous leukemia were administered drug-LDL formulation containing ^{14}C-sucrose labeled LDL. From the results of this study it was concluded that LDL could potentially be used as drug carrier for targeting lipophilic anti-cancer drugs to leukemia cells.

FUTURE DEVELOPMENT

As indicated in the literature, it is feasible to deliver therapeutic compounds specifically to malignant tumors through the LDL-receptor mediated route. Significant progress has been made in many laboratories in both fundamental research and practical applications. To enhance the efficacy of LDL-receptor mediated drug targeting, new compounds mimicking the physical and chemical properties of native cholesteryl esters, either cholesterol-based or non-cholesterol-based compounds, need to be further developed. Suitable pharmaceutical formulations for these compounds are essential for effective interactions with lipoproteins and subsequent drug loading into lipoproteins in either *in vivo* or *in vitro* environment. Based on the experimental results at the molecular level and the cellular level, preclinical animal studies as well as clinical studies need to be carefully arranged to evaluate the efficacy of the novel therapeutic compounds carried by various pharmaceutical formulations for LDL-receptor mediated drug targeting to malignant tumors.

REFERENCES

1. Danik M, Champagne D, Petit-Turcotte C, Beffert U and Poirier J. Brain lipoprotein metabolism and its relation to neurodegenerative disease. Crit. Rev. Neur. 1999; 13(4): 357-407
2. Hussain M M, Strickland D K and Bakillah A. The mammalian low-density lipoprotein receptor family. Annu Rev Nutr 1999; 19: 141-172

3. Murakami M, Ushio Y, Mihara Y, Kuratsu J, Horiuchi S, Morino Y. Cholesterol uptake by human glioma cells via receptor-mediated endocytosis of low-density lipoprotein J Neurosurg 1990 73(5): 760-767

4. Maletinska L, Blakely EA, Bjornstad KA, Deen DF, Knoff LJ, Forte TM. Human glioblastoma cell lines: levels of low-density lipoprotein receptor and low-density lipoprotein receptor-related protein. Cancer Res 2000; 60(8): 2300-2303

5. Gueddari N, Favre G, Hachem H, Marek E, Le Gaillard F, Soula G. Evidence for up-regulated low density lipoprotein receptor in human lung adenocarcinoma cell line A549. Biochimie 1993; 75(9): 811-819

6. Yen CF, Kalunta CI, Chen FS, Kaptein JS, Lin CK, Lad PM. Regulation of low-density lipoprotein receptors and assessment of their functional role in Burkitt's lymphoma cells. Biochim Biophys Acta 1995; 1257(1): 47-57

7. Chen Y, Hughes-Fulford M. Human prostate cancer cells lack feedback regulation of low-density lipoprotein receptor and its regulator, SREBP2. Int J Cancer 2001; 91(1): 41-45

8. Lombardi P, Norata G, Maggi F M, Canti G, Franco P, Nicolin A and Catapano A L. Assimilation of LDL by experimental tumors in mice. Biochim Biophys Acta 1989; 1003(3): 301-306

9. Vitols S, Gahrton G, Bjorkholm M and Peterson C. Hypocholesterolaemia in malignancy due to elevated low-density-lipoprotein-receptor activity in tumor cells: evidence from studies in patients with leukemia. Lancet 1985; 2: 1150-1154

10. Nakagawa T, Ueyama Y, Nozaki S, Yamashita S, Menju M, Funahashi T, Kameda-Takemura K, Kubo M, Tokunaga K, Tanaka T, et al. Marked hypocholesterolemia in a case with adrenal adenoma--enhanced catabolism of low density lipoprotein (LDL) via the LDL receptors of tumor cells. J Clin Endocrinol Metab 1995; 80(1): 92-96

11. Meresse S, Delbart C, Fruchart JC, Cecchelli R. Low-density lipoprotein receptor on endothelium of brain capillaries. J Neurochem 1989; 53(2): 340-345

12. Lucarelli M, Gennarelli M, Cardelli P, Novelli G, Scarpa S, Dallapiccola B and Strom R. Expression of receptors for native and chemically modified low-density lipoproteins in brain microvessels,. FEBS Letters 1997; 401(1): 53-58

13. Dehouck B, Fenart, L, Dehouck M, Pierce A, Torpier G and Cecchelli R. A new function for the LDL receptor: transcytosis of LDL across the Blood Brain Barrier. J Cell Biol 1997; 138(4): 877-889

14. Gutman RL, Peacock G. Lu D.R. Targeted drug delivery for brain cancer treatment. J. Controlled Release, 2000; 65: 31-41.

15. Lu DR and Ji B. Carborane containing cholesterol, a new type of molecule for targeted boron drug delivery. U.S. Patent No. 09/609,957, (2001)

16. Feakes DA, Spinler JK and Harris FR. Synthesis of Boron containing cholesterol derivatives for incorporation into unilamellar liposomes and evaluation as potential agents for BNCT. Tetrahedron 1999; 55: 11177–11186

17. Chen W, Mehta S and Lu DR. Selective boron drug delivery to brain tumors for boron neutron capture therapy. Adv. Drug Delivery Reviews 1997; 26: 231-247.

18. Shawer M, Greenspan P, Øie S and Lu DR. VLDL-resembling phospholipid-submicron emulsion for cholesterol-based drug targeting. J. Pharm. Sci. 2002 (In press)

19. Ji B, Chen W, Halpern DS and Lu DR. Cell culture and animal studies for intracerebral delivery of borocaptate in liposomal formulation. Drug Delivery 2001; 8: 13-17

20. Lundberg S. Preparation of drug-low density lipoprotein complexes for delivery of antitumoral drugs via the low density lipoprotein pathway. Cancer Res 1987; 47: 4105-4108

21. Lestavel-Delattre S, Martin-Nizard F, Clavey V, Testard P, Favre G, Doualin G et. al. Low Density Lipoprotein for delivery of an acrylophenone antineoplastic molecule into malignant cells. Cancer Res 1992; 52: 3629-3635

22. Kerr D J, Hynds S A, Shepherd J, Packard C J and Kaye S B. Comparative cellular uptake and cytotoxicity of a complex of daunomycin-low density lipoprotein in human squamous lung tumor cell monolayer. Biochem Pharmacol 1988; 37(20): 3981-3986

23. Samadi-Baboli M, Favre G, Canal P and Soula G. Low Density Lipoprotein for cytotoxic drug targeting: improved activity of elliptinium derivative against B16 melanoma in mice. Br J Cancer 1993; 68(2): 319-326

24. Reddi E. Role of delivery vehicles for photosensitizers in the photodynamic therapy of tumors. J Photochem Photobiol B: Biology 1997; 37: 189-195

25. Reddi E, Zhou C, Biolo R, Menegaldo E and Jori G. Liposome or LDL-administered Zn (II)-phthalocyanine as a photodynamic agent for tumors. I. Pharmacokinetic properties and phototherapeutic efficiency. Br J Cancer 1990; 61: 407-411

26. Laster B H, Kahl S B, Popenoe E A, Pate D W and Fairchild R G. Biological efficacy of boronated low-density lipoprotein for boron neutron capture therapy as measured in cell culture. Cancer Res 1991; 51: 4588-4593

27. De Smidt P C and van Berkel T J. Prolonged serum half life of antineoplastic drugs by incorporation into the low density lipoprotein. Cancer Res 1990; 50: 7476-7482

28. Vitols S, Soderberg-Reid K, Masquelier M, Sjostrom B and Peterson C. Low density lipoprotein for delivery of a water-insoluble alkylating agent to malignant cells. *In vitro* and *in vivo* studies of a drug-lipoprotein complex. Br J Cancer 1990; 62(5): 724-729

29. Versluis AJ, Rensen PC, Rump ET, Van Berkel TJ and Bijsterbosch MK. Low-density lipoprotein receptor-mediated delivery of a lipophilic daunorubicin derivative to B16 tumours in mice using apolipoprotein E-enriched liposomes. Br J Cancer 1998; 78(12): 1607-1614

30. Vitols S, Angelin B, Ericsson S, Gahrton G, Juliusson G, Masquelier M. Uptake of low-density lipoproteins by human leukemic cells *in vivo*: relation to plasma lipoprotein levels and possible relevance for selective chemotherapy. Proc Natl Acad Sci USA 1990b; 87: 2598-2602.

GLOSSARY

Apolipoprotein or apoprotein: Specific proteins found on the surface of lipoproteins that serve as recognition sites for different lipoprotein receptors.

BNCT (Boron Neutron Capture Therapy): An experimental therapy that has been used to treat glioma, melanoma and other malignant tumors.

Cholesterol: It is a steroid that is the principal component of animal cell membranes.

Emulsion: It is a biphasic liquid dosage form.

Gliomas: These are brain tumors and malignant gliomas are the most common primary tumors of the central nervous system

LDL (Low Density Lipoproteins): This type lipoprotein is the major circulatory form of cholesterol and cholesteryl esters in the blood.

LDL receptor: LDL receptors are transmembrane receptors present on cell surfaces that recognize and internalize LDL to obtain cholesterol from blood

Lipoprotein: Primary transport form of lipids like phospholipids, triacyglycerols, cholesterol and cholesteryl esters in the body.

Liposome: It is a type of drug delivery system composed of a phospholipids vesicle.

Malignant tumors: These tumors have a tendency to spread to other organs or areas of the body and are difficult to treat.

18

TARGETING BRAIN TRAUMA AND STROKE

Margaret A. Petty* and Eng H. Lo[+]
*CNS Pharmacology, Aventis Pharmaceuticals Inc. Route 202-206, P.O. Box 6800, Bridgewater, New Jersey 08807. [+] Neuroprotection Research Laboratory, Dept. of Neurology and Radiology, Massachusetts General Hospital, and Program in Neuroscience, Harvard Medical School

INTRODUCTION

Acute stroke can be classified as ischemic, hemorrhagic, or both and result in the occurrence of multiple pathophysiological processes. These pathophysiological events develop over the subsequent hours to days, as the original core of the infarct develops into the surrounding penumbral area (1, 2). Initial cell death results from the deprivation of blood supply to the brain. However, a significant portion of the brain damage occurs later when secondary deleterious mechanisms come into play (2). The recent progress made in defining the mechanisms involved in the pathophysiology of stroke will probably lead to the identification of new strategies for intervention in the ischemic cascade. Therefore, it becomes increasingly important to initially consider how these new therapeutics may be delivered into the target tissue in brain and secondly to speculate on new strategies that would target ischemic brain tissue.

Drug delivery into normal brain and its constraints

Blood-brain barrier

Direct administration of drugs to the brain is difficult, the most obvious route of delivery being via the blood. Although blood flow to the brain is high, blood is not in free diffusional communication with the interstitium of brain. Endothelial cells in brain capillaries form a barrier to maintain the fragile extracellular microenvironment in the neuronal parenchyma, which is essential for normal brain function and precise synaptic signaling (3). The blood brain barrier (BBB) of higher vertebrates is made up of brain microvessel endothelial cells, unlike the barrier of invertebrates, which is derived from glia. BBB endothelial cells are distinct from other peripheral endothelial cells in that they possess a low number of vesicles, no fenestrae, a higher mitochondrial volume fraction, a higher electrical resistance (in the range of 1000-5000Ω cm^2), and specialized transport systems (4). The local brain environment (including astrocytes, pericytes, and neurons) likely confers these characteristics. The BBB, therefore, severely restricts direct exchange between the vascular compartment and cerebral parenchyma. Gases and small lipophilic molecules can diffuse through; all other substances require transport via carrier mediated or vesicular mechanisms (5).

Vascular delivery

The BBB is responsible for protecting the brain against noxious chemicals, variation in blood composition and breakdown of the concentration gradient, which may damage the brains fragile extracellular environment. The BBB impedes the entry of most substances from the blood by two methods. The transcellular pathway permits entry by passive diffusion only by those substances that are small, have a molecular weight of less than 450, are neutral, and lipophilic. There are, however, groups of small and large hydrophilic molecules that can penetrate the brain by means of transcellular active transport. Ions and solutes diffuse between adjacent endothelial cells down their concentration gradient. However, this paracellular space is almost completely obstructed by tight junctions, which are cell-cell junctional complexes in the apical region of cell membranes. Tight junctions prevent substances with a molecular weight of greater than 180 from paracellular diffusion (6).

One can temporally open the BBB to assist in drug administration. One approach is via osmotic opening with hyperosmolar substances (e.g., mannitol injected into the cerebral circulation) (7). Pharmacological opening of the BBB has been proposed by means of bradykinin or nitric oxide analogues (8). Manipulation of endogenous transport systems in the BBB; for example, transferrin and insulin receptors have been targeted using antibody conjugation and chimeric peptide methods (9) as a means of penetrating the BBB. However, after successfully traversing the endothelial cell layer another barrier exists, the basal lamina, which reduces the efficacy of the BBB opening strategies (10).

Intracerebral delivery

Alternatively, one can bypass the BBB by introducing the drug directly into brain parenchyma. Drugs can be injected directly via intrathecal catheters or by means of controlled release matrices (16), microencapsulated chemicals (17), or recombinant cells (18). However, a fundamental problem with this approach is that because brain cells are tightly packed and the interstitial volume only occupies about 20% of total brain volume, the diffusion coefficients associated with drug movement within brain tissue are low. This results in limited movement of drugs away from the initial injection site.

Intraventricular delivery

Another possibility to bypass the BBB is to instill the therapeutic agent into the cerebral ventricular system. The cerebrospinal fluid (CSF) is in free communication with the brains interstitial fluid, thus allowing free movement into the brain parenchyma. However, once a compound has been introduced into the ventricular system it must diffuse into the target area. As previously mentioned, diffusion rates can be very slow for compounds in the brain. These slow diffusion rates would have to compete with the faster rates of CSF clearance via the foramina and subarachnoid space into the venous system. Hence, intraventricular drug injections rapidly drain into the venous system resembling a slow intravenous infusion (19, 20).

Drug delivery into ischemic brain

Therapeutic targets in stroke

Stroke is associated with a drastic fall in cerebral blood flow in the core of the ischemic territory, which results in rapid cell death. The secondary processes of cell death then follow in the ischemic penumbra. Although not mutually exclusive, these secondary processes can be broadly categorized into mechanisms of excitotoxicity, oxidative stress, inflammation and apoptosis. Based on the multiple mechanisms involved in stroke, potential therapeutic agents cover a broad spectrum of compounds including sodium and calcium channel blockers, glutamate receptor antagonists, GABA and adenosine receptor modifiers, free radical scavengers and spin traps, anti-inflammatory agents, inhibitors of deleterious enzymes, neuroprotective growth factors, antisense oligonucleotides and genes that enhance endogenous protective responses and suppress the activation of damaging processes. Gene cassettes, oligonucleotides, peptides, and recombinant proteins are not lipid soluble and are unable to penetrate the BBB. Therefore, efficient drug delivery of potential neuroprotectants into brain cannot be assured.

An additional aspect to be taken into consideration is the therapeutic time window of opportunity. This window for effective stroke treatment is narrow, in most therapeutic regimes the target times for intervention is in the order of hours (1, 2). Although with a clearer understanding of apoptotic-like mechanisms this window may be extended. This is an important issue, when considering the types of drug delivery strategies discussed in the previous sections (e.g., intraventricular and intracerebral), which may be limited because of very slow diffusion times.

In addition to the drug delivery strategy and the window of opportunity, it is also necessary to consider issues regarding delivery to specific brain regions. Restricting drug delivery to specific damaged areas of brain is challenging. To limit a drug to a certain damaged brain area is an important goal since a major limitation of certain candidate neuroprotective drugs has been their side effects that are mostly manifest in normal brain. If issues (discussed below) compromise delivery to damaged brain, then general delivery schemes, without targeting, would result in therapeutic indices that are too low.

Blood-brain barrier disruptions

Disruption of the BBB occurs following acute stroke. However, alterations in BBB permeability can follow a heterogeneous spatial and temporal pattern. Following transient cerebral ischemia, for example, there is an immediate BBB opening, but the barrier closes within minutes to hours depending on the severity and duration of the ischemic insult (15). Hence, BBB opening as a method of drug delivery is not reliable, as complete penetration of a particular compound cannot be assured.

Reductions in blood delivery

When considering intravascular delivery of therapeutic agents, alterations in cerebral blood flow must be taken into account. In the ischemic core blood flow can rapidly decrease to 5 – 10% of normal baseline (16). Even in the surrounding penumbra, blood flow has been estimated to be only about 30 – 40% of normal value (16). Therefore, vascular delivery of drugs into these target regions is limited. This issue is of tremendous importance since the therapeutic index of potential neuroprotective agents depends on their differential delivery to injured versus normal brain tissue.

Edema and interstitial pressure

Acute stroke is invariably associated with edema, which increases intracranial pressure and tissue resistance (i.e., resistance to blood flow). In the context of brain drug delivery, the elevated intracranial pressure presents an obstacle to efficient delivery of drugs by both the intravascular and intraventricular routes. Hence, cerebral edema and elevated intracranial pressure should be considered in the context of drug delivery to damaged brain.

Speculative strategies for targeting ischemic brain

There is no effective current means for stroke targeting; even animal studies are at a relatively early stage. However, several potential strategies can be theoretically tested for this purpose.

Pro-drugs

The rationale for pro-drugs is the idea of delivering compounds that are inactive until activated by local conditions. One obvious local condition that changes in cerebral ischemia is pH. Measurements in ischemic brain show that pH rapidly falls from a normal baseline of about 7.0 to about 6.2 after loss of perfusion (17). Compounds have been synthesized that are active only under acidic pH conditions, for example sodium/hydrogen exchange inhibitors, which permits the possibility of achieving relatively selective effects only in ischemic brain tissue.

Another possible approach might be to design compounds that are cleaved or activated by local enzymes. It is interesting to note that many intra and extracellular proteases become upregulated after stroke. An example of extracellular proteases that are increased is the family of matrix metalloproteinases or MMPs (18). Recently, MMP-sensitive vectors have been constructed that show selective targeting in tumors with elevated MMP activity (19). It is conceivable that similar approaches may work in stroke.

Immunoliposomes

Liposomes have long been considered as possible drug delivery methods for penetrating BBB (20). In this context, it may also be reasonable to consider the use of liposomes as carriers of stroke therapeutics. For example, liposome-encased superoxide dismutase has been used successfully in models of focal cerebral ischemia and brain trauma (21, 22). To further build on the liposome approach, one might envision using liposomes that are targeted (i.e., immunoliposomes). By tagging the outside of the liposomes with antibodies that may recognize certain antigens upregulated or exposed in stroke, one may achieve additional targeting towards ischemic tissue. A proof-of-concept study used cultured cardiomyocytes subjected to hypoxia (23) and a model of myocardial ischemia in rabbits (24). Immunoliposomes constructed with anti-myosin antibodies were able to target ischemic cells where leaky cell membranes presumably exposed intracellular myosin antigens. In the brain, it is conceivable that immunoliposomes targeted against neuronal, astrocytic, or oligodendrocytic antigens may also be used.

Gene therapy using viral vectors

Recent advances in molecular biology and virus genetics have permitted the possibility of gene therapy using viral vectors for a variety of neurological diseases including stroke. A number of such vectors have been constructed, including those derived from herpes simplex virus (HSV), which is particularly appropriate for delivering genes to the adult central nervous system since the virus is neurotropic (25).

Several studies have shown that cerebral ischemia alters gene expression and some of the induced genes, although not produced in large enough amounts, are protective at least using various *in vivo* models of cerebral ischemia. Of the various candidate genes, enhanced neuronal survival has been reported following transient focal ischemia through energy restoration with the over-expression of the glucose transporter (GLUT-1) (26) and buffering calcium excess by means of calbindin D28K over expression (27). Similarly prevention of protein malfolding or aggregation by the heat shock protein HSP72 over expression is protective in ischemic conditions (28) as is the inhibition of apoptotic cell death with BCL-2 (29). Unfortunately, the sparing of neurons from insult induced death does not necessarily translate into the sparing of function (30).

Although gene therapy in experimental cerebral ischemia is feasible, the technical problems are formidable and are not easily solved. These problems include the limited number of cells that the vector is able to transfect which result lesion volume cannot be altered by the current approach. Secondly, the route of administration is also a limiting factor since in the above-mentioned studies replication defective herpes viral vectors that transduce the genes are administered into a brain ventricle or directly into cerebral tissue. However, even if the viral vector transfects the ependyma following intraventricular injection, the problem remains of a gene product with very slow rates of diffusion. The maintenance and control of foreign gene expression and the control of unwanted host immune responses also pose significant concerns concerning the safety of viral vectors.

Protein transduction

Schwarze et al. (31) have recently reported *in vivo* protein transduction as a potential method of delivering biologically active protein in mice. The authors used fusion proteins containing the protein transduction domain from the immunodeficiency virus TAT protein. Protein transduction occurs independently of receptors and transporters and is thought to target the lipid biolayer component of cell membranes. Thus all cell types should be susceptible to protein transduction and when injected intraperitoneally in mice the active fusion protein is delivered to all tissues including the brain. This methodology opens the possibility for direct delivery of proteins to the brain while circumventing the problems associated with BBB penetration.

Stem cell therapy

Neural transplantation has been used to study and promote the regenerative potential of the brain after ischemic insult. Fetal neural stem cells can reduce behavioral deficits and take on a neurochemical phenotype that resembles normal neocortex following ischemic hypoxic brain injury in neonate rats (32). However, transplantation of embryonic grafts is plagued with problems and other stem cell sources are being considered as an alternative for transplantation therapy. Recently, Li et al. (33) reported that whole bone marrow stromal cell transplantation, which has the characteristics of stem and progenitor cells, into the ischemic boundary of adult rat brain 1 day after stroke induce plasticity in ischemic brain. Such treatment resulted in BrudU-reactive cells (used as a marker for newly formed DNA) expressing neuronal and astrocytic proteins, neuronal nuclei protein and glial fibrillary acidic protein immunoreactivities. In addition bone marrow transplantation promoted proliferation of ependymal and subependymal cells, identified by means of nestin (a neuroepitheal stem cell marker) within the ventricular and subventricular zones. Bone marrow stromal cell transplantation into the ischemic boundary survived, and differentiated following middle cerebral artery occlusion (33). Further, intra-arterial transplantation of the bone marrow stromal cells appears superior to intracerebral transplantation. They appear to distribute over a wider area of the ischemic core and penumbra and not only did they survive but improved functional recovery was reported (34). Similar findings have more recently been reported after the intravenous administration of bone marrow stromal cells (36) and also human umbilical cord blood, a rich source of stem and progenitor cells (35). The mechanism by which these cells are able to cross the BBB is unknown, although the authors speculate that they may be using the vascular adhesion molecules, like inflammatory cells, to penetrate the brain.

Hence, stem cells are able to survive, migrate, differentiate and reduce functional deficits after stroke and such stem cells have a therapeutic window of days. But what are the mechanisms involved? One possibility is that these cells integrate into the tissue, replace damaged cells, and reconstruct neuronal circuitry. At present there is no evidence to support this hypothesis. A feasible explanation is that the interaction of the transplanted stem cells with the host brain leads to the production of trophic factors that may contribute to the recovery of function (36).

CONCLUSION

Recent advances in non-invasive imaging technologies have allowed the rapid diagnosis of acute stroke brain injury and the identification of potentially salvageable target tissue. This penumbral tissue presents a tremendous challenge for delivering effective therapies. Cerebral drug delivery is faced with many obstacles due to the unique anatomic and physiological characteristics of the brain. Deprivation of the blood supply to the brain initiates several pathophysiological features that may additionally affect drug delivery. Several of these features have been discussed in this review, including altered BBB permeability, decreased cerebral blood flow, edema and increased interstitial pressure, decreased cerebral metabolism, changes in proteolytic and degradative enzymes, altered gene expression and reduced protein synthesis. Careful consideration of these issues should provide a framework for the optimization of drug delivery strategies for damaged brain. Such optimization of delivery strategies will play a major role in determining therapeutic gain.

REFERENCES

1. Dirnagl U, Iadecola, C, Moskowitz, MA, Pathobiology of ischemic stroke: an integrated view, Trends Neurosci 1999; 22: 391-397.
2. Lee JM, Zipfel GJ, Choi DW, The changing landscape of ischemic brain injury mechanisms, Nature 1999; 399: A7-A14.
3. Suckling AJ, Rumsby MG, Bradbury M.W.B., Eds., The blood-brain barier in health and disease (Ellis Horwood, Chichester,) 1986.
4. Brightman MW, Ultrastructure of brain endothelium. In M. W. B. Bradbury, Physiology and pharmacology of the blood-brain barrier, Springer-Verlag, Berlin, 1992: pp. 1-22.
5. Pardridge W, Peptide drug delivery to the brain. (Raven Press, New York) 1991.
6. Mitic LL, Anderson JM, Molecular architecture of tight junctions. Annu. Rev. Physiol. 1998; 60: 121-142.
7. Kroll RA, Neuwelt EA, Outwitting the blood-brain barrier for therapeutic purposes: osmotic opening and other means, Neurosurgery 1998; 42: 1083-1099.
8. Pardridge W, Peptide drug delivery to the brain. J Cereb Blood Flow Metab 1997: 17; 713-731.
9. Pardridge WM, Vector mediated drug delivery to the brain, Adv Drug Deliv Rev 1999; 36: 299-321.
10. Muldoon LL, Pagel MA, Kroll RA, Roman-Goldstein S, Jones RS, Neuwelt EA, A physiological barrier distal to the anatomic blood-brain barrier in a model of transvascular delivery, Am J Neuroradiol 1999; 20: 217-222.
11. Mahoney MJ, Saltzman WM, Controlled release of proteins to tissue transplants for treatment of neurodegenerative disorders, J Pharm Sci 1996; 85: 1276-1281.
12. Benoit JP, Faisant N, Venier-Julienne MC, Menei P, Development of microspheres for neurological disorders: basics to clinical applications, J Controlled Release 65 (2000) 285-296.
13. Chang PL, Van Raamsdonk JM, Hortelano G, Barsoum SC MacDonald NC, Stockley TL, *In vivo* delivery of heterologous proteins by microencapsulated recombinant cells, Trends Biotechnology 1999; 17: 78-83.
14. Yan Q, Matheson C, Sun J, Radeke MJ, Feinstein SC, Miller JA, Distribution of intracerebral ventricularly administered neurotrophins in rat brain and its correlation with Trk receptor expression, Exp Neurol 1994; 127: 23-36.
15. Kuroiwa T, Ting P, Martinez H, Klatzo I, The biphasic opening of the blood-brain barrier to proteins following temporary middle cerebral artery occlusion, Acta Neuropathol 1985; 68: 122-129.
16. Jones TH, Morawetz RB, Crowell RM, Marcoux FW, Fitzgibbon SJ, De Girolami U, Ojemann RG, Threshold of focal cerebral ischemia in awake monkeys, J Neurosurg 1981;54: 773-782.
17. Kraig RP, Petito CK, Plum F, Pulsinelli WA, Hydrogen ions kill at concentrations reached in ischemia. J Cereb Blood Flow Metab 1987;7: 379-386.
18. Mun-Bryce S, Rosenberg GA, Matrix metalloproteinases in cerebrovascular disease, J Cereb Blood Flow Metab 1998; 18: 1163-1172.
19. Peng KW, Morling FJ, Cosset FL, Murphy G, Russell SJ, A gene delivery system activatable by disease-associated matrix metalloproteinases. Hum Gene Ther 1997; 8:729-783.
20. Maysinger D, Morinville A, Drug delivery to the nervous system. Trends Biotechnol 1997;15: 410-418.
21. Imaizumi S, Woolworth V, Fishman RA, Chan PH, Liposome-entrapped superoxide dismutase reduces cerebral infarction in cerebral ischemia in rats. Stroke 1990; 21:1312-1317.

22. Stanimirovic DB, Markovic M, Micic DV, Spatz M, Mrsulja BB, Liposome-entrapped superoxide dismutase reduces ischemia/reperfusion oxidative stress in gerbil brain. Neurochem Res 1994; 19:1473-1478.

23. Khaw BA, Torchilin VP, Vural I, Narula J, Plug and seal: prevention of hypoxic cardiocyte death by sealing membrane lesions with antimyosin-liposomes. Nat Med 1995; 1:1195-1198.

24. Torchilin VP, Narula J, Halpern E, Khaw BA, Poly(ethylene glycol)-coated anti-cardiac myosin immunoliposome: factors influencing targeted accumulation in the infarcted myocardium. Biochim Biophys Acta 1996; 1279:75-83.

25. Glorioso, JC, Goins WF, Meaney CA, Fink DJ, DeLuca NA, Gene transfer to brain using herpes simplex virus vectors. Ann Neurol 1994; 35 Suppl: S28-S34.

26. Lawrence MS, Sun GH, Kunis DM, Saydam TC, Dash R, Ho DY, Sapolsky RM, Steinberg GK, Overexpression of the glucose transporter gene with a herpes simplex viral vestor protects striatal neurones against stroke. J Cereb Blood Flow Metab 1996; 16: 181-185.

27. Yenari MA, Minami M, Sun GH, Meier TJ, Kunis DM, McLauglin JR, Ho DY, Sapolsky RM, Steinberg GK, Calbindin d28k Over-expression protects striatal neurones from transient focal cerebral ischemia. Stroke 2001; 32: 1028-1035.

28. Hoehn B, Ringer, TM, WU L, Giffard RG, Sapolsky RM, Steinberg GK, Yenari MA, Overexpression of HSP72 after induction of experimental stroke protects neurones from ischemic damage. J. Cereb Blood Flow Metab. 2001; 21: 1303-1309.

29. Linnick MD, Zahos P, Geschwnd MD, Federhoff HJ, Expression of bcl-2 from a defective herpes simplex virus-1 vector limits neuronal death in focal cerebral ischemia. Stroke 1995; 26: 1670-1674.

30. Phillips RG, Lawrence MS, Ho DY, Sapolsky RM, Limitations in the neuroprotective potential of gene therapy with BCL-2. Brain Res 2000; 859: 202-206.

31. Schwarze SR, Ho A, Vocero-Akbani A, Dowdy SF, *In vivo* protein transduction: Delivery of a biologically active protein into the mouse. Science 1999; 285: 1569-1572.

32. Jansen EM, Solberg L, Underhill S, Wilson S, Cozzari C, Hartman BK, Faris PL, Low WC, Transplantation of fetal neocortex ameliorates sensorimotor and locomotor deficits following neonatal ischemic-hypoxic brain injury in rats. Exp Neurol 1997; 147: 487-497.

33. Li Y, Chen J, Chopp M, Adult bone marrow transplantation after stroke in adult rats. Cell Transplantation 2001; 10: 31-40.

34. Li Y, Chen J, Wang L, Lu M, Chopp M, Treatment of stroke in rat with intracarotid administration of marrow stromal cells. Neurology 2001; 56: 1666-1672.

35. Chen J, Li Y, Wang L, Zhang Z, Lu D, Lu M, Chopp M, Therapeutic benefit of intravenous administration of bone marrow stromal cells after cerebral ischemia in rats. Stroke 2001; 32: 1005-1011.

36. Chen J, Sanberg PR, Li Y, Wang L, Lu M, Willing AE, Sanchez-Ramos J, Chopp M, Intravenous administration of human umbilical cord blood reduces behavioral deficits after stroke in rats. Stroke 2001; 32: 2682-2688.

GLOSSARY

BBB, blood brain barrier: A tight, high-resistance lining of endothelial cells in the cerebral vasculature that lacks fenestrae and transcytotic vesicles and has specific molecular transporters that repel xenobiotics and many other molecules from the cells to blood. BBB restricts diffusion of molecules to the brain.

Direct drug delivery to the brain: An infusion of drugs directly into brain parenchyma using intrathecal catheters or via cerebral ventricles using cerebrospinal injection.

Ischemic penumbra: An area at risk surrounding zone of the primary ischemic necrosis in the brain.

19

TARGETING DRUGS INTO THE CENTRAL NERVOUS SYSTEM

Laszlo Prokai
Center for Drug Discovery and Department of Pharmaceutics, College of Pharmacy, and the McKnight Brain Institute, University of Florida, Gainesville, FL 32610-0497, USA

INTRODUCTION

Drugs face a formidable obstacle in reaching the central nervous systems (CNS) due to the existence and specific properties of the blood-brain barrier (BBB) that is a vital element in the regulation of the internal environment of the brain and the spinal cord. This chapter summarizes the principles and perspective of strategies that offer invasive and non-invasive approaches to overcome this major hurdle to the pharmacotherapy of the CNS.

THE BLOOD-BRAIN BARRIER

The schematic model for the cerebral microcirculation is shown in Figure 1 (1). The endothelium of the CNS (brain and spinal cord) vasculature exhibits structural differences from that of other organs, as highlighted in Figure 2.

Fenestrations between the vascular endothelial cells (which contribute to the exchange of water, nutrients and metabolites in most organs) are not found within the normal mammalian brain and spinal cord. The capillary endothelial cells of the brain feature tight junctions that abolish any aqueous paracellular pathways into the internal environment of the brain (2). Fluid-phase pinocytosis (a nonspecific, continuous process believed to be a general way of transporting macromolecular constructs through epithelia, into various blood cells and through some endothelia) is scant because endocytotic vesicles also are practically absent in the endothelial cells of the cerebral and spinal cord microvessels. Endocytotic vesicles also are practically absent in the endothelial cells of the cerebral microvessels. These properties of the CNS have led to the notion of blood-brain barrier (BBB).

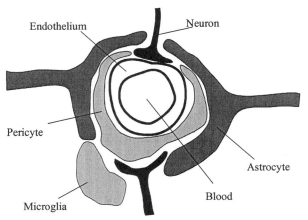

Figure 1. Cerebral microcirculation model. The capillary endothelium is endowed with tight junctions; endothelial cells share microvascular basement membrane with pericytes and astrocyte foot processes invest more than 90% of the capillaries. Neuronal endings also innervate brain endothelial cells directly and microglia are located in the vicinity of pericytes. (Reproduced from Reference 1 with permission of Birkhäuser, Basel.)

The BBB of the brain also has two major parts: endothelial (between blood and interstitial fluid) and ependymal (between blood and cerebrospinal fluid) (3). At the spinal cord, the BBB consists only of the endothelial barrier. Systemically injected molecules may reach the cellular elements of the tissue in the circumventricular organs (CVOs) of the brain, which are perfused by capillaries without endothelial tight junctions. However, the surface area of the BBB is about 5,000-fold greater than that of the CVOs (4) and the latter usually contributes to the overall drug transport into the CNS only to a negligible extent. Therefore, intracellular or transcellular transport (transport directly through the endothelial cell membrane) is the principal route into and out of the CNS.

The morphological component of the BBB is represented by the lumenal and antilumenal membranes of the endothelial cells (two plasma membranes in series) separated by 0.3 μm of endothelial cytosol. The BBB, thus, behaves as a continuous lipid bilayer and, as such, exhibits a low permeability to hydrophilic substances (ions and polar compounds) that do not have specific transport mechanisms. Passive transport (diffusion) of many drugs is restricted. The degree of restriction the BBB imposes on passive transport is variable and many lipid-insoluble drugs are effectively excluded from the CNS. However, lipid-soluble substances are generally transported across the BBB by diffusion (passive transport, mechanism A) as shown in Figure 3 below.

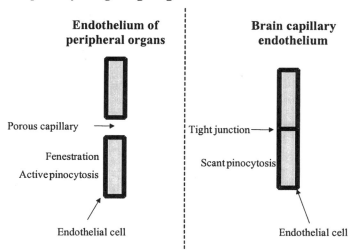

Figure 2. Illustration of the principal differences between peripheral vasculature and the capillary endothelium of the CNS (brain and spinal cord). (Reproduced from Reference 1 with permission of Birkhäuser, Basel.)

Specific transport mechanisms exist in the BBB to supply the CNS with polar nutrients such as essential amino acids and glucose (5). The amino acid transporters system-L and system-ASC are expressed in both the luminal and abluminal membranes of the endothelium and are principally directed from the blood to the endothelial cell and from the endothelial cell to the interstitial fluid of the CNS (mechanism B, Fig. 3). System-A is present on the abluminal membrane and is directed mainly out of the brain. These amino acid transporters are energy-dependent; system-ASC and system-A also are sodium-dependent. Glucose enters the brain via a facilitated carrier (GLUT-1) present in the endothelial cells. GLUT-1 is expressed at a relatively high level and it is insulin insensitive, but upregulated in chronic hypoglycemia and downregulated in chronic hyperglycemia. Carrier-mediated transport of several dipeptides and other small peptides (leucine, enkephalin, delta sleep-inducing factor, etc.) also occurs into the brain, and brain-to-blood carrier-mediated transport systems for small peptides have also been identified (6). Nonspecific, absorptive-mediated transcytosis (mechanism C, Fig. 3), where endocytosis is initiated by the binding of a polycationic substance on the plasma membrane, may also be involved in the BBB transport of peptides and proteins that have multiple positive charges under physiological conditions (1). Certain larger peptides and proteins (IGF-I, IGF-II, insulin and transferrin) are known to have receptors on the BBB. These receptors are identified on the luminal surface of the brain capillaries and may act as transcytosis systems (mechanism D, Fig. 3) because they are present both on luminal and antiluminal borders of the endothelial cells (7).

Besides the morphological elements, highly active enzymes present in the brain endothelial cells and in the cerebral pericytes represent a metabolic component that contributes to the homeostatic balance regulated by the BBB (8). Metabolically unstable substances may become rapidly degraded before reaching the CNS. For example, most peptides are metabolically unstable and attacked by highly active metabolizing enzymes in CNS compartments such as in the cytosolic endothelial space, the luminal surface of the endothelial cells, cerebral pericytes, and/or synaptic regions juxtaposed to the brain microvessels even if they have certain permeability across the BBB.

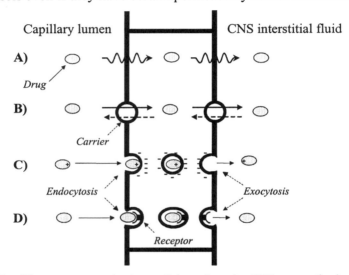

Figure 3. Possible transport mechanisms of drugs into the CNS across the brain capillary endothelial cells: A) Diffusion, when the molecule has adequate lipophilicity; B) carrier-mediated transport due to the presence of a transporter on the luminal and abluminal membrane; C) adsorptive-mediated transcytosis in which endocytosis is induced by non-specific binding to the membrane, and D) receptor-mediated transcytosis. (Adapted from Reference 1 with permission of Birkhäuser, Basel.)

The transmembrane glycoprotein known as the P-glycoprotein (P-gp) is also expressed in the BBB (9). This 170-kDa macromolecule is a member of the large ATP-binding cassette superfamily of transport proteins also called traffic ATPases. It is composed of two homologous halves, each containing six transmembrane domains and an ATP binding/utilization domain, separated by a flexible linker polypeptide, as shown schematically in Figure 4. ATP binding and hydrolysis appear to be essential for the proper functioning of P-gp, including drug transport. P-gp has been shown to operate as an active (ATP-dependent) efflux system, and it generally transports back into the blood a variety of lipophilic molecules that enter the endothelial cells or penetrate into the brain. The classical model confines P-gp in the brain microvasculature to the luminal membrane of the brain capillary endothelial cells, but a revised model localizing its presence to the astrocyte foot processes investing the brain microvascular endothelium (actually, behind the BBB) has also been proposed recently (10). Nevertheless, this membrane

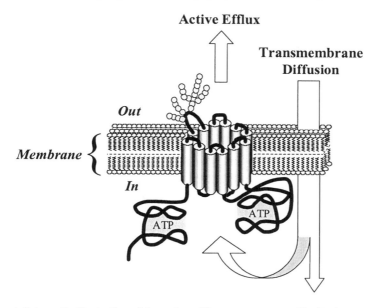

Figure 4. Schematic illustration of the active efflux process exerted by P-glycoprotein, which may reduce drug transport into the CNS.

glycoprotein is a functional part of the BBB because P-gp knock-out mice show enhanced sensitivity to circulating drugs and potential toxins that accumulate in the brain at higher-than-normal levels. Several other transporters such as the monocarboxylic acid transporter (MCT1) may also contribute to the exclusion of certain drugs from the CNS because they work in the CNS interstitial fluid to endothelial cell and/or endothelial cell to blood direction (5).

In summary, hydrophilic drugs do not cross the BBB in pharmacologically significant amount and various drugs are subject to active efflux processes that limit their transport into the CNS. Therefore, drug targeting to the CNS must be addressed. Delivery of a drug into the CNS is considered effective and efficient when the pharmacological effect of the compound is localized, stable for the duration of action, and a sustained and effective dose is achieved at the site of action. Various delivery strategies to achieve this aim have been developed, and they can be grouped into two general categories: invasive procedures and noninvasive methods. Invasive strategies go around the BBB or alter/modify the BBB to provide entry into the interstitial fluid compartment of the brain or spinal cord. Noninvasive techniques exploit various transport processes that exist in the brain capillary endothelium to ferry therapeutic agents into the CNS after systemic administration.

INVASIVE STRATEGIES

Direct delivery to the tissue

Injection directly into the brain has been suggested for avoiding problems associated with systemic delivery of biologically active substances. Lumbar punctures, Ommaya reservoir for intracerebroventricular (ICV) injections, and epidural catheter systems are being used clinically for delivery of anesthetics and narcotics, but frequent multiple injections may be necessary to maintain therapeutic drug concentrations. Thus, they are associated with increased risk of infections and uncomfortable for the patients. Implanted infusion pumps that deliver drugs through an ICV or intrathecal (IT) catheter have been evaluated. For intrathecal (IT) delivery, infusion pumps are simple to implant and remove under local anesthesia and are safe, reliable, and tolerated well by patients (11). For example, predictable steady-state CSF levels of thyrotropin-releasing hormone (TRH) were produced in a clinical trial, avoiding peaks and troughs of parenteral dosing, and also resulted in considerable savings in drug expenses. However, the same symptoms of shivering, chills, and bladder fullness were noted during a 6-h infusion into the CNS as during intravenous (IV) infusion of TRH. A rapid appearance of intaventricularly administered peptides in the systemic circulation also has been shown in animal studies (12).

Limitations of ICV or IT delivery into the CNS are considerable. The diffusion in the brain is limited by the decreased extracellular space, by physical barriers such as synaptic regions protected by ensheathing glial processes, by many catabolizing enzymes, high- and low-affinity uptake sites that reduce extracellular concentrations. The continuous production of CSF constructs a 'sink' for the injected agent, and the existence of brain-to-blood active transport systems has been revealed for certain peptides. Low diffusion coefficients that result in steep concentration between the parenchyma and the ependymal surface has been revealed upon ICV or IT administration of high molecular weight agents such as peptides which would allow for delivery of the compound only to the surface of the brain (1). This may be beneficial when target receptors are found on the surface, but is a poor mode of delivery to the brain parenchyma.

Controlled-release polymer implants can deliver drugs directly to brain tissue (13). Bioerodible polymer implants, containing poly(1,3-pcarboxyphenoxypropane-sebacic acid) and poly(fatty acid dimer-sebacic acid) matrices, have been biocompatible for CNS application (14). A nondegradable poly(ethylene-co-vinyl acetate) matrix has been evaluated for potential direct CNS-delivery of nerve-growth factor (NGF) (15). Nondegradable polymer implants can be recovered from the site of implantation, if necessary, have no toxic degradation products to distribute, and may release the protein on a longer time-scale than degradable polymers. Biodegradable microspheres (16) and multivesicular liposomes (17) have been suggested for direct CNS-delivery.

An invasive method has also been developed that relies on CNS-implantation of cells supported in a cross-linked hydrophilic polymer (hydrogel) and encapsulated by a semipermeable matrix. This minimizes deleterious effects of the host's immune system on the cells within the capsule to produce specific peptides and proteins (opioid peptides, NGF, etc.) genetically at their intended site of action (18).

Altering the blood-brain barrier

Another invasive method relies on a reversible BBB disruption (19). Intracarotid infusion of hypertonic solutions of mannitol, arabinose, lactamide, saline, urea, glycerol and radiographic contrast agents causes vasodilation and shrinks the brain capillary endothelial cells resulting in transient opening of the tight junctions to an estimated 200 Å in radius. This allows for the transport of molecules that otherwise cannot cross the BBB. The effect may be facilitated by calcium-mediated contraction of the endothelial cytoskeleton. Increased permeability to intravascular small molecules, large biomolecules, and even virus-sized iron oxide particles is experienced transiently following infusion of hypertonic mannitol, after which it returns to pre-infusion levels within 2 h. The marked increase in BBB permeability is due to both increased diffusion and bulk fluid flow across the transiently opened junctions of the endothelial cells. Thus far, osmotic modification of the BBB has been employed most commonly as a method for improving brain-tumor chemotherapy. However, the considerable toxic effects of osmotic BBB opening should be taken into account; it can lead to inflammation, encephalitis, and seizures (as high as 20% of the applications). In experimental animals, the osmotic method has been used to provide access to the brain of water-soluble drugs, peptides, antibodies, boron compounds for neutron-capture therapy, and viral vectors for gene therapy.

Internal carotid artery infusion of bradykinin also causes extensive breakdown of the BBB and an intense increase in the number of pinocytotic vesicles in the permeable segments, but no change in the interendothelial junctions (20). Various synthetic analogues of bradykinin may be promising candidates for various parenteral and nonparenteral routes of administration because of their increased metabolic stability. Passage of neuropharmaceutical agents into abnormal brain tissue without increasing the permeability of the normal BBB has also been indicated upon intracarotid infusion of low doses of bradykinin. However, repeated BBB breakdown carries the risk of undesirable influx of blood constituents such as serum proteins into the interstitial fluid of the CNS, which may induce neuropathological events.

In conclusion, invasive procedures are only justified for life-threatening CNS maladies such as brain cancer, but these (often costly) surgical routes are not preferred for less dramatic illnesses.

NON-INVASIVE METHODS

Modifying Physicochemical Properties of Drugs to Enhance Transport

Diffusion (passive transport) into the CNS is governed primarily by the lipid-solubility of the drug. Hydrophobic substances, because of their high lipid solubility, can generally diffuse freely across the BBB. However, partitioning between n-octanol and water (expressed as the logarithm of the partition coefficient (logP) which is generally considered the measure of lipophilicity) alone may be a poor indicator of the drug's ability to penetrate the BBB. Additional factors should often be considered (21). The increase in dipole moment, polarizability, and hydrogen-bonding capacity tends to reduce, while the increase of molar refractivity and molecular size generally tends to augment a drug's BBB permeability. In turn, size exclusion may hinder BBB transport, and is considered by some researchers a confining factor in the transport of large lipophilic molecules. No consensus exists regarding the limit of the molecular size that may prevent passive transport. Nevertheless, encapsulating a drug in liposomes results in no measurable transport across the BBB, although liposomes may be taken up by cells lining the reticuloendothelial system of liver and spleen (22).

Improving transport properties of drugs through chemical modification generally targets an improvement of lipid solubility. The objective of these approaches is to turn water-soluble substances into lipid-soluble ones by chemical modifications that thereby increase passive transport across biological membranes. However, P-gp-mediated efflux may be involved in restricting the access of various lipophilic drugs (cyclosporin A, doxorubicin, phenytoin, etc.) to the brain. Competitive inhibition of this outwardly directed active transport mechanism and ATP-depletion (because P-gp-mediated transport requires ATP) can significantly increase the accumulation of these drugs within the CNS (5). Thus, saturation of the efflux pump by co-administration of a P-gp inhibitor with the therapeutic agent may be an approach to improve CNS delivery. One of the confounding factors is the extremely high total capacity of the efflux system, which may require toxic concentrations of currently available inhibitors to be effective *in vivo*. A new generation of inhibitors with reduced toxicity or the use of an inhibitor cocktail (in which the respective concentration of the individual components does not reach toxic levels) would be required for potential clinical applications of this strategy. On the other hand, P-gp and related active efflux systems are part of the BBB with essential protective function(s). Their inhibition will prevent them from providing protection to the CNS and the safety of the strategy to exploit them for enhanced brain targeting can be of concern.

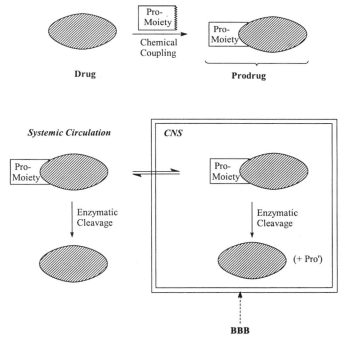

Figure 5. The pro-drug approach to improve drug access to the CNS.

In pro-drug approaches shown schematically in Figure 5, generally lipophilic drug derivatives are synthesized (23). Because of its increased lipid-solubility, the pro-drug may penetrate biological membranes (including the BBB) and may reach organs (including the brain and spinal cord) that are otherwise inaccessible to the non-modified compound. Enzymatic or chemical transformation then converts the inactive pro-drug to the pharmacologically active species in the CNS. Pro-drugs are often designed to limit metabolism of the parent molecule. In addition, the approach to enhance the CNS-access of therapeutic agents that are substrates to P-gp may involve pro-moieties whose attachment reduces affinity to the efflux system.

Although the acquired lipophilicity through chemical modifications or pro-drug creation may assure penetration to the BBB (and to other membranes), this is not the sole factor to be considered in the transportability of drugs into the CNS. The enzymatic degradation and the consequent attenuation or loss of biological activity should also be prevented during the passage of the substance from the general circulation to the brain tissue. In addition, lipid-soluble pro-drugs that can cross the BBB will only sustain active concentrations in the CNS if their blood concentrations are maintained at adequately high levels. In other words, efflux from the CNS by passive transport is not prevented.

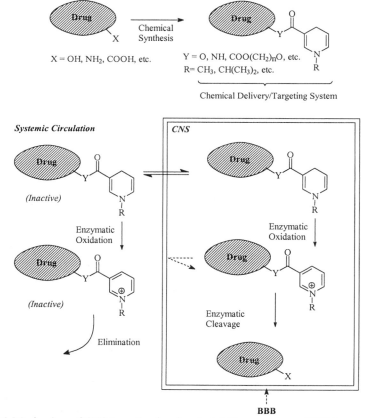

Figure 6. Mechanism of CNS targeting by chemical delivery systems (CDSs).

The chemical delivery system (CDS) strategy (24) is an extension of a simple pro-drug approach in which a specific pro-moiety is attached to the drug, as shown in Figure 6 above. The attachment of 1,4-dihydrotrigonellyl or other suitable redox functional group as a pro-moiety provides not only an increase in lipid solubility, but also promotes retention in the CNS. This is due to an *in situ* metabolic conversion of the non-ionic dihydropyridine to a membrane-impermeable pyridinium ion as an intermediate before the release of the active agent. Essentially, it is a "pro-pro-drug" approach.

The oxidative conversion of a dihydropiridine to pyridinium occurs ubiquitously and it is analogous to the oxidation of NAD(P)H, a coenzyme associated with many oxidoreductases and cellular respiration. Any of the oxidized form in the periphery will be rapidly lost as it is now polar and an excellent candidate for elimination by the kidney and bile. Thus, concentration of the active drug should remain low in the periphery, which reduces systemic, dose-related toxicities. Therefore, the CDS strategy is designed to function as a targeting system, because a preferential delivery of the active agent to the CNS versus the rest of the body may be achieved. Additional metabolic process (or processes) achieves a controlled, post-delivery release of the drug. The attachment of the redox moiety alone may result in brain targeting of small molecules such as dopamine; CDSs designed to deliver peptides to the CNS require additional structural modifications. Finally, the CNS-retained compounds are designed to release the active compound through subsequent metabolic processes (usually enzymatic hydrolysis) in a sustained manner.

Representative examples to the brain-enhanced delivery by this redox brain-targeting approach include steroids, neurotransmitters, anticonvulsants, antibiotics, antiviral, anticancer and antidementia agents, neuropeptides and their analogues (24). The efficacy of CDSs varies according to the structural complexity and size of the therapeutic agent concerned and may increase the access of drugs to the CNS significantly (>1% of the injected dose in experimental animals). *In vivo* and *in vitro* studies and preliminary clinical data of several novel derivatives have been promising, which could lead to a practical use of the redox chemical delivery systems after proper pharmaceutical development. The conceptual success of the strategy accentuates the need for considering physicochemical, metabolic and pharmacokinetic properties in designing of carrier systems that are able to target drugs into the CNS.

Strategies Based on Biological Carriers

Another approach of CNS delivery of drugs may rely on specific transport systems existing in the BBB. The plausible method of designing drug conjugates that exploit carrier-mediated uptake mechanisms present in the endothelial cells of the CNS vasculature for specific biomolecules (Fig. 3, process B) suffers from a critical kinetic feature of these systems; they are often of low capacity, albeit of high affinity. Besides, current knowledge about the structural requirement of a drug capable of fully utilizing these specific transporters is limited. Efforts to exploit biological carriers have, thus, concentrated on auxiliary transport systems. The target molecule is linked to the carrier, so that the conjugate may cross the BBB by carrier-, adsorptive- or receptor-mediated transport (Fig. 3, mechanism B-D). Upon reaching the CNS, the conjugate may interact with the cognate receptor of the drug as an analogue (no separation from the transporter required), or may be enzymatically cleaved to release the therapeutic agent at the site of action (i.e., the conjugate functions as a pro-drug).

The glucose carrier GLUT-1 of the BBB endothelial cells has very large capacity to transport β-D-glucose into the CNS. L-serinyl-β-D-glycoside analogues of peptides have shown to reach the CNS in pharmacologically significant amount after intraperitoneal administration of relatively large doses to produce dose-related CNS-action in animal models; the corresponding non-glycosylated analogues did not have CNS-activity (25). These glycopeptides have reduced lipophilicity compared to the L-serinyl analogues, which indicates their entry into the CNS via a mechanism other than diffusion. The brain transport via GLUT-1 appears to be specific for 3-O-linked glycosides, and not for -linked or N-linked glycosides. To take advantage of carbohydrate recognition and transport processes to deliver drugs into the brain, structural modification of a lead compound to include the appropriate functional groups must be made while paying attention that CNS-activity and/or desired receptor selectivity are preserved. Other biological carriers exploiting transporters for essential nutrients or vitamins (mechanism B, Fig. 3) have also been employed (6).

Strategies that utilize adsorptive-mediated transcytosis (mechanism C, Fig. 3) are based on cationic proteins or peptides as "vectors" to cross the BBB. Cationized albumin has been suggested as a transport vector, but it is more efficiently extracted from the blood by the kidney than by the brain. Protein cationization may also increase immunogenicity. To overcome this problem, the use of peptide vectors has been suggested (26). Pegelin and penetratin peptides efficiently translocate through biological membranes and they provide the basis for the development of the strategy. Pegelin peptides such as SynB1 (RGGRLSYSRRRFSTSTGR) are obtained by replacing disulfide-bridge-forming cysteine residues with serines (S) to remove the cytolytic effect of the natural protegrins. Penetratin peptides are derived from the transcription factor antennapedia. The all D-amino acid analogue of the third helix from antennapedia (rqikiwfqnrrmkwkk; D-penetratin) is also transported across the BBB by adsorptive-mediated transcytosis. Covalent coupling of doxorubicin (which is subject to P-gp-mediated efflux) through an appropriate chemical linker to these peptide vectors resulted in a 6- to 20-fold increase (depending on the experimental technique used) in the brain uptake/transport compared to the "vectorized" drug in experimental animals. The conjugated doxorubicin apparently bypassed P-gp upon its transport into the CNS. After administration, the conjugate behaved as a pro-drug (Fig. 5) by releasing doxorubicin, although this release was not site (brain) specific. On the other hand, a significant decrease in the drug concentration in the heart pointed to the existence of a targeting mechanism upon using this strategy. Despite these promising advantages, the peptide-vector method faces obstacles in acceptance as a practical approach, partly due to difficulties in peptide manufacture and in conjugation chemistry.

The observed paucity of endocytotic activity of the brain capillary endothelium does not imply the complete lack of various transcytosis mechanisms, but points to their rather low capacity. (In comparison, the capacity of receptor-mediated transcytosis is by far smaller than that of a typical adsorptive-mediated process). Nevertheless, CNS-targeting methods that rely on the existence of such systems (mechanism D, Fig 3.) for various large peptides and proteins in the BBB have been developed (27). This method based on the coupling of the drug that is not normally transported through the BBB to protein vectors that undergo receptor-mediated transcytosis. These so-called chimeric peptides may then be transported through the BBB via these vectors into the brain. Potential therapeutic peptides have been the typical targets for CNS-delivery by this strategy. After entering the brain interstitial space, the biologically active peptide interacts with its cognate CNS-receptor to initiate pharmacological action while still attached to the chimeric peptide itself or its release from the conjugate. Design considerations in the development of effective chimeric peptides include vector specificity for the brain, vector pharmacokinetics, coupling between vector and peptide, cleavability of the vector-peptide linkage (if necessary), and intrinsic receptor affinity for the peptide released from the transport vector.

Receptor ligands such as insulin and insulin fragment, IGF and transferrin are, however, not CNS-specific; uptake by non-neural cells or by cells outside the CNS also has been revealed. Competing serum transferrin also inhibits the transport of radiolabeled tranferrin. Besides, the affinity of the chimeric peptide for the receptor is consistently 1 to 2 log orders lower than it is for the native peptide, which may result in a limited endocytosis of the chimeric peptide. The use of native peptides or proteins as vectors has often limited by their very rapid clearance from the bloodstream. Recently, anti-transferrin receptor (OX26) and anti-insulin (Mab83-7 and Mab83-14) receptor antibodies have been proposed as efficient and selective BBB transport vectors. Overall, receptor-specific antibodies have been proposed to be better delivery vectors than cationic proteins because they have higher BBB permeability–surface (P·S) products. The coupling of a therapeutic protein or peptide to transport vectors has been achieved by covalent chemical conjugation that targets surface amino, carboxyl, or thiol groups in proteins, as exemplified in Figure 7.

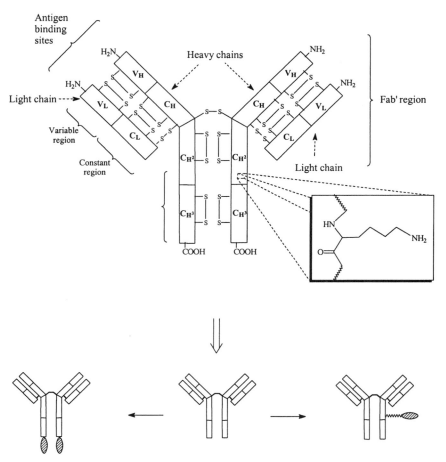

Figure 7. The schematic structure of an antibody, such as OX26, raised against BBB transferrin and illustration of possible covalent linking of therapeutic agents (represented by the shaded ovals) to this carrier macromolecule. (Adapted from Reference 1 with permission of Birkhäuser, Basel.)

Cross-linking reactions may, however, proceed with unsatisfactory (10-15%) yields. High-affinity non-covalent binding of the biotinylated peptide to an avidin/vector covalent conjugate has also been developed to overcome this shortcoming. In this avidin-biotin method, first neutral avidin is covalently attached to the vector, for example, by a thiol-ether linkage to the ε-amino groups of lysine residues of the protein. Avidin is an avian protein that binds biotin with extremely high affinity (dissociation constant of about 10^{-15} M and half-time of 89 days). Then, a biotinylated agent is used to attach the therapeutic molecule to the avidin/vector conjugate. The target therapeutic peptide must be monobiotinylated to prevent the formation of high molecular weight aggregates because of the multiple binding sites for biotin in avidin. The use of the neutral form of avidin (streptavidin) is recommended to prevent rapid removal from blood after IV injection. Monobiotinylated peptides conjugated to OX26/streptavidin with a noncleavable amide linker have shown about 10-fold increase of brain uptake upon IV injection compared to the unconjugated peptide, but only reached about 0.1% uptake (of the injected dose)/g brain.

Although certain chimeric peptides may retain full biological activity of the therapeutic agent, its release from the transport vector to receptor sites within the CNS is necessary to produce pharmacological activity. However, cleavage of a disulfide-bound in a chimeric peptide may not to yield a biologically inactive peptide as a product. A pharmacologically active, biotinylated thiol derivative of a metabolically stable peptide analogue has been proposed as an ideal candidate for incorporation into a disulfide-linked chimeric peptide based on the avidin-biotin binding strategy. Enzymatic reduction of the disulfide bond is presumed to take place in the brain to yield a desbio-analogue that is the pharmacologically active species. Nevertheless, the fraction of administered dose of the chimeric peptide entering the brain tissue beyond the BBB has shown a moderate (two- to three-fold) increase upon intracarotid infusion of the avidin complex of a biotinylated peptide analogue when compared to the peptide analogue injected without the transport vector. A noninvasive administration such as IV injection may result in a significantly less efficient delivery.

The concept of brain delivery by immunoliposomes was also developed based on the principle of receptor-mediated transcytosis. The drug is packaged in the interior of neutral liposomes, which are stabilized for *in vivo* use by surface conjugation with polyethyleglycol (PEG). The tips of about 1% of the PEG strands are attached to the targeting monoclonal antibody such as OX26 to ferry the liposome carrying the drug across the biological barriers of the brain, but also to other organs. For example, a widespread expression of an exogenous gene in brain and peripheral tissues was induced with a single intravenous administration of plasmid DNA packaged in the interior of PEGylated immunoliposomes (28).

Several serious drawbacks may arise from an antibody-based transport approach. The poor stoichiometry of the cargo to the carrier molecule limits the mass transport even of a large peptide. (Relative to the entire avidin/vector-peptide conjugate, a large peptide such as a biotinylated

VIPa in a chimeric peptide represents less than 3% of conjugate's molecular mass.) In rats, less than 2 pmol of about 500 pmol of the usually injected dose reaches the brain based on the reported data. Injecting larger doses can hardly increase this quantity, because carrier- or receptor-mediated cellular transport has physiologically limited transported capacity (saturation) that may prevent pharmacologically significant amounts from entering the brain for most therapeutic peptides or drugs. The low amount delivered to the CNS stresses the need for extremely potent therapeutic agent. This objective has not been met by specifically developed and CNS-cleavable chimeric peptides with pharmacological activity demonstrated at or above 100 pmol quantities injected ICV. Other strict requirements, such as monobiotinylation of the therapeutic peptide, *in vivo* cleavability of the linker and retention of biological activity after release, make this method very restrictive. Already discovered and potentially useful CNS-agents have to be radically redesigned to incorporate them into chimeric peptides for CNS-delivery by this strategy.

Another method to overcome the BBB in delivering drugs to the CNS is based on the use of nanoparticles (29). Although the mechanism of nanoparticle-mediated transport is not fully understood, the most likely mechanism involves endocytosis by the brain capillary endothelial cells. The method relies on the coating the surface of 200- to 300-nm poly(butylcyanoacrylate) particles with nonionic (polysorbate-type) surfactants. Polysorbate-coated nanoparticles mimic low-density lipoprotein (LDL) particles and can bind to LDL receptors expressed in the endothelial cells. This binding may eventually induce endocytosis (mechanism D, Fig. 3). A subsequent exocytosis or drug release in the endothelial cells followed by diffusion into the interstitial fluid may be responsible for the transport of therapeutic agents into the interstitial fluid of the CNS. However, the high systemic nanoparticle concentrations necessary to achieve the delivery of pharmacologically significant amount of drug into the brain are accompanied by toxicity that limits the therapeutic usefulness of this approach (30).

CONCLUSION

Various ways of drug delivery into the CNS by invasive procedures and noninvasive techniques have been conceived to overcome the major obstacle — the BBB. However, much remains to be learned about their merits and limitations before their promise to target drugs safely and efficiently into the brain and spinal cord can be realized. However, progress is steady which clearly warrants continued exploration and development of the methods outlined in this chapter.

ACKNOWLEDGEMENT

The author wishes to acknowledge support of his research in the area of brain drug targeting, in part, by grants from the National Institute on Mental Health (MH59380) and the National Institute on Aging (AG10485).

REFERENCES

1. Prokai, Laszlo. "Peptide drug delivery into the central nervous system." In *Progress in Drug Research,* Vol. 51, E.M. Jucker, ed. Basel: Birkhäuser, 1998.
2. Brightman, Milton W. "Ultrastructure of brain endothelium," In *Physiology and Pharmacology of the Blood-Brain Barrier,* Michael W.B. Bradbury, ed. Berlin: Springer-Verlag, 1992.
3. Davson, H., Welch, K., Segal, M.B., *The Physiology and Pathophysiology of the Cerebrospinal Fluid,* Edinburgh, UK: Churchill Livingstone, 1987; pp. 105-118.
4. Crone, Christian. "The blood-brain barrier - facts and questions." In *Ion Homeostasis of the Brain,* B.K. Siesjo, S.C. Sorensen, eds. Copenhagen: Munksgaard, 1971.
5. Tamai, I., Tsuji, A. Transporter-mediated permeation of drugs across the blood-brain barrier. J Pharm Sci 2000; 89:1371-1388.
6. Maness, L.M., Banks, W.A., Zadina, J.E., Kastin, A.J. Periventricular penetration and disappearance of ICV Tyr-MIF-1, DAMGO, tyrosine, and albumin. Peptides 1995; 17:247-250.
7. Pardridge, William M. Receptor-mediated peptide transport through the blood-brain barrier. Endocrine Rev 1986; 7:314-330.
8. Brownlees, J., Williams, C.H. Peptidases, peptides, and the mammalian blood-brain barrier. J Neurochem 1993; 60:793-803.
9. Tatsuta, T., Naito, M., Oh-Hara, T., Sugawara, I., Tsuruo, T. Functional involvement of P-glycoprotein in blood-brain barrier. J Biol Chem 1992; 28: 20383-20391.
10. Golden, P.L., Pardridge, W.M. Brain microvascular P-glycoprotein and a revised model of multidrug resistance in brain. Cell Mol Neurobiol 2000; 20: 165-81
11. Munsat, T.L., Taft, J., Jackson, I.M.D., Andres, P.L., Hollander, D., Skerry, L., Ordman, M., Kasdon, D., Finison, L. Intrathecal thyrotropin-releasing hormone does not alter the progressive course of ALS: Experience with an intrathecal drug delivery system. Neurology 1992; 42: 1049-1053.
12. Passaro, E., Jr., Debas, H., Oldendorf, W., Yamada, T. Rapid appearance of intraventricularly administered neuropeptides in the peripheral circulation. Brain Res 1982; 241:335-340.
13. Domb, A.J., Ringel, I. Polymeric drug carrier systems in the brain. Methods Neurosci 1994; 21:169-183.
14. Brem, J., Domb, A.J., Lenartz, D., Dureza, C., Olivi, A., Epstein, J.I. Brain biocompatibility of a biodegradable controlled release polymer consisting of anhydride copolymer of fatty acid dimer and sebacic acid. J Controlled Release 1992; 19:325-329.
15. Krewson, C.E., Saltzman, M. W. "Targeting of proteins in the brain following release from a polymer." In *Trends and Future Perspectives in Peptide and Protein Drug Delivery,* V.H.L. Lee, M. Hashida, Y. Mizushima, eds. Chur (Switzerland): Harwood Academic Publishers, 1995.
16. Mendez, A., Camarata, P.J., Suryanarayanan, R., Ebner, T.J. Sustained intracerebral delivery of nerve growth factor with biodegradable polymer microspheres. Methods Neurosci 1994; 21:150-168.

17. Bonetti, A., Kim, S. Pharmacokinetics of an extended-release human interferon alpha-2b formulation. Cancer Chemother Pharmacol 1993; 33:258-261.

18. Lysaght, M.J., Frydel, B., Gentile, F., Emerich, D., Winn, S. Recent progress in immunoisolated cell therapy. J Cell Biochem 1994; 196-203.

19. Rapoport, Stanley I. Osmotic opening of the blood-brain barrier: Principles, mechanism, and therapeutic applications. Cell Mol Neurobiol 2000; 20:217-30.

20. Raymond, J.J., Robertson, D.M., Dinsdale, H.B. Pharmacological modification of bradykinin induced breakdown of the blood-brain barrier. Can J Neurol Sci 1986; 13:214-220.

21. Habgood, M.D., Begley, D.J., Abbott, N.J. Determinants of passive drug entry into the central nervous system. Cell Mol Neurobiol 2000; 20: 231-253.

22. Patel, Harish M. Liposomes: bags of challenge. Biochem Soc Trans 1984; 12:333-335.

23. Bundgaard, Hans, *Design of Pro-drugs.* Amsterdam: Elsevier, 1985.

24. Prokai, L., Prokai-Tatrai, K., Bodor, N. Targeting drugs to the brain by redox chemical delivery systems. Med Res Rev 2000; 20:367-416.

25. Polt, R., Porreca, F., Szabó, L.Z., Bilsky, E.J., Davis, P., Abbruscato, T.J., Davis, T.P., Horvath, R., Yamamura, H.I., Hruby, V.J. Glycopeptide enkephalin analogs produce analgesia in mice - evidence for penetration of the blood-brain-barrier. Proc Natl Acad Sci USA 1994; 91:7114-7118.

26. Rousselle, C., Clair, P., Lefauconnier, J.-M., Kaczorek, M., Scherrmann, J.-M., Temsamani, J. New advances in the transport of doxorubicin through the blood-brain barrier by a peptide vector-mediated strategy. Mol Pharmacol 2000; 57: 679-686.

27. Pardridge, William M. Vector-mediated drug delivery to the brain. Adv Drug Deliv Rev. 1999; 36:299-321.

28. Shi, N.Y., Boado, R.J., Pardridge, W.M. Receptor-mediated gene targeting to tissues *in vivo* following intravenous administration of pegylated immunoliposomes. Pharm Res 2001; 18:1091-1095.

29. Kreuter, Jörg. Nanoparticulate systems for brain delivery of drugs. Adv Drug Deliv Rev 2001; 47:65-81.

30. Olivier, J.-C., Fenart, L., Chauvert, R., Pariat, C., Cecchelli, R., Couet, W. Indirect evidence that drug brain targeting using polysorbate 80-coated polybutylcyanoacrylate nanoparticles is related to toxicity. Pharm Res 1999; 16:1836-1842.

GLOSSARY

Active efflux (P-glycoprotein): A variety of (lipophilic) molecules that enter the endothelial cells or penetrate into the brain. Transports back into the blood via the ATP-dependent transmembrane glycoprotein known as the P-glycoprotein (P-gp).

Adsorptive-mediated transcytosis: A transport process initiated by endocytosis via non-specific binding to the (luminal) membrane.

Blood-brain barrier (BBB): Morphological, metabolic and active-efflux components of the brain microcapillary endothelial cells, which prevents transport of molecules present in the systemic circulation into the interstitial fluid of the central nervous system; a vital element in the regulation of the internal environment of the brain and the spinal cord.

Carrier-mediated transport: Entry into the central nervous system via a transporter (protein) expressed on the luminal and abluminal membrane of the brain capillary endothelial cells.

Cerebral microcirculation: Blood vessels that infuse the brain.

Diffusion: Transport process ("passive") initiated by a concentration gradient (difference).

Endothelial cells (brain capillary): Part of the vascular system of the brain and spinal cord featuring tight junctions that abolish paracellular pathways into the internal environment of the central nervous system.

Invasive strategies: Injection into the central nervous system via surgical bypassing of the blood-brain barrier, or by opening the tight junctions of the endothelial cells.

Nanoparticle: Particle with diameter of less than 1-μm.

Pro-drug: An inactive derivative that is converted to an active drug *in vivo*.

Receptor-mediated transcytosis: Transport process initiated by binding to a specific receptor expressed on the (luminal) surface of the endothelium.

SECTION 5:

MISCELLANEOUS,
NEW HORIZONS IN TARGETING

20

STRATEGIES FOR TARGETING INFECTION

John W. Babich, Ph.D.
Biostream, Inc., Cambridge, Massachusetts

INTRODUCTION

Currently the need to target infection has been driven by the need to visualize inflammation and infection in patients who do not present clinically with localizing symptoms. In this case, identification of site and causative agent is a critical step in implementing appropriate medical treatment. This is particularly critical in immune compromised patients, since signs and symptoms of infection may be minimized in patients with neutropenia (1). This review will focus on the targeted visualization of infection and inflammation, although such targeting may likely play a role in the delivery of therapeutic agents in the future.

The body's response to tissue injury, regardless of cause or anatomical site, results in a complex series of physiologic changes that we recognize as the inflammatory response. The classical physical findings of inflammation, which were described at the time of Hippocrates, are dolor (pain), rubor (redness), calor (heat), tumor (swelling), and loss of function (functio laesa). The latter was added by Virchow centuries later.

The ability to localize infection is dependent on how conspicuous the various tissue changes are which accompany the host response to infectious insult. Generally speaking, the classic signs of inflammation can be exploited to help localize injury at superficial sites or in the extremities. In deeper internal structures such as in the abdomen, brain and chest, inflammation can be difficult to localize without additional diagnostic procedures. Medical imaging procedures that allow visualization of deep structures in the body can be used to detect the presence of inflammation. Magnetic resonance imaging (MRI), X-ray computed tomography (CT) and ultrasound (US) can localize the area of inflammation only when the lesion has progressed to the stage of tissue necrosis and abscess formation. However, early in the course of this process, when tissue changes associated with necrosis have not yet occurred, lesion localization may be extremely difficult. Targeted imaging agents become an important means of enhancing the visualization of inflammation prior to the development of anatomically distinct changes. Of the currently available imaging techniques, nuclear medicine procedures could be said to be superior to X-ray CT and magnetic resonance imaging (MRI) for whole-body surveys. It is likely that the ability to visualize infected tissue spurred development of numerous radiopharmaceuticals.

A variety of approaches for localizing sites of inflammation have been developed. New approaches are being investigated with the hope of developing agents with increased sensitivity and specificity, as well as speed of detection. These approaches have attempted to exploit various components, both biochemical and physiological, which are present in the inflammatory process. Such approaches have included: (a) the targeting of receptors present on cells involved in the inflammatory process, (b) labeling of constituents of the protein pool which are available to enter the inflamed tissue as exudate due to increased vascular stasis and pressure and (c) using labeled blood cells or pseudo-cell macroparticulates, such as liposomes, which are eventually attracted to the site of infection by chemical or mechanical factors.

Clinical imaging makes use of the following radiopharmaceuticals for infection/inflammation imaging: ^{67}Ga-citrate (2), ^{111}In-labeled leukocytes (3), ^{99m}Tc-labeled leukocytes (4), ^{111}In-labeled human polyclonal IgG (5), and anti-leukocyte monoclonal antibodies (6). In order to appreciate why each of these radiopharmaceuticals localizes at sites of infection/inflammation, it is important to understand the underlying pathophysiology of inflammation. As we shall see, each infection/inflammation imaging agent relies on one or more attributes of the inflammatory response in order to accumulate at the site of infection.

PATHOPHYSIOLOGY OF INFLAMMATION

The main purpose of inflammation appears to be to minimize tissue damage and defend against invaders by bringing fluid, proteins, and cells from the blood into the insulted tissues. The main features of the inflammatory response are: (a) vasodilation, i.e., widening of the blood vessels to increase the blood flow to the infected area; (b) increased vascular permeability, which allows diffusible components to enter the site of insult; and (c) cellular infiltration by the chemically directed movement (chemotaxis) of inflammatory cells through the walls of blood vessels into the site of injury. In reviewing the various approaches to infection imaging, it is clear that these three findings represent gross pathological changes that have been exploited to create methods of detection.

The influx of neutrophils, which are antigen non-specific, is one of the earliest stages of the inflammatory response. These cells mount a rapid, non-specific phagocytic response. Hence, neutrophils are a primary target for imaging. Following the infiltration of neutrophils is the recruitment of more antigen specific cells and cells that can provide further regulation of the immune response. These include monocyte-macrophages and lymphocytes (specific T-cell and B-cell lymphocytes). These cells, once activated, produce molecules that modulate further the immune response.

Table 1. Examples of major pro-inflammatory biomolecules

Endogenous	Receptor binding affinity	
Interleukin 1	3-8	pM
Interleukin 2	10	pM
Interleukin 8	0.3 - 4	nM
Platelet factor 4	5	nM
Tuftsin	-	
Complement (C5a)	1-2	nM
Leukotriene B4	0.46	nM
Exogenous		
Bacterial chemotactic peptide	10-30	nM

The infiltrating cells express on their surfaces an increasing number of receptors, as well as glycoproteins known as cell adhesion molecules. Activated endothelial cells of the vasculature attract and slow down white blood cells in circulation by expressing receptors for the cell adhesion molecules as well as other receptors. This recruitment at the site of activated vasculature is a critical step required for the subsequent extravascular migration of these cells into the inflamed tissue.

Cellular influx to inflammatory sites is orchestrated by a large number of mediator substances. These mediators are found in the serum or tissue fluids, released by degranulating cells, and also secreted by activated inflammatory cells, or activated endothelial cells in blood vessels at the site of inflammation. Evolution has further allowed for the host to respond directly to invading microorganisms. Bacterial by-products such as N-formylated peptides also act as chemoattractants for leukocytes which possess high affinity receptors for these peptides on their surfaces. These peptides and proteins serve as muscle-active and edema-promoting substances, chemotaxins, cellular activators, and inducers of all kinds of effector cells engaged in the inflammatory response.

Inflammatory mediators include compounds such as anaphylatoxins of the complement cascade (C5a), kinins of the coagulation system, leukotriens, prostaglandins (LTB4), and many other lipid mediators. Another group of mediators is neuropeptides, such as tachykinins, vasoactive intestinal peptide and vascular permeability factor. These substances enhance capillary permeability and have vasodilatatory and bronchoconstrictory activity.

A number of cytokines, known collectively as pro-inflammatory cytokines because they accelerate inflammation, also regulate inflammatory reactions either directly or by their ability to induce the synthesis of cellular adhesion molecules or other cytokines in certain cell types. Cytokines are a unique family of growth factors. Secreted primarily from leukocytes, cytokines stimulate both the humoral and cellular immune responses, as well as the activation of phagocytic cells. Cytokines that are secreted from lymphocytes are termed lymphokines, whereas those secreted by monocytes or macrophages are termed monokines. A large family of cytokines exists that are produced by various cells of the body. Many of the lymphokines are also known as interleukins (ILs), since they not only are secreted by leukocytes but also are able to affect the cellular responses of leukocytes. Specifically, interleukins are growth factors targeted to cells of hematopoietic origin.

It is safe to say that the inflammatory process provides a rich variety of vectors and phenomena to exploit for targeting purposes. Targeting strategies can be developed that exploit both the signaling processes and the subsequent physiological changes of the inflammatory response as a means of delineating inflammation. The following sections will highlight agents used clinically and those being investigated as enhanced targeting agents.

CHARACTERISTICS OF AN IDEAL INFECTION IMAGING AGENT

The characteristics of an ideal infection imaging agent should include selective and irreversible localization at areas of infection, and rapid clearance from normal tissues. Although these "magic bullets" have not yet materialized, more realistic characteristics of an ideal agent include: rapid localization and blood clearance, prolonged retention in sites of infection/inflammation, and a stable, predictable, low level of accumulation in normal tissues. Low levels of accumulation in bowel and blood pool are particularly important characteristics. Focal accumulation or transient activity in the bowel would make detection of infections in this area difficult. Similarly, high blood pool activity increases background and complicates the visualization of vascular infections or highly vascularized tissues.

CLINICAL RADIOPHARMACEUTICALS

While the aim of this chapter is to provide a perspective on strategies for targeting infection, it seems appropriate to include a review of some of the agents currently in clinical use in context of the strategy employed to detect inflammation, as well as the pros and cons of such an approach and how it may point to new approaches.

Table 2. Examples of clinically used radiopharmaceuticals for imaging infection and inflammation

Agent	Radioisotope	Target
Gallium citrate	Ga-67	Transferrin
White blood cells	In-111, Tc-99m	Cellular infiltrate
Immunoglobulin G	In-111, Tc-99m	Protein leakage
Anti-granulocyte Antibodies	In-111, Tc-99m	Protein leakage/ Leukocytes

^{67}Ga-Citrate

The first radiopharmaceutical to be widely used for infection imaging was ^{67}Ga-citrate. This agent was originally used as a tumor imaging agent, primarily due to its high affinity for transferrin and the increased expression of transferrin receptors on certain tumors (7). Subsequently, its avidity for the inflammatory process was identified. The ability of ^{67}Ga to localize at inflammatory processes is due to a series of phenomena that suggest several strategies for targeting infection and inflammation. Due to the similarities of gallium and iron (III) chemistry, gallium can enter many of the metabolic pathways of iron and bind to several carrier molecules that bind iron with high affinity (i.e., transferrin, lactoferrin, and ferritin). While ionic ^{67}Ga itself does not represent a targeting strategy outside of its imaging applications, the pathways by which it ultimately accumulates in infection offer several.

After intravenous injection, there is a rapid transfer of gallium from citrate to serum apotransferrin (an iron transport protein, molecular weight: 100kDa). The labeled protein then can be delivered to sites of inflammation as a result of hemodynamic changes and increased vascular permeability associated with the inflammatory process. This event may be the primary mechanism responsible for the ability of ^{67}Ga to delineate infection.

Rennen and co-workers have studied the localization of a series of "non-specific" proteins into sites of infection. In an attempt to determine the role of molecular weight in the accumulation in infectious inflammation, a series of 11 proteins with molecular weights ranging from 2.5 kDa to 800 kDa were studied (8). Each protein was labeled with Tc-99m using a standard method and evaluated in rats that were inoculated with E. coli intramuscularly. The results indicated that not molecular weight but blood residence time is the principal factor that determines localization of a non-specific tracer protein in infectious foci. Proteins of intermediate size (MW 66 kDa–206 kDa) demonstrated relatively slow blood clearance with moderate uptake in liver and spleen. Hence, the molecular weight of transferrin appears to be ideal for non-specific localization based on the results of this study.

If ^{67}Ga-transferrin can accumulate in an inflammation as a result of leaky vasculature, circulating ionic ^{67}Ga or ^{67}Ga-citrate should pass through leaky vessels even more readily. Gallium can bind to circulating neutrophils by associating with lactoferrin, which is abundant in these cells. As leukocytes migrate to the site of infection, ^{67}Ga is transported and localized with the cells. This mode of accumulation in infection suggests labeled cells as a means of delineating infection. This can be approached by ex vivo labeling and in situ labeling, as will be discussed below.

Since lactoferrin is contained in secondary granules of neutrophils, this protein may also be involved in ^{67}Ga sequestration at the site of infection. After neutrophils localize at sites of infection, lactoferrin is released and retained by interaction with receptors on macrophages. This suggests an approach that targets cellular debris and proteins at the site of the infectious inflammation. The enzyme elastase has been suggested as such a target (9).

Clinically, ^{67}Ga-citrate has the advantage of localizing in infections produced by a variety of organisms, and this has led to its use in patients presenting with fevers of unknown origin (FUO) and in immune-compromised patients. Although ^{67}Ga-citrate has been used extensively for infection/inflammation imaging, the high degree of nonspecific accumulation of ^{67}Ga-citrate has led to a reduction of its use in favor of more inflammation-specific agents and agents that lack such a myriad of interactions with the iron transport and metabolic pathways. Clearly, the multiple ways in which ^{67}Ga can accumulate in the infectious inflammation has stimulated further development of more specific approaches to targeting infectious inflammation.

RADIOLABELED LEUKOCYTES

The migration of white blood cells (WBCs) out of the vasculature and into injured tissue is a hallmark of the inflammatory process (10) and has made leukocytes an excellent candidate for radiolabeling. Methodologies for cell labeling vary with the choice of radionuclide, the cell population to be labeled, and the clinical condition under investigation. In general, the radionuclide must localize within the cells and bind to an intracellular target. Ideally it should remain bound for the duration of imaging so as not to confound the interpretation of the image.

Methods for labeling leukocytes using ^{111}In-oxine or ^{99m}Tc-exemetazine have been reviewed previously in detail (11). Briefly, whole venous blood, obtained from a patient suspected of infection, is treated with anticoagulant (heparin or acid-citrate dextrose). White blood cells are isolated by gravity sedimentation, which may be facilitated by the addition of a sedimenting agent such as hydroxymethylcellulose or hetastarch. The leukocyte-rich layer of cells is isolated and the plasma is removed by dilution with saline followed by centrifugation. The isolated cells are then re-suspended in saline followed by the addition of radiolabel and incubation with the cells for 30 to 60 minutes. Radiolabel that does not attach to the cells is washed off and the cells are re-suspended for injection, usually in platelet-poor plasma.

^{111}In labeled leukocytes have been a highly successful imaging agent and currently represent the "gold standard" for infection imaging. Unfortunately, significant preparation time and blood handling are required for the radiolabeling of ^{111}In-labeled leukocytes. Study times are prolonged because radiolabeled cells require several hours to localize after injection, since they must detect a chemoattractant signal and then migrate to the site of inflammation. Other considerations such as radiation dosimetry limit the amount of radioactivity that can be administered, frequently resulting in less than optimal image quality for clinical detection of the infectious inflammation.

RADIOLABELED IMMUNOGLOBULINS

A characteristic of the acute inflammatory response is a change in hydrostatic pressure, which is followed by the development of transudates (ultrafiltrate of plasma, with low protein concentration) and exudates (ultrafiltrate of plasma, rich in protein). This influx of proteins is an early aspect of the humoral response to injury. For these reasons, it is not surprising that infection imaging agents based upon labeled proteins have evolved. These include both non-specific proteins and proteins directed toward a target within the inflammatory milieu.

Radiolabeled Monoclonal IgG

In 1957, Pressman et al. (12) described the first use of antibodies for detecting tumor localization. These observations stimulated considerable interest in the use of antigen-specific antibodies for detecting tumors and other disease states. The development of the hybridoma technique heightened this interest as it became possible to produce large quantities of epitope-specific monoclonal antibodies (mAb) (13).

The development of antigranulocyte mAbs was stimulated by studies characterizing polyclonal antisera to carcinoembryonic antigen (CEA). These investigations demonstrated that substances that cross-reacted with CEA, such as nonspecific cross-reacting antigens (NCA), were present at high concentrations on the surfaces of granulocytes and other tissues. In selecting for monoclonal antibodies to CEA, two mAbs (AK-47 and BW 250/183) which immunoprecipitated a 95-kDa glycoprotein (NCA-95) present in perchloric extracts of normal lung and granulocytes were identified. When screened with human tissue sections, these mAbs stained only granulocytes (14).

Immunohistochemical studies performed to characterize the binding of AK-47 to the granulocyte precursors demonstrated significant binding to metamyelocytes and granulocytes. Although there was some binding to myelocytes, no binding to early granulocyte precursor cells were detected. After intravenous injection, approximately 8 to 20% of the injected dose of these antibodies was bound to circulating granulocytes. The distribution of these antibodies in humans was similar, with the majority of the activity in bone marrow, liver, spleen, and blood. This distribution reflects reticuloendothelial system (RES) accumulation of labeled leukocytes and circulating free IgG. Clinically, antigranulocyte antibodies have been used for the detection of bone infection, soft tissue infection, abdominal abscesses, and vascular graft infection. Anti-granulocyte antibodies have been useful for the detection of soft tissue infections, but localization is slow (20-40 hours) (14).

The mechanism of infection localization with antigranulocyte antibodies depends on two processes: (a) diffusion of free antibody into the expanded protein space of the lesion, as described for nonspecific IgG, with or without subsequent granulocyte binding, and (b) labeling of circulating and marginated leukocytes which eventually migrate to the site of infection via chemotaxis.

Radiolabeled Polyclonal IgG

The ability to detect tumors by radioimmunoimaging suggested that this technique might also be useful for infection imaging. Studies with monoclonal antibodies directed to capsular antigens of *Pseudomonas aeruginosa* type I demonstrated the feasibility of this approach (15). In this study, both specific and non-specific control IgG localized at the site of infection within 24 hours after injection. However, the specific antibody was retained for a longer period of time. These observations led the way to further studies with nonspecific polyclonal human IgG. Radioiodinated and ^{111}In-labeled IgG were shown to be effective for visualizing infections caused by a variety of organisms as well as sterile abscesses produced with turpentine[33]. Comparisons with ^{67}Ga-citrate demonstrated that IgG produced clearer and better localization (16). These results suggested that scintigraphic imaging after intravenous injection of radiolabeled IgG could form the basis of an inflammation scan suitable for use in humans. Subsequent studies have established that ^{111}In-labeled human polyclonal IgG is a safe and highly effective reagent for imaging a variety of types of infection and inflammation in humans.

The mechanisms of ^{111}In-IgG localization at sites of inflammation was originally postulated to involve binding of the Fc portion of IgG to specific receptors on inflammatory cells. Microautoradiography studies, however, have revealed that there is minimal association of radiolabel with inflammatory cells. Also, it has been recently demonstrated that, although digestion of IgG with endoglycosidase-F markedly reduced Fc receptor binding, inflammation imaging was not altered. These observations suggest a role for other, less specific mechanisms, as suggested by the work of Rennen et al (13). It appears that nonspecific protein leakage into the greatly expanded space of inflammatory lesions plays a significant role in the early localization of ^{111}In-IgG (17).

Despite the success of ^{111}In-IgG imaging, localization usually requires 24 hours before many lesions can be visualized. The explanation for the lengthy time required for infection localization with ^{111}In-labeled IgG is similar to ^{67}Ga-citrate/transferrin, where long circulation times are needed in order to allow for accumulation in the inflamed tissue. Although inflammatory lesions usually have increased vascular permeability, the diffusion barrier to molecules of this size range is still substantial, resulting in slow delivery of the radiopharmaceutical to the lesion. In addition, since blood levels remain high for several hours, background activity remains high, resulting in obscured visualization during the first several hours of such a study. From a practical perspective, this is a serious deficiency, since clinical decision-making frequently requires a rapid assessment of patients with possible focal infection.

ALTERNATIVE STRATEGIES FOR TARGETING INFECTION

Underlying new targeting approaches is the concept that radiolabeled leukocytes actively migrate to and accumulate at sites of infectious inflammation. This phenomenon opens up two interesting possibilities: (a) label the leukocytes in situ and/or (b) create a pseudo-leukocyte that is labeled prior to administration. These two concepts have been the driving force behind the development of a series of new agents that will be discussed below. In addition, the infection/inflammation process presents other avenues for exploitation such as directing labeling to the invading microorganism or to constituents (soluble or insoluble) of the inflammatory milieu.

Some candidate molecules that possess high affinity for leukocytes include the interleukins (IL-1, IL-1 antagonist and IL-8) and the peptide N-formyl-methionyl-leucyl-phenylalanine (For-MLF). Alternatively, agents that can effectively extravasate into inflamed tissue while demonstrating rapid blood clearance may also present an attractive approach to imaging inflammation. Liposomes represent one such class. The following discussion will highlight how some of these agents are being investigated for imaging infection.

TARGETING NON-SPECIFIC VASCULAR CHANGES

Liposomes

Liposomes are microparticulate lipoidal vesicles that represent a non-specific approach to infection imaging by exploiting the increased vascular permeability at the site of an infection and inflammation. The ability of liposomes to carry large amounts of relatively insoluble drug has resulted in the FDA approval of several liposomal-based drug formulations. It was also recognized that liposomes might serve as imaging agents to visualize pathological processes by carrying gamma-emitting radioisotopes, x-ray or magnetic resonance contrast materials (18).

Initial attempts to target liposomes to pathologic sites such as tumors or infections showed promise, however, the majority of the particles rapidly accumulated in liver and spleen [via phagocytosis] after intravenous injection (19). Subsequent advances in liposome technology showed that a variety of physical and chemical factors effect circulation kinetics and tissue distribution of liposomes after intravenous injection. These include vesicle size, lipid composition and dose, and vesicle surface characteristics such as charge and hydrophilicity. In particular, surface modification with water-soluble polymers, such as polyethylene glycol (PEG), decreases phagocytic uptake of liposomes by inhibiting interaction with plasma opsonins. This ability to create long circulating liposomes has greatly broadened their potential in vivo application.

Radiolabeled PEG-liposomes have been shown to be effective for detection of infectious processes in animals. The size of these PEG-ylated liposomes was also studied for its effect on imaging. Liposomes smaller than 100 nm were shown to have greater accumulation in infected processes than those of 120 nm or greater. This is likely due to the fact that the size of the endothelial gaps in inflamed tissue is on the order of 100 nm or less. Methods of labeling showed that covalent attachment of radiolabel to the lipid components rendered an improved imaging agent as compared with loading of the liposomal cargo space (20). In comparison with other imaging agents, radiolabeled liposomes compared favorably with ^{111}In-labeled IgG and ^{111}In-leukocytes in animal models of infection and inflammation. Microscopic observations indicate that uptake and retention of PEG-liposomes in the infectious focus is a result of enhanced extravasation due to increased vascular permeability and subsequent phagocytosis of PEG-liposomes by macrophages in the infected tissue.

Clinically, ^{99m}Tc-labeled PEG-ylated liposomes compared favorably with ^{111}In-IgG in patients presenting with a variety of pathologies. A role for liposomes as imaging agents in the future is suggested by the ease of preparation and the rapidity with which scanning can take place.

TARGETING LEUKOCYTES

The recruitment of inflammatory cells to sites of injury is a concerted interaction of several types of soluble mediators in addition to cell adhesion molecules. These include complement factor C5a, platelet activating factor (PAF), and leukotriene B4. All act as chemotactic agonists. Interleukin-1 and tumor necrosis factor (TNF) play important roles in the inflammatory process. IL-1 and TNF are derived from monocytes and macrophages and promote the synthesis of proteins that contribute to the inflammatory process. Pro-inflammatory cytokines such as interleukin-8 (IL-8), which is also known as neutrophil activating factor, is also a potent chemoattractant. IL-8 synergizes with other cytokines and growth factors to amplify various neutrophil cytotoxic functions. Bacteria also aid in the recruitment of leukocytes through the ability of the leukocytes to respond to formylated peptides that are shed from bacteria. These formylated peptides are strong chemoattractants and also modulate oxidative burst.

These mediators of inflammation and immune response create an interesting class of soluble and specific ligands that demonstrate high affinity binding to specific components of the inflammatory and immune responses. Several of these ligands have been investigated as imaging probes for infectious inflammation. Both cytokines and bacterial chemotactic peptides offer examples of attractive strategies for imaging infectious inflammations and will be discussed below.

CYTOKINES

A promising class of vectors for targeting infection is cytokines. Cytokines are a unique family of growth factors that are secreted primarily from leukocytes. Cytokines stimulate the humoral and cellular immune responses, as well as the activation of phagocytic cells. Cytokines usually bind to their respective receptors with high affinity in the sub-nanomolar to low nanomolar range.

IL-1

IL-1 binds with high affinity to receptors expressed mainly on granulocytes, monocytes and lymphocytes. Using radioiodinated IL-1, Van Der Laken and co-workers demonstrated specific uptake of IL-1 into *S. aureus* infections in mice (21). Target to background ratios exceeded 40:1 at 48 hours post injection, suggesting cytokines provided a potential strategy for imaging infection. However, the systemic biological effects of IL-1, even at very low doses, make IL-1 an unsuitable candidate to advance into the clinic.

IL-1ra

A naturally occurring IL-1 receptor antagonist (IL-1ra) competes for binding and is capable of blocking IL-1 binding both in vitro and in vivo. IL-1ra binds IL-1 receptor with similar affinity but lacks the biological activity. IL-1ra is found in high levels in patients with various infections and inflammations. Hence, van der Laken, et al, tested the equally sized (17kDa) protein as an infection imaging agent (22). In a comparative study in rabbits with *E. coli* infection, the radiolabeled IL-1ra was shown to be comparable to IL-1. In patient studies however, significant bowel excretion was demonstrated, severely limiting the clinical utility of this agent (23).

IL-8

Interleukin-8 (IL-8) is a chemoattractant cytokine (chemokine) produced by a variety of tissues and blood cells and, significantly, endothelial cells. IL-8 is a polypeptide consisting of 72 amino acids in its native form. The biological profile is similar to that of the classical chemotactic peptides C5a and formyl-Met-Leu-Phe. It is able to induce the full pattern of responses observed in chemotactically stimulated neutrophils and the production of reactive oxygen metabolites. IL-8 is not species specific and is a potent angiogenic factor. IL-8 belongs to the CXC sub-family of chemokines, in which the first two cysteine residues are separated by one amino acid residue.

IL-8 binds to receptors on neutrophils with high affinity (0.3-4 nM). The ability to image inflammation with directly radioiodinated IL-8 was first described by Hay et al (24). Transient uptake in sterile inflammation was reported. In further studies, radioiodinated IL-8 was able to visualize inflammation in a pilot study of eight patients.

Further investigation explored the behavior and kinetics of radioiodinated IL-8 in various models of infection and sterile inflammation in rabbits. These studies found that the choice of radioiodination method had a significant effect on the imaging results, likely due to the rapid de-iodination of the directly iodinated IL-8 at the site of infection. Using labeling approaches, such as the Bolton-Hunter (BH) method, which are more resistant to de-iodination in vivo, resulted in superior imaging characteristics, however one must recall that the BH method is complex and yields lower specific activity preparations (25). In infected rabbits, abscess visualization was rapid and abscess accumulation at 8 hours post injection was high. Subsequently, ^{99m}Tc-labeled IL-8 use was investigated for imaging infections in a rabbit model. A labeling technique incorporating the metal complexing agent, hydrazino nicotinamide (HYNIC), was used that resulted in a radiopharmaceutical with high specific activity. This allowed a decrease in the IL-8 dose administered, thus reducing unwanted biologic activity. A non-specific size matched protein (lysozyme; 14.3 kDa) was used as a control. The study showed that ^{99m}Tc-labeled IL-8 rapidly accumulated in infectious foci, while it rapidly cleared from non-target tissues. Except for uptake in the kidneys and bladder, no uptake was noted in any non-inflamed tissue.

These results suggest IL-8 is a potential imaging agent for infection. The limitations on IL-8 are related to its biological activity, which involves a number of effects on a variety of circulating leukocytes. The mild transient drop of leukocyte counts without subsequent leukocytosis suggests that ^{99m}Tc-labeled IL-8 may be a clinically useful imaging agent without significant side effects. These effects may be mitigated further by a radiolabeled preparation with very high specific activity, allowing the injection of smaller amounts of IL-8.

CHEMOTACTIC PEPTIDES

For-MLF is a bacterial product that initiates leukocyte chemotaxis by binding to high-affinity receptors on white blood cell membranes. These receptors are present on both PMNs and mononuclear phagocytes. Granulocytes respond to a chemoattractant gradient migrating toward the site of inflammation, where the concentration of chemoattractant is greatest. Previous studies have demonstrated that many synthetic analogs of For-MLF bind to neutrophils and macrophages with equal or greater affinity compared to the native peptide (26).

The possibility of using radiolabeled chemotactic peptides for leukocyte labeling was initially explored more than ten years ago (27). At the time of these studies, the radiolableing methods available yielded agents of relatively low specific activity, requiring pharmacological amounts of peptide for imaging which were shown to produce transient neutropenia in rabbits.

Since previous structure-activity studies have established that the C-terminus of chemotactic peptide analogs can be extensively modified without significantly altering bioactivity or receptor binding, this is a potentially useful site for introducing a radiolabel. A series of chemotactic peptides have been prepared which include metal chelators at the C-terminus. C-terminal DTPA-derivatized chemotactic peptide analogs have been prepared by standard methods of solid-phase peptide synthesis and radiolabeled with [111]In (28). These DTPA-derivatized chemotactic peptide analogs maintained biological activity (EC_{50} for O_2 production by human PMNs: 3 to 150 nM) and the ability to bind to the chemoattractant receptor on human PMNs (EC_{50} for binding: 7.5 to 50 nM); biological activity and receptor binding were highly correlated (r =0.99). When labeled with ^{111}In, these peptides showed rapid blood clearance in animals and low levels of accumulation in heart, lung, liver, spleen, and GI tract. These studies indicated that ^{111}In-labeled chemotactic peptide analogs are effective agents for the external imaging of focal sites of infection.

Introduction of the chelating agent, hydrazino nicotinamide (HYNIC), at the C-termninus of the chemotactic peptide analogs formyl-Nle-Leu-Phe-Lys, formyl-Nle-Leu-Phe-Lys, formyl-Met-Leu-Phe-NH(CH$_2$)$_6$NH$_2$, and formyl-Met-Leu-Phe-$_D$-Lys, allowing for Tc-99m-labeling. All peptides maintained biological activity (EC_{50} for O_2- production by humans PMNs: 12 to 500 nM) and the ability to bind to the chemoattractant receptor on human PMNs (EC_{50} for binding: 0.12 to 40 nM). [99m]Tc -labeled peptides could be isolated by high-performance liquid chromatography (HPLC) at high specific activity (>10,000 mCi/umol).

[99m]Tc-labeled peptides retained receptor binding to human neutrophils with EC_{50}s of <10 nM. Blood clearance of all four peptides was rapid. The in vivo distribution of the individual peptides was similar, with low levels of accumulation in most normal tissues. In rats, all of the peptides concentrated

at sites of infection as determined by gamma camera imaging (target-to-background [T/B] ratio: 2.5-3.1) within 1 hour of injection. In rabbits, outstanding images of infection sites were obtained, with T/B ratios obtained from imaging data of >20:1 at 15 hours after injection (Fig. 1).

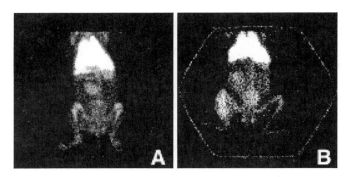

Figure 1. Gamma camera images of a rabbit with intramuscular bacterial infection in the thigh injected with Tc-99m chemotactic peptide antagonist; 3h (A) and 18h (B) after injection.

In an effort to more clearly define the mechanisms of localization and the relative ability of ^{99m}Tc-labeled chemotactic peptides to image infection, the biodistribution and infection imaging properties of ^{99m}Tc-chemotactic peptide (Tc-HP) were compared with ^{111}In-labeled leukocytes (^{111}In-WBCs) in rabbits with intramuscular *E. coli* infections.

When compared to ^{111}In-labeled leukocytes (^{111}In-WBCs) in the same animal, the distributions of ^{99m}Tc-labeled chemotactic peptides (Tc-HP) and ^{111}In-WBCs were similar and the sites of infection were well visualized with both radiopharmaceuticals. The target (infected muscle) to background (contralateral normal muscle) ratios (T/B) were greater for the Tc-HP than the leukocytes at each time point studied. The average T/B ratio (^{99m}Tc-HP to ^{111}In-WBCs) was 2.99 $\pm$ 1.88 with no value less than unity. T/B ratios calculated from direct tissue sampling were significantly higher for ^{99m}Tc-HP than for ^{111}In-WBCs (33.6:1 vs. 8.1:1, p < 0.01). These differences were primarily due to a four-fold increase in the absolute accumulation of ^{99m}Tc-HP in infected muscle rather than a difference in accumulation in normal muscle (29).

COMPARISON WITH ^{111}In-IgG

In an effort to determine the role of nonspecific uptake mechanisms in peptide localization, Tc-HP was compared to ^{111}In-IgG in the rabbits with intramuscular bacterial infection. Imaging demonstrated markedly different biodistributions of the two reagents over the times studied. The highest concentrations of ^{111}In-DTPA-IgG were detected in blood pool structures, liver, and kidney. In contrast, localization of ^{99m}Tc-labeled peptide was greatest in spleen, lung, and liver (consistent with binding to leukocytes).

In general, the sites of infection were better visualized with the Tc-HP, and T/B ratios increased with time (p < 0.01). At both early (3-4 h) and late (16-18h) times, the T/B ratios obtained from gamma camera imaging of ^{99m}Tc-peptide were higher (p <0.01). No significant correlation was found between the accumulations of ^{99m}Tc-HP and ^{111}In-DTPA-IgG at the site of infection, suggesting that nonspecific mechanisms do not play a major role in accumulation of ^{99m}Tc-peptide at sites of infection. At all imaging times, the T/B ratio for the peptide was significantly higher than for IgG. Furthermore, the biodistribution studies demonstrated much lower levels of peptide accumulation in non-target tissues. These characteristics suggest that ^{99m}Tc-chemotactic peptides should be superior to ^{111}In-IgG in many complicated clinical situations, such as the detection of infections of the cardiovascular system (29).

RECEPTOR AFFINITY AND INFECTION LOCALIZATION

The relationship between receptor affinity and infection localization has also been investigated, along with a comparison of non-specific markers of extracellular space (^{111}In-DTPA) and blood volume (^{111}In-RBC) in rabbits with *E. coli* infection. Three Tc-99m labeled HYNIC derivatized chemotactic peptide analogs of varying receptor affinity were chosen for study (Formyl-MLFK(HYNIC), i-Boc-MLFK(HYNIC), Acetyl-MLFK(HYNIC); EC_{50}; 0.2 nM, 150 nM, 300 nM, respectively). To correct for variation in infection intensity, all animals were also injected with ^{111}In-WBC's.

At all times, imaging demonstrated that the T/B was greatest for the peptide with the highest affinity (p<0.01) and the T/B for the peptide with the lowest affinity was not significantly different from the non-specific controls. These results indicate that the infection localization properties of chemotactic peptides are strongly correlated with ForMLF receptor affinity, and nonspecific accumulation makes a small contribution to infection localization (29).

This finding was recently confirmed by van der Laken and co-workers (30), who prepared a chemotactic peptide agonist (formyl-methionyl-leucyl-phenylalanyl-lysine-hydrazinonicotinamide (^{99m}Tc-labeled fMLFK-HYNIC)) and a peptide of similar size that displayed low affinity binding (N-hydrazinonicotinamide-methionyl-leucyl-phenylalanyl-OMe (^{99m}Tc-labeled N-HYNIC-MLF-OMe)). The results of their study showed that, although blood clearances of ^{99m}Tc-labeled fMLFK-HYNIC and ^{99m}Tc-labeled N-HYNIC-MLF-OMe were similar, ^{99m}Tc-labeled fMLFK-HYNIC was retained in the abscess (E. coli) approximately at 10 fold greater levels than the control peptide. These authors concluded that ^{99m}Tc-labeled fMLFK-HYNIC is retained in both acute infection and sterile inflammation by means of specific receptor binding if sufficient cellular infiltration is present.

SUMMARY AND FUTURE DIRECTIONS

Currently, reagents for targeting infection represent cellular or protein components involved in the inflammatory process. Such approaches have met with some success, as they comprise integral parts of the inflammatory process. The notion of exploiting exudative changes, while dramatic at the microscopic level, fail to provide a large signal on the macroscopic level or that equivalent to the spatial resolution of most imaging devices. Circulation times must be prolonged to facilitate diffusion out of the vasculature, creating a large and constant pool of background signal. Targeting with labeled cells requires the migration of the cells from the vasculature to the site of infection. Initially, leukocytes must detect a chemoattractant signal to migrate to the lesion. Subsequent passage of these relatively large vectors through leaking vasculature takes several hours. For these reasons, it is unlikely that a radiolabeled cell preparation or large molecular weight protein will be developed with more rapid localization than those currently available. Also, preparation of such labeled cells is laborious.

Improved agents for targeting infection likely will be based on small molecules whose diffusion into the lesion is not hindered by molecular size constraints and which bind to molecular targets at the site of infection/inflammation. In general, the lower molecular weight should also lead to enhanced blood clearance, avoiding elevated blood pool activity that contributes to background. New agents should also obviate the need to handle blood, as this represents potential hazards to both patient and medical personnel alike.

The future "gold standard" for infection imaging remains to be determined. There are many alternatives, some based on similar specific mechanisms such as the interleukins, formylated chemotactic peptides, LTB4, and some on non-specific mechanisms such as liposomes. Ultimately, the clinical situation and advances in imaging hardware may determine the ideal agent. As we learn more about the inflammatory process at the molecular level, new targets will be defined, prompting the design of new vectors. With increasing sophistication in drug design and drug delivery systems, we will formulate strategies that will allow detection of and potential drug delivery to the inflammatory process.

REFERENCES

1. Pizzo PA. Evaluation of fever in the patient with cancer. Eur J Cancer Clin Oncol 25:Suppl 2:S9-S16. 1989.
2. Lavender, J.P., Lowe, J., Barker, J.R., Burn, J.I., and Chaudri, M.A. Ga-67 citrate scanning in neoplastic and inflammatory disease. *Br. J. Radiol.* 44:361-366, 1971.
3. Peters, A..M., Saverymuttu, S.H. Reavy, H.J. Danpure, H.J. Osman, S., and Lavender, J.P. Imaging of inflammation with indium-111 tropolonate labeled leukocytes. *J. Nucl. Med.* 24(1):39-44, 1983.
4. Peters, A.M., Danpure, H.J., Osman, S., Hawker, R.J., Henderson, B.L., Hodgson, H.J., Kelly, J.D., Neirinckx, R.D., and Lavender, J.P. Clinical experience with ^{99m}Tc-hexamethylpropyleneamineoxime for labeling leukocytes and imaging inflammation. *Lancet* 2:946-949, 1986.
5. Fischman, A.J., Rubin, R.H., Khaw, B.A., Callahan, R.J., Wilkinson, R., Keech, F., Dragotakes, S., Kramer, P., LaMuraglia, G.M., Lind, S., Strauss, H.W., Detection of acute inflammation with ^{111}In-labeled non-specific polyclonal IgG. *Semin. Nucl. Med.* 18:335-344, 1998.
6. Locher, J.T., Seybold, K., Andres, R.Y., and Schubiger, A. Imaging of inflammatory lesions after injection of radioiodinated monoclonal antigranulocyte antibodies. *Nucl. Med. Commun.* 7:659-670, 1986.
7. Edwards, C.L., and Hayes, R.L. Tumor scanning with ^{67}Ga citrate. *J. Nucl. Med..* 10:103-105, 1969.
8. Rennen HJ, Makarewicz J, Oyen WJ, Laverman P, Corstens FH, Boerman OC. The effect of molecular weight on nonspecific accumulation of (99m)T-labeled proteins in inflammatory foci. Nucl Med Biol 2001 May;28(4):401-8
9. Rusckowski M, Qu T, Pullman J, Marcel R, Ley AC, Ladner RC, Hnatowich DJ. Inflammation and infection imaging with a 99mTc-neutrophil elastase inhibitor in monkeys. J Nucl Med 2000 Feb;41(2):363-74
10. Snyderman, R. and Uhing, R.J. Chemoattractant stimulus-response coupling, in Inflammation: Basic Principles and Clinical Correlates. 2nd ed. Gallin, J.I., Goldstein, I.M., and Snyderman, R., Eds., Raven Press, New York, 1992, p.421.
11. Srivastava, S.C. and Chervu, L.R. Radionuclide labeled red blood cells: Current status and future prospects. Semin. Nucl. Med. 14(2):68-82, 1984.
12. Pressman, D., Day, E.D., and Blau, M. The use of paired labeling in the determination of tumor localizing antibodies. Cancer Res. 17:845-850, 1957.

13.   Kohler, G., and Milstein, C. Continuous cultures of fused cells secreting antibody of predefined specificity. Nature 256:495-497, 1975.

14.   Becker W, Goldenberg DM,Wolf F. The use of monoclonal antibodies and antibody fragments in the imaging of infectious lesions. Semin Nucl Med 24(2):142-53, 1994

15.   Rubin, R.H., Young, L.S., Hansen, W.P., Nedelman, M., Wilkinson, R., Nelles, M.J., Callahan, R., Khaw, B.A., and Strauss, H.W. Specific and non-specific imaging of localized Fisher Immunotype I Pseudomonas aeruginosa infection with radiolabeled monoclonal antibody. J. Nucl. Med. 29:651-656, 1988.

16.   Rubin, R.H., Fischman, A.J., Nedelman, M., Wilkinson, R., Callahan, R.J., Khaw, B.A., Hansen, W.P., Kramer, P.B., and Strauss, H.W. Radiolabeled non-specific polyclonal human immunoglobulin in the detection of focal inflammation by scintigraphy: comparison with Ga-67-citrate and Tc-99m-labeled albumin. J. Nucl. Med. 30:385-389, 1989.

17.   Rubin RH Fischman AJ. The use of radiolabeled non-specific immunoglobulin in the detection of focal inflammation. Semin Nucl Med 24(2):169-79, 1994

18.   Torchilin VP. Polymeric contrast agents for medical imaging. Curr Pharm Biotechnol 2000 Sep;1(2):183-215

19.   Morgan JR, Williams LA, Howard CB. Technetium-labelled liposome imaging for deep-seated infection. Br J Radiol 1985 Jan;58(685):35-9

20.   Laverman P, Dams ET, Oyen WJ, Storm G, Koenders EB, Prevost R, van der Meer JW, Corstens FH, Boerman OC. A novel method to label liposomes with 99mTc by the hydrazino nicotinyl derivative. J Nucl Med 1999 40(1):192-7

21.   van der Laken CJ, Boerman OC, Oyen WJ, van de Ven MT, Claessens RA, van der Meer JW, Corstens FH. Specific targeting of infectious foci with radioiodinated human recombinant interleukin-1 in an experimental model. Eur J Nucl Med 1995 22(11):1249-55

22.   van der Laken CJ, Boerman OC, Oyen WJ, van de Ven MT, Claessens RA, van der Meer JW, Corstens FH. Different behaviour of radioiodinated human recombinant interleukin-1 and its receptor antagonist in an animal model of infection. Eur J Nucl Med 1996 23(11):1531-5

23.   Barrera P, van der Laken CJ, Boerman OC, Oyen WJ, van de Ven MT, van Lent PL, van de Putte LB, Corstens FH. Radiolabelled interleukin-1 receptor antagonist for detection of synovitis in patients with rheumatoid arthritis. Rheumatology (Oxford) 2000 39(8):870-4

24.   Hay RV, Skinner RS, Newman OC, Kunkel SL, Lyle LR, Shapiro B, Gross MD. Scintigraphy of acute inflammatory lesions in rats with radiolabelled recombinant human interleukin-8. Nucl Med Commun 1997 18(4):367-78

25.   Van der Laken CJ, Boerman OC, Oyen WJ, Van de Ven MT, Ven der Meer JW, Corstens FH. The kinetics of radiolabelled interleukin-8 in infection and sterile inflammation. Nucl Med Commun 1998 Mar;19(3):271-81

26.   Showell, H.J., Freer, R.J., Zigmond, S.H., Schiffman, E., Aswanikumar, S., Corcoran, B., and Becker, E.L. The structural relations of synthetic peptides as chemotactic factors and inducers of lysosomal enzyme secretion for neutrophils. J. Exp. Med. 143:1154-1169, 1976

27.   Zogbhi, S.S., Thakur, M.L., and Gottschalk, A. A potential radioactive agent for labeling of human neutrophils. J. Nucl. Med. 22(Abstr.):32, 1981.

28.   Fischman, A.J., Pike, M.C., Kroon, D., Fucello, A.J., Rexinger, D., ten Kate, C., Wilkinson, R., Rubin, R.H., and Strauss, H.W. Imaging of focal sites of bacterial infection in rats with 111In-labeled chemotactic peptide analogs. J. Nucl. Med. 1991;32:483-491.

29.   Fischman AJ, babich JW, Rubin RH. Infection imaging with Technetium-99m labeled chemotactic peptide analogs. Semin Nucl Med 24(2):154-68, 1994.

30. van der Laken CJ, Boerman OC, Oyen WJ, van de Ven MT, Edwards DS, Barrett JA, van der Meer JW, Corstens FH. Technetium-99m-labeled chemotactic peptides in acute infection and sterile inflammation. J Nucl Med. 1997 Aug;38(8):1310-5.

GLOSSARY

Chemoattractant: A compound that produces positive directed migration of one or more kinds of leukocytes. The cells follow a chemical gradient. Chemotactic factors are of three general sources: bacterial (N-formylated peptides, which are unique to the initiation of bacterial proteins), plasma proteins (e.g., C5a, one of the activated products of either the classical or alternative pathways of complement activation), and cells (e.g., the cytokine, TGF-beta).

Chemokines: Related family of proteins produced by many mammalian cell types that mediate chemotaxis and organize activities of cells of specific and non-specific defenses.

Cytokine: A vast array of relatively low molecular weight, pharmacologically active proteins that are secreted by one cell for the purpose of altering either its own functions (autocrine effect) or those of adjacent cells (paracrine effect). In many instances, individual cytokines have multiple biological activities.

Inflammatory response: A part of innate immunity. Inflammation occurs when tissues are injured by viruses, bacteria, trauma, chemicals, heat, cold, or any other harmful stimulus.

Liposome: Microparticulate, fluid-filled vesicle whose walls are made of layers of phospholipids identical to the phospholipids that make up cell membranes. Liposomes are used to deliver certain vaccines, enzymes, contrast materials or drugs to the body.

Nuclear medicine: The branch of medicine that uses very small amounts of radioactive materials or radiopharmaceuticals to diagnose and treat disease.

Radiopharmaceuticals: A radioactive pharmaceutical (biomolecule or drug) that is administered to patient for the purpose of diagnosis or therapy.

21

ANTI-HIV IMMUNOTOXINS

Seth H. Pincus, Hua Fang, and Royce Wilkinson
Department of Microbiology, Montana State University, Bozeman MT 59717, and Research Institute for Children, Children's Hospital, LSU Health Sciences Center, New Orleans LA 70118.

INTRODUCTION

The use of targeted therapies to treat infectious diseases is a novel application that requires a persistent infection that cannot be cleared by other means and the expression of microbial antigens on the surface of productively-infected cells. Although some bacterial or parasitic infections may meet these criteria, chronic viral infections and microbe-induced neoplasia are the most likely targets. In this chapter we will discuss the use of immunotoxins to treat human immunodeficiency virus (HIV) infection. The results demonstrate the importance of targeting the appropriate molecules and utilizing the cell biology of the microorganism.

In the past decade a number of antiviral agents have been developed. When used in combination, these are very effective in limiting the replication of HIV. The virus enzymes reverse transcriptase and protease are the main targets of current therapies. The introduction of this highly active antiretroviral therapy (HAART) has led, in developed countries, to a significant drop in mortality and morbidity associated with HIV infection. Nevertheless there is still need to develop new approaches. The treatments are associated with severe side effects and many patients cannot tolerate current therapies. Virus resistance to antiviral drugs is becoming more prevalent. Even when therapies are optimally used, many patients fail to achieve virus suppression and in no patients has HAART completely eradicated HIV. Thus there is need to develop new anti-HIV therapeutics.

Targeted therapies offer a number of advantages. They attack HIV at a different stage of its lifecycle than current agents. They may be delivered to reservoirs where the virus is sequestered. Drug resistance is less likely to develop if the agents are targeted to well-conserved portions of virus proteins, since these have been subject to immunologic selection during the entire evolutionary history of HIV and thus conservation must be necessary for virus function. The cells of the immune system are highly accessible to targeted drug delivery. The rationale for the use of targeted therapies in HIV infection is discussed in detail elsewhere (1).

Targeted agents may be delivered either to cell subsets that are known sites of HIV replication or to cells that are productively infected and expressing HIV antigens. We will discuss the latter approach in detail. The HIV envelope protein(s) gp160 (precursor), gp120 (extracellular domain), and gp41 (transmembrane domain) are the only HIV proteins expressed intact on the surface of infected cells. These molecules may be targeted by CD4 (the HIV-receptor) or by anti-Env monoclonal antibodies (Mabs). In vitro studies demonstrate that in the absence of enhancement either approach is equally effective, but that the activity of anti-gp41 Mab-based immunotoxins may be enhanced 30-100 fold by the addition of soluble CD4. A clinical trial with a chimeric CD4-pseudomonas exotoxin construct (CD4-PE40) demonstrated a high degree of toxicity and no therapeutic effect at the maximum tolerated dose (MTD). We have argued that CD4-PE40 is a flawed immunotoxin because of its high degree of toxicity, short plasma residence time, and targeting to gp120 rather than gp41. We present data in severe combined immunodeficiency (SCID) mice and in simian/human immunodeficiency virus (SHIV)-infected macaques that support this contention. We conclude that anti-HIV immunotoxins are a potentially useful form of therapy whose utility has not yet been tested.

TARGETING HIV-INFECTED CELLS

The object of using immunotoxins to treat AIDS is to eliminate HIV-infected cells that are actively secreting virus and spreading infection. HIV infects CD4+ T lymphocytes and cells of the macrophage/monocyte lineage. Other cell types may also be infected. The immunodeficiency is caused by a depletion of the number of CD4+ T cells, which makes the patient susceptible to a variety of opportunistic infections. The dynamic nature of HIV infection has been demonstrated (2). The lifespan of a productively HIV-infected CD4+ lymphocyte has been estimated to be 2.2 days, with a daily cell turnover of 10^9 cells. Because of the short lifespan of productively infected cells, it may seem that killing them with immunotoxins would be unnecessary. However, before dying, these cells produce 10^{10} virions per day. These virions in turn infect other cells, with the mean time of 1.2 days from production of virion to initiation of productive infection in the next cell. Because immunotoxins eliminate productively infected cells before they have had an opportunity to produce virions, such therapy should break this cycle, limit the production of new virions and thus protect uninfected cells from becoming infected. This may be accomplished either by targeting cell subsets in which HIV is known to proliferate or by specifically eliminating cells once they have become productively infected (Figure 1). Molecular targets are listed in Table 1.

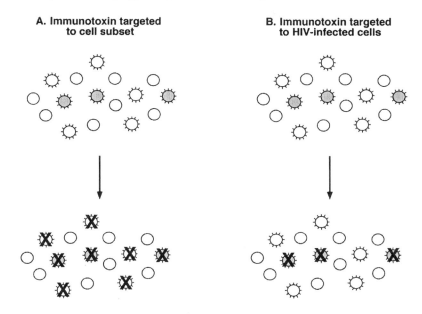

Figure 1. Targeting of immunotoxins to cell subsets in which HIV resides (indicated by bars on cell surface) or to infected cells expressing HIV antigens (shaded). Targeting cell subsets (A) runs the risk of eliminating functionally important cells. Eliminating only productively-infected cells (B) will not eliminate those cells that are latently infected and carry the HIV provirus.

Targeting to cell subsets

HIV exists within a limited number of different cell subsets. Because the same cellular processes that activate T cells also turn on HIV transcription, replicating virus may be found within the subset of lymphocytes that expresses the IL2 receptor, a known marker of activated T cells (3, 4). Immunotoxins that eliminate cells expressing the IL2 receptor, whether targeted by IL2 itself or by Mabs directed against the receptor, are effective in eliminating HIV tissue culture infection in vitro. More recently, it was shown that, in peripheral blood mononuclear cells explanted in vitro, the majority of latently-infected cells exist within the subset of memory T cells defined by the marker CD45RO (5). If this is true in vivo as well, then this may be the first form of therapy that can target latent HIV with any degree of specificity. A Mab to CD7, a T cell marker, has been conjugated to pokeweed antiviral protein and found to have anti-HIV activity when administered to HIV-infected chimpanzees and humans (6). It is unclear whether the antiviral effect was due to killing of CD7+ cells in which HIV replicates or to a specific antiviral effect of the pokeweed protein. Although the elimination of subsets of cells in which HIV resides has some promise and advantages over specific targeting of HIV-infected cells, there exists substantial concern that the elimination of entire subsets of T cells in immunocompromised patients may create an iatrogenic immunodeficiency of severity equal to that seen in AIDS. Another concern is the existence of productively-infected cells outside of the targeted cell subset.

Table 1. Targets of immunotoxins or immunoconjugates.

Target Molecule	Targeting Agents	References
Cell subsets in which HIV resides:		
IL2 receptor	IL2, anti-CD25 Mabs	3,4
CD45RO	Anti-CD45 Mabs	5
CD7	Anti-CD7 Mabs	6
Cells productively infected with HIV:		
gp120	CD4, anti-gp120 Mabs	7-10
gp41	anti-gp41 Mabs	9,10

HIV-infected cells

The envelope proteins are the only HIV-encoded proteins that are expressed intact on the surface of infected cells, despite reports that Gag is present (1). The extracellular portion of Env, gp120, binds to the HIV receptor, CD4, and to the chemokine receptors that act as the HIV coreceptor, among them CXCR4 and CCR5. In the course of infection, gp120 is then removed, exposing gp41. A coiled-coil region of gp41 is then freed from its initial constraints and allows the fusion domain of gp41 to spear the target cell and begin cell fusion. We have used the ability of CD4 to strip off gp120, and expose gp41, as a means to enhance the efficacy of anti-gp41 immunotoxins.

Gp41, the transmembrane portion of Env, may be targeted with Mabs (9, 10). The fusion domain of gp41 normally forms multimers under conditions of infection. A peptide representing this domain has been found to bind to gp41, inhibit multimerization, and prevent infection (11). Although experiments have not been performed, it is possible that this peptide could be used to deliver therapeutics to HIV-infected cells. Therapeutics have been delivered to gp120 using Mabs and using CD4 (7-10). A combination of CD4 and coreceptor has been used to deliver lytic viruses to cells expressing gp120 (12), and such an approach might be applied to soluble molecules as well.

For a number of reasons gp41 is likely to be a better target of immunotoxin therapy than gp120 (13). Gp41 is an integral transmembrane protein, whereas gp120 is non-covalently attached to gp41. Soluble gp120 can be released from the target cell and inhibit the binding of anti-gp120 immunotoxins. But most importantly, the activity of anti-gp41 immunotoxins can be markedly enhanced in the presence of soluble CD4 so that they are 30-100 times more effective than anti-gp120 immunotoxins (Figure 2).

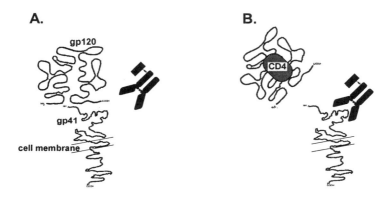

Figure 2. CD4-mediated enhancement of anti-gp41 immunotoxins. Gp120 and gp41 are non-covalently associated on the surface of HIV-infected cells and the accessibility of anti-gp41 immunotoxins to their target is hindered (panel A). In the presence of CD4, gp120 undergoes a conformational alteration and dissociates from gp41 allowing immunotoxins access to their targets (panel B). In addition, the internalization rates of immunotoxins are enhanced in the presence of CD4. The net effect is that the presence of soluble CD4 markedly enhances the efficacy of anti-gp41 immunotoxins.

Therapeutic molecules delivered to HIV-infected cells

Although our own studies, and this review, will focus on toxins delivered to infected cells, it is worthwhile noting that a variety of different agents have been delivered by targeted therapies, either attached directly to the targeting molecule or encapsulated within virions or liposomes (1). These agents include specific antiviral agents such as the reverse transcriptase inhibitor AZT, pokeweed antiviral protein that has both cytotoxic and antiviral effects, cytotoxic drugs, gene therapies, and lytic viruses. Toxins appear to be the most effective of these agents.

IN VITRO ANALYSES OF ANTI-HIV IMMUNOTOXINS

A number of different immunotoxins directed against HIV Env have been made. The most extensively tested include a series of anti-gp120 and anti-gp41 Mabs conjugated to ricin A chain (RAC), made in our laboratory (1, 9, 10, 14, 15), and the chimeric IT containing CD4 attached to the toxic portion of pseudomonas exotoxin A, CD4-PE40 (7, 16-18).

The efficacy of anti-HIV immunotoxins has been tested in a variety of different cell culture systems, including T cell lines acutely or persistently infected with laboratory isolates of HIV, activated T-cell cultures infected with either laboratory or primary clinical isolates of different tropism, and in macrophage cultures. The immunotoxins were highly effective in killing infected cells and halting the spread of infection at therapeutically obtainable concentrations. Cytotoxic action was rapid (< 1 hour) and was accompanied by an immediate cessation in the secretion of infectious virions (14). One report has indicated complete elimination of HIV from a cell culture with a combination of an immunotoxin and reverse transcriptase inhibitors (16), although others have found that the immunotoxin must be continually present to suppress HIV. Not all Mabs that bind cell-surface Env yield equally efficacious immunotoxins, and the degree of cell-surface binding does not necessarily correlate with the ability to kill (10, 15). We have screened over 100 anti-gp160 mabs and have identified the most effective for further study.

Several maneuvers have been demonstrated to enhance the efficacy of anti-HIV immunotoxins. These include: (a) combining immunotoxins with other anti-retrovirals (16, 19); (b) using drugs that inhibit the lysosomal degradation of immunotoxins, such as chloroquine, monensin, NH_4Cl, brefeldin A, or bafilomycin A1(10, 20, 21); and (c) by the addition of soluble CD4 (9, 10). CD4-mediated enhancement of immunotoxin action is restricted to anti-gp41 immunotoxins, but has been seen with immunotoxins directed against at least four different, well-conserved epitopes on gp41. The addition of CD4 lowers the concentration of immunotoxin required for increasing cytotoxicity 30 to 100-fold without increasing nonspecific toxicity. Enhancement occurs at concentrations of CD4 that are readily obtainable in human tissues and is the result of two different effects: increased surface exposure of gp41 epitopes and increased rates of internalization from the cell surface (9). CD4-mediated immunotoxin enhancement occurs even in primary clinical isolates resistant to neutralization by soluble CD4 (10).

When we test Mab-RAC and CD4-PE40 side-by-side using the same in vitro assays, we find that the efficacy curves are the same (9, 10). When anti-gp41 immunotoxins were combined with soluble CD4, we found cytotoxicity of immunotoxins on HIV-infected cells at concentrations lower than 0.01 µg/ml with no non-specific toxicity on uninfected cells at 100 µg/ml (9), an in vitro therapeutic index of >10,000. This index is far greater than that reported for any other anti-HIV drug.

POTENTIAL PROBLEMS WITH IMMUNOTOXIN THERAPY FOR HIV INFECTION

All patients infected with HIV produce antibodies to the virus, including the envelope proteins. These antibodies may bind to viral structures on infected cells and prevent the immunotoxins from reaching their target (10, 14, and 15). In vitro, we have shown that, with time, an equilibrium may be reached so that the immunotoxin may eventually bind to the target cell. There are several approaches to this problem of blocking antibodies. It is possible to target the immunotoxins with antibodies directed against immunorecessive regions (e.g., the neutralizing anti-gp41 antibody 2F5 is directed against an epitope that elicits little antibody response in patients) or with high affinity antibodies that can compete favorably with the patient derived antibodies. An alternative approach may be to remove circulating antibodies, such as with specific ex vivo adsorption or to induce transient drops in the antibody response by administering anti-CD20, or other B cell-specific antibodies.

The release of soluble or virion associated gp120 or gp41 can have several potential deleterious effects. Antigen may bind to the immunotoxin and prevent it from reaching the target cell. Alternatively, the immunotoxin may bind to soluble gp120, which in turn binds to an uninfected CD4+ cell, is internalized, and kills the uninfected cell. These effects may be eliminated or minimized using anti-gp41 immunotoxins.

The failure of a subpopulation of HIV-infected cells to express viral antigens on their surfaces would limit the utility of anti-HIV immunotoxins. This lack of expression may either be due to viral latency or to the fact that the infected cell type does not secrete virions at the cell surface. No existing anti-HIV therapies have an effect on latently infected cells. In most cases, it is unlikely that cells lacking surface expression of HIV antigens are serving as important centers for the spread of infection. Although the ability of immunotoxins to eliminate HIV-infected macrophages has been demonstrated, it is possible that a subpopulation of macrophages or dendritic cells may be a reservoir of immunotoxin-resistant cells.

Finally, the difficulty and cost of immunotoxin administration must be considered. Immunotoxins are given in a hospital setting, by IV routes. If these agents are effective, then the costs of administration will be offset by the decreased cost of hospitalization for AIDS. But even so, the costs and the facilities required will undoubtedly prevent the use of immunotoxins in developing countries, where the AIDS epidemic is most devastating.

CLINICAL TRIAL WITH CD4-PE40

For a number of reasons, CD4-PE40 appeared to be an ideal candidate for clinical testing. These included scientific rationale, such as the broad reactivity of CD4-PE40 with all HIV isolates and potent in vitro activity (7, 16-18), as well as economic concerns, such as patent coverage and production in bacterial fermentation cultures. Pharmaceutical grade CD4-PE40 was manufactured and clinical trials were carried out at the National Institutes of Health Clinical Center and by the AIDS Clinical Trials Group.

Phase I trials were performed to define dosing, toxicity, and pharmacokinetics (22, 23). The maximum tolerated dose was found to be 10µg/kg, with higher doses inducing a dose-dependent elevation in hepatic aminotransferases. In contrast, ricin immunotoxins used in clinical trials in cancer have been tolerated at levels of 300-500 µg/kg (24-26). The serum half-life of CD4-PE40 was 2-4 hours. Antibodies and immunotoxins made with intact antibodies have $t_{1/2}$ values of several days, although these values are lower if there is a large tumor burden to which the administered antibody or immunotoxin adheres (27). Over half of the patients developed antibodies to CD4-PE40. In the phase I trials there was no evidence of anti-HIV effect, although the trials were not designed to detect clinical efficacy. A phase II trial has been performed; results have not yet been published. There was no evidence of clinical effect. On the basis of these results, development of CD4-PE40 was abandoned.

In considering the failure of this clinical trial, several factors seem prominent. The first is the nonspecific toxicity seen at disappointingly low doses of CD4-PE40. Efficacy in treating autoimmune diseases (where the target population of lymphoid cells may be considered comparable) was only seen at tenfold higher doses of immunotoxin. In fact, the maximum dose in the CD4-PE40 trial was less than one third that found to be ineffective in treating rheumatoid arthritis, and less than 1/20 the dose of other immunotoxins used in cancer trials. The second factor is the short $t_{1/2}$ of CD4-PE40, 2-4 hours. Antibody-based immunotoxins can have $t_{1/2}$ of 2-4 days, similar to that of exogenously administered intact Ig. In trials of immunotoxins for cancer therapy, the best clinical effects were seen in patients with the greatest $t_{1/2}$. (For these reasons, we are proposing development of immunotoxins based on intact antibodies, rather than on single chain Fv molecules). Finally, the target of CD4-PE40 is gp120, the disadvantages of which compared to gp41 have already been discussed. In summary, it is likely that therapeutic concentrations of immunotoxin were never reached in the clinical trial and CD4-PE40 may be directed against the wrong target molecule.

IN VIVO COMPARISONS OF CD4-PE40 WITH ANTIBODY TARGETED IMMUNOTOXINS PLUS SOLUBLE CD4

Because we have argued that CD4-PE40 is a flawed immunotoxin, and that the true efficacy of anti-HIV immunotoxins has not yet been tested, we have designed in vivo trials to compare the efficacy of CD4-PE40 with other approaches to immunotoxin therapy. In particular, we have examined the combined efficacy of anti-gp41 immunotoxins co-administered with a soluble form of CD4, termed CD4-IgG2. This tetrameric molecule binds to gp120 with high avidity, and because it is a chimera with Ig, it will have a $t_{1/2}$ comparable to that of an immunotoxin utilizing an intact antibody (28). We have studied the in vivo effects of anti-HIV immunotoxins both in a novel SCID mouse model that we have developed and in macaques infected with the chimeric SIV/HIV termed SHIV.

There is no fully adequate small animal model for HIV infection because HIV only infects the cells of humans and some primates. Mice carrying the SCID mutation have been used because they may be engrafted with cells of the human immune system. These cells can then be infected with HIV. However, because of limited availability of cells, marginal engraftment, and donor-to-donor variation, the utility of SCID mouse models for the testing potential HIV therapies is limited. We therefore sought to develop a model that would provide a sufficient number of mice with a reproducible infection that may be used to perform comparative analyses of different immunotoxins. We have developed a model that allows us to test the efficacy, toxicity, and pharmacokinetics of anti-HIV immunotoxins and other antiviral therapies. However, this model does not reflect the true pathophysiology of HIV infection.

Figure 3 outlines the experimental protocol for testing immunotoxins in HIV-infected mice and details are published elsewhere (29). Irradiated SCID/NOD (non-obese diabetic mutation, also induces defects in complement and natural killer activity) mice are injected with two distinct tumors, one consisting of CD4+ human lymphoma cells that are susceptible to HIV infection, the other consisting of HIV-infected cells actively secreting virus. Mice are treated over a ten day period following injection of the tumors. At the completion of this time, mice are sacrificed and the degree of infection measured as the level of the HIV Gag protein, p24, in the plasma and the presence of HIV-infected cells (ICs) in the spleen. In the absence of either tumor, there is no evidence of HIV infection.

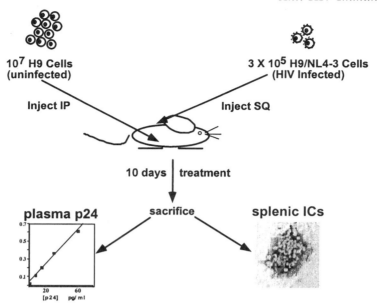

Figure 3. A mouse model for testing the efficacy of anti-HIV immunotoxins

We have validated this mouse model using approved antiviral therapies and neutralizing monoclonal antibodies. We then performed a series of experiments to compare different anti-HIV immunotoxins. Each experiment involved experimental groups of 8-10 mice. The results are summarized in Table 2. Two different anti-gp120 immunotoxins were tested, each at their maximum tolerated dose. However, for the monoclonal antibody 924 conjugated to ricin A chain (RAC), this dose was 30 µg/mouse, whereas for CD4-PE40 the maximum dose was 3 µg/mouse. The dose-limiting toxicity of CD4-PE40 was hepatic, the same as in the human clinical trial. Thus the main reason that 924-RAC was so much more effective than CD4-PE40 was that it could be used in much higher doses. But even when administered at the same dose, 924-RAC achieved much higher plasma concentrations than CD4-PE40 and persisted for two days, whereas CD4-PE40 was completely cleared within 3 hours. The anti-gp41 immunotoxin and CD4-IgG2 were administered in much lower doses, a maximum of 3 µg/mouse. Complete antiviral efficacy was seen at doses as low as 0.5 µg/mouse. Thus the combination of anti-gp41 immunotoxin and CD4-IgG2 was highly effective when compared to either anti-gp120 immunotoxin.

Table 2. Efficacy of immunotoxins in the SCID mouse model of HIV infection

Immunotoxin	Number of Experiments	Mean % Inhibition
924-RAC	7	80.09
CD4-PE40	7	35.00
41.1-RAC	3	71.02
41.1-RAC + CD4IgG2	6	96.52

Because the murine experiments so clearly support our basic contentions that CD4-PE40 is a flawed immunotoxin, we wanted to compare immunotoxins in a more relevant model of infection. We have chosen to do so in macaques that have been infected with SHIV. Because the immunotoxins are directed against epitopes on the HIV envelope, and these are not present on the SIV envelope, it was necessary to use this chimeric virus. All animals had a profound depletion of CD4+ cells and high levels of plasma viremia. We performed a dose escalation study to determine maximum tolerated doses of immunotoxins in groups of three animals, one receiving an anti-gp41 Mab conjugated to RAC combined with CD4-IgG2, while the other received CD4-PE40. Monkeys received weekly IV doses of immunotoxin starting at 4 μg/kg and doubling each week until a final dose of 64 μg/kg was given. There was no toxicity with the Mab-RAC immunotoxin, whereas, similar to the human trial, transient elevations of hepatic enzymes were observed for doses of CD4-PE40 of 16 μg/kg or greater. Elevations were dose related and returned to normal within one week. In monkeys receiving anti-gp41 Mab-RAC plus CD4-PE40, there was suppression of plasma virus load of approximately 0.5 to 1.3 logs, with efficacy seen at the lowest doses. There was no evidence of efficacy in CD4-PE40 treated animals at any dose. There was little anti-immunotoxin immune response, which was not surprising given the advanced immunodeficiency in these animals.

CONCLUSIONS AND FUTURE DIRECTIONS

Immunotoxins targeted to the HIV envelope proteins are among the most effective anti-HIV agents in vitro. The efficacy of anti-gp41 immunotoxins, but not anti-gp120, may be enhanced 30-100X in vitro by the addition of soluble CD4. A human clinical trial was performed with the anti-gp120 immunotoxin CD4-PE40. This agent proved to be highly toxic and ineffective at tolerable doses. Moreover it had an exceedingly short plasma retention time. Because of this clinical failure, there was a loss of interest in developing anti-HIV immunotoxins.

We have argued that CD4-PE40 is a flawed immunotoxin because of its targeting to the wrong region of Env, its high toxicity, and its short plasma residence. We further argue that the true efficacy of anti-HIV immunotoxins has not yet been fully tested. To confirm this hypothesis, we have performed a series of experiments in both SCID mice and in macaques in which we compared CD4-PE40 to other immunotoxins. We have found that the combination of anti-gp41 immunotoxins with CD4-IgG2, a tetrameric CD4-immunoglobulin chimera, is highly effective at very low doses, whereas CD4-PE40 had marginal, if any, effects at the maximum tolerated dose. Moreover, the toxicity and pharmacokinetics of CD4-PE40 was similar in both animal models to that seen in the human clinical trial. These results support our contentions that CD4-PE40 is the wrong immunotoxin, and that chances of obtaining a therapeutic effect with an anti-gp41 immunotoxin combined with a soluble CD4 derivative are considerably greater.

On the basis of these results, we have proposed a more thorough evaluation of immunotoxins in SHIV-infected macaques. Optimal immunotoxin preparations, the best dosing schedules, and effects of combinations with antivirals need to be determined. If a pronounced therapeutic effect can be obtained in SHIV-infected macaques, and broadly reactive immunotoxin preparations can be made, then the stage will be set for a human clinical trial in which the chances for success are optimized.

ACKNOWLEDGEMENTS

We wish to thank Tami Marcotte and Leta Eng for expert animal care; the staff of the Bozeman Deaconess Cancer Center for irradiation of mice, and Bill Olsen and Progenics Pharmaceuticals for the provision of CD4-IgG2. We are especially indebted to Shiu-Lok Hu, Nadeem Sheikh, and the staff of the Washington Regional Primate Research Center for performing experiments in SHIV-infected macaques.

REFERENCES

1.   Pincus, S. H., and V. V. Tolstikov.   Anti-human immunodeficiency virus immunoconjugates. *Adv. Pharmacol.* 1995;*32:205.*
2.   Perelson, A. S., A. U. Neumann, M. Markowitz, J. M. Leonard, and D. D. Ho. HIV-1 dynamics in vivo: Virion clearance rate, infected cell lifespan, and viral generation time. *Science* 1996;*271:1582.*
3.   Finberg, R. W., S. M. Wahl, J. B. Allen, G. Soman, T. B. Strom, J. R. Murphy, and J. C. Nichols.   Selective elimination of HIV-1-infected cells with an interleukin-2 receptor-specific cytotoxin. *Science* 1991;*252:1703.*

4. Borvak, J., C.-S. Chou, K. Bell, G. Van Dyke, H. Zola, O. Ramilio, and E. S. Vitetta. Expression of CD25 defines peripheral blood mononuclear cells with productive versus latent HIV infection. *J. Immunol.* 1995;*155:3196*.

5. McCoig, C., G. Van Dyke, C.-S. Chou, L. J. Picker, O. Ramilo, and E. S. Vitetta. An anti-CD45RO immunotoxin eliminates T cells latently infected with HIV-1 in vitro. *Proc. Natl. Acad. Sci. USA* 1999;*96:11482*.

6. Uckun, F. M., K. Bellomy, K. O'Neill, Y. Messinger, T. Johnson, and C.-L. Chen. Toxicity, biological activity, and pharmacokinetics of TXU (Anti-CD7)-pokeweed antiviral protein in chimpanzees and adult patients infected with HIV-1. *J. Pharmacol. Exp. Ther.* 1999;*291:1301*.

7. Chaudhary, V. K., T. Mizukami, T. R. Fuerst, D. J. FitzGerald, B. Moss, I. Pastan, and E. A. Berger. Selective killing of HIV-infected cells by recombinant human CD4-*Pseudomonas* exotoxin hybrid protein. *Nature* 1988;*335:369*.

8. Berger, E. A., B. Moss, and I. Pastan. Reconsidering targeted toxins to eliminate HIV infection: You gotta have HAART. *Proc Natl Acad Sci USA* 1998;*95:11511*.

9. Pincus, S. H., and J. McClure. Soluble CD4 enhances the efficacy of immunotoxins directed against gp41 of the human immunodeficiency virus. *Proc. Natl. Acad. Sci. USA* 1993;*90:332*.

10. Pincus, S. H., K. Wehrly, R. Cole, H. Fang, G. K. Lewis, J. McClure, A. J. Conley, B. Wahren, M. R. Posner, A. L. Notkins, S. A. Tilley, A. Pinter, L. Eiden, M. Teintze, D. Dorward, and V. V. Tolstikov. In vitro effects of anti-HIV immunotoxins directed against multiple epitopes on the HIV-1 envelope glycoprotein gp160. *AIDS Res. Hum. Retrovirus* 1996;*12:1041*.

11. Wild, C., T. Oas, C. McDanal, D. Bolognesi, and T. Matthews. A synthetic peptide inhibitor of human immunodeficiency virus replication: correlation between solution structure and viral inhibition. *Proc. Nat. Acad. Sci. (USA)* 1992;*89:10537*.

12. Mebatsion, T., S. Finke, F. Weiland, and K. K. Conzelmann. A CXCR4/CD4 pseudotype rhabdovirus that selectively infects HIV-1 envelope protein-expressing cells. *Cell* 1997;*90:841*.

13. Pincus, S. H. Anti-HIV immunotoxins: gp41 rather than gp120 should be the target. *Int. Antiviral News* 1994;*2:147*.

14. Pincus, S. H., K. Wehrly, and B. Chesebro. Treatment of HIV tissue culture infection with monoclonal antibody-ricin A chain conjugates. *J. Immunol.* 1989;*142:3070*.

15. Pincus, S. H., R. L. Cole, E. M. Hersh, D. Lake, Y. Masuho, P. J. Durda, and J. McClure. In vitro efficacy of anti-HIV immunotoxins targeted by various antibodies to the envelope protein. *J. Immunol.* 1991;*146:4315*.

16. Ashorn, P., B. Moss, J. N. Weinstein, V. K. Chaudhary, D. J. FitzGerald, I. Pastan, and E. A. Berger. Elimination of infectious human immunodeficiency virus from human T-cell cultures by synergistic action of CD4-Pseudomonas exotoxin and reverse transcriptase inhibitors. *Proc. Natl. Acad. Sci. USA* 1990;*87:8889*.

17. Ashorn, P., G. Englund, M. A. Martin, B. Moss, and E. A. Berger. Anti-HIV activity of CD4-*Pseudomonas* exotoxin on infected primary human lymphocytes and monocyte/macrophages. *J. Infect. Dis* 1991;*163:703*.

18. Kennedy, P. E., B. Moss, and E. A. Berger. Primary HIV-1 refractory to neutralization by soluble CD4 are potently inhibited by CD4-*Pseudomonas* exotoxin. *Virology* 1993;*192:375*.

19. Pincus, S. H., and K. Wehrly. AZT demonstrates anti-HIV-1 activity in persistently infected cell lines: implications for combination chemotherapy and immunotherapy. *J. Infect. Dis.* 1990;*162:1233*.

20. Till, M. A., S. Zolla-Pazner, M. K. Gorny, J. S. Patton, J. W. Uhr, and E. S. Vitetta. Human immunodeficiency virus-infected T cells and monocytes are killed by monoclonal human anti-gp41 antibodies coupled to ricin A chain. *Proc. Natl. Acad. Sci. USA* 1989;*86:1987*.

21. Pincus, S. H., J. McClure, and H. Fang. Use of anti-HIV immunotoxins as probes of the biology of HIV-infected cells. *Can. J. Infect. Dis.* 1994;*5(suppl. A):23A.*

22. Davey, R. T., C. M. Boenning, B. R. Herpin, D. H. Batts, J. A. Metcalf, L. Wathen, S. R. Cox, M. A. Polis, J. A. Kovacs, J. Falloon, R. E. Walker, N. Salzman, H. Masur, and H. C. Lane. Recombinant soluble CD4-pseudomonas exotoxin, a novel immunotoxin, in the treatment of individuals infected with HIV. *J. Inf. Dis.* 1994;*170:1180.*

23. Ramachandran, R. V., D. A. Katzenstein, R. Wood, D. H. Batts, and T. C. Merigan. Failure of short-term CD4-PE40 infusions to reduce viral load in HIV infected individuals. *J. Inf. Dis.* 1994;*170:1009.*

24. LeMaistre, C. F., S. Rosen, A. Frankel, S. Kornfeld, E. Saria, C. Meneghetti, J. Drajesk, D. Fishwild, P. Scannon, and V. Byers. Phase I trial of H65-RTA immunoconjugate in patients with cutaneous T-cell lymphoma. *Blood* 1991;*78:1173.*

25. Strand, V., P. E. Lipsky, G. W. Cannon, L. H. Calabrese, C. Weisenhutter, S. B. Cohen, N. J. Olsen, M. L. Lee, T. J. Lorenz, and B. Nelson. Effects of administration of an anti-CD5 plus immunoconjugate in rheumatoid arthritis: results of two phase two studies. *Arthritis Rheum.* 1993;*36:620.*

26. Amlot, P. L., M. J. Stone, D. Cunningham, J. Fay, J. Newman, R. Collins, R. May, M. McCarthy, V. Ghetie, O. Ramilo, P. E. Thorpe, J. W. Uhr, and E. S. Vitetta. A phase I study of an anti-CD22-deglycosylated ricin A chain immunotoxin in the treatment of B-cell lymphomas resistant to conventional therapy. *Blood* 1993;*82:2624.*

27. Press, O. W., J. F. Eary, F. R. Appelbaum, P. J. Martin, C. G. Badger, W. B. Nelp, S. Glenn, G. Butchko, D. Fisher, B. Porter, D. C. Matthews, L. D. Fisher, and I. D. Bernstein. Radiolabeled-antibody therapy of B-cell lymphoma with autologous bone marrow support. *N. Engl. J. Med.* 1993;*329:1219.*

28. Allaway, G. P., K. L. Davis-Bruno, G. A. Beaudry, E. B. Garcia, E. L. Wong, A. M. Ryder, K. W. Hasel, M.-C. Gauduin, R. A. Koup, S. McDougal, and P. J. Maddon. Expression and characterization of CD4-IgG2, a novel heteroteramer that neutralizes primary HIV-1 isolates. *AIDS Res. Hum. Retroviruses* 1995;*11:533.*

29. Pincus, S. H., T. K. Marcotte, B. M. Forsyth, and H. Fang. In vivo testing of anti-HIV immunotoxins. In *Immunotoxin Methods and Protocols*, Vol. 166.Methods in Molecular Biology, W. A. Hall, ed. Humana Press, 2001.

GLOSSARY

CD4: An immune interaction molecule expressed on the surface of some T lymphocytes and macrophages. It serves as the primary receptor for HIV.

CD4-PE40: A chimeric immunotoxin based upon CD4 and the translocation and toxic domains of pseudomonas exotoxin A. This toxin targets HIV gp120 expressed on the surface of HIV-infected cells.

Chemokine receptors: Chemokines are cell attractant molecules involved in the generation of immune and inflammatory responses. Some of the receptors for these molecules also serve as the coreceptor for HIV infection, most notably CXCR4 and CCR5. The coreceptor usage defines the cellular tropism of HIV.

gp41: The transmembrane domain of the HIV envelope protein, gp41 is involved in fusion of the virus to the cell it infects. It is the most promising target of anti-HIV immunotoxins.

gp120: The extracellular domain of the HIV envelope protein, gp120 binds to the receptor (CD4) and coreceptor (chemokine receptor) on the surface of target cells.

HIV: The human immunodeficiency virus, the cause of AIDS.

HIV envelope protein(s): The envelope proteins are secreted as a precursor molecule (gp160), which is cleaved by a cellular protease to the extracellular domain (gp120) and transmembrane domain (gp41).

Mab-RAC: An immunotoxin consisting of a ricin A chain targeted by a monoclonal antibody.

SCID mice: Mice carrying the severe combined immunodeficiency mutation that aborts development of both T and B cells. These mice may be engrafted with human cells and used for studies of HIV infection and of tumor development.

SHIV: A chimeric virus consisting of the envelope protein derived from HIV and the remainder from SIV (the simian immunodeficiency virus). This virus is used in primate studies of vaccine efficacy and other studies of the pathogenesis and treatment of AIDS.

22

LIGAND-MEDIATED GASTROINTESTINAL TARGETING

John Woodley
Faculté des Sciences Pharmaceutiques, 31500 Toulouse, France

INTRODUCTION

This chapter will describe the rationale for drug targeting to the gastrointestinal (GI) tract, why it is important, and what the objectives of such targeting are. The approaches used to achieve these targeting objectives using ligands will be considered and discussed in detail. It it is important to consider some of the pharmaceutical issues involved, such as the type of vehicles to which ligands can be usefully attached. It should be stressed that at the current time, much of the work in this area is theoretical and experimental, with studies in cell culture systems or animals, and has yet to be transferred to man, let alone into pharmaceutical products on the market. In many cases, costs and regulatory considerations may make it prohibitive for the pharmaceutical industry to adopt some of the most interesting ideas emanating from the research laboratories.

THE REASONS FOR TARGETING THE GI TRACT

The first questions to consider are: why target the gastrointestinal tract? What are the objectives of such targeting? Below are listed what might be considered to be main reasons for wishing to achieve such targeting.

Increasing the Gastrointestinal Residence Time

The major site of drug absorption for orally administered drugs is the small intestine, which in man is 5-6 meters long and has a surface area of around 200 square meters. In man, the transit of pharmaceutical formulations through the small intestine is relatively constant between normal individuals (unlike the colon transit) and is 3-4 hours. This means that if a drug is not fully dissolved or released from whatever formulation is used within this time frame, absorption will not take place and the drug will be lost. There may be some absorption in the colon, but it is not normally on the same scale as in the small intestine. Thus, for poorly absorbed drugs, it is of great interest to increase the amount of time that they stay in the small intestine. Even for well-absorbed drugs, the concept of a controlled release formulation that has prolonged residence time at the major site of absorption is also therapeutically attractive. This can improve the pharmacokinetic profile with, for example, a prolongation of plasma peak levels. It can consequently lead to an increase in the time between doses with better patient compliance. The quantity of drug needed to achieve the therapeutic effect can be reduced along, therefore, with any undesirable side effects and costs.

Targeting Specific Regions of the GI Tract

The targeting of drug formulations to specific regions of the GI tract may be advantageous for a number of reasons. For example, there may be 'absorption' windows for drugs, ie: they may be preferentially absorbed in some regions more than in others. In fact, there is not a lot of evidence for specific regions of absorption, it is more a matter of degree, and is probably more linked to metabolic rather than to absorption phenomena as such. Many drugs are absorbed into the intestinal cells and then can be 're-exported' back into the intestinal lumen by the action of the membrane transporter P-glycoprotein (P-gp). The effect of this can be to reduce the net absorption of the drug at the level of the intestine, which is a potentially important consideration given that as many as 50% of drugs currently administered orally may be P-gp substrates. The levels of P-glycoprotein increase moving down the length of the gut. Thus, in the case of drugs which are known to be substrates of the P-gp, the bioavailabilty may be enhanced if they can be targeted to the proximal parts of the small intestine where the level of P-gp expression is lower. Conversely, the drug metabolizing enzyme cytochrome P450 subtype 3A4 (CYP3A4) decreases in expression down the length of the gut. This enzyme is important in contributing to first pass metabolism of many drugs during their passage across the intestinal epithelium. Thus it may be advantageous to target such drugs to the more distal parts of the intestine to limit the effect on bioavailability of the CYP3A4.

Another reason for targeting drugs to the lower small intestine would be to avoid the high levels of digestive enzymes present in the proximal small intestine. Such is the case for peptide drugs which, if unprotected, are rapidly metabolized by the peptidase enzymes in the pancreatic secretions that enter the upper intestine. Although still present in the distal small intestine, these enzymes will be more dilute and partly autodigested and thus may pose a reduced threat to peptides present in the lumen.

As discussed below, there are also good reasons for targeting to the colon to try to target diseased tissues. There has also been some enthusiasm for targeting therapeutic peptides to the colon in the belief that there are lower amounts of peptidase enzymes present that degrade peptides. While this may be true, the long residence time in the colon means that the peptides will be exposed to the enzymes present for a longer time, particularly as the cells of the colon are poor at absorbing such molecules, and so the idea may be self-defeating.

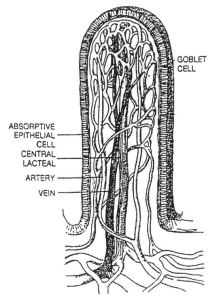

GOBLET
CELL

ABSORPTIVE
EPITHELIAL
CELL
CENTRAL
LACTEAL
ARTERY
VEIN

Figure 1 Schematic representation of an intestinal villus showing the single layer of enterocytes or absorprtive epithelial cells. Goblet cells are also are present which secrete mucus.

Targeting to Specific Cells in the GI Tract

The majority of cells in the intestinal epithelium are enterocytes or columnar epithelial cells (also known as absorptive epithelial cells). As can be seen in Figure 1 above, these cells form a single layer covering the whole of the intestine surface. The enterocytes are the absorbing cells and their surfaces are greatly enhanced by the folding of their apical membranes to form the microvilli, as shown in the Figure 2. These cells have a number of highly specialised transport systems in their membranes to ensure the absorption of hydrophilic molecules. Other hydrophilic molecules may pass between the cells through the tight junctions. Lipophilic molecules diffuse across the microvilli. By targeting these cells, ie: taking drugs to the cell membrane without loss or dilution, it should be possible to enhance the intestinal absorption of drugs. This, indeed, has been the goal of many of the experimental ligand-based systems described.

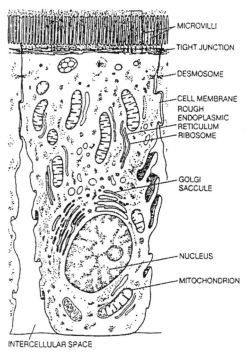

Figure 2. Schematic representation of an enterocyte. Note the convoluted apical membrane which forms the microvilli and enhances the surface area.

In theory, one can imagine the possibility of targeting such transport systems with appropriate ligands to 'persuade' the transport system to carry a molecule of choice such as a low molecular weight drug. As will be seen later, one such system has been developed (cobalamin transporter).

In addition to the enterocytes, there are groups of specialized cells which have attracted much attention from the point of view of intestinal targeting. These are the discrete groups of cells which constitute the gut associated lymphoid tissue (GALT). Anatomically known as Peyer's patches, they are scattered down the length of the small intestine. Figure 3 shows a schematic representation of a Peyers patch.

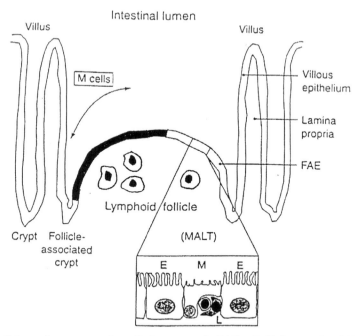

Figure 3. Schematic representation of a Peyers patch; FAE = Follicle-associated Epithelium; MALT = Mucosa-associated lymphoid tissue; E= Enterocytes; M = M-cells

The predominant cell type exposed to the intestinal lumen is the 'M-cells', while deeper in the Peyer's patches lymphocytes and macrophages are found. M-cells do not have microvilli and can endocytose and phagocytose macromolecules and particulate matter. It is generally accepted that these structures play an important role in sampling lumen proteins as part of the protective function of the immune system. These sampled proteins will then be processed and generate an immune response, most notably a mucosal immune response which will prevent the entry of foreign proteins into the mucosa. This is a very important mechanism in protecting the body against the many infectious microorganisms and viruses that gain entry to the body via the intestinal mucosa. It is for this reason that there is considerable interest in targeting these cells with orally administered vaccines. Effective oral vaccines would be of great medical benefit, especially for disease prevention in the developing world.

Targeting to Diseased Tissues

The general concept of 'drug targeting' is the idea of directing drugs specifically to disease sites. This is also true of GI targeting where attempts are being made to target to disease sites. Inflammatory diseases of the GI tract, particularly of the colon, are a major medical problem, and colonic cancer is an ever-increasing disease. The idea of orally administering drugs which can be targeted specifically to inflamed tissue or cancer cells is very seductive, but like many of these areas, is proving hard to achieve in reality. A form of targeting to the colon is already on the market with such anti-inflammatory drugs as Azocol, where the active principles are released by the action of enzymes which are present in the colon but not in other parts of the GI tract. Another interesting system would be to target drugs specifically against infectious organisms which may enter the GI tract, but little work seems to have been done in this area.

Thus there are a number of very good reasons for trying to target to the gastrointestinal tract and, as in other examples of drug targeting, the belief is that this is best achieved by the use of ligands that will recognise and bind specifically to appropriate sites. However, not only do the ligands have to be considered, but normally any ligand-based drug delivery system has to have another component, namely the carrier or vehicle to which the putative ligand is to be attached. In some cases it may be appropriate to conjugate the ligand directly to the drug. Therefore, before considering the ligands, the next section briefly describes the types of vehicles that are being investigated at the present time.

CARRIERS FOR LIGAND ATTACHMENT

The choice of carriers for ligand attachement depends to some extent on the targeting objective sought. For example, if the objective is to achieve prolonged residency in the small intestine for the controlled release of a drug, then some form of microcapsule will be appropriate. On the other hand, if the objective is for the active molecule to target and enter M-cells, then nanocapsules/nanoparticles or liposomes are likely to be more appropriate as these stand a greater chance of being phagocytosed by the target cells. Most of the studies on the use of ligands for targeting in the GI tract have used micro- or nanoparticles/capsules as carriers. These may be non-degradable for example polystyrene or latex, or made from biodegradable polymers such as poly-(lactic-co-glycolic) acid (PLGA). However, the disadvantage of many of the nano-systems is the low drug loading capacity. Liposomes have also been used and have the advantages that higher drug loading is possible and attaching ligands is generally not difficult. While liposomes fell somewhat out of favor for GI drug delivery because of their instability in the GI milieu, new generations of polymerised liposomes are more stable and have been used in targeting studies. Figure 4 (below) illustrates some types of drug carriers useful for GI targeting.

Nanoparticles   < 1 μm, Microparticles   1-1000 μm. D = drug; L = ligand

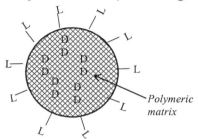

Nanocapsules   < 1 μm, Microcapsules   1-1000 μm

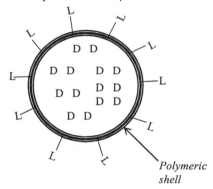

Liposomes   100-500 nm

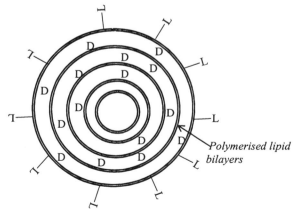

Figure 4A. Polymeric carriers and liposomes for GI drug delivery (see explanations in the text).

The use of synthetic polymers as drug carriers has also been explored following the success in clinical trials of parenterally administered polymers which have both targeting ligands and drugs covalently attached to the polymer backbone. The attractiveness of these polymers is the versatility which enables a range of different targeting ligands and drugs to be attached to the polymer backbone by different types of chemical bonds for triggered released by enzymes, pH, reducing agents, etc. Most of the studies to date concern the synthetic polymer N-(2-hydroxypropyl)methacrylamide (HPMA), with drug being liberated at the target site by enzymatic activity (Fig. 4B). For example, a conjugate has been produced with an attached anticancer drug which is specifically released from the polymer in the colon.

Drug carrying polymers (eg HPMA)

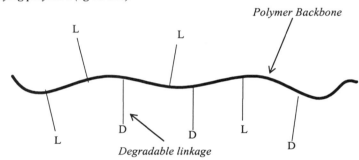

Mucin-targeted polymers, SH = sulfhydryl group

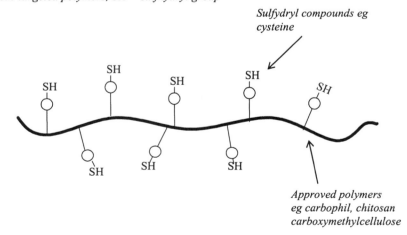

Figure 4B. HPMA and sulfhydrul polymer drug carriers (see explanations in the text).

In terms of more conventional pharmaceutical formulations, there is little described, but as will be described later, an interesting approach is being researched by a group in Austria that works with a range of approved pharmaceutical polymers for targeting. They have modified the polymers by the addition of sulfhydryl groups, which makes them target to mucin, and unlike other targeting systems, involves the formation of covalent bonds between the carrier and the target. The polymers have then been made into tablets for oral administration of drugs.

LIGANDS USED FOR GASTROINTESTINAL TARGETING

One of the basic premises of drug targeting is that of specificity, ie: the use of a ligand that will recognise only the target site. This is not easy to attain, and no more so in the GI tract than elsewhere in the body. One of the problems in the GI tract is an ever-present layer of mucus, which is constantly produced by the Goblet cells in the epithelial layer and covers the entire surface of the GI tract. In man this layer is 50 – 450 μm thick. Mucus contains the large complex glycoprotein mucin, which has many terminal sugars on its surface as well as negatively charged groups. This has several consequences. Firstly, ligand-carrying formulations must somehow penetrate the mucus layer to reach the target cell surfaces. Secondly, the mucin may also contain competitive sites for ligand attachment. In fact, many of the ligands tested interact with mucin, and this has lead to the concept of 'muco-adhesion': the binding of ligand carriers to mucin as a target itself. In fact, as will be seen, this is a form of targeting which can result in prolonged GI residency. Below we analyze some of the ligands that are being investigated for GI tract targeting. (Table 1)

Table 1. Summary of ligands and carriers used for gastrointestinal targeting

Ligands	Carriers	Targets
Antibodies	Microparticles	M cells
Lectins	Nanoparticles Microparticles Liposomes	Enterocytes M cells
	Polymers (HPMA)	Cancers Inflammation
Adhesins Invasins	Nanoparticles	M cells
Cobalamin	Nanoparticles Peptide drugs	Cobalamin transporter (ileum)
Sulfydryl compounds	Polycarbophil Carboxymethylcellulose Chitosan	Mucin

Antibodies

Antibodies are nature's supreme molecules for specificy, showing exquisite ability to recognise individual types of molecules. Not surprisingly, therefore, their use for cell-specific GI targeting has been investigated, notably for targeting to M cells in Peyer's patches in the quest for oral vaccines, as described earlier. The difficulty is to show the existence of cell surface components which are present on the M cell surface and not on the other major cell type the enterocytes (The M cell surface represents only about 1% of the total surface area of the gut). There are some reports of differences in the surface glycoproteins expressed between species. In 1991, Pappo et al. bound an M cell specific antibody to polystyrene microspheres and showed a 3.5-fold increase in uptake by rabbit M cells, compared with control microspheres coated with non-specific antibodies (1). The use of antibodies in GI targeting has not been further investigated despite the promise of specificity. The problem with antibodies is that being proteins, they are unstable in the hostile gut lumen. The intestinal lumen abounds with large quantities of peptidase enzymes both secreted in the pancreatic fluid and located on the cell surface membranes. These degrade proteins very rapidly and so the life-time of an antibody is likely to be too short for it to act in a targeting role.

Lectins

Lectins are glycoproteins found in abundance mostly, but not exclusively, in the plant world. The unique feature of lectins is that they recognise and bind to arrays of sugars on cell surfaces. These sugars may be part of the carbohydrate side chains attached to integral membrane glycoproteins, or they may be attached to lipids that constitute the membrane structure (glycolipids). Lectins themselves are large glycoproteins, and each lectin shows specificity for particular sugars and/or multiples of sugars. For example, tomato lectin (TL) recognises structures containing the sugar N-acetyl glucosamine, whereas a lectin from *Ulex europeaus* (UAE 1) specifically recognizes L-fucose in glycoproteins and glycolipids.

The idea of using lectins for gastrointestinal targeting was first proposed in 1988 by Woodley, who showed that tomato lectin bound to at least 6 different membrane proteins on the surface of rat intestinal absorptive cells. He suggested that this might thus increase GI residence time of the lectin (2). In addition, it had been shown that TL was relatively resistant to digestion in the gut, thus overcoming the problem of stability described above for antibodies. Given also the high consumption of raw tomatoes by the general population it seemed unlikely that the tomato lectin was toxic. Tomato lectin was endocytosed by rat intestinal cells *in vitro* and transported across the epithelial layer to the serosal side. However, when *in vivo* experiments were carried out in rats, the results were disappointing in that the gastrointestinal transit time of the lectin was similar to that of non-specific control macromolecules (3). These studies were done with unconjugated lectin, but other studies have been carried out with the lectin bound to microspheres. These ligand-bearing microspheres bound to epithelial cells and to mucin, but also *in vivo* failed to show any significant increase in the intestinal transit time. However, more recently Montisci et al. showed that TL-conjugated to polylactide microspheres showed delayed GI transit compared with non-conjugated controls (4). They attributed stomach retardation as the main factor in causing the delay in transit, and noted that much of the interaction of the conjugate with the GI tract was not specific, as it could not be inhibited by lectin blocking sugars. In other studies, microparticles conjugated with Phaseolus vulgaris agglutin (PHA) spread more broadly down the intestine, with considerable evidence of retardation (5). PHA is specific for galactose and N-acetyl glucosamine.

Thus, it may be possible to increase GI residence time, but the lectins would have to be carefully chosen. The failure to increase transit times by many of these systems may be due to the interaction of the lectin with the mucus and the constant flow of mucus down the gut. Very little is known about the mucus turnover time, but it would appear to be rapid with the time in rats reported to be between 47 and 270 minutes (6). It must be said that the role of mucus and its influence on ligand conjugates is very unclear. As will be seen later, formulations which have been designed to specifically target mucin can apparently significantly increase GI residence time and enhance drug absorption.

While these studies were largely conceived as an approach to increasing the GI tract residence time of formulations, others have used TL to target the cell surfaces to increase drug uptake using particulate systems. The idea is that particles bound to cell surfaces would be phagocytosed by the cells and transported across the epithelium, or the contents released at the membrane and thus favor absorption. TL has been coupled to micro- and nanoparticles, and they have been shown to cross the intestinal mucosa both *in vitro* and *in vivo*. An interesting study showed that when rats were dosed orally over a 5 day period with TL-bearing 500 nm polystyrene nanoparticles, there was a 23% systemic uptake of the dose compared with 0.5% for controls where the lectin had been blocked by a competing sugar (7). If these results were to be attainable in man there is potential for a novel oral drug delivery system.

Lectins have also been tried in experimental systems to achieve the objective of targeting to specific cell types, ie: targeting to the M cells in the gut associated lymphoid tissue (GALT). For example, Hirst and colleagues have coupled the lectin UAE 1, which is specific for the sugar fucose, to microparticles for M cell targeting. The lectin appears to be specific for M cells in mice. When these microparticles were administered into ligated intestines of mice, they showed a rapid binding to M cells, which was 100-fold greater than control microparticles with albumin as the ligand (8). The lectin-induced binding also resulted in the uptake of the microparticles by the M cells. Recently, the same group coupled the UAE 1 lectin to polymerised liposomes and showed effective M cell targeting in mouse intestines (9). Other workers have also bound this lectin to stabilised liposomes and showed that 10.5 % of the dose was taken up from the GI tract of mice, compared with 3.2 % for the lectin-free control liposomes. The lectin-conjugated liposomes showed effective Peyer's patch targeting (10).

The objective of targeting to diseased tissue has also been the subject of a number of studies using lectins. Interesting work has been carried out with lectins bound to a synthetic polymer (HPMA) with a view to targeting to inflamed tissue and cancer cells, notably in the colon. Anticancer drugs have been attached to this polymer for release in the colon. The lectin peanut agglutinin PNA is of interest as the polymer carrying the lectin was associated more with diseased tissue in a colitis model than with normal (11). The binding sites for this lectin are also expressed on the colon cancer cell lines HT 29 and Caco-2. Another lectin, wheat germ agglutinin (WGA), has been conjugated to microspheres and these showed a high binding to Caco-2 cells. When it was directly conjugated to the anti-cancer drug doxorubicin, the conjugate exhibited considerable cytostatic activity towards these cells in culture (12). However, studies with polymer-bound WGA showed that this conjugate bound to normal tissue in rat intestine, so specificity towards cancerous tissue may be compromised (11). Recently, these investigations have been extended to include human biopsies from precancerous tissue and shown, for example, that the PNA lectin binds to the metaplastic glandular tissue of Barrett's esophagus (13).

Thus lectins have been tried in a range of experimental systems to attain different targeting objectives in the GI tract. It must be stressed that most of these systems are still very much at the experimental stage. One of the difficulties, as with many ligand-based delivery sytems, is that of achieving the specificity required. Lectins interact with binding sites which are widely distributed, notably in the mucin in the gut and in normal dietary components, so competition for binding sites may be present. Many questions remain unanswered and problems exist, some of which are discussed in further detail at the end of the chapter. (For recent comprehensive reviews on lectin-mediated targeting, see (9, 14))

Bacterial Adhesins and Enterocytes

Pathogenic bacteria have evolved mechanisms by which they attach themselves to human cell surfaces as part of the process of pathogenicity. In some cases, there is also a triggering of phagocytosis by the host cells to ensure that the microorganisms gain entry into the cells. These two processes occur because the bacteria produce specific functional proteins to achieve these goals. In the case of adhering to cells, these proteins are called 'adhesins' and consist of long filamentous proteins called fimbriae. The interaction with the cells is by sugar recognition (mannose), as is the case with lectins. Fimbrins have been tried for GI delivery systems, and fimbrin-coated particles transited down the intestine more slowly than control particles. More interesting results have been obtained using the phagocytosis triggering protein, invasin, from a *Yersinia* species. This protein recognises receptors containing the protein ß1 integrin, which is expressed on M cells but not on enterocytes. Its potential use as a targeting ligand in the GI tract is attractive all the more so because, while it is a large protein, its binding capacity lies in a reduced-sized fragment of 192 amino acids. In addition, it is amenable to large-scale production by biotechnology. This fragment has been bound as a ligand to nanoparticles and administered orally to rats. After 24 hours, 13% of the intial dose was recovered in the cardiovascular compartment compared with less than 2% for the controls (15). Such *in vivo* experiments give no indication of the site of targeting of the formulation, and it is unlikely that this difference could have been achieved by the nanoparticles targeting only the M cells. Indeed, in this study, histology showed that the nanoparticles abundantly deposited in the serosal layer of the distal ileum.

Sugars

Just as exogenous lectins interact with sugar molecules on cell surfaces, the reverse situation also exists: there are molecules on cell surfaces that have lectin properties (endogenous lectins) and will interact with exogenous sugars. One of the best-known examples is the receptor on the surface of hepatocytes that recognises the sugar galactose. This has led to the development of a polymeric drug carrier that has galactose attached to it to target to liver cells and doxorubicin attached as a drug to treat liver cancer. This system has entered clinical trials in the UK. Work with similar polymeric structures suggested that polymers with either fucose or galactose as attached ligands could interact with receptors in the gut. In particular, fucose-bearing polymers showed a higher affinity for the colon than the small intestine and have been further investigated as vehicles for targeted drug delivery to the colon.

Recently, a family (10 to date) of galactose binding endogenous lectins has been described, known as 'galectins.' Several of these are expressed on the surface of the gastrointestinal tract. One of them, galectin-3, is found on colon tumor cells and its expression is reported to correlate with tumor progression. It is hence an attractive target, and work is in progress to develop HPMA polymer conjugates to target this cell marker. Polymers with attached galactose show binding to 3 differerent colon cancer cell lines in culture. Increasing the amount of galactose on the polymers increases the binding. When an anticancer drug was attached to these polymers cytotoxicty towards these cells in culture could be shown (16).

Cobalamin (Vitamin B$_{12}$)

Cobalamin (vitamin B$_{12}$) is a large hydrophilic molecule; distal intestinal enterocytes have on their surface a specific receptor and endocytic transport system to enable the body to absorb the vitamin from dietary sources. To exploit this system for oral drug delivery, an interesting and highly specific ligand-based targeting system has been developed by Biotech Australia Pty. The cobalamin has been attached to nanoparticles and these have been shown to have an enhanced uptake by Caco-2 cells in culture compared with controls. Most interestingly, the ligand has recently been conjugated to therapeutic peptides, directly or via an aliphatic spacer. These peptide-ligand conjugates were then administered orally to rats. Impressive absorption of the peptides was seen. This was nearly completely inhibited by an excess of competing free cobalamin, showing that the highly specific B$_{12}$ route was being utilised by the ligand-peptide complexes (17). This system is an interesting application of a highly specific targeting system. However, it may be limited to select very highly active drugs because of the inherent low capacity.

Cysteine and Sulfhydryl Compounds

As noted earlier, the intestinal mucosa is covered with a layer of mucus which protects the surface of the epithelium. The mucus layer may also be a barrier to the arrival of large molecular complexes or particulate formulations at cell surfaces. The major macromolecular component of mucus, namely mucin, is a high molecular weight glycoprotein with many sulfhydryl groups (-SH). In an interesting and innovative approach to intestinal targeting, Andreas Bernkop-Schnürch and his colleagues in Vienna have attached the amino acid cysteine and other sulfhydryl compounds as targeting ligands to various polymers (christened 'thiomers') (18). These compounds contain free sulphydryl groups (-SH) that can react with the -SH groups in the mucin to form a covalent -S-S- linkage between the ligand and the mucin, thus in a sense 'anchoring' the formulation. *In vitro* tests show that the conjugates have increased adhesion to excised intestinal mucosa. One of the advantages of the system is that the ligands have been attached to the standard polymers polycarbophil, carboxymethyl cellulose, chitosan and alginate. These are approved for human use and can be made into conventional tablet which have very good stability. In addition, the researchers have also conjugated inhibitors of peptidase enzymes onto polymers to create formulations suitable for the oral administration of therapeutic peptides. The group has made microtablets using the mucin-targeting polymer polycarbophil-cysteine, and carboxymethylcellulose with attached peptidase inhibitors. They put insulin into these tablets and administered them to diabetic mice. The effect of the adhesion and the inhibitors lead to a prolonged and sustained insulin effect (reduction of blood glucose) (19). This mucin-targeting system therefore looks very promising for controlled delivery of drugs in the intestine.

DIFFICULTIES TO OVERCOME

It is clear from looking at the work described in this chapter that ligand-mediated gastrointestinal targeting is very much in its infancy. Before serious gastrointestinal targeting becomes a reality there are many difficulties to overcome. These are scientific, particularly biochemical, toxicological, regulatory and industrial. Some of these difficulties are discussed below.

In Vitro versus In Vivo and Species Variations

Many of the studies have been carried out with cell culture systems, notably the Caco-2 cell monolayer as a model for the small intestine epithelium. This is a cell line derived from a colon carcinoma which has morphological and biochemical characteristics similar to the cells of the small intestinal eptihelium. However the Caco-2 cells may also differ in important ways from the normal small intestine cells in terms of proteins expressed on their cell surfaces. Thus data obtained from studies with Caco-2 may be different from those obtained when studies are carried out *in vivo*. However, for evaluating targeting to cancer cells, Caco-2 is a useful model as it is cancer derived.

A step up from Caco-2 takes us to tests of ligand-based targeting systems in animals. Here there may be biochemical differences between the species used and man. For example, in a number of studies cited earlier, lectins have been used to try to target to M cells, in particular fucose-specific lectins, because mouse M cells are high in sites displaying this sugar. When mouse M cells were stained with a panel of lectins, they labelled exclusively with fucose-specific lectins. Unfortunately, this was not the case in man, where no distinct M cell staining pattern was observed. Thus transferring experimental studies from rodent species to man may not give the same results.

Competition with Food and Mucus

Glycoproteins and glycolipids are ubiquitous in nature. Most animal proteins are glycosylated: animal cell membranes are rich in glycolipids; plants contain many complex carbohydrates. All these will be present in the normal diet, and even if animal products are excluded, the complex carbohydrates in plants will be present. In addition, the human intestine contains large numbers of microorganisms, with up to 10^5 organisms per gram of wet weight in the proximal regions and 10^6 to 10^7 in the distal regions. The surface envelopes of microorganisms also contain complexes of sugars. All these sources will be competitive binding sites for lectins, and so the impact of food and resident microorganisms on a lectin-based drug delivery system may be quite considerable. This will only become apparent when any putative lectin-based delivery systems are tested *in vivo* with different dietary regimes.

As discussed earlier, the GI mucin is also a major site of competition for lectin binding, and so it is important that studies move from the *in vitro* to the *in vivo* as soon as possible. The binding of bacterial invasin to cell surfaces has shown to be inhibited by mucin, but it is encouraging that the *in vivo* experiments using invasin conjugated nano-particles (15) gave very positive results. It should be noted that targeting to mucus may in itself consitute a useful approach as demonstrated by the work of Bernkop-Schnürch discussed earlier.

Toxicity and Immunogenicity of Ligands

Plant lectins have a long history of toxicity, and the use of many plant lectins in drug delivery systems may be limited because of their toxicity. For example, both WGA and PHA (cited earlier) are reported to be toxic, albeit at higher doses than might be envisaged for use in drug delivery. On the other hand, circumstantial evidence, ie: the fact that raw tomatoes are widely consumed (annual average tomato lectin consumption in USA estimated at 100–200 mg) suggests *a priori* that tomato lectin is unlikely to be toxic. The amounts likely to be administered in a potential drug delivery system are in the microgram range so should pose no toxicity problems.

However, while TL may not be toxic, it is highly immunogenic, with small single oral doses eliciting immune responses in mice. These included a secretory immune response whereby the intestinal cells secrete immunoglobulin A to bind the offending antigen. Anti-TL antibodies have been detected in the blood of a normal individual. This suggests that, as it is part of the diet, individuals may be immunised against the lectin and this will be manifested as a secretory immune response. This would render any TL-based delivery system useless. This phenomenon would not be seen in laboratory animals unless, of course, they had been fed a diet containing tomatoes! Obviously, these problems would need to be thoroughly investigated before any targeting system using lectins as ligands became a reality.

Non-scientific Problems

Many of the 'biological' ligands described in this chapter, notably lectins, would be difficult and expensive to produce on an industrial scale. Thus, unless major benefits were seen to accrue from their use, it unlikely that the pharmaceutical industry would undertake their mass production, so they are destined to remain very much experimental systems. The exception may be if they could be seen to work in oral vaccines which could potentially have a very large market if the costs were appropriate. Lectins are very large complex glycoproteins, but through genetic engineering techniques, it may be possible to produce smaller fragments which retain the specific binding activity.

Given also the problems of potential toxicity and/or immunogenicity, the regulatory issues will be complex and the need for toxicity testing extensive. All these factors may limit such ligand-based GI targeting systems appearing in the market place for some time to come. Other systems, such as the use of cobalamin as a ligand or the cysteine targeting to mucin, may fare better.

CONCLUSIONS

In this chapter, the rational bases for developing targeted drug delivery systems targeted at the GI tract has been outlined. The reasons and objectives are clear: achieving them is the challenge. A considerable number of extremely interesting and innovative systems have been described, especially using natural macromolecules such as lectins and ligands. As with all forms of targeted drug delivery the specificity of the ligand for the target remains a difficult challenge. Lectins, sugars, and adhesins have rather broad specificities, so they will meet competition for binding to the target site. As has been pointed out, one also has to be pragmatic and assess the reality of the situation from a practical point of view. Of the ligand-based systems described, it seems that the least problematic are the use of cobalamin as a ligand and of sulfydryl compounds. Both are showing promise for the drug delivery of bioactive peptides, a highly sought-after therapeutic goal. In the former case, the advantage of the idea is the use of a totally specific transport system, which obviates the problem of competition. On the down side, the carrying capacity is possibly rather limited, but many putative therapeutic peptides have very high biological activities and small quantities may suffice to achieve the desired pharmacological effect. In the case of the use of sulfydryl compounds as ligands, there are a number of advantages. Approved polymers are used and they can be formulated into conventional tablets. A strong interaction with mucin appears to be achieving the objective of increasing residence time with a consequent enhancement of drug bioavailability. Systems with protein ligands may well in the future achieve some of the other objectives described, particularly targeting to diseased tissues, which could have medical benefits. For oral vaccines, opinion may be shifting away from the importance of the role of Peyer's patches as the necessary site to target; increased uptake of antigens by all the cells of the small intestine, achieved using enterocyte-targeted ligand-bearing nanoparticles, may be effective.

REFERENCES

1. J. Pappo, T.H. Ermak and H.J. Steger. Monoclonal antibody-directed targeting of fluorescent polystyrene microspheres to Peyer's patch M cells. *Immunology* **73**: 277-280 (1991).

2. J.F. Woodley and B. Naisbett. The potential of lectins for delaying the intestinal transit of drugs. *Proc. Int. Symp. Contr. Rel. Bioact. Mater.* **15**: 125-126 (1988).

3. B. Naisbett and J. Woodley. The potential use of tomato lectin for oral drug delivery. 3. Bioadhesion in vivo. *Int. J. Pharm.* **114**: 227-236 (1995).

4. M.J. Montisci, A. Dembri, G. Giovannuci, H. Chacun, D. Duchene and G. Ponchel. Gastrointestinal transit and mucoadhesion of colloidal suspensions of Lycopersicon esculentum L. and Lotus tetragonolobus lectin-PLA microsphere conjugates in rats. *Pharm. Res.* **18**: 829-837 (2001).

5. Lehr, C.-M,. A. Pustzai. "The potential of bioadhesive lectins for the delivery of peptide and protein drugs to the gastrointestinal tract." In *Lectins:Biomedical perspectives,* A.Pusztai, S.Bardocz, ed. London and Bristol: Taylor and Francis, 1995.

6. C.-M. Lehr, F.G.J. Poelma, H.E. Junginger and J.J. Tukker. An estimate of turnover time of intestinal mucus gel layer in the rat in situ loop. *Int. J. Pharm.* **70**: 235-240 (1991).

7. N. Hussain, P.U. Jani and A.T. Florence. Enhanced oral uptake of tomato lectin-conjugated nanoparticles in the rat. *Pharm. Res.* **14**: 613-618 (1997).

8. N. Foster, M.A. Clark, M.A. Jepson and B.H. Hirst. Ulex europaeus 1 lectin targets microspheres to mouse Peyer's patch M- cells in vivo. *Vaccine* **16**: 536-541 (1998).

9.   M.A. Clark, B.H. Hirst and M.A. Jepson. Lectin-mediated mucosal delivery of drugs and microparticles. *Adv. Drug Deliv. Rev.* **43**: 207-223 (2000).

10.   H. Chen, V. Torchilin and R. Langer. Polymerized liposomes as potential oral vaccine carriers: stability and bioavailability. *J. Cont. Rel.* **42**: 263-272 (1996).

11.   S. Wróblewski, P. Kopěckova, B. Říhová and J. Kopeček. Lectin-HPMA copolymer conjugates- drug carriers for gastrointestinal tract targeting. *Proc. Int. Symp. Contr. Rel. Bioact. Mater.* **25**: 768-769 (1998).

12.   M. Wirth, A. Fuchs, M. Wolf, B. Ertl and F. Gabor. Lectin-mediated drug targeting: preparation, binding characteristics, and antiproliferative activity of wheat germ agglutinin conjugated doxorubicin on Caco-2 cells. *Pharm. Res.* **15**: 1031-1037 (1998).

13.   S. Wroblewski, M. Berenson, P. Kopeckova and J. Kopecek. Potential of lectin-*N*-(2-hydroxypropyl)methacrylamide copolymer-drug conjugates for the treatment of pre-cancerous conditions. *J. Cont. Rel.* **74**: 283-293 (2001).

14.   E.C. Lavelle. Targeted delivery of drugs to the gastrointestinal tract. *Crit. Rev. Ther. Drug Car. Syst.* **18**: 341-386 (2001).

15.   N. Hussain and A.T. Florence. Utilizing bacterial mechanisms of epithelial cell entry: invasin-induced oral uptake of latex nanoparticles. *Pharm. Res.* **15**: 153-156 (1998).

16.   D. Ayelet, P. Kopecková, T. Minko, A. Rubinstein and J. Kopeček. The involvement of endogenous lectins in mediating the antitumor activity of targetable HPMA copolymer-doxorubicin conjugates in human colon adenocarcinoma and hepatoma cells. *Pharm. Res.* In press: (2002).

17.   J. Alsenz, G.J. Russell-Jones, S. Westwood, B. Levet-Trafit and P.C. de Smidt. Oral absorption of peptides through the cobalamin (vitamin B12) pathway in the rat intestine. *J. Cont. Rel.* **17**: 825-832 (2000).

18.   A. Bernkop-Schnürch, V. Schwarz and S. Steininger. Polymers with thiol groups: a new generation of mucoadhesive polymers? *Pharm. Res.* **16**: 876-881 (1999).

19.   M.K. Marschütz, P. Caliceti and A. Bernkop-Schnürch. Design and *in vitro* evaluation of an oral delivery system for insulin. *Pharm. Res.* **17**: 1468-1474 (2000).

GLOSSARY

Caco-2:   A colonic cancer-derived cell line which, when grown as a monolayer, gives has the appearance and many (but not all) of the biochemical characteristics of enterocytes. Widely used to study drug absorption and ligand-mediated targeting, as well as a screen for the anticancer activity of drugs and conjugates.

Enterocytes: Columnar epithelial cells lining the small intestine. The cell membrane is folded into microvilli and contains digestive enzymes and transporters. Lipophilic drugs diffuse across the membrane, whereas hydrophilic molecules are transported or pass between the cells via the paracellular route. Proteins may be slowly transported by endocytosis.

Invasins: Specialised proteins produced by pathogenic bacteria, which enable the microbes to bind to mamalian cell surfaces and enhance their penetration into the cells.

Lectins: Glycoproteins widespread and abundant in plants and microbes, but also found in animal cells. They recognise and bind with high specificity to sugar molecules exposed on cell surfaces.

M cells: Specialised cells of the gut associated lymphoid tissue (GALT) that endocytose and phagocytose macromolecules and particles from the intestinal lumen.

Microparticles: Particles in the size range 1-1000 μm usually made of synthetic polymers such as polystyrene or poly-(lactic-co-glycolic) acid, though proteins and chitosan have been used. Drugs can be incorporated in the polymer matrix.

Mucus: Viscous gel-like secretion which covers and protects the entire surface of the gastrointestinal tract. The major component is mucin, a high molecular weight sulfated glycoprotein.

Nanoparticles: As microparticles but with size less than 1 μm.

23

TRANSMEMBRANE TARGETING OF DNA WITH MEMBRANE ACTIVE PEPTIDES

Sabine Boeckle, Ernst Wagner and Manfred Ogris
Department of Pharmacy, Chair of Pharmaceutical Biology – Biotechnology, Ludwig-Maximilians-Universität München, Butenandtstraße 5-13, D-81377 Munich, Germany

INTRODUCTION

Within recent years, the delivery of therapeutically active genes for the treatment of different diseases, such as cancer, and hereditary diseases, has become a major issue in the development of new therapies. In this case, DNA acts as a kind of pro-drug; it is completely inactive until it is translated into the therapeutically active protein within target cells by the cellular transcription/translation machinery. When applying such therapeutic genes into an organism, a manifold of hurdles has to be circumvented until the transgene reaches its final goal, the cells nucleus. The transgene has to bind to the cell's surface, cross the plasma membrane, or become internalized into intracellular vesicles by endocytic mechanisms. In the latter case, release from intracellular compartments into the cytoplasm is an important step in order to prevent degradation of the transgene within lysosomes. In the case of mitotically active cells, reaching the cytoplasm is close to the final station in such a journey. During the next round of mitosis the nuclear membrane will be dismantled and thereafter the transgene incorporated into the nucleus during the next steps of the cell cycle. A further hurdle is awaiting the gene to be delivered in non- or only slowly dividing cells, since access to the nucleus is tightly controlled by the complex machinery of the nuclear pore complex. Viruses have developed clever mechanisms during their evolution to overcome these barriers and to deliver their own nucleic acid. Binding can occur via specific cell surface receptors, depending on host- and tissue type and trigger subsequent internalization or membrane fusion. Internalized virus particles can disrupt endosomal membranes (i.e. after certain viral proteins are activated by a change in the microenvironment within the intracellular vesicles). After reaching the cytoplasm, the utilization of other intracellular mechanism helps the virus to reach the nucleus (i.e. by carrying specific nuclear localization sequences).

All these mechanisms can be mimicked by generating synthetic gene delivery systems that include these certain features for enhanced intracellular gene delivery. These so called "artificial viruses" comprise these functions in the form of distinct chemical compounds carrying different functions. Intracellular active compounds, i.e. for endosomal release or nuclear targeting can be incorporated into an artificial virus by utilizing peptide sequences either derived from viral proteins or naturally occurring venoms. Usually these peptides are relatively short (below 50 AA) and can be chemically synthesized.

In this chapter, we give a short overview of intracellular active peptides that can be used to develop highly active synthetic gene transfer systems for optimal DNA delivery into mammalian cells.

OVERCOMING CELLULAR MEMBRANES

Several natural transport mechanisms exist for crossing biomembranes. The first membrane to be overcome is the cell surface membrane. Diffusion, facilitated or active transport and transport through ion-channels are all very restricted transport mechanisms. Larger molecules such as proteins, DNA, or DNA containing particles cannot utilize these mechanisms to permeate cellular membranes because of their size. Cells employ distinct biological mechanisms for the uptake of macromolecules and viruses. After physical binding to the cell surface (through unspecific or receptor-specific processes), the macromolecular substrate usually is internalized by engulfment into an intracellular vesicle. Alternatively, direct transport into the cytoplasm may happen in special cases (such as several enveloped viruses).

The actual crossing of a lipid membrane can proceed either by membrane fusion, pore formation, and/or membrane disruption. Fusion may take place at the plasma membrane or after endocytosis. Pore formation and/or membrane disruption occur after internalization into vesicles at the endosomal/lysosomal membrane, as cells hardly would tolerate disruption of their plasma membrane. The distinct biological processes and their importance for the intracellular delivery of a DNA vector into the nucleus of a cell will be described in the next sections.

Cell Surface Membrane Fusion

Generally biological membranes show a high rupture tension and they do not undergo rapid fusion processes. However, there are specific circumstances in which membranes spontaneously fuse. These include fusion of intracellular organelles to the plasma membrane, the fusion of sperm and egg cells in the process of fertilization and the fusion of enveloped viruses to target membranes. In the case of some enveloped viruses, cell surface fusion may lead to direct delivery of the viral nucleic acid into the cytosol.

Enveloped viruses are characterized by an additional lipid coating surrounding its nucleocapsid. After close contact of the viral envelope with the cell membrane upon binding to cell surface receptors, viral fusion proteins induce membrane fusion, and release the nucleocapsid into the cytoplasm. In the case of Sendai virus (also termed hemagglutinating virus of Japan, HVJ) for example membrane fusion is induced following the interaction of protein HN (binds to cell surface sialic acid residues) and protein F (interacts with lipids, such as cholesterol). Efforts have been made to adapt this viral pathway for delivery of therapeutic DNA. Envelopes of inactivated HVJ viruses can be used for the preparation of liposomes encapsulating DNA ("virosome approach"). Alternatively, HVJ viruses are mixed with cationic liposome-DNA complexes. These chimerical vectors can thereafter deliver the transgene to a broad range of target cells (for review, see (1)).

Endocytosis

Endocytosis is a collective term to describe vesicular uptake mechanisms of extracellular material into mammalian cells. Endocytic mechanisms serve many important cellular functions including the uptake of extracellular nutrients, regulation of cell-surface receptor expression, maintenance of cell polarity, and antigen presentation. Endocytic pathways are also utilized by viruses, toxins, and symbiotic microorganisms to gain entry into cells.

Basically two mechanisms of endocytosis exist: receptor-mediated endocytosis via clathrin-coated pits and clathrin-independent endocytosis including phagocytosis, pinocytosis, and potocytosis. Phagocytosis is the ability of specialized cells (macrophages and neutrophil leukocytes) to incorporate large particles and microorganisms by endocytosis and to destroy them by enzymatic degradation. Potocytosis represents a mechanism by which small and large molecules as well as macromolecular complexes are sequestered and transported by caveolae. Caveolae are flask-shaped ("omega-shaped") plasma membrane invaginations. They can internalize ligand-receptor complexes to deliver them to specific locations in the cell, by-passing the lysosome.

One of the best characterized endocytic mechanisms is receptor-mediated endocytosis via clathrin-coated pits. Upon binding of a ligand to a specific cell surface receptor, the activated receptors are targeted to clathrin-coated membrane invaginations (clustering of the ligand-receptor complex), which through a series of highly regulated biochemical events, pinch off (vesicle budding) to form intracellular clathrin-coated vesicles. Subsequent maturation (uncoating and fusion of vesicles) delivers the contents into endosomes. During progression along the endocytic pathway, the endosomes are modified in protein composition and pH; ligands and receptors are sent to the appropriate cellular destination (e.g. lysosome, Golgi apparatus, nucleus, or cell surface membrane). If the endocytic pathway leads to the formation of lysosomes, acidification of the lysosomal compartment can be observed (pH 4.5-5.0) facilitating enzymatic degradation of the content.

Researchers have used the transferrin receptor for receptor mediated targeted gene delivery by incorporating transferrin into our non-viral gene delivery systems. Covalent linkage to polycationic carrier molecules and subsequent condensation with DNA allowed efficient targeting and elevated levels of transgene expression on a broad range of cell types *in vitro*. Gene delivery into distant tumors after systemic application via the blood stream was observed (for review, see (2)).

Endosomal Escape

The idea of coupling ligands to a gene transfer system can lead to enhanced uptake by receptor mediated endocytosis. Nevertheless, complexes are still captured within the endosomes and have to be released before enzymatic degradation. Viruses that enter cells by receptor-mediated endocytosis (RME) possess mechanisms of endosomal escape to avoid enzymatic degradation in the lysosomes. Adenovirus, a vector frequently used for gene delivery, binds to the cell surface by interacting with the coxsackie and adenovirus (CAR) receptor. After its internalization into endosomes, the acidification of the vesicles triggers the activation of certain viral proteins resulting in vesicle disruption and the release of the virus capsid into the cytoplasm. Besides the use of recombinant adenovirus for gene delivery protocols, the inactivated virus particle can be used solely for its endosomolytic function. Inactivation of adenovirus by cross-linking the viral genome with psoralen/UV irradiation and subsequent attachment to DNA/polycation complexes greatly enhances the release of transferred DNA into the cytoplasm and transgene expression (for review see (3)).

An alternative endosomal escape mechanism is provided by virosomes based on influenza virus, which triggers membrane fusion with the endosomal membrane after endocytosis. Such systems also have been found effective for gene delivery.

The Nuclear Membrane

The next step of DNA delivery towards the cell nucleus is to overcome the nuclear membrane. Transport across the nuclear membrane is controlled by nuclear pores with the involvement of cytoplasmic receptors and accessory molecules. Passive transport (diffusion) of small (up to diameters of 9 nm) molecules through nuclear pores is unrestricted, but nuclear import of macromolecules or particles is a highly regulated process (see review (4)).

To induce uptake of macromolecules into the nucleus, they have to interact with the nuclear active transport system. The transport system comprises both nuclear membrane proteins and soluble proteins that are found within the cytoplasm. The membrane proteins form a highly organized supramolecular assembly known as the nuclear pore complex (NPC). The NPC interacts with a group of cytoplasmic proteins that recognize macromolecules destined for the nucleus, and provide the energy for translocation into the nucleus. Recognition of nucleoproteins is mediated by oligopeptide sequences termed nuclear localization sequences (NLSs), which bind to the cytoplasmic receptors. NLSs do not show strict consensus sequences, but there are clear similarities between most NLSs. Typically, they include clusters of four or more cationic residues.

One of the best-known NLS sequence is that of SV40 large tumor antigen (large T-antigen). This sequence enables binding to cellular shuttling proteins, termed importins, and translocation into the nucleus. The SV40 NLS has been used extensively to study nuclear import mechanisms by attaching the peptide to different proteins. Several attempts have been made to enhance nuclear delivery of transgenes by incorporating NLS sequences into gene transfer particles (for review, see (5)). Figure 1 summarizes the different steps in intracellular delivery of DNA.

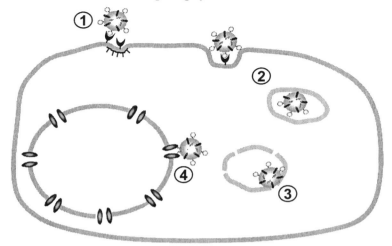

Figure 1. Cellular barriers for non viral gene delivery:
The DNA containing particle binds to cell surface receptors (1) and is internalized into endosomes (2). Thereafter, release from the endosome into the cytoplasm (3) and subsequent transport into the nucleus (4) are limiting steps in gene delivery.

TRANSMEMBRANE TARGETING OF DNA

One approach to deliver transgenes into cells is to use biophysical or chemical methods. These non-natural pathways for the transmembrane transport of synthetic DNA-vectors include the transient permeabilization of cellular membranes by chemical compounds (i.e. dimethylsulfoxide, (poly)ethyleneglycol or glycerol). Due to the high concentration of the chemicals needed, this application is limited to cultured cells and cannot be applied *in vivo*. Biophysical methods, i.e. electroporation or particle bombardment, can either be applied in cell culture or locally *in vivo*. The so called "gene gun" uses gold particles coated with the DNA to be transferred. After their acceleration with pressurized air these particles can penetrate cellular membranes due to their kinetic energy and deliver DNA even into the nucleus. In the case of electroporation, the DNA to be delivered and the target cells are incubated within an electrical field. After applying a few millisecond pulses ranging from 100 to 300 V/cm, the DNA can enter the cell. The basic mechanism of this method is not yet completely clarified. One possible explanation is the transient destabilization of cellular membranes within the electric field allowing the DNA to cross through temporary pores. As this effect is not limited to the type of membrane, DNA can be delivered directly into the nucleus. This results in efficient transfection of cells independent of the cycling status (6).

Particulate gene transfer systems have been the first step in the development of artificial viruses. Cationic lipids designed for that purpose consist of a cationic head group and a lipophilic tail. Usually, liposomes are formed by sonication/filtration and incubated with DNA to form so called lipoplexes. A different strategy for DNA condensation was developed by mimicking the function of DNA condensing histones within the cellular nucleus. Polycationic carrier molecules, e.g. polyaminoacids, purified histones or synthetic cationic polymers can strongly bind to DNA and lead to a hydrophobic collapse of the assembly followed by particle formation (= polyplexes).

More recently, a combination thereof, termed "lipopolyplexes" was developed. The system comprises a core of DNA complexes with polycations surrounded by a lipid layer.

Usually, lipid and polycation based gene delivery vectors are generated with an excess of positive charge. This enables the unspecific binding of these positively charged particles with the negatively charged plasma membrane followed by adsorptive endocytosis. Alternatively, cell binding and internalizing ligands can be combined with such gene delivery systems, thus enabling specific targeting to certain cell types and/or facilitated internalization. After internalization, a major bottleneck occurs as a result of the release of polyplexes or lipoplexes from the endosome into the cytoplasm. Cationic lipids usually interact with the negatively charged lipids from the endosomal membrane and this lipid intermixing can finally lead to membrane disruption and the subsequent release of transferred DNA into the cytoplasm. This mechanism significantly differs from polyplexes. In the case of (poly)ethylenimine (PEI), the polymer-structure bears an intrinsic endosomolytic mechanism: the amino groups of PEI are only partially protonated at neutral pH. After the intracellular proton pump starts to acidify these vesicles, PEI can act as a kind of proton sponge. The buffering effect combined with subsequent osmotic effect and swelling of the polymer can finally lead to vesicle disruption and release of polyplexes into the cytosol (7).

Particulate synthetic gene delivery systems offer several advantages compared to viral based ones. The DNA and the carrier molecule can be produced at large scale with rather low costs. The size of the therapeutic gene that can be inserted in the synthetic DNA complex is not restricted and there are no biohazards related to the viral genome. Their synthetic design allows high flexibility of the formulation that can be easily modified by diverse chemical reactions and physical interactions. Polycationic carrier molecules can act as a kind of a template where biologically active molecules carrying different functions can be covalently attached (see Figure 2 below). As described below, this can help to overcome intracellular membrane barriers in non-viral gene delivery.

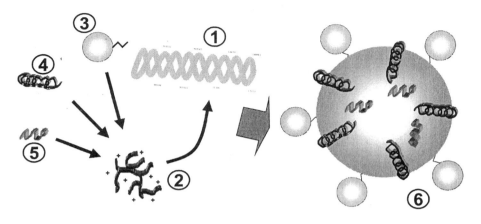

Figure 2. Different functions can be incorporated into artificial viruses.
Plasmid DNA (1) can be condensed by polycationinc carrier molecules (2). Cell-binding ligands (3) and intracellular active compounds, e.g. membrane active peptides for endosomal release (4) or nuclear homing sequences (5) can be attached to the polycationic carrier molecule. The resulting particles (6) contain all this multiple functions.

Membrane Active Peptides for DNA Delivery

In most cases, DNA vectors enter the cell by the endocytic pathway. The major barrier on this pathway that impairs transfection efficiency is the entrapment and degradation of the DNA complex within intracellular vesicles (endosomes and lysosomes). Thus, efforts have been made to protect DNA vectors against enzymatic degradation within the endosome-lysosome and to increase the release from the intracellular vesicles.

Viruses, Viral Peptides, and Bacterial Toxins

It was shown that the endosomolytic activity of viruses could be employed for non-viral gene delivery by directly coupling inactivated adenovirus, rhinovirus, or HVJ particles to the complex. A major drawback in using viruses is their immunogenicity as well as inflammatory responses. Therefore an alternative approach to achieve endosomal escape is to use only specific peptide sequences of viral coat proteins. Short synthetic membrane active peptides (N-terminus of influenza virus haemagglutinin = HA_2 subunit or rhinovirus VP-1 protein) have been incorporated into DNA complexes. These complexes still show fusion and leakage of liposomal contents and were able to enhance gene transfer efficiency. The gene transfer enhancing activities of membrane active peptides were found to correlate with their efficiencies in releasing hemoglobin from erythrocytes. Instead of being derived from viral sequences, peptides may also be designed synthetically by molecular modeling, for example, the GALA, KALA, or JTS1 peptides (8,9).

Another approach of increasing endosomal release to enhance non-viral gene transfer is the use of bacterial toxins. Exotoxins, like diphtheria toxin or pseudomonas exotoxin, consist of two polypeptide chains. The A chain contains the toxic activity which inhibits essential cellular steps in the cytosol (like protein synthesis); the B chain contains functions that trigger uptake into cellular vesicles and translocation of the toxin A chain from the endosome to the cytosol. The efficient translocation process of the B chain has been exploited for targeted immunotoxins and also for gene delivery by designing fusion proteins containing specific cell-binding and DNA binding domains (10).

The cytolysins staphylococcal α-toxin or streptolysin O belong to a class of bacterial proteins that lyse cells (or cell vacuoles) by formation of large aqueous pores. This process requires multimerization of the proteins within the membrane. Streptolysin O and staphylococcal α-toxin have been used as standard reagents for intracellular delivery of reagents by permeabilization of the cells. A related cytolysin, perfingolysine O, was used to efficiently deliver DNA into cultured cells (9).

In addition, membrane-lytic peptides derived from naturally occurring toxins could be used to disrupt the endosomal membrane. Although the group of cytolytic peptides include various peptides from totally different hosts (amphibiae, insects, fish and arthropods), there is a number of common characteristics that are outlined below (11). Table 1 below gives an overview about membrane active peptides derived from different sources.

Characteristics of Membrane-Lytic Peptides

Membrane-lytic peptides interact with bilayers, resulting in the alteration of the cell's membrane permeability, which leads to cell death. Their function is either antimicrobial activity or lytic activity. Cytolytic peptides have the common feature of being cationic under physiological conditions (lysine and arginine residues) and of forming structures. The amphipathic character enables membrane permeabilization and/or perturbation. The net positive charge of these peptides is generally +2 or more, which is believed to facilitate their interactions with negatively charged membrane phospholipids (e.g. lipopolysaccharides of Gram-negative bacteria or sialic acid molecules of erythrocytes). The D-enantiomers of a number of membrane-lytic peptides were found to exhibit similar activity to their L-counterpart. This lack of stereo specificity suggests that the peptides interact with achiral components of the cell membrane.

The two main conformations induced upon binding to membranes are the α-helix and β-sheet. Cytolytic α-helical peptides include melittin (from the venom of the honeybee), magainin (from frog skin), lycotoxins (from the venom of the jumper ant), and pardaxin (shark repellent from fish); (for review, see (12)). Defensins isolated from mammalian leukocytes are among the best-characterized β-sheet-forming antimicrobial peptides. Other cytotoxic peptides include gramicidin A which adopts a left handed, double-stranded β-helix and cyclic peptides such as gramicidin S (gramicidins are antimicrobial peptides from bacillus brevis) (13).

Mechanism of Membrane-Lytic Peptides

While the structure of most membrane-lytic peptides is well established, the orientation of these peptides in the membrane remains controversial. The peptides can either adsorb onto the membrane surface or insert into the membrane, which may result in the formation of pores.

Two alternative mechanisms were proposed to describe the detailed steps involved in membrane permeation and pore-formation by cytolytic peptides. In the "barrel-stave" model, amphipathic α-helices insert into the hydrophobic core of the membrane and form transmembrane pores. The "toroidal" model (or "carpet" model), the peptides, which do not necessarily need to adopt amphipathic α-helical structure, are in contact with the lipid head groups during the whole process of membrane permeation and do not insert into the hydrophobic core of the membrane (14-16).

Table 1. Membrane active peptides

Viral and synthetic peptides	Source	Sequence
HA-2 subunit of Influenza (X31) HA-2 subunit of Influenza (C)	N-terminus of influenza virus haemagglutinin	GLFGAIAGFIENGWEGMI DGWYG- IFGIDDLIIGLLFVAIVEAG IG-
Rhino HRV-14 VP-1 Rhino HRV-2 VP-1	N-terminus of rhinovirus VP-1 protein	GLGDELEEVIVEKTKQTV ASISSGNPVENYIDEVLN EVLVVPNINSSN–
JTS1	peptide derived from the sequence of Influenza virus	GLFEALLELLESLWELLL EAC
GALA	anionic peptide, based upon a Glu-Ala-Leu-Ala motif	WEAALAEALAEALAEHL AEALAEALEALAA
KALA	cationic peptide, based upon a Lys-Ala-Leu-Ala motif	WEAKLAKALAKALAKH LAKALAKALKACEA
Cytolytic peptides		
DEFENSINS	mammalian granulozytes NP-1 (rabbit) HNP-1 (human)	VVCACRRALCLPRERRA GFCRIRGRIHPLCCRRAC YCRIPACIAGERRYGTCI YQGRLWAFCC
GRAMICIDIN A GRAMICIDIN S	antimicrobial peptides from bacillus brevis	VGAδLAδVVδVTδLTδLδL *cyclo*-(LδFPVOrn)2
LYCOTOXIN I LYCOTOXIN II	venom of the jumper ant	IWLTALKFLGKHAAKHL AKQQLSKL KIKWFKTMKSIAKFIAKE QMKKHLGGE
MAGAININ II	venom of the frog skin	GLGKFLHSAKKFGKAFV GEIMNS
MELLITIN	venom of the honeybee	GIGAVLKVLTTGLPALIS WIKRKRQQ
PARDAXIN	shark repellent from fish	GFFALIPKIISSPLFKTLLS AVGSALSSSGGQE

The Barrel Stave Mechanism

A large number of pore-forming agents are supposed to create channels through a barrel-stave mechanism (see Figure 3 top). Three discrete steps have been defined for this process: 1) water soluble monomers bind to the membrane; 2) they insert into the membrane; 3) they aggregate like barrel staves surrounding a central pore that increases in diameter through progressive recruitment of additional monomers. The pore is formed by aggregation of the monomers with their hydrophilic sides lined up in the middle of the pore and their hydrophobic sides turned to the membrane acyl chains. Stable transmembrane pores are formed that allow passive flux of ions and small molecules across the bilayer. This may result in ionic imbalance and colloid osmotic lysis.

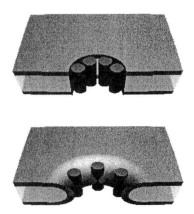

Figure 3. Schematics of the barrel-stave model (top) and the toroidal model (bottom). The dark layers represent the headgroup regions of bilayers. Peptide monomers are represented by the cylinders. Adapted from Yang et al (15).

A minimum of 20 residues is needed to form a membrane spanning α-helix and at least ten residues to form a membrane-spanning β-sheet. It has been suggested that α-helices must be amphipathic and that they need to have a high enough degree of hydrophobicity to allow partitioning into the bilayer in a vertical orientation.

The Toroidal Pore Model

Whereas the barrel-stave model seems a reasonable model for predominantly hydrophobic peptides, the toroidal model was proposed for cationic peptides that are more hydrophilic (see Figure 3 bottom). In toroidal pores, the lipid monolayer bends continuously from the top to the bottom in the fashion of a toroidal hole. The pore is lined by both the peptides and the lipid headgroups. The positive charges of the peptides may therefore interact with the negatively charged headgroups of the phospholipids. The orientation of membrane-lytic peptides varies with the physico-chemical condition of the bilayer and with the peptide concentration. A peptide is bound parallel to a lipid bilayer when the ratio between peptide and lipid is below a certain threshold value. As the ratio of peptide to lipid increases, an increasing fraction of the peptide molecules change to the perpendicular orientation until above another threshold concentration; all of the peptide molecules become oriented perpendicularly.

MELITTIN - A CATIONIC AMPHIPATHIC PEPTIDE FOR DNA DELIVERY

Melittin is the major peptide component of the venom of the honey bee Apis melifera cerana that is responsible for lysis of the cell membrane (17). The cationic amphipathic polypeptide consists of 26 amino acids with the sequence Gly1- Ile2- Gly3- Ala4- Val5- Leu6- Lys7- Val8- Leu9- Thr10- Thr11- Gly12- Leu13- Pro14- Ala15- Leu16- Ile17- Ser18- Trp19- Ile20- Lys21- Arg22- Lys23- Arg24- Gln25- Gln26. The overall charge of melittin is +6 (four charges at the C-terminal sequence Lys-Arg-Lys-Arg, two at Lys-7 and the N-terminal NH_2-group with no acidic groups), which results in high water solubility. Its tertiary structure has been determined in detergent micelles and in non-polar solvents where melittin is present as a monomeric form. In melittin-crystals grown from solution of high ionic strength melittin molecules form tetramers. The secondary structure of melittin depends on the solvent but also on various other parameters like concentration, pH, ionic strength, or nature of counter ions. In water, both random coil conformation and α-helical conformation have been observed. In solvents with a low dielectric constant (like methanol) and in detergent micelles, the α-helical conformation predominated. The prolin residue at position 14 is responsible for a bend separating two segments of the helical structure: a hydrophobic segment, going from residue Gly-1 to Leu-13, and an amphipathic segment going from residue Ala-15 to Lys-21, with non-polar amino acids segregated on one face of the α-helix and polar amino acids on the opposite side. The COOH-terminal residues 22-26 form a non-helical hydrophilic domain. The "hinge" effect of central prolin increases flexibility at the center of the molecule and allows bending to accommodate conformational constraints induced by intermolecular interactions. The flexibility seems to be important for some actions of melittin in membranes. Because no significant structural variations are observed in the different environments, it is likely that the α-helical structure is a good model for the membrane bound conformation. Figure 4 below shows structural features of melittin.

The characteristic effect of melittin on cell membranes is its hemolytic activity. At concentrations ≥ 1µg/ml melittin binds rapidly to erythrocytes and induces the release of hemoglobin. It is likely that melittin

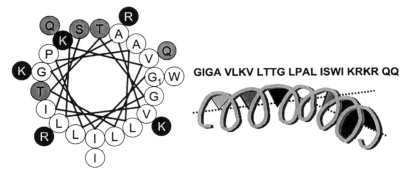

GIGA VLKV LTTG LPAL ISWI KRKR QQ

Figure 4. Helical wheel projections (left) and schematic drawings of the amphipathic helix of melittin, illustrating its structural features (right). Hydrophobic residues are shown in white, polar residues in gray and cationic residues in black circles. Adapted from Dathe & Wieprecht (18).

monomers or dimers are necessary for the initial step of hemolysis. It has been shown that larger melittin aggregates do not show lytic activity. Phosphate suppresses hemolysis to an extent that correlates with its effect on inducing tetramerization. Complete suppression occurs at 0.5 M phosphate. Melittin peptides bind to erythrocytes within seconds. There are about 1.8 x 10^7 binding sites per erythrocyte (probably unspecific interactions with membrane lipids). When about 1% of the melittin binding sites are occupied, cell lysis can be observed. 50% lysis occurs when there are about 2 x 10^6 molecules bound to the cell membrane (19).

The association of melittin with bilayers and the mechanism involved in the initiation of membrane lysis have been extensively studied (20,21). Obviously melittin's action on membranes is dependent on its concentration and on the physico-chemical condition of the bilayer. At low concentrations, helical melittin is oriented parallel to the membrane interface with its non-polar surface facing toward the bilayer interior. With increases in the surface concentration of melittin, dimerization appears to be an important step and an increasing fraction of the peptide molecules change to the perpendicular orientation. The lipid bilayer will be subject of a fast perturbation with an apparent lipid flip-flop that allows melittin to penetrate deeper into the bilayer. In the next step, a pore opening is formed (possibly with additional monomers). The size of the pores is not fixed; it likely increases with increase in membrane concentration. Melittin pores do not conform to the barrel-stave model. Instead, they are consistent with the toroidal model as described above.

Melittin-Enhanced Gene Transfer

Researchers have already evaluated the usability of melittin for non-viral gene delivery. Legendre and colleagues compared the transfection activity of melittin with other natural cationic peptides (22). However, melittin/DNA complexes only enabled low gene transfer efficiency. Concomitant high toxicity was observed due to the fast partitioning of the peptide from the complex. In order to increase the stability of such a peptide/DNA complex, melittin was covalently bound to a lipophilic residue. This hybrid molecule dioleoyl-melittin enabled efficient binding to DNA and high levels of reporter gene expression with the absence of cellular toxicity (23). Our own work focused on the covalent attachment of the peptide to the cationic polymer (poly)ethylenimine (PEI). Initial studies with melittin and DNA alone revealed that the interaction of melittin with DNA was too weak to enable a stable complex formation (unpublished results, see also (23)). In the case of the melittin-PEI conjugate, this interaction was significantly increased due to the high number of positive charges in the PEI molecule. Within a broad range of cell lines and types tested, reporter gene expression was significantly increased; even slowly dividing or non-dividing primary cells were susceptible to transfection (24).

A detailed view on the transfection mechanism pointed out a dual functionality of the peptide. After internalization of melittin containing polyplexes, the release of the transferred DNA from intracellular vesicle into the cytoplasm was highly efficient compared to polyplexes without the peptide. This effect enhanced gene delivery, especially in mitotic cells. Additionally, we observed a further effect of melittin on gene delivery after helping the polyplex to reach the cytoplasm. In the case of cells with low mitotic activity or even non-dividing cells, melittin also enabled efficient reporter gene expression. When injecting polyplexes with and without melittin directly into the cytoplasm of cells, we observed increased access of the transgene to the nucleus due to higher frequency of reporter gene expression. Co-injection with a specific inhibitor of the nuclear pore complex (e.g., wheat germ agglutinin) reduced reporter gene expression to a level obtained with melittin free polyplexes. Therefore we concluded that melittin might bear a so far unknown nuclear localization activity. The cationic cluster [21]KRKR[24] could be the reason for this effect, as similar amino acid sequences on different nuclear and nuclear proteins directs them into the nucleus/nucleolus (25,26).

A delivery system for RNA was developed by Bettinger and colleagues utilizing melittin's ability to release polyplexes into the cytoplasm. In this case, melittin was attached to a low molecular weight PEI and subsequently complexes with mRNA were formed. This delivery system enabled highly efficient mRNA delivery into the cytoplasm of non dividing cells, like primary endothelial cells, where mRNA was released and subsequently translated into the encoded protein (27).

CONCLUSION

This chapter should outline the importance of intracellular membranes acting as barriers for efficient transfer of therapeutic DNA into the cell. Each step in intracellular delivery of DNA can be a bottleneck reducing the final amount of DNA reaching the cell's nucleus to a minimal fraction. When designing systems for DNA delivery, natural mechanisms for membrane crossing can be utilized. Highly potent membrane active peptides have evolved in viruses (to deliver their genome into the cell) or in other organisms (i.e. cytolytic peptides in venoms). We and several other groups have exploited these powerful substances by incorporating them into synthetic gene delivery systems. Chemical synthesis allows the design of artificial viruses comprising functions to overcome major intracellular barriers like the release from the endosome or the entry into the nucleus. Melittin, one of the most active membrane-lytic peptides known, is an example for the usability of such a system as efficient transfer of transgene from the endosome into the cytoplasm and further into the nucleus can be achieved.

REFERENCES

1.   Kaneda, Y., Y. Saeki, and R. Morishita. Gene therapy using HVJ-liposomes: the   best of both worlds? Molecular Medicine Today 1999;5:298
2.   Kircheis, R., L. Wightman, and E. Wagner. Design and gene delivery activity of modified polyethylenimines Adv. Drug Deliv. Rev. 2001;53:341
3.   Cotten, M., E. Wagner, and M. L. Birnstiel. Receptor-mediated transport of DNA into eukaryotic cells Methods Enzymol 1993;217:618
4.   Pouton, C. W. Nuclear import of polypeptides, polynucleotides and supramolecular complexes Adv. Drug Deliv. Rev. 1998;34:51
5.   Bremner, K. H., L. W. Seymour, and C. W. Pouton. Harnessing nuclear localization pathways for transgene delivery Curr Opin Mol Ther 2001;3:170
6.   Brunner, S., E. Furtbauer, T. Sauer, M. Kursa, and E. Wagner. Overcoming the nuclear barrier: cell cycle independent non-viral gene transfer with linear polyethylenimineor electroporation Mol. Ther. 2002;5:80
7.   Zuber, G., E. Dauty, M. Nothisen, P. Belguise, and J. P. Behr. Towards synthetic viruses Adv. Drug Deliv. Rev. 2001;52:245
8.   Sparrow, J. T., V. Edwards, V, C. Tung, M. J. Logan, M. S. Wadhwa, J. Duguid, and L. C. Smith. Synthetic peptide-based DNA complexes for non-viral gene delivery Adv. Drug Deliv. Rev. 1998;30:115
9.   Plank, C., W. Zauner, and E. Wagner. Application of membrane-active peptides for drug and gene delivery across cellular membranes Adv. Drug Deliv. Rev. 1998;34:21

10.   Uherek, C., J. Fominaya, and W. Wels. A modular DNA carrier protein based on the structure of diphtheria toxin mediates target cell-specific gene delivery J. Biol. Chem. 1998;273:8835

11.   Blondelle, S. E., K. Lohner, and M. Aguilar. Lipid-induced conformation and lipid-binding properties of cytolytic and antimicrobial peptides: determination and biological specificity Biochim. Biophys. Acta 1999;1462:89

12.   Kourie, J. I. and A. A. Shorthouse. Properties of cytotoxic peptide-formed ion channelsAm J Physiol Cell Physiol 2000;278:C1063-C1087

13.   Marsh, D. Peptide models for membrane channels Biochem. J. 1996;315 (Pt 2):345

14.   Shai, Y. Mechanism of the binding, insertion and destabilization of phospholipid bilayer membranes by alpha-helical antimicrobial and cell non-selective membrane-lytic peptides Biochim. Biophys. Acta 1999;1462:55

15.   Yang, L., T. A. Harroun, T. M. Weiss, L. Ding, and H. W. Huang. Barrel-stave model or toroidal model? A case study on melittin pores Biophys. J. 2001;81:1475

16.   Bechinger, B. The structure, dynamics and orientation of antimicrobial peptides in membranes by multidimensional solid-state NMR spectroscopy Biochim. Biophys. Acta 1999;1462:157

17.   Dempsey, C. E. The actions of melittin on membranes Biochim Biophys Acta 1990;1031:143

18.   Dathe, M. and T. Wieprecht. Structural features of helical antimicrobial peptides: their potential to modulate activity on model membranes and biological cells Biochim. Biophys. Acta 1999;1462:71

19.   Tosteson, M. T., S. J. Holmes, M. Razin, and D. C. Tosteson. Melittin lysis of red cells J. Membr. Biol. 1985;87:35

20.   Rex, S. and G. Schwarz. Quantitative studies on the melittin-induced leakage mechanism of lipid vesicles Biochemistry 1998;37:2336

21.   Ladokhin, A. S. and S. H. White. 'Detergent-like' permeabilization of anionic lipid vesicles by melittin Biochim. Biophys. Acta 2001;1514:253

22.   Legendre, J. Y. and F. C. Szoka, Jr. Cyclic amphipathic peptide-DNA complexes mediate high-efficiency transfection of adherent mammalian cells Proc Natl Acad Sci U S A 1993;90:893

23.   Legendre, J. Y., A. Trzeciak, B. Bohrmann, U. Deuschle, E. Kitas, and A. Supersaxo. Dioleoylmelittin as a novel serum-insensitive reagent for efficient transfection of mammalian cells Bioconjug Chem 1997;8:57

24.   Ogris, M., R. C. Carlisle, T. Bettinger, and L. W. Seymour. Melittin enables efficient vesicular escape and enhanced nuclear access of non-viral gene delivery vectors J Biol Chem 2001;12:12

25.   Subramaniam, P. S., M. G. Mujtaba, M. R. Paddy, and H. M. Johnson. The carboxyl terminus of interferon-gamma contains a functional polybasic nuclear localization sequence J Biol Chem 1999;274:403

26.   Eilbracht, J. and M. S. Schmidt-Zachmann. Identification of a sequence element directing a protein to nuclear speckles Proc Natl Acad Sci U S A 2001;98:3849

27.   Bettinger, T., R. C. Carlisle, M. L. Read, M. Ogris, and L. W. Seymour. Peptide-mediated RNA delivery: a novel approach for enhanced transfection of primary and post-mitotic cells Nucleic Acids Res. 2001; 29:3882

GLOSSARY

Amphipathic: Having both hydrophobic and hydrophilic regions, as in phospholipids or a detergent molecule.

Lipoplex: Cationic lipid – nucleic acid complex

Liposome: An artificial phospholipids bilayer vesicle formed from an aqueous suspension of phospholipids molecules.

Membrane fusion: The process in which two membranes break down at the point of contact between them allowing the two contents to mingle.

Polyplex: Cationic polymer – nucleic acid complex

Reporter gene: A gene that encodes for a quantifiable protein that can be easily assayed and is used also in transfection studies (see also, transfection).

SV40: Simian virus 40, a monkey virus

Transfection: The introduction of a foreign nucleic acid molecule into a eukaryotic cell that is usually followed by expression of one or more genes from the newly introduced nucleic acid (see reporter gene).

Transgene: A foreign gene from another cell or organism that should be introduced into a cell.

Vector: In cell biology, an agent (virus or plasmid) used to transmit genetic material to a cell or organism.

24

POLYMERSOMES: A NEW PLATFORM FOR DRUG TARGETING

Dennis E. Discher, Peter Photos, Fariyal Ahmed, Ranganath Parthasrathy, and Frank S. Bates

Department of Chemical and Biomolecular Engineering, Departments of Bioengineering and Mechanical Engineering and Applied Mechanics, Institute for Medicine and Engineering, University of Pennsylvania, Philadelphia, PA 19104; and Department of Chemical Engineering and Material Science, University of Minnesota, Minneapolis, MN 55455.

INTRODUCTION

Liposomes were first described in literature more than 30 years ago by Bangham (1). They have since been used widely in many fundamental studies of amphiphilic systems as well as in applications to extend and control the delivery of a broad variety of drugs (Fig. 1A). Thousands of publications, reviews, and monographs (e.g., (2)) now exist on liposomes. A handful of the documents have expressed ideas that emerge as the clearest backdrop for outlining the motivation, formation, properties, and compatibility of novel polymer-based vesicle platforms called "polymersomes" (3) (Fig. 1B).

The defining basis for liposomes is, of course, that lipids are near symmetric amphiphiles with a sufficiently low critical micelle concentration (CMC) for 'kinetically stable' formation of semi-permeable vesicles (2). As such, drug molecules can be either encapsulated within, or, if the drug is hydrophobic, intercalated into the membrane's core. In addition, targeting moieties, especially antibodies, can be stably added to the membrane. Despite the presumed bio-stability/compatibility of the constituent phospholipids and cholesterol, pure or "conventional" liposomes – of any formulation – were found some time ago to be cleared from the circulation in minutes to hours. Polymers have provided a solution to this problem of short circulation time; conjugation of kilodalton-sized, hydrophilic synthetics such as polyethylene glycol/oxide (PEG or PEO) to a small percentage of the lipids was shown about 10 years ago to prolong the circulation times of 'stealth' liposomes to tens of hours or days and thereby improving, for example, antitumor therapies (reviewed in (2)).

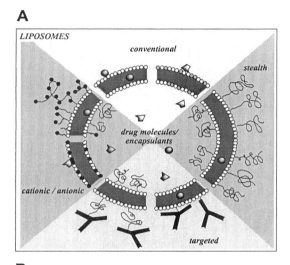

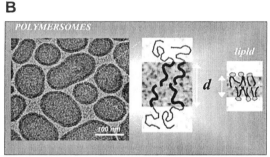

Figure 1. Vesicle systems. (A) Liposomes for drug delivery. (Clockwise) Conventional liposomes are composed of one or more lipids, typically phospholipids and cholesterol. Stealth liposomes possess, in addition, polymer chains grafted to a relatively small proportion (<10%) of lipid headgroups. These prove to be more bio-stable in the blood circulation. Targeted liposomes use grafted antibodies and other ligands to direct encapsulated drugs to specific cell-surface receptors. Cationic/anionic liposomes use surface charge to electrostatically interact with oppositely charged therapeutics such as DNA. Macromolecular encapsulants include oxygen-binding globins (Liposome Encapsulated Hemoglobin, or LEH) and metabolic enzymes. 'Drug' molecules can be of both water-soluble type (e.g., anti-cancer drugs like doxorubicin-hydrochloride as well as imaging agents) and membrane-soluble or lipophilic type. (B) Polymersomes. The cryo-TEM image shows 100-200 nm diameter vesicles of diblock copolymer. The schematics illustrate the difference in membrane thickness, (d), that can be engineered into polymersomes by controlling the molecular weight.

Grafting of PEO to organic surfaces has long been known to generically delay the adsorption, denaturation, and/or activation of plasma proteins as well as inhibit platelet adhesion (Figure 1). Tens of hours or days is nonetheless much shorter than the circulation times of many nascent blood components such as erythrocytes, which circulate in rats for weeks or for months in humans. Furthermore, second injections of stealth liposomes (5–21 days after the first) have been shown to be cleared much more rapidly, in less than 30 minutes, due to binding of plasma components recognized by hepatic and splenic macrophages (4). Nevertheless, one of the clearest successes in liposomal drug delivery is being found with stealth liposome-encapsulated doxorubicin which minimizes macrophage and cardiac toxicity by circulating long enough to non-specifically find its way into the leaky vasculature of tumors (2) [www.alza.com (Doxil®)]. In comparison, "conventional liposomes have been unsuccessful in delivering drugs preferentially to tumors" (5). Unique pharmacokinetics still motivate alternatives to such vesicles since a considerable fraction of human patients (up to 50%) display hand-foot ulcerations among other toxic side effects such as stomatitis which ultimately limits dose (6).

Since polymers such as PEO impart biocompatibility to lipids and can also be incorporated into near symmetric (hydrophobic versus hydrophilic) synthetic amphiphiles, polymersomes seem to be the next logical design. It is important, however, to first distinguish polymer-only vesicles that are made and processible in aqueous media, like liposomes, from closely related copolymer shell systems, which require organic solvents to facilitate their formation (reviewed in (7)). Several such organic requisite copolymers have been made with most based on a hydrophobic block of polystyrene (PS), which has a high bulk glass transition temperature or T_g. A recent example is a diblock of PEO-PS made by Yu and Eisenberg (8), EOx-PSy (x = 15, y = 240); the pharmacological utility of this and cognate copolymers, beyond compatibility issues, would seem limited by the need for solvents such as N,N-dimethylformamide (DMF) and tetrahydrofuran (THF). Since proteins generally denature under such solvent conditions, the needed solvents largely eliminate use of proteins that might be desirable either therapeutically (encapsulated growth hormones or insulin for example) or for targeting (e.g., antibodies). Residual solvents can also be difficult to extract from the hydrophobic cores of formed microstructures and could thus lead to further toxicity.

The second distinction to be made is with a growing class of altered biomolecules which also self-assemble into vesicles. For example, chitosan, a natural carbohydrate, has been modified with fatty-acids to make vesicles that ultimately prove both bio- and hemo- compatible (9). Distinct from this and related examples is another sub-class of polymer vesicle systems based on polymerizable lipids. In such systems, studied for decades now, lateral polymerization occurs after membrane assembly. Enhanced stability of at least small vesicles sometimes results (10) and provides a basis for emerging applications such as oral drug delivery (11). Further opportunities in polymer-based membranes where assembly is not requisite to polymerization (i.e., polymersomes) are generally suggested by these systems. Moreover, an ability to make polymersomes with crosslinkable copolymers (12) should present new opportunities in vesicle stabilization and overcome limits widely encountered but seldom reported with polymerized liposomes.

Distinctions: Lipid versus Polymersome-forming Copolymers

Given the above distinctions with other polymeric vesicle systems, the first important comparisons to be made between polymersome-forming diblock copolymers and lipids are molecular weight and amphiphilic character. PEG-lipids, mentioned above, with molecular weights of several kilodaltons (typically 2 – 5 kDa) establish initial design ideas. Inclusion of 5% PEG-lipid clearly reduces by several-fold or more the binding of plasma proteins that likely mediate clearance (13). Increasing PEG-lipid content from 5% to 10% reduces such binding (in two minute incubations) even further, if less dramatically. However, because of the comparatively large hydrophilic mass fraction of the attached PEG chain relative to the hydophobic portion of any lipid (see Table 1), PEG-lipids tend to segregate into spherical micelles above a relative concentration of about 10% (14). Such segregation severely limits the amount of PEG-lipid that can be added to liposomes. In order to counter this micellization tendency and make pure component vesicles, the hydrophobic volume fraction of such an amphiphile must be made larger. Synthetic block copolymers allow this. Table 1 lists a number of polymersome-forming diblock copolymers that all contain a lipid-like fraction of hydrophilic ($f_{\text{hydrophilic}}$) versus hydrophobic mass.

Currently, the various polymersome-forming copolymers made differ in hydrophobic block type and certainly raise issues of compatibility (partially addressed below). However, all have molecular weights of at least a few kilodaltons. This increased molecular weight has consequences on aggregate stability: the CMC, as one measure of stability, ought to decrease with molecular weight (e.g., (15)). Other measures of membrane stability prove more accessible and show, as elaborated later, that polymersome stability does indeed increase with increasing molecular weight. This may prove to be an important advantage over liposomes in pharmacological application since "Numerous studies (for reviews see (16, 17)) have established that destabilization of liposome membranes resulting in loss of membrane integrity may significantly contribute to liposome clearance" as summarized by Cullis and coworkers (13). The same review further points out that liposome interactions with a long list of plasma components, including lipoproteins, result in increased leakage of entrapped solutes and/or net transfer/release of phospholipids. Polymersome membranes with a higher

PEO density plus a greater stability conferred by larger amphiphiles (i.e., membrane patency) should clearly address, if not strictly overcome, some of the apparent limitations of PEG-lipid stealth liposomes.

Table 1 Properties of vesicle-forming amphiphiles and the membranes they form in aqueous solution ((3, 25); Bermudez, personal communication]. DMPC and SOPC are common phosphotidylcholine lipids. Diblock copolymers are designated with two letters for each type of block plus a number that presently indicates a synthesis order. M_n denotes the number-average molecular weight and $f_{hydrophilic}$ the weight or volume fraction of the hydrophilic segments. The membrane core thickness is d and the maximum tension sustainable by the membrane is τ_{max}. EO is ethylene oxide; BD is butadiene; and LA is lactic acid.

Molecule	Structure	M_n (kDa)	$f_{hydrophilic}$	d (nm)	τ_{max} (mN/m)
DMPC	...	0.68	0.36	2.5	6
SOPC	...	0.79	0.31	3.0	9
OE7	$EO_{40} - EE_{37}$	3.9	0.39	8.0	20
OB2	$EO_{26} - BD_{46}$	3.6	0.28	9.6	22
OB16	$EO_{50} - BD_{55}$	5.2	0.37	10.6	19
OB18	$EO_{80} - BD_{125}$	10.4	0.29	14.8	33 ± 5
OB19	$EO_{150} - BD_{250}$	20.0	0.28	21.0	...
OL1	$\sim EO_{50} - LA_{55}$	~6.0	~0.33	...	...

In addition to enabling pure copolymer membranes, the increased molecular weight of the copolymers (Table 1) leads to an increased membrane thickness up to tens of nanometers for the self-assembled vesicles. As a reference, a universal feature of all biomembranes is a hydrophobic core thickness, d_{lipid}, in a very narrow range of 3 – 4 nm. This narrow range occurs despite great diversity in lipids from diacyl phospholipids with typical chains of 14 – 26 carbons to compact cholesterol and ring-like archaelipids (for review, see (18) and references therein). The uniformity of d_{lipid} across phyla may be quite well suited for the insertion of membrane proteins derived from a common (albeit diverse) genetic code, but this universal thickness is not otherwise dictated by any obvious physical necessity for assembly. Moreover, while the enhanced thickness of polymersomes affects properties ranging from membrane permeability and stability to bending rigidity, it also allows for more hydrophobic drugs to intercalate (see Fig. 1A).

Importantly, the increased thickness of polymersome membranes does not restrict the ability to make 100 – 200 nm diameter vesicles as well as giant, many micron-diameter vesicles (Fig. 2 below) (3, 19, and 20). Electron microscopy images (Fig. 1B) plus dynamic light scattering (DLS) results (19) highlight the quality of the smaller unilamellar vesicles that have previously been found, with liposomes, to be optimal for long circulation times. In fact many of the processing methods used for liposomes (e.g., film hydration, sonication, freeze/thaw, and filtered extrusioncan) can also be used to fission a polydisperse population of polymersomes with many spontaneous giants down to a more monodisperse sub-micron size range (19). Finally, although the polymersomes' thicker membranes with thicker PEO brushes will tend to displace encapsulated drugs, the increased thickness is only tens of nanometers or less; this could be easily accommodated by increasing polymersome diameters with suitable modifications of extrusion filters and methods. Ultimately, a minimal difference in drug delivery is expected between, for example, 100 nm and 120 nm vesicles.

Micro-physical characterizations of Polymersomes

Membrane properties such as interfacial elasticity (3), electromechanical cohesiveness (21), and lateral fluidity (22) are all directly accessible through measurements on giant vesicles. Figure 2 shows a giant vesicle being aspirated into a micropipette.

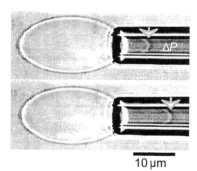

10 µm

Figure 2. Giant polymersome characterization by micromanipulation. A single vesicle is pulled into a micropipette by increasingly negative pressure, ΔP. Phase contrast imaging of such a process shows a sustained refractive difference between a typical encapsulated medium (250 mM sucrose) and the external medium (phosphate buffered saline).

A negative pressure ΔP increases the membrane area by ΔA relative to the original vesicle surface area, A_0. Although the larger the molecular weight, the more viscous the copolymer systems appear in aspiration, all membranes are clearly fluid (unless intentionally crosslinked (12)) and respond to a pressure-imposed Laplace tension, τ. This is found to be proportional to the relative area dilation, $\alpha = \Delta A/A_0$, where the constant of proportionality is an area elastic modulus, $K_a = \tau/\alpha$, with units of interfacial tension. For the OE and OB copolymers of Table 1 we find $K_a \approx 100$ mN/m independent of molecular weight or membrane thickness ((19); Bermudez, personal communication). In contrast, the bending elastic constant reported for our first generation OE7 vesicles, $K_b \sim 35 \, k_B T$ (3), appears extremely well approximated by an elastic plate model prediction of $\frac{1}{48} K_a \, d^2$ which is derivable for a bilayer of two uncoupled monolayers (23). Such determinations clearly provide important insights into the structure of polymersome membranes.

Based on simple ideas of area elasticity, K_a provides further insight into the membrane assembly. The cohesive interfacial tension that is set up at the hydrophobic-hydrophilic interface separating the blocks can be estimated to be $\gamma = \frac{1}{4} K_a$ (15). A value of $\gamma \approx 25$ mN/m is not only consistent with expectations for an oil-water (hydrophobic–hydrophilic) interface but also corresponds, within about 20%, to a simple upper bound on the maximum tension that these membranes can sustain (Table 1) (21). This sets an extremely important design limit. Pure component membranes made from large molecular weight copolymers cannot be made any stronger than the block-determined interfacial tension γ. Interestingly, copolymers in the 10–20 kDa range already run up against this bound. Lower molecular weight systems, such as liposomes, have lower strengths simply because defects and fluctuations permeate these thinner membranes much more readily when stressed. Higher molecular weight copolymers might give thicker and less permeable membranes, but they will not prove more stable than the more intermediate weight systems.

At this point, one might wonder why cell membranes are not thicker for reasons of greater stability. Cells certainly can and do synthesize many larger, more complex self-associating molecules than lipids, and membrane proteins could, in principle, be made larger in order to integrate into thicker, more stable membranes. Perhaps the answer lies in the reduced diffusivity that arises with increased molecular weight. Recent measurements show that incipient entanglements between chains can dominate at surprisingly low molecular weights; thereby reducing self-diffusivities within polymersome membranes by orders of magnitude (22). In cell membranes, lipids are too short to entangle and few cell biologists would object to the idea that rapid lateral diffusion is generally a requirement for cell membrane function. However, there is no obvious need for great fluidity in vesicle-based drug delivery systems except for the importance of some membrane fluidity in processing steps such as extrusion where large vesicles must fission and re-seal post-filtration in order to generate a monodisperse population of vesicles. Glassy copolymer and solid systems are limited in this respect in that they tend to fracture and are generally unable to heal by re-sealing.

Encapsulants & Stability in Complex Media

Complex solutions ranging from plasma to drug mixtures can modulate and, in particular, undermine the stability of self-assembled systems through mechanisms that include minimizing the cohesive γ or the spontaneous curvature. However, the hydrated PEO brush of the present polymersomes tends to reduce, in proportion to copolymer molecular weight, the interfacial access to external model surfactants such as Triton X-100. Although difficulties in the encapsulation of proteins can likewise arise with the surfactant-like character of denatured proteins, encapsulation of proteins within polymersomes can be as straightforward as adding solid pieces of bulk diblock to an aqueous solution of desired protein and waiting 24 hours (19). To develop a sense of encapsulation efficiency, three proteins have so far been examined without optimization: myoglobin, hemoglobin, and albumin. All three proteins were shown to be entrapped during vesicle formation, but the efficiency of encapsulation of these as well as a molecular weight series of dextrans up to 500 kilodalton clearly decreases with increasing molecular size. As implied, encapsulation of small molecule solutions is readily achieved. Sucrose, glucose, and PBS buffer can be entrapped during vesicle formation at concentrations that approximate external concentrations up to ~ 2 M. Even doxorubicin can be loaded into polymersomes by efficient and widely used methods that exploit pH or salt gradients across the vesicle membrane (e.g., (5)).

As alluded to above, blood plasma has a number of components including surface active agents and white cell-recognizable proteins that are implicated in the removal of liposomes from the circulation. *In vitro* stability of polymersomes in plasma thus has at least two aspects: membrane patency and colloidal stability. Polymersome membranes do not become leaky when suspended in plasma and also kept well-mixed in a quasi-physiological manner at room temperature (19). Colloidal stability was also found in quiescent plasma over several days with frank aggregation of settled-out vesicles occurring at longer times in plasma (though not in PBS). However, polymersomes in the plasma-mediated aggregates do not appear to coarsen into giant vesicles or other structures; this is despite the close proximity and elevated density in the aggregates. This indicates that polymer membrane fusion is not readily achieved -- an important finding most likely attributable to repulsion by the PEO brush. Nonetheless, the dense aggregates are not exceedingly fragile assemblies either since they cannot easily be sheared apart. Although the likelihood of forming such aggregates *in vivo* seems remote due to incessant fluid motion, these simple observations do indicate some eventual level of plasma protein adsorption/precipitation on the polymersome membranes.

Interactions with cells: Phagocyte Challenge *in vitro*

Tissue-resident macrophages, especially those in the liver, have been shown to take up liposomes in a plasma protein dependent fashion (24, 25). Neutrophils, which can be very rapidly isolated (hence less perturbed), express many of the same surface receptors as macrophages and thus serve as a convenient primary cell type for first screens of interactions. Neutrophils are also, of course, the predominant circulating phagocyte and probably in frequent contact with injected vesicles.

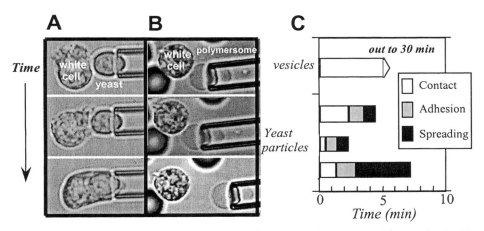

Figure 3. Phagocyte challenge *in vitro*. Yeast cells (A) or polymersomes (B) are mixed with freshly isolated red and white blood cells in plasma. The yeast cells or polymersomes are then manipulated, one at a time, into contact with the phagocytic white blood cells or the more inert red blood cells. (C) Within about 5 minutes, white cells are seen to adhere to and engulf the yeast cells. Polymersomes appeared inert in contact with a white cell for as long as 30 min. Interactions with red cells were non-existent as well. The micropipette inner diameter is 5 μm. Experiments shown were done at room temperature and lasted 30 – 60 min in total duration.

The basic *in vitro* experiment is illustrated in the video excerpts of Fig. 3A, B which show either a yeast cell or a polymersome being brought into contact with blood cells. When placed in contact with a red cell, neither a polymersome nor a yeast cell exhibits any adhesion or other clear cellular response. In comparison, 1 – 2 min of contact between a yeast cell and the neutrophil leads to strong adhesion. This generally develops further as the white cell spreads and actively engulfs the yeast particle (Fig. 3A). This type of control experiment was generally complete within 3 – 4 minutes and occurred much faster at physiological 37 °C. By contrast, over the same length of time and much longer, polymersomes appear inert to these phagocytic cells (Fig. 3B). Several such experiments are summarized in the timelines of Fig. 3C. Ongoing experiments are focused on interactions after longer pre-incubations of polymersomes in plasma.

Similar *in vitro* tests of polymersomes with macrophage cell lines as well as more quiescent cells, including endothelial cells and smooth muscle cells, further indicate the inertness of the polymersome surface. On short time scales, the dense PEO brush of the polymersomes seems to act like the glycocalyx on cellular exofaces, preventing the deposition of phagocytic ligands on the vesicle surface and/or repelling phagocyte adhesion. Ultimately, the lack of polymersome recognition by phagocytes seems important to prolonged circulation upon intravital injection and also suggests promise in targeted delivery.   Emerging studies involving intravenous injections of ~100 nm vesicles into rats appear to substantiate a prolonged circulation.

Targeting, release, and molecular compatibility

As mentioned in the Introduction, liposome-loaded doxorubicin is "passively" targeted to the leaky vasculature of tumors simply by prolonging its circulation and increasing its chance of extravasating within the tumor. More specific mechanisms of targeting are also now being engineered since PEO's terminal hydroxy group is the same on PEG-lipids where it has been widely used to attach ligands ranging from antibodies (26) to avidin and small compounds (e.g., (27, 28)). Fluorescent dyes have already been attached to this weakly reactive –OH on several of the copolymers in order to make probe molecules for various purposes including membrane diffusion measurements (22).

Once targeted to a tissue, organ, or tumor, polymersomes will next have to release their encapsulated drug contents. Release is a potential problem with current stealth liposomes as it seems clear that the presence of large molecules on the liposomal surface reduces the interactions of liposomes with cells (as intended) and thus hinders entry (29). Fusion with cell membranes appears unlikely for polymersomes, but internalization of small polymersomes should occur just as readily as with liposomes. Release of encapsulated contents can then be designed by a number of means. One mechanism being explored is osmotically poised rupture where vesicles are first loaded and stored in mildly hypertonic solutions. When transferred to isotonic media, the osmotic pressure difference generates a membrane tension which is less than the instantaneous lytic tension τ_{max} (Table 1) but sustained over time to increase the release probability: $\sim exp(\tau)$. Among the many variations envisioned for this is the encapsulation of hydrolysable poly-drugs that augment the osmotic pressure as they degrade. A separate mechanism of release being developed involves synthesis of polymersome-forming block copolymers that are hydrolysable. Table 1 lists the first of these copolymers, PEO-PLA (polylactic acid).   Blending such copolymers with non-hydrolysable copolymers provides one means of controlling membrane degradation rate. Alternatively, since hydrolysis rates of polyesters tend to be modulated by pH, polymersomes might also be made with different interior pH's to control membrane destabilization. In sum, there are a number of ways by which drug release can be controllably designed into polymersomes.

Lastly, new polymers and different applications raise new questions of molecular biocompatibility or toxicity. Among the copolymers of Table 1, degradable PEO-PLA is certainly compatible. For the PEO-PBD copolymers, several injections of these polymer systems into rats already suggest that they are likely to prove as safe as naturally occurring dolichols that contain both similar tertiary carbons and double bond structures.

CONCLUSION

Polymersomes are, arguably, a logical next step in vesicular delivery since the current liposomes of choice have evolved away from pure lipid systems to lipid plus polymer hybrids. As shown here, a range of copolymers can be synthesized which build upon key ideas in the development of liposome therapeutics, from processing to targeting. At the same time, novel membrane properties such as increased stability, reduced permeability, and controlled release can be introduced by controlling composition and molecular weight without compromising compatibility.

ACKNOWLEDGEMENTS

The authors gratefully acknowledge critical contributions to the synthesis of copolymers and characterization of vesicles by several graduate students and post-doctoral fellows, most notably Aaron Brannan and Irene Omaswa (University of Minnesota), Harry Bermudez, Dr. Helim Aranda-Espinoza, and Dr. Bohdana Discher (University of Pennsylvania), as well as Dr. You-Yeon Won (now at Harvard University), and Dr. James C-M. Lee (now at Lawrence Berkeley Laboratory). The authors also thank Professor D.A. Hammer and Professor Vladimir Muzykantov for many important discussions. Support for the evaluation of polymersome properties was provided by the NSF-sponsored Materials Research Science and Engineering Centers (MRSEC) at the University of Pennsylvania and the University of Minnesota. Development toward carrier systems has been supported under an NSF-PECASE grant to D.E. Discher.

REFERENCES

1. Bangham AD. Surrogate cells or Trojan horses. The discovery of liposomes. *Bioessays* 1995.17:1081-8.
2. Lasic DD, Papahadjopoulos D (Ed.): *Medical applications of liposomes*. Elsevier, 1998.
3. Discher BM, Won YY, Ege DS, Lee JC, Bates FS, Discher DE, Hammer DA: Polymersomes: tough vesicles made from diblock copolymers. *Science* 1999, 284 (5417): 1143-1146.
4. Laverman P. Carstens MG. Boerman OC. Dams ET. Oyen WJ. van Rooijen N. Corstens FH. Storm G. Factors affecting the accelerated blood clearance of polyethylene glycol-liposomes upon repeated injection. *Journal of Pharmacology & Experimental Therapeutics* 2001. 298(2):607-12.
5. Williams SS. Alosco TR. Mayhew E. Lasic DD. Martin FJ. Bankert RB. Arrest of human lung tumor xenograft growth in severe combined immunodeficient mice using doxorubicin encapsulated in sterically stabilized liposomes. *Cancer Research* 1993. 53:3964-7.
6. Lotem M. Hubert A. Lyass O. Goldenhersh MA. Ingber A. Peretz T. Gabizon A. Skin toxic effects of polyethylene glycol-coated liposomal doxorubicin. *Archives of Dermatology* 2000. 136:1475-80.
7. Discher BM, Hammer DA, Bates FS, and Discher DE. Polymer vesicles in various media. *Current Opinion in Colloid & Interface Science* 2000. 5: 125-131.
8. Yu K, Eisenberg A. Bilayer morphologies of self-assembled crew-cut aggregates of amphiphilic PS-b-PEO diblock copolymers in solution. *Macromolecules* 1998, 31: 3509-3518.
9. Uchegbu IF, Schatzlein AG, Tetley L, Gray AI, Sludden J, Siddique S, Mosha E. Polymeric chitosan-based vesicles for drug delivery. *Journal of Pharmacy and Pharmacology* 1998. 50 (5): 453-458.
10. Liu S, O'Brien DF. Cross-Linking polymerization in two-dimensional assemblies: Effect of the reactive group site. *Macromolecules* 1999. 32: 5519-5524.
11. Okada J, Cohen S, Langer R. *In vitro* evaluation of polymerized liposomes as an oral drug delivery system. *Pharmaceutical Research* 1995. 12:576-82.
12. Discher BM, Bermudez H, Hammer DA, Discher DE., Won Y-Y, and Bates FS. *J. Phys. Chem. B* 2002 (published online in February).
13. Semple SC, Chonn A, and Cullis PG. Interactions of liposomes and lipid-based carrier systems with blood proteins: Relation to clearance behavior *in vivo*. *Advanced Drug Delivery Reviews* 1998, 32: 3-17.
14. Bedu-Addo FK, Tang P, Xu Y, Huang L. Effects of polyethyleneglycol chain length and phospholipid acyl chain composition on the interaction of polyethyleneglycol phospholipid conjugates with phospholipid: implications in liposomal drug delivery. *Pharmaceutical Research* 1996. 13: 718-724.
15. Israelachvili J. *Intermolecular and Surface Forces*, 2nd ed., Academic Press, 1991.
16. Gregoriadis G. Fate of injected liposomes: Observations on entrapped solute retention, vesicle clearance and tissue distribution *in vivo*. In G. Gregoriadis (Ed.) *Liposomes as Drug Carriers: Recent Trends and Progress*, Wiley. New York, 1988, pp.19-27.
17. Hwang KJ, and Beaumier PL. Disposition of liposomes *in vivo*. In G. Gregoriadis (Ed.) *Liposomes as Drug Carriers: Recent Trends and Progress*, Wiley. New York, 1988, pp.19-27.
18. Lipowsky R, Sackmann E (Ed.). *Structure and dynamics of membranes. Vol. 1A: From cells to vesicles.* Elsevier Science, 1995.

19.   Lee JC-M, Bermudez H, Discher BM, Sheehan MA, Won Y-Y, Bates FS, and Discher DE. Preparation, stability, and *in vitro* performance of vesicles made with diblock copolymers. *Biotechnology and Bioengineering* 2001a. 73: 135-145

20.   Lee JC-M, Law R, and Discher DE. Bending contributions to the hydration of phospholipid and block copolymer membranes: Unifying correlations between probe fluorescence and vesicle thermoelasticity 2001b. *Langmuir* 17: 3592-3597.

21.   Aranda-Espinoza H, Bermudez H, Bates FS, and Discher DE. Electromechanical limits of polymersomes. *Physical Review Letters* 2001. 87: 208301(1-4).

22.   Lee JC-M, Santore M, Bates FS, and Discher DE. From membranes to melts, Rouse to reptation: diffusion in polymersome versus lipid bilayers. *Macromolecules* 2002. 35: 323-326.

23.   Bloom M, Evans E, Mouritsen OG. Physical Properties of the fluid lipid-bilayer component of cell membranes: a perspective. *Q. Rev. Biopohys* 1991. 24, 293-397.

24.   Kiwada H. Obara S. Nishiwaki H. Kato Y. Studies on the uptake mechanism of liposomes by perfused rat liver. I. An investigation of effluent profiles with perfusate containing no blood component. *Chemical & Pharmaceutical Bulletin* 1986. 34:1249-56.

25.   Kiwada H. Miyajima T. Kato Y. Studies on the uptake mechanism of liposomes by perfused rat liver. II. An indispensable factor for liver uptake in serum. *Chemical & Pharmaceutical Bulletin* 1987. 35:1189-95.

26.   Torchilin VP. Levchenko TS. Lukyanov AN. Khaw BA. Klibanov AL. Rammohan R. Samokhin GP. Whiteman KR. p-Nitrophenylcarbonyl-PEG-PE-liposomes: fast and simple attachment of specific ligands, including monoclonal antibodies, to distal ends of PEG chains via p-nitrophenylcarbonyl groups. *Biochimica et Biophysica Acta* 2001. 1511:397-411.

27.   Nilsson K, and Mosbach K. Immobilization of ligands with organic sulfonyl chlorides. *Methods in Enzymology* 1984. 104:56-69.

28.   Zalipsky S. Functionalized poly(ethylene glycol) for preparation of biologically relevant conjugates. *Bioconjugate Chemistry* 1995, 6:150-162.

29.   Hong RL. Huang CJ. Tseng YL. Pang VF. Chen ST. Liu JJ. Chang FH. Direct comparison of liposomal doxorubicin with or without polyethylene glycol coating in C-26 tumor-bearing mice: is surface coating with polyethylene glycol beneficial? *Clinical Cancer Research* 1999. 5:3645-52.

GLOSSARY

Diblock: A two-part polymer with one block in series with the other block. Amphiphilic diblock copolymers have a hydrophobic part covalently linked at one end to a hydrophilic part.

Liposome: A spherical shell or membrane, which self assembles in water and is composed of lipids. The membrane is, by definition, semi-permeable.

Polymersome: A spherical shell or membrane, which self-assembles in water and is composed of amphiphilic polymers. The membrane is again, by definition, semi-permeable.

25

TARGETING MITOCHONDRIA

Volkmar Weissig[*], Gerard D'Souza and Vladimir P. Torchilin
Northeastern University, Bouve College of Health Sciences, School of Pharmacy, Department of Pharmaceutics, Boston, MA 02115. [*]Corresponding author: vweissig@hotmail.com

INTRODUCTION

The field of mitochondrial research is currently one of the fastest growing disciplines in biomedicine. During the last decade alone, more than 26,000 articles on mitochondria have been published in over 1000 scientific journals. What brings mitochondria into the limelight of the scientific community? Since the end of the '80s, a series of key discoveries have been made which have rekindled the scientific interest in this long-known cell organelle. It has become increasingly evident that mitochondrial dysfunction contributes to a variety of human disorders, ranging from neurodegenerative and neuromuscular diseases, obesity, and diabetes to ischemia-reperfusion injury and cancer. Moreover, since the middle of the '90s, mitochondria, the "power houses" of the cell, have also become accepted as the "motor of cell death" (1), which reflects their increasingly acknowledged key role during apoptosis (programmed cell death).

Based on these recent developments in mitochondrial research, increased pharmacological and pharmaceutical efforts have lead to the emergence of "Mitochondrial Medicine" as a whole new field of biomedical research (2). Targeting of biologically active molecules to mitochondria in living cells will open up avenues for manipulating mitochondrial functions, which may result in the selective protection, repair or eradication of cells. This chapter describes the current strategies of mitochondrial targeting and some of their possible therapeutic applications.

MITOCHONDRIA AS CELL ORGANELLES

The major function of mitochondria is the conversion of food energy into chemical energy (ATP) that can be used to drive the cellular reactions essential in keeping the cell alive ("power house" of the cell). In addition, mitochondria are involved in several other central metabolic pathways such as the oxidation of fatty acids, the citrate cycle, the synthesis of steroid hormones and gluconeogenesis. Although present in all eukaryotic cells, the number of mitochondria per single cell largely depends on the cell's energy demand. Metabolically active organs such as the liver, the brain and cardiac and skeletal muscle tissues may contain up to several thousands of mitochondria per cell, while somatic tissues with a lower demand for energy contain only a few dozen of these organelles. Human spermatozoa have a constant number of 16 mitochondria, while oocytes contain up to 100,000.

Each mitochondrion is composed of two membranes which together create two separate compartments, the internal matrix space and the narrow intermembrane space. The outer membrane is permeable to molecules smaller than 5 kDa making the intermembrane space chemically equivalent to the cytosol with respect to small molecules. In contrast, the inner membrane is highly impermeable and characterized by an unusually high content of membrane proteins as well as a unique lipid composition. The mitochondrial inner membrane proteins are components of the respiratory chain including the ATP synthase and a wide variety of transport proteins. The impermeability of the inner membrane is a prerequisite for the establishment of an imbalance in the distribution of protons between the mitochondrial matrix and the cytosol. The imbalance in turn is the driving force for the synthesis of ATP. In order to increase its total surface, the inner mitochondrial membrane is convoluted into cristae.

Mitochondria are very mobile and plastic organelles. The movement of mitochondria within cells appears to be controlled by association with cellular microtubules and motor proteins like myosin, dyneins and kinesins, reviewed in (3).

Mitochondria contain their own genome (mtDNA), and transcription and translation systems. Human mtDNA is a circular molecule 16,569 bp in size, sequenced more than 20 years ago. A striking feature of human mtDNA is the lack of introns; all genes are joined end-to-end or separated by only a few nucleotides, and noncoding stretches are missing. Human mtDNA encodes two ribosomal RNAs, all 22 tRNAs necessary for protein synthesis at mitochondrial ribosomes, and 13 polypeptides that are all subunits of the oxidative phosphorylation (OXPHOS) enzyme complexes. In summary, human mitochondrial DNA exclusively encodes only genes responsible for the production of ATP.

WHY TARGETING MITOCHONDRIA?

In this section, the role of mitochondrial dysfunction in human diseases and the therapeutic potential of targeting biologically active molecules to and into mitochondria will be discussed.

Delivery of DNA to Mitochondria for the Treatment of Mitochondrial DNA Diseases

A connection between human diseases and defects of the mitochondrial genome was revealed for the first time in 1988 with the publication of two papers, one in *Science* (4) and the other in *Nature* (5). The first one demonstrates an association between a mitochondrial missense mutation and maternally transmitted Leber's hereditary optic neuropathy. The second paper shows the presence of mitochondrial DNA deletions in patients with spontaneous mitochondrial encephalomyopathies. Large deletions of mtDNA were found to lead to mitochondrial myopathies such as progressive external ophthalmoplegia and Kearns-Sayre syndrome. Other mitochondrial myopathies, such as myoclonus epilepsy with ragged red fibers, mitochondrial encephalopathy with lactic acidosis, and stroke-like episodes, are caused by point mutations of mtDNA.

Table 1. Organ manifestations of mitochondrial DNA diseases, adapted from (6).

ORGAN	CLINICAL MANIFESTATION
Skeletal muscle	Progressive external ophthalmoplegia; proximal myopathy; intolerance to exercise; hypotonia; pulmonary insufficiency
Heart	Hypertrophic myocardia; disorder of impulse conduction
CNS	Cerebellar ataxia; epilepsy; myoclonic convulsion; mental retardation; dementia; ischemia
Neurosensory systems	Optic atrophy; retinitis pigmentosa; deafness
Endocrine glands	Diabetes mellitus; hypothyroidism; hypoparathyroidism; adrenal insufficiency; sexual and growth retardation; sterility
Kidney	Tubulopathy: glucosuria; aminoaciduria
Liver	Hepatic insufficiency
Pancreas	Insufficiency of exocrine glands
Intestine	Malabsorption; diarrhea
Blood	Pancytopenia; anemia

Since 1988, the number of diseases found to be associated with defects of the mitochondrial genome has grown significantly (7). However, clinical profiles remain difficult to identify. Currently, tissue-specific syndromes associated with mtDNA defects, are recognized. Decrease of cellular respiration is poorly tolerated by tissues that are metabolically active. These organ systems include, in decreasing order of vulnerability, the brain, skeletal muscle, heart, kidney and liver. Therefore, "typical" groups of mtDNA diseases are neuromuscular diseases and neurodegenerative diseases. Also, prominent clinical signs often involve the visual system. Ptosis, restriction of eye movement, optic atrophy, pigmentary retinopathy, sudden or subacute visual loss, and hemianopia are particularly noteworthy. Table 1 shows typical organ-specific manifestations of mitochondrial DNA diseases.

Despite major advances in understanding mtDNA defects at the genetic and biochemical level, there is no satisfactory treatment available to a vast majority of patients. This is largely due to the fact that most of these patients have respiratory chain defects, i.e. defects that involve the final common pathway of oxidative metabolism, making it impossible to bypass the defect by administering alternative metabolic carriers of energy. These objective limitations of conventional biochemical treatment for patients with defects of mtDNA warrant the exploration of gene therapy approaches. Two different approaches to mitochondrial gene therapy are imaginable (Figure 1).

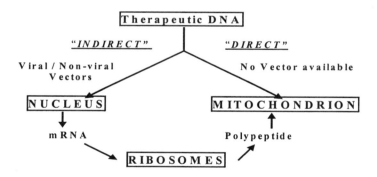

Figure 1. Schematic illustration of the two principal strategies for mitochondrial gene therapy, adapted from (8)

The first approach involves expressing a wild-type copy of the defective gene in the nucleus, with cytoplasmic synthesis and subsequent targeting of the gene product to the mitochondria. However, besides the different codon usage in mitochondria, there are three major difficulties in adapting this nuclear-cytosolic approach to mitochondrial gene therapy of mammalian cells, reviewed in (8). First, the majority of mtDNA defects involve tRNAs and to date, no natural mechanism for the mitochondrial uptake of cytosolic tRNAs in mammalian cells has been reported. Second, the 13 mtDNA-encoded proteins are highly hydrophobic. It has therefore been suggested that these proteins need to be synthesized at the location of their function. Third, it has been hypothesized that some of the proteins encoded by the mitochondrion may potentially toxic if synthesized in the cytosol. Considering these problems associated with the nuclear-cytosolic approach, the direct transfection of mitochondria appears to be the better alternative. As a necessary prerequisite, technology has to be developed which allows the delivery of DNA into the matrix of mitochondria in living cells (8).

Protecting Mitochondria from Oxidative Stress

Mitochondria are the major source of highly reactive oxygen species (ROS). About 1-2% of the electrons passing through the respiratory chain complexes "escape" from the OXPHOS pathway and react with oxygen to form superoxide $O_2^{\cdot(-)}$, reviewed in (2). Superoxide itself causes non-specific oxidative damage to mitochondrial lipids, proteins and DNA. It also reacts further to form other ROS like hydrogen peroxide, which can decompose to form reactive hydroxyl radicals. Consequently, mitochondria are continuously being exposed to oxidative stress and are prone to accumulate oxidative damage to a higher extent than any other cell organelle. ROS mediated oxidative damage of the respiratory chain may lead to an increased formation of ROS, thereby starting a vicious cycle that may be related to a number of "late-onset", i.e. age-related dysfunctions.

Under normal conditions, ROS and their peroxidation products are neutralized by a natural defense system consisting of mitochondrial and cytosolic superoxide dismutases and several peroxidases. However, under conditions of an impaired antioxidant defense system and/or under conditions of an increased ROS formation, e.g., in ischemia-reperfusion, upon the action of xenobiotics, during inflammation and under ionizing irradiation, reactive oxygen species can accumulate which in turn may lead to severe damage to the cell and the whole organism, reviewed in (9).

In conclusion, it has been hypothesized that the selective prevention of mitochondrial oxidative damage may be an effective therapeutic approach for a wide range of human diseases (10). This hypothesis has already been verified by the over-expression of mitochondrial superoxide dismutase, which leads to a decrease of liver reperfusion injury (11).

Delivery of Proapoptotic Drugs to Mitochondria

Apoptosis (programmed cell death) is an energy requiring, tightly regulated and genetically encoded process of cell suicide that leads to the clearance of cells without provoking any damaging inflammatory response. Apoptosis plays a fundamental role for the maintenance and regulation of tissues within a multicellular organism and is therefore crucial for the normal development of an organism. In particular, apoptosis occurs in embryogenesis and metamorphosis, i.e. during the growth and maturation of organs, but has also been demonstrated to be associated with pathologic conditions of the nervous system (Alzheimer's disease, Parkinson's disease, brain trauma, stroke and others).

The role of apoptosis during carcinogenic processes is most intriguing. The inhibition of programmed cell death is widely accepted as an important part of cancer development (12). Malign transformations are generally believed to be rather common in animal and human cells. Under non-pathological conditions, however, such cells are efficiently eliminated by the organism via programmed cell death. Only cells that have learned to avoid apoptosis, give rise to malignant growth (9). Thus, the diminished apoptotic capacity of cancer cells is assumed to be essential for the progression of a tumor (13).

Although the detailed mechanism of apoptosis is still the subject of intense research, it has become clear that two separate pathways may be involved. One pathway is induced by receptor-mediated signaling at the plasma membrane (cell surface "death receptors"), and the other is triggered by leakage of proapoptotic factors like cytochrome C, apoptosis inducing factor (AIF) and procaspase-3 from the intermembrane space of mitochondria. Once activated, both pathways lead to the activation of several cysteine-dependent proteases (caspases), which in turn hydrolyze a multitude of substrates to give rise to the characteristic morphological changes like cell and nuclear shrinkage. The cell eventually disintegrates into smaller membrane-bound bodies, which are ingested by adjacent cells.

The two apoptosis-triggering pathways are not mutually exclusive. Following its death receptor-mediated activation, caspase 8 can cleave a member of the pro-apoptotic Bcl-2 family into two fragments, one of which translocates to mitochondria and triggers the release of cytochrome C. Thus, mitochondria seem to act, in some cell lines, as amplifiers of the receptor-induced cell death (9).

The molecular mechanism of the release of cytochrome C and the other apoptosis inducing factors from the mitochondrial intermembrane space is currently under intense investigation. Mitochondrial permeability transition (MPT) has been identified as a critical event in this process, an event in which the inner mitochondrial membrane becomes rapidly permeable to solutes under 1.5kD in size. MPT appears to be under the control of the mitochondrial permeabilization transition pore complex (mPTPC), a "megapore" spanning through both mitochondrial membranes. The components of the PTPC as well as proteins associated with it have not yet been completely identified. The Adenine Nucleotide Translocase (ANT), mitochondrial cyclophilin D, the Voltage Dependent Anion Channel (VDAC) and hexokinase are believed to be major parts of the PTPC, reviewed in (13).

It was widely believed that opening of the PTPC leads to hyperosmolarity of the mitochondrial matrix, which causes it to swell. Since the inner mitochondrial membrane has a larger surface area than its outer counterpart, the expanding matrix will rupture the outer membrane, releasing cytochrome C from the inner membrane space. However, more recent investigations have indicated that cytochrome C is liberated from mitochondria by a mechanism that preserves outer mitochondrial membrane integrity, reviewed in (9). The PTPC is thought to associate with the pro-apoptotic Bcl-2 family member Bax forming a channel large enough to release cytochrome C. Association of Bax with PTPC is inhibited by the antiapoptotic oncoprotein Bcl-2. Consequently, a delicate balance between proapoptotic and antiapoptotic proteins and their interaction with the PTPC are decisive for apoptotic death or survival of the cell (9).

In tumor cells it has been found that several changes interrupt the death receptor pathway, reviewed in (12). Mechanisms that have been reported include the reduced expression of death receptors and the overexpression of so-called decoy receptors that compete for ligand. Inactivation of the death receptor pathway renders cells less susceptible to death signals from cytotoxic lymphocytes that express ligands for the death receptors (FasL) on their surface. Thus, the surface of tumor cells "becomes immune" against the immune system, which results in an unhindered progression of the tumor.

While several conventional chemotherapeutic drugs indirectly trigger mitochondrial membrane permeabilization by activation of endogenous factors involved in the physiological control of apoptosis, an increasing number of new compounds have been identified, which are able to act directly on mitochondrial membranes and/or on the mPTPC, reviewed in (14). These agents may induce apoptosis under circumstances in which endogenous apoptosis inducing mechanisms, such as the death receptor pathway and others, are disrupted, i.e. when conventional drugs fail to act.

Stabilization of the mitochondrial membrane by antiapoptotic Bcl-2-like proteins tends to reduce the cytotoxicity of these new apoptosis-triggering agents. Therefore, the targeting of specific components of the mPTPC has been suggested as a means to overcome this Bcl-2-mediated inhibition of apoptosis (14). Target candidates suggested so far are redox-sensitive thiol groups within the mPTPC and the mitochondrial benzodiazepine receptor

(BzPR), which is believed to be associated with outer membrane components of the mPTPC.

In summary, the mitochondrial PTPC, due to its central and possibly decisive role in apoptosis, represents a privileged pharmacological target for cytotoxic as well as for cytoprotective therapies.

Targeting of Uncoupling Proteins in the Inner Mitochondrial Membrane

During oxidative phosphorylation at the inner mitochondrial membrane, "food energy" is converted into the "energy currency" (ATP) of the cell. Enzymes and low molecular weight redox intermediates transport electrons from the hydrogens in the respiratory substrates (NADH and $FADH_2$) down the redox potential to molecular oxygen, the final electron acceptor. The considerable amount of free energy released during this "down-hill" flow of electrons is used to translocate protons against a gradient from the mitochondrial matrix, across the inner mitochondrial membrane, into the inner membrane space. This process creates an electrochemical gradient at the inner mitochondrial membrane, which includes contributions from both, a membrane potential (negative inside) and a pH difference (acidic outside). The energy stored in this transmembrane proton electrochemical gradient is then used to drive the synthesis of ATP via the flow of protons from the inner membrane space through the ATPsynthase complex back into the mitochondrial matrix.

In brief, the electron flow down the redox potential is coupled with the synthesis of ATP via a proton gradient along the inner mitochondrial membrane.

Any damage of the inner mitochondrial membrane resulting in a back flow of protons that bypasses the ATPsynthase complex results in the release of the energy as heat, i.e. the electron flow and the ATP synthesis become uncoupled. This reduces the efficiency of mitochondrial ATP synthesis and ultimately leads to a decrease in the storage of triglycerides in fat depots.

The energy stored in the proton electrochemical gradient can also be dissipated in the form of heat by the presence of naturally occurring uncoupling proteins (UCPs). The first uncoupling protein, UCP-1, was discovered in brown adipose tissue, UCP-2 is expressed in a variety of tissues, UCP-3 is largely expressed in skeletal muscle and UCP-4 is expressed preferentially in the brain, reviewed in (2). These uncoupling proteins generally increase the proton permeability of the mitochondrial inner membrane, thus allowing the proton gradient to bypass ATP synthesis. Although the mechanism of UCP regulation is still poorly understood, it seems likely that their expression levels are altered in response to cold, diet and hormones (2).

Intriguingly, it has been found that the activity of UCP-1 can be modulated by chemical agents. Free fatty acids increase, while purine di- and trinucleotides decrease the UCP-1 activity (15). This finding opens up the possibility to modulate pharmacologically the activity of UCPs at the inner mitochondrial membrane by targeting these uncoupling proteins with yet to be determined drug molecules. Eventually, this approach may lead to new treatments of obesity.

Mitochondrial Toxins

Mitochondrial bioenergetics, i.e. the production of ATP, can be affected by a large variety of natural, commercial, pharmaceutical and environmental chemicals, comprehensively reviewed in (16). For example, more than 60 different types of natural and synthetic compounds are known to inhibit the activity of mitochondrial NADH:ubiquinone oxidoreductase (complex I), the first enzyme complex of the respiratory chain at the inner mitochondrial membrane (16). One of the classical inhibitors is rotenone, a naturally occurring isoflavonoid produced by plants of the genus Leguminosae. In isolated bovine heart or liver mitochondria, the median inhibitory concentration (IC_{50}) for rotenone is 0.07 nmol/mg of protein with a K_i of 4 nM, reviewed in (16). Even more powerful is rolliniastatin-1, an acetogenin derivative produced by Annonacea plants. For complex I, its K_i is 0.3 nM (16).

Most of the corresponding enzyme kinetic studies have so far been conducted either using isolated mitochondria or on the isolated respiratory chain complex itself.

Likewise, antipsychotic and antidepressant drugs, some antitumor drugs, a number of plasticizers, lipid-lowering drugs, antimycotics, numerous antihelmintics and various herbicides and insecticides have all been reported to uncouple oxidative phosphorylation in isolated mitochondria, reviewed in (16).

Given the vast amount of information about the interaction of drugs and xenobiotics with isolated mitochondria and/or isolated mitochondrial enzyme complexes, it appears reasonable to conclude that, upon development of mitochondria-specific drug delivery systems (drug carriers), the re-evaluation of the cytotoxic potential of a large number of compounds on living cells and *in vivo* might lead to new and powerful cytotoxic therapies.

Targeting of Potassium Channel Openers to Mitochondria

Potassium channel openers (KCOs) act by stimulating ion flux through K^+ channels. They were first identified in the early '90s by their antianginal or antihypertensive mechanism of action. Currently KCOs are at various stages of development as antiasthmatic and cardioprotective agents, reviewed in (9). It was believed that KCOs act only on K^+ channels in cell surface membranes (9). Evidence has been accumulated, however, for the existence of targets at mitochondrial sites. The interaction of KCOs with mitochondria might even be the basis for the cardioprotective action of these compounds (9).

Mitochondrial Targets for Anti-ischemic Drugs

Mitochondrial targets for anti-ischemic drugs have recently been reviewed comprehensively in (17). The cessation of blood flow followed by reperfusion causes severe cellular damages by inducing a complex cascade of events which involve, among others, an alteration of ionic homeostasis promoting H^+ and Ca^{2+} accumulation and the generation of free radicals. In this context, mitochondria appear to be highly vulnerable and seem to play a decisive role in the cell signaling leading to cell death. Therefore, recent efforts to find an effective therapy for ischemia-reperfusion injury have focused on mitochondrial drug targets (17).

Mitochondrial DNA metabolism targeting drugs

A wide range of structurally diverse drugs has been identified which selectively deplete mammalian cells of mtDNA, reviewed in (18). Among them are nucleoside analogs used as antiviral drugs such as AZT, the agent widely used to inhibit the HIV virus. For many of these drugs, the specific mechanisms underlying their effect are poorly understood. However, the wide variation of chemical structures of these agents suggests that very different aspects of mtDNA metabolism are being targeted. Identification of their molecular targets will aid in the design of new and more effective cytotoxic (anticancer) drugs, which might either target mitochondria in living cells by virtue of their chemical nature or have to be delivered to mitochondria utilizing a mitochondria-specific drug delivery system.

Mitochondrial Targets for Photosensitizers

As photodynamic therapy (PDT) becomes established as a treatment for cancer, the interest in identifying the underlying mechanisms of PDT-based cell killing is increasing. The subcellular localization of many photosensitizers and the early response to light activation indicate that mitochondria play a major role in photodynamic cell death, reviewed in (19). It has been found that mitochondrial photosensitizers can target several critical proteins within or associated with the mitochondrion (19).

Delivery of tRNA into the Mitochondrial Matrix

Many defects in mitochondrial protein synthesis which give rise to numerous neuromuscular diseases are due to mutations in mitochondrial tRNA. The replacement of the defective tRNA inside the mitochondrion could provide a possible cure for such mutations. Based on extensive studies about the tRNA mitochondrial import in yeast, it was recently demonstrated that human isolated mitochondria are able to import tRNA in the presence of yeast import directing factors (20). Moreover, it was shown that the imported yeast tRNA derivative can correctly participate in the protein synthesis in human mitochondria.

Targeting of Antitumor Sulfonylureas to Mitochondria

Diarylsulfonylureas are antitumor agents that have been shown to be effective against xenografts of human tumors in mice, reviewed in (9). Though their mechanism of action is still under investigation, it has been established that certain sulfonylureas uncouple oxidative phosphorylation in isolated mouse mitochondria (9).

Targeting the Mitochondrial Benzodiazepine Receptor

Benzodiazepines are widely prescribed drugs for relieving anxiety; they are also used as anticonvulsants, muscle relaxants and sedative hypnotics. These effects are mediated in the CNS through postsynaptic plasma membrane receptors specific for the neurotransmitter GABA. In addition to these central-type benzodiazepine receptors, binding sites have also been identified in peripheral tissues, reviewed in (9). Such so-called peripheral benzodiazepine receptors (PBR) have been localized in mitochondrial membranes. Protoporphyrin IX has been identified as an endogenous ligand to the PBR, suggesting an involvement of PBR in mitochondrial heme synthesis. A synthetic agonist to the PBR was found to strongly protect against apoptosis induced by the death receptor pathway. In vitro studies also demonstrated the involvement of PBR in the regulation of cholesterol transport from the outer to the inner mitochondrial membrane, a known rate-limiting step in the biosynthesis of steroids, reviewed in (9). In conclusion, the mitochondrial PBR appears as a pharmacological target for a variety of cytoprotective and cytotoxic therapies.

Delivery of Imunosuppressant Drugs to Mitochondria

Cyclosporin A (CsA) is a potent immunosuppressive drug known to block the transcription of cytokine genes in activated T cells. CsA has also been found to block the opening of the mPTPC by binding to cyclophilin D, which is part of the mPTPC. The blocking of the mPTP opening is thought to be the mechanism underlying the protective action of CsA against ischemic injuries. Such beneficial effects have recently been described in ischemic and traumatic brain injury (TBI) in animals, reviewed in (9). It has been suggested that agents such as CsA, which improve mitochondrial function, may be effective in the treatment of TBI (9).

Mitochondrial Targets for Nonsteroidal Anti-inflammatory Drugs

Nonsteroidal anti-inflammatory drugs (NSAIDs) such as aspirin and ibuprofen are among the most frequently used drugs. NSAIDs act via the inhibition of cyclooxygenases and thereby reduce the synthesis of prostaglandin. Increasing evidence suggests that aspirin and other NSAIDs also reduce the risk of colorectal cancer, reviewed in (9). Although the molecular mechanism for this action is unclear, NSAIDs have been found to uncouple oxidative phosphorylation and to decrease ATP synthesis, i.e. to act on mitochondria. It has been proposed that the uncoupling effect of NSAIDs is mediated by inducing the opening of the mPTPC. For example, incubation of isolated mitochondria with ibuprofen induces mitochondrial membrane depolarization and mitochondrial swelling, which is blocked by CsA (9).

Mitochondrial Targets for Local Anesthetics

Many local anesthetics are lipophilic tertiary amines with pK_a values between 7 and 9. Besides, at their basic site of action, which is the plasma membrane of nerve cells, they have also long been known to act at mitochondrial sites, reviewed in (9). It has been demonstrated that local anesthetics interfere with mitochondrial ion transport, with the adenine nucleotide translocase and with metabolic activities in mitochondria. Recently, it has been shown that the local anesthetic dibucaine is able to inhibit the growth of promyelocytic leukemia cells. The induction of apoptosis through release of cytochrome C from the inner mitochondrial membrane space has been suggested as a mechanism of action (9).

Mitochondria and Lipid Metabolism Targeting Drugs

Mitochondria play a central role for several metabolic pathways in which lipids are involved and therefore may present a sensitive target for pharmacological intervention (9). For example, in noninsulin-dependent diabetes mellitus, hyperglycemia can potentially be prevented by reducing the oxidation of fatty acids in the mitochondrial matrix. This can be achieved by inhibiting carnitine acyl transferase I located at the outer mitochondrial membrane, i.e. the shuttle system responsible for the transport of activated fatty acids from the cytosol into the inner space of mitochondria (9).

HOW CAN MITOCHONDRIA BE TARGETED?

The current strategies for the delivery of biologically active molecules to and into mitochondria are based mainly on two distinct properties of this organelle: the high membrane potential across the inner mitochondrial membrane and the complex apparatus for the transport of proteins across both mitochondrial membranes.

Mitochondrial Membrane Potential and Mitochondriotropic Molecules

One of the major metabolic roles of mitochondria is the synthesis of ATP by oxidative phosphorylation via the respiratory chain. According to Mitchell's chemiosmotic hypothesis, electrons from the hydrogens on NADH and $FADH_2$ are carried along the respiratory chain at the mitochondrial inner membrane, thereby releasing energy that is used to "pump" protons across the inner membrane from the mitochondrial matrix into the intermembrane space. This process creates a transmembrane electrochemical gradient, which includes contributions from both, a membrane potential (negative inside) and a pH difference (acidic outside).

The membrane potential of mitochondria is, at 130-150 mV, by far the largest within cells. Therefore, positively charged molecules are attracted by mitochondria in response to the highly negative membrane potential. Although most charged molecules cannot enter the mitochondrial matrix because the inner mitochondrial membrane is impermeable to polar molecules, certain amphiphile compounds ("mitochondriotropics," Figure 2) are able to cross both mitochondrial membranes and to accumulate in the mitochondrial matrix in response to the negative membrane potential.

(A)   (B)   (C)

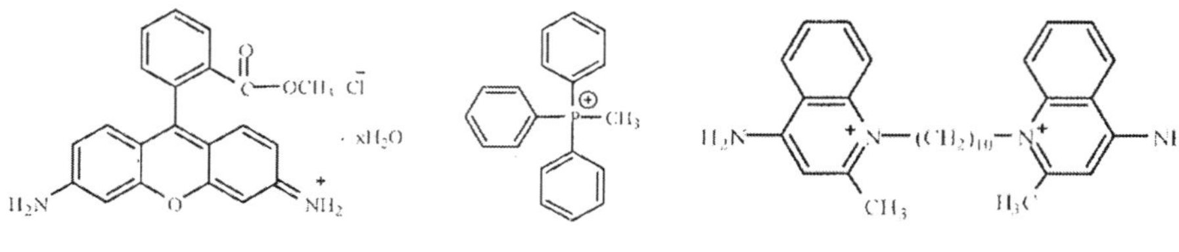

Figure 2. Chemical structures of representative mitochondriotropic molecules: A: Rhodamine 123; B: Methyl-triphenylphosphonium; C: Dequalinium chloride

Among the first described mitochondriotropic cationic amphiphiles were phosphonium salts such as methyltriphenylphosphonium (Fig. 2, compound B). Probably the most "popular" mitochondriotropic compound is Rhodamine 123 (Fig. 2, compound A), which has been used extensively for the last two decades as a specific stain for mitochondria in living cells.

It is evident that these mitochondriotropic molecules have two structural features in common. Firstly, they are all amphiphilic in nature, i.e. they combine a hydrophilic charge center with a hydrophobic core. Secondly, the Π-electron charge density in all structures extends over at least three atoms or more instead of being limited to the internuclear region between the heteroatom and the adjacent carbon atom. This causes a distribution of the positive charge density between two or more atoms, i.e. the positive charge is delocalized. Both structural features have been recognized to be crucial for the accumulation of these organic cations inside the matrix of mitochondria.

Mitochondriotropics for Therapy

The ability of this type of molecule to specifically accumulate in mitochondria of living cells has been explored for the transport of small therapeutic molecules into mitochondria, reviewed in (2, 8). Two principally different therapeutic strategies are being developed. One approach aims at killing cancer cells by interfering with mitochondrial functions; the other approach is aimed at protecting mitochondria in normal and healthy cells from oxidative damage.

The use of lipophilic mitochondriotropic molecules to kill cancer cells is based on the elevated mitochondrial membrane potential that many cancer cells have in comparison to untransformed cells, reviewed in (21). The higher membrane potential leads to greater accumulation of lipophilic cations in mitochondria causing cell death by disruption of mitochondrial functions.

For instance, dequalinium demonstrated a 100-fold greater inhibition of the clonal growth of carcinoma vs. control epithelial cells in culture and displayed activity against human colon adenocarcinoma cells injected subcutaneously in nude mice (21).

In contrast to targeting toxic molecules to mitochondria, the delivery of antioxidants into the mitochondrial matrix may protect mitochondria from oxidative stress. For example, the antioxidant phenolic residue of vitamin E was covalently linked to triphenylphosphonium and found to accumulate several-hundred fold within the mitochondrial matrix, driven by the organelle's large membrane potential (22). When cells were incubated with micromolar concentrations of this vitamin E conjugate, they accumulated millimolar concentrations within their mitochondria. Consequently, the targeted derivative of vitamin E protected mitochondrial function from oxidative damage far more effectively than free vitamin E itself (22).

Self-assembling Mitochondriotropics: "Mitochondriotropic Vesicles"

Dequalinium (Fig. 2, compound C) is a dicationic compound resembling bolaform electrolytes, i.e. it is a symmetrical molecule with two charge centers separated at a relatively large distance by a single hydrophobic hydrocarbon chain. Symmetric bola-like structures, known from archaeal lipids, consist of two glycerol backbones connected by two hydrophobic chains. Such lipids and their ability to self-associate into mechanically very stable monolayer membranes have been extensively studied.

Analogous to the bola-like archaeal lipids, it was shown that dequalinium, a single-chain bola amphiphile, is able to self-assemble into membrane-like structures (23). Based on transmission electron microscopy, freeze-fracture electron microscopy, size distribution measurements via dynamic laser light scattering and on Monte Carlo Computer Simulations, it was determined that dequalinium chloride, as well as dequalinium acetate, form spherical, liposome-like vesicles (Fig. 3) upon sonication, reviewed in (8). The diameter of these so-called "DQAsomes" lies in the range between about 70 and 700 nm.

DQAsomes are unique vesicles, considering that they combine the most useful features of three different drug delivery systems. Just as liposomes, which are in clinical use as a delivery system for anticancer drugs, DQAsomes have an aqueous inner space suited for the encapsulation of water-soluble drug molecules. Just as cationic lipids, which are the basis for a large variety of non-viral transfection systems, DQAsomes are cationic vesicles able to bind DNA. Finally, DQAsomes are composed entirely of mitochondriotropic molecules, which have been shown to accumulate

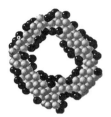 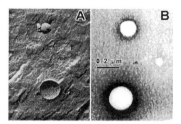

Figure 3. Left panel: Monte Carlo Computer Simulation, self-assembled vesicular aggregate (cross-section). Right panel: Electron photomicrograph of vesicles prepared from dequalinium. (A) Freeze fractured. (B) Negatively stained; adapted from (23).

exclusively in mitochondria in living cells (24). All three properties taken together, DQAsomes potentially constitute the first universal mitochondria-specific drug and DNA delivery system. While the delivery of small molecules to mitochondria using DQAsomes still has to be fully explored, it has already been shown that DQAsomes meet all criteria for a mitochondria-specific DNA delivery vector, recently reviewed in (8). The strategy for the use of DQAsomes as a mitochondria-specific DNA delivery system is based on the mitochondrial protein import machinery. Therefore, mitochondrial protein import shall be discussed next in this chapter, followed by a brief description of DQAsome mediated DNA delivery to mitochondria in living cells.

Hitch-hiking on the Mitochondrial Protein-import Machinery

The biogenesis of mitochondria and their function depends on the coordinated import of precursor proteins from the cytosol. Only a very small set of all mitochondrial proteins, 13 polypeptides that are all part of the protein complexes involved in the oxidative phosphorylation, are being synthesized inside mitochondria. All other proteins must be imported. To this end, both mitochondrial membranes contain an elaborate network of protein translocases together with a variety of chaperones and processing enzymes in the matrix and intermembrane space to mediate protein import. A clear picture of this highly complex mechanism, greatly simplified in Figure 4, has emerged over the past years.

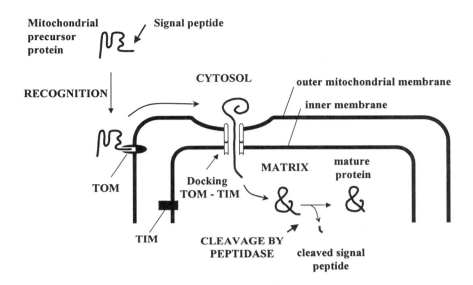

Figure 4. Major steps during the import of proteins from the cytosol into the mitochondrial matrix (for details, see text).

Generally, proteins bearing an amino-terminal targeting sequence, a so-called mitochondrial leader (or signal) peptide (MLS peptide), are escorted through the cytosol by chaperones to the TOM complex, which is a translocase localized in the outer mitochondrial membrane. After crossing the outer membrane, so-called TIM complexes, i.e. translocases of the inner membrane, mediate the further transport into the mitochondrial matrix. Finally, inside the mitochondrial matrix, the leader peptide is cleaved off by a matrix processing protease.

The mitochondrial TIM-TOM machinery has been utilized for the transport of exogeneous DNA into the inner space of mitochondria, reviewed in (8). Already in 1989 it was shown that both, single- and double-stranded 24bp oligonucleotides can be taken up by isolated yeast mitochondria after the oligonucleotides have been conjugated to a precursor protein consisting of the yeast cytochrome C oxidase subunit IV presequence fused to a modified mouse dihydrofolate reductase. In 1995, the import of double stranded DNA molecules (17 bp or 322 bp, conjugated to the amino-terminal leader peptide of the rat ornithine transcarbamylase) into the matrix of isolated mouse mitochondria was reported. The same laboratory also studied the recognition and cleavage of DNA-peptide conjugates by the endogenous mitochondrial signal peptide processing machinery. It could be demonstrated that such artificial peptide-DNA conjugates are recognized by the mitochondrial proteolytic machinery, reviewed in (8).

More recently, it was shown that Peptide Nucleic Acids (PNAs), i.e. synthetic DNA-like molecules in which the chains of pyrimidine and purine bases are linked by an amino ethyl backbone, can be partially directed to mitochondria in living cells when conjugated to mitochondria-specific targeting peptides, reviewed in (25). Intriguingly, this approach may launch the development of anti-sense therapy for disorders of the mitochondrial genome, since the same laboratory has shown earlier that sequence-specific PNAs selectively inhibit the replication of mutated mtDNA *in vitro* (25).

All data taken together demonstrate clearly the feasibility of delivering exogenous DNA-peptide conjugates into the mitochondrial matrix by hitch-hiking on the mitochondrial protein import pathway. However, with the probable exception of hydrolysis-resistant oligonucleotide derivatives (like PNA), the transport of peptide-DNA conjugates to mitochondria in living cells requires a mitochondria-specific delivery system that charge-neutralizes the DNA, protects the DNA from nuclease digestion, and mediates its cellular uptake and transport to mitochondria. At the mitochondrial membrane, the DNA-peptide conjugate has to dissociate from the carrier system in order to be able to be taken up by the TOM-TIM machinery. As mentioned earlier, DQAsomes appear to be the prime candidate for such a carrier system that is able to deliver DNA to mitochondria of living cells.

DQAsomes as the First Mitochondrial Transfection Vector

The proposed strategy for the delivery of DNA into the matrix of mitochondria is based upon the DQAsome mediated transport of a DNA-MLS peptide conjugate to the site of mitochondria, and the liberation of this conjugate from DQAsomes at the mitochondrial outer membrane followed by uptake of the DNA-MLS peptide conjugate via the mitochondrial protein import machinery (comprehensively reviewed in (8)). It was shown that DQAsomes, just like any other cationic transfection vector (i.e. cationic lipids or polymere), bind the DNA, protect it from nuclease digestion and mediate the uptake of DNA into mammalian cells (8). Once inside the cell, the DNA ultimately has to dissociate from its carrier to make the nucleic acid accessible to the transcription machinery. It was demonstrated that anionic phospholipids, typically localized at the inner layer of cytosolic membranes, can displace the anionic DNA from cationic lipids, suggesting that the DNA may be liberated from its delivery system already during the endocytotic uptake of the lipid/DNA complex (30).

However, to achieve delivery of the DNA-MLS peptide conjugate to the site of mitochondria, i.e. to utilize the natural mitochondriotropism of the carrier system (DQAsomes), the DNA conjugate must remain stably associated with DQAsomes during cell entry. Only after the DNA-peptide conjugate has been transported to the site of mitochondria can the cationic carrier release the DNA conjugate, thus making it accessible to the mitochondrial protein import machinery.

The selective release of DNA from the DQAsome/DNA complex at mitochondrial membranes has been demonstrated using three different experimental approaches: first by employing model membranes, i.e. artificial phospholipid vesicles (liposomes) (27), second by using isolated mouse liver mitochondria (28) and third with mammalian cells *in vitro* (29).

For the first DNA release study, anionic liposomes, the lipid composition of which mimicked cytoplasmic (CPM), inner mitochondrial (IMM) and outer mitochondrial membranes (OMM) were incubated with DQAsome/DNA complex and with DNA bound to a commercially available nuclear transfection vector (Lipofectin™), respectively. It was found that, in striking contrast to DNA/Lipofectin complexes, DQAsomes/DNA complexes do not release any DNA in the presence of CPM liposomes, i.e. liposomes resembling the cytosolic membrane, in the vicinity of a 1:1 charge ratio, not even at about 150% excess of anionic charge. However, with a similar small charge excess of anionic liposomes to cationic DQAsomes, IMM and OMM liposomes, i.e. liposomes resembling both mitochondrial membranes, are able to displace up to 75% of the DNA from its DQAsomal carrier (27). In agreement with these data, it was found independently that for the complete liberation of DNA from DNA/DQAsome complex, an eight-fold excess of phosphatidylserine (typical anionic lipid of the cytosolic membrane), is necessary (J. Lasch, A. Meye, personal communication).

In the second study, the release of DNA from DQAsome/DNA complexes upon contact with the mitochondrial outer membrane was confirmed using isolated mitochondria in vitro (28). Mitochondria were prepared from mouse liver and characterized by electron microscopy and the determination of mitochondrial marker enzyme activity. DQAsomes were added to DNA in the presence of SYBR Green I (a fluorescence dye, which stains specifically free DNA only), resulting in the formation of DQAsome/DNA complex and the complete loss of fluorescence (Figure 5). Following the addition of isolated mitochondria to DQAsome/DNA complex, the fluorescence signal was recovered due to the dissociation of DNA from its cationic carrier.

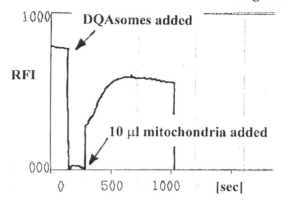

Figure 5. Effect of isolated mouse liver mitochondria on the DNA release from DQAsome/DNA complexes, adapted from (28)

Finally, it was shown most recently by confocal fluorescence microscopy (29) that DQAsome/DNA complexes not only transport the DNA to mitochondria in living mammalian cells, but also release the DNA upon contact with these organelles (Figure 6).

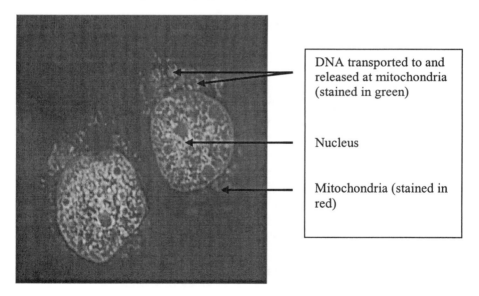

Figure 6: Confocal fluorescence microscopic image of cells incubated with pDNA/DQAsome complex, adapted from (29)

Cells were incubated with DQAsome/DNA complex followed by specifically staining mitochondria and free DNA with two different fluorescence dyes. After overlaying both images, i.e. the image with stained mitochondria and the image with stained free DNA, a perfect colocalization of free DNA with mitochondria could be observed.

CONCLUSION

Significant progress has been made in the area of "Mitochondrial Pharmacology" (9) and in the area of "Mitochondrial Delivery Systems" (26). As result of the successful merging of both fields of research, "Mitochondrial Medicine" (2) will open up avenues for the treatment of human diseases, which stem from the dysfunction of mitochondria.

ACKNOWLDEGMENT

The work of the author (VW) was supported in part by a Research Development Grant from the Muscular Dystrophy Association, Tucson, AZ.

REFERENCES

1. Brown, G.C., Niccholls, D.G., Cooper, C.E. (Eds.), Mitochondria and Cell Death. Princton University press, Princton, New Jersey (1999) pp.. vii-viii
2. Murphy, M.P., Smith, R.A., Drug delivery to mitochondria: The key to mitochondrial medicine. *Adv.Drug.Deliv.Rev.* 2000; *41: 325.*
3. Scheffler, I.E., Mitochondria make a come back. *Adv. Drug Deliv. Rev.* 2001;*49:3.*
4. Wallace, D. C., Singh, G., Lott, M. T., Hodge, J. A., Schurr, T. G., Lezza, A. M., Elsas, L. J. 2d, Nikoskelainen, E. K., Mitochondrial DNA mutation associated with Leber's hereditary optic neuropathy. *Science* 1988; *242: 1427.*
5. Holt, I. J., Harding, A. E. and Morgan-Hughes, J. A., Deletions of muscle mitochondrial DNA in patients with mitochondrial myopathies. *Nature* 1988;*331:717.*
6. Collombet, J. M. and Coutelle, C. Towards gene therapy of mitochondrial disorders. *Molecular Medicine Today* 1998;*4:31.*
7. Wallace, D. C., Mitochondrial diseases in man and mouse. *Science* 1999;*283:1482.*
8. Weissig, V. and Torchilin, V.P., Cationic bolasomes with delocalized charge centers as mitochondria-specific DNA delivery systems. *Advanced Drug Delivery Reviews* 2001;*49:127.*
9. Szewczyk, A., Wojtczak, L., Mitochondria as a Pharmacological Target. *Pharmacological Reviews* 2002;*54:101.*
10. Smith, R.A.J., Porteous, C.M., Coulter, C.V., Murphy, M.P., Selective targeting of an antioxidant to mitochondria. *Eur.J.Biochem.* 1999;*263:709.*
11. Zwacka, R.A., Zhou, W., Zhand, Y., Darby, C.J., Dudus, C.J., Halldorson, J., Oberly, L., Engelhardt, J.F., Redox gene therapy for ischemia/reperfusion injury of the liver reduces AP-1 and NF-KB activation. *Nat.Med.* 1998;4:698.
12. Kaufmann, S.H., Gores, G.J., Apoptosis in cancer: cause and cure. BioEssays 2000;*22:1007.*
13. Preston, T.J., Abadi, A., Wilson, L., Singh, G., Mitochondrial contribution to cancer cell physiology: potential for drug development. Advanced Drug Delivery reviews 2001;*49:45.*
14. Costantini, P., Jacotot, E., Decaudin, D., Kroemer, G., Mitochondrion as a novel target of anticancer chemotherapy. *J.Natl.Cancer Inst.* 2000;*92:1042.*

15. Enerback, S., A. Jacobson, E.M. Simpson, C. Guerra, H. Yamashita, M.E. Harper and L.P. Kozak, Mice lacking mitochondrial uncoupling protein are cold-sensitive but not obese. *Nature* 1997;*387:90*.

16. Wallace, K.B., Starkov, A.A., Mitochondrial targets of drug toxicity. *Annu.Rev.Pharmacol.Toxicol.* 2000;*40:353*.

17. Morin, D., Hauet, T., Spedding, M., Tillement, J.-P., Mitochondria as targets for antiischemic drugs. *Advanced Drug Delivery Reviews* 2001;*49:151*.

18. Rowe, T.C., Weissig, V., Lawrence, J.W., Mitochondrial DNA metabolism targeting drugs. *Advanced Drug Delivery Reviews* 2001;*49:175*.

19. Morgan, J., Oseroff, A.R., Mitochondria-based photodynamic anti-cancer therapy. *Advanced Drug Delivery Review* 2001;*49:71*.

20. Kolesnikova, O.A., Entelis, N.S., Mireau, H., Fox, T.D., Martin, R.P., Tarassov, I.A., Suppression of mutations in mitochondrial DNA by tRNA imported from the cytoplasm. *Science* 2000;*289:1931*

21. Modica-Napolitano, J.S., Aprille, J.R., Delocalized lipophilic cations selectively target the mitochondria of carcinoma cells. *Advanced Drug Delivery Reviews* 2001;*49:63*.

22. Smith, R.A.J., Porteous, C.M., Coulter, C.V., Murphy, M.P., Selective targeting of an antioxidant to mitochondria. *Eur.J.Biochem.* 1999;*263:709*.

23. Weissig, V., Lasch, J., Erdos, G., Meyer, H., Rowe, T.C., Hughes, J., DQAsomes: A novel potential drug and gene delivery system made from dequalinium. *Pharmaceut.Res.* 1998;*15:334*.

24. Weiss, M.J., Wong, J.R., Ha, C.S., Bleday, R., Salem, R.R., Steel, Jr., G.D., Chen, L.B., Dequalinium, a topical antimicrobial agent, displays anticarcinoma activity based on selective mitochondrial accumulation. *Proc.Natl.Acad.Sci.USA* 1987;*84:5444*.

25. Taylor, R.W., Wardell, T.M., Smith, P.M., Muratovska, A., Murphy, M.P., Turnbull, D.M., Lightowlers, R.N., An antigenomic strategy for treating heteroplasmic mtDNA disorders. *Advanced Drug Delivery Reviews* 2001;*49*:121.

26. Weissig, V., Torchilin, V.P. (Eds.), Drug and DNA delivery to mitochondria. *Advanced Drug Delivery Reviews* – Theme Issue 2001;*49:Nos. 1-2*

27. Weissig, V., Lizano, C., Torchilin, V.P., Selective DNA release from DQAsome/DNA complexes at mitochondria-like membranes. *Drug Deliv.* 2000;*7*:1.

28. Weissig, V., D'Souza, G.G.M., Torchilin, V.P., DQAsome/DNA complexes release DNA upon contact with isolated mouse liver mitochondria. *J.Controlled Release* 2001;*75*:401.

29. D'Souza, G.G.M., Rammohan, R., Torchilin, V.P., Weissig, V., DQAsome mediated delivery of pDNA to mitochondria in living cells. 2002, submitted for publication

30. Xu, Y., Szoka Jr., F.C., Mechanism of DNA release from cationic liposome/DNA complexes used in cell transfection. *Biochemistry* 1996;*35*:5616.

GLOSSARY

Apoptosis: Programmed cell death. Energy-dependent mechanism for cells to "commit suicide."

ATP: Adenosine 5'-triphosphate. Principal carrier of energy in cells.

Cytochrome C: Colored, heme containing protein. Transfers electrons during cellular respiration (see OXPHOS) and is involved in apoptosis.

Dequalinium: Symmetric cationic amphiphilic molecule, which accumulates specifically in mitochondria of living cells.

DQAsomes: Tiny vesicles formed from dequalinium.

Mitochondrion (plural **mitochondria**): Membrane-bounded organelle, about the size of a bacterium. Central function is the production of ATP ("powerhouse" of the cell). Plays crucial role in apoptosis ("arsenal" of the cell).

MPT: Mitochondrial permeability transition. Event in which the inner mitochondrial membrane becomes rapidly permeable to solutes under 1.5kD in size. Crucial role during apoptosis.

mPTPC: Mitochondrial Permeabilization Transition Pore Complex (mPTPC), a "megapore" spanning through both mitochondrial membranes. The components of the PTPC as well as proteins associated with it have not yet been completely identified. The Adenine Nucleotide Translocase (ANT), mitochondrial cyclophilin D, the Voltage Dependent Anion Channel (VDAC), and hexokinase are believed to be major parts of the PTPC.

mtDNA diseases: Diseases caused by defects in the mitochondrial genome.

OXPHOS: Oxidative phosphorylation. Pathway in mitochondria for the generation of ATP. During OXPHOS, electrons are transferred from "food molecules" to oxygen.

ROS: Reactive Oxygen Species. Formed by the transfer of a single electron to molecular oxygen. Highly reactive molecules able to oxidize a wide variety of biological molecules like lipids, proteins and nucleic acids.

INDEX

A

C

Caco-2 cell line: 431
Carcinoembryonic antigen (CEA): 180, 388
Caspases: 479
Catalase targeting: 137, 140
Cationization: 370
Caveoli/Caveolae: 39, 113, 143, 443
Caveoli-associated antigen, gp 90: 39, 143
Cerebrospinal fluid: 314, 349
Chemical Delivery Systems (CDS): 386
Chemotactic peptides: 383, 394
Chemokines and chemokine receptors: 323, 405
Chemotherapy: 202, 221, 269
Cholesterol: 330
Clathrin-coated pits endocytosis: 444
Clinical studies: 51, 54, 72, 77, 86, 201, 203, 276, 292, 387, 410
Coagulation: 32, 100, 231
Complement: 31, 384
Complement receptors: 33
Coxackie-Adenovirus Receptor (CAR): 176, 182, 444
Cross-linking agents:
      Cleavable cross-linkers, 292, 372
      SPDP: 89
      (Strept)Avidin-biodin: 133, 373
Cytochrome C: 478
Cytokines: 33, 138, 152, 234, 266, 383, 392
Cytolysins: 449
Cytomegalovirus (CMV) promoter: 184
Cytotoxic agents: 197, 205, 291, 298, 408

D

Decay accelerating factor (DAF): 31, 37
Dextran carrier: 194, 293
Diblock copolymers: 461
DNA delivery, non-viral: 60, 352, 447, 455
DNA mitochondrial: 474
DNA polyplexes: 444
DNA targeting to mitochondria: 476, 490
Diphteria toxin: 294
Doxorubicin: 200, 292, 461
DTPA: 58, 163, 219, 395

G

Gallium citrate radioimaging: 385
Glioma: 335
Glucaric acid Tc^{99m}-labeled: 54
Gene targeting: 62
        Gene targeting to ischemic myocardium: 59
        Gene targeting to endothelium: 168, 174
        Gene delivery to brain: 352
Glucose oxidase: 139
Growth factors: 239, 283
Gut associated lymphoid tissue (GALT): 422

H

Hirudin: 100
HIV: 322, 403
        Envelop glycoproteins gp 160, gp120, gp 41: 404, 406
        CD4+cells: 407
        Immunotoxins: 404, 413
Hodgkin's disease, 234
HPMA polymer carrier: 194, 216, 426
Human anti-mouse antibodies (HAMA): 252
Hydrogen peroxide: 139

I

Immunogenicity: 425
Immunoglobulins (see also antibodies)
        Interactions with cells: 31
        Radiolabeled: 389
Immunotoxins: 9, 240, 284, 294, 403
Immunomicelle: 18,
Inflammation: 32, 130, 149, 382
Infection: 385
Insulin and insulin receptor: 371, 320
Intercellular Adhesion Molecule-1 (ICAM-1): 140, 153, 161
Interleukins: 266, 383, 393, 405
Interferon: 217, 233
Integrins: 154, 177, 242
Invasins: 431
Intestines: 420